Holistic Approach to Breast Disease

Bhawna Dev • Leena Dennis Joseph
Editors

Holistic Approach to Breast Disease

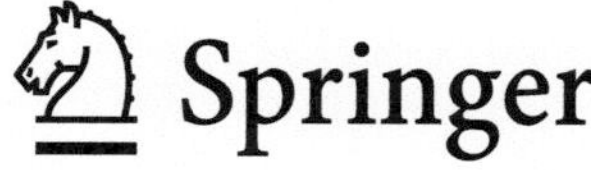

Editors
Bhawna Dev
Department of Radiology
Sri Ramachandra Institute of Higher
Education and Research
Chennai, Tamil Nadu, India

Leena Dennis Joseph
Department of Pathology
Sri Ramachandra Institute of Higher
Education and Research
Chennai, Tamil Nadu, India

ISBN 978-981-99-0037-4 ISBN 978-981-99-0035-0 (eBook)
https://doi.org/10.1007/978-981-99-0035-0

This Springer imprint is published by the registered company Springer Nature Singapore Pte Ltd.
The registered company address is: 152 Beach Road, #21-01/04 Gateway East, Singapore 189721, Singapore

Preface

A few years ago, our "normal way of life" was altered drastically. All over the world, people learnt that we needed to adapt to this sudden disruption. Originating as an offhand suggestion, the medical workforce at SRIHER chose to use this challenging time constructively and that has resulted in *Holistic Approach to Breast Disease*.

Breast disease is a common entity in everyday practice for all physicians, and breast cancer has become the most common cancer in women. In this book, we have endeavoured to provide clinically useful information to all doctors who are involved in the multidisciplinary management of breast disease.

We have included chapters on basic anatomy, physiology and histology and radiology of the normal breast. Subsequent chapters outline the characteristic features of the particular disease followed by the triple assessment features and management of the condition. This book has few unique chapters like utility of Artificial Intelligence (AI) in breast imaging and pathology, ocular manifestations in breast cancer, liquid biopsy, etc.

The book is an example of all the good and collaborative work done by a team of dedicated doctors to showcase their unique insights in the field of breast disease. As the name suggests, this book uses a comprehensive and holistic approach to the subject by covering viewpoints from Radiology, Oncology, Pathology, Surgery, and more. The roster of contributors is unfinished without undergraduate student Niharika Praveen, who demonstrated her creative skills through her artistic illustrations.

We wish to thank our University Officials and the management for facilitating the creation of this book.

This book offers useful perspectives and will serve as a ready reckoner to postgraduate students, educators, young practitioners as well as experienced clinicians in the related fields.

We hope that you will enjoy reading our book and use it in your practice, especially when you need a quick look into the management approaches to breast disease.

Chennai, Tamil Nadu, India — Bhawna Dev
Chennai, Tamil Nadu, India — Leena Dennis Joseph

Contents

Part XI Recent Advances

About the Authors

Bhawna Dev is Professor in radiology, lead consultant—breast imaging and interventions, at Sri Ramachandra Institute of Higher Education and Research, Chennai, India with 20 years of undergraduate and postgraduate teaching experience. She is one of the few who have obtained EDBI—European Diploma in Breast Imaging in India. She also holds FICR—Fellowship of "Indian College of Radiology & Imaging". Her academic interests include breast imaging and interventions, non-vascular imaging-guided interventions, intra-operative ultrasound-guided interventions and MR-guided focused ultrasound. She is involved with numerous interdisciplinary research projects; along with guiding breast fellows and postgraduate students. Dr. Bhawna has many ongoing research projects pertaining to breast diseases. She has won multiple awards including Dr. Ashok Mukherjee Award in 2004, onco-imaging "Innovative Research" award in 2005 and Professor Ida Scudder Citation award in the year 2021. She has more than 70 publications in various national and international peer-reviewed journals. She has been conducting hands-on workshops and CMEs as an organizing secretary and chairperson since 2003. She is a founder member of Indian Academy of CT guided interventions (IACTI), Society of Interventional Oncology (SIO), India Chapter, Society of Oncologic Imaging India (SOII). She is also a life/active member of various national and international professional organizations. Presently, she is President of Society of Gynecological Imaging and Interventions India. In the past, she had held the position of council member (2019–2021) and joint secretary (2017–2019) of Breast Imaging Society, India (BISI), treasurer (2016–2018), IRIA (Tamil Nadu and Pondicherry Chapter).

Leena Dennis Joseph is Professor in pathology at Sri Ramachandra Institute of Higher Education and Research, Chennai, India with 20 years of undergraduate and postgraduate teaching experience. She is a fellow of Indian College of Pathologists (FICP). Her academic interests include breast pathology, dermatopathology and gastro-intestinal pathology. She is also passionate about medical education and mentorship for medical undergraduates.

Dr. Leena is the associate dean of student affairs in her university and also member of various committees including the internal quality assurance cell, the innovation council, etc. She has many publications in various national and international peer-reviewed journals. She is a peer reviewer and editorial board member of few national journals. She is a resource person in faculty development programmes in medical education and has also completed her advanced course in medical education. She is a life member of several professional organizations.

Dr. Leena is involved with lot of interdisciplinary research projects, along with guiding her own postgraduate students. She has served as a resource faculty in over 150 conferences, CMES, and workshops. She has many ongoing research projects in breast.

Part I

Surgical Anatomy, Radiological Anatomy, Histology of the breast

Surgical Anatomy

1

Ramya Ramakrishnan

Abstract

This chapter outlines the basic anatomy of the breast and axilla with reference to the pathology and management of breast disease. The surgical anatomy is described in detail with appropriate illustrations and relevant clinical applications. The location, extent, gross and microscopic structure, vascular supply, venous and lymphatic drainage are explored in depth. The applied anatomy with respect to clinical features and surgical management of breast cancer is highlighted towards the end of this chapter.

Keywords

Surgical anatomy · Lymphatic drainage · Breast

The breasts are paired organs located on the anterior thoracic wall, in the pectoral region. They are present in both the genders, yet are more prominent in females following puberty.

The horizontal extension of the breast is from the lateral border of the sternum to the midaxillary line. Vertically, it extends between the second and sixth costal cartilages. It lies superficial to the pectoralis major and serratus anterior muscles (Fig. 1.1).

R. Ramakrishnan (✉)
Sri Ramachandra Institute of Higher Education & Research (Deemed University), Chennai, India
e-mail: ramya.r@sriramachandra.edu.in

B. Dev, L. D. Joseph (eds.), *Holistic Approach to Breast Disease*,
https://doi.org/10.1007/978-981-99-0035-0_1

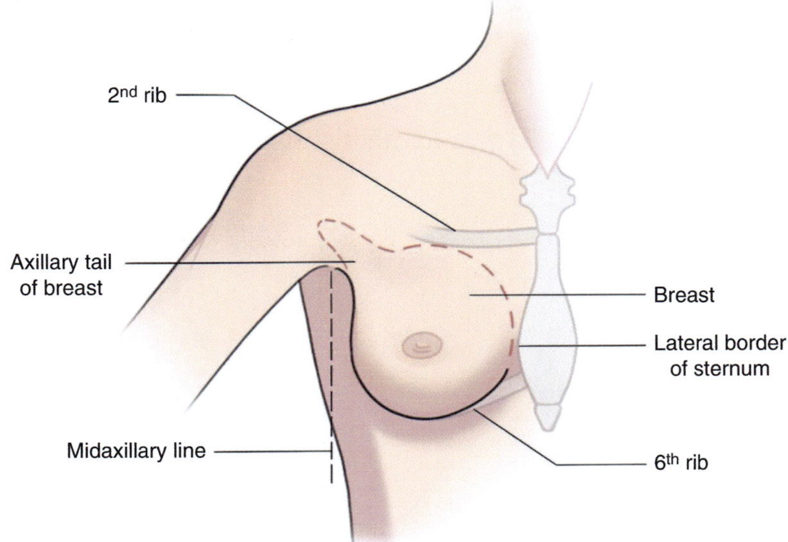

Fig. 1.1 Location and extent of the breast

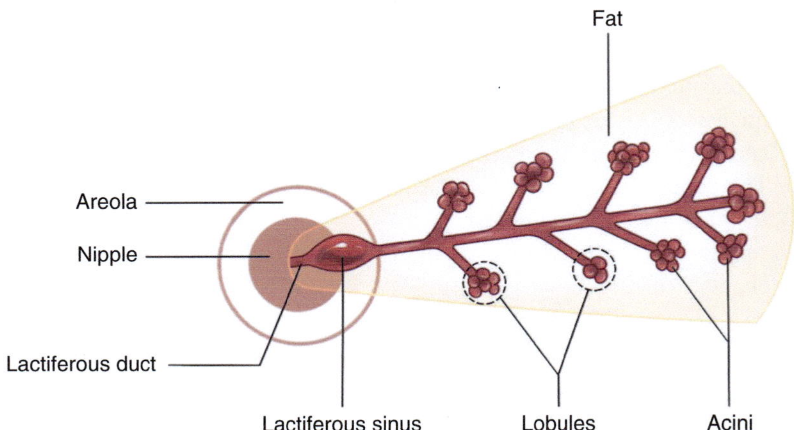

Fig. 1.2 Structure of the lobe of the mammary gland

1.1 Structure of the Breast

The breasts contain the mammary glands in females. These mammary glands are modified sweat glands and are the cardinal structures involved in lactation [1]. They consist of a series of ducts and secretory lobules—15–20 in number. Each lobule consists of many alveoli drained by a single *lactiferous duct*. Each duct branches until they form what is called a Terminal Ductal Lobular Unit (TDLU) or an acinus. Ducts and acini are lined by luminal cells that produce milk in TDLUs (Fig. 1.2). Luminal cells express estrogen and/or progesterone receptors and thus are thought to be the precursor cells for most breast carcinomas.

These ducts converge on the *nipple* like the spokes of a wheel. The nipple is at the center of the breast and is composed mostly of smooth muscle fibers. Surrounding the nipple is a pigmented area of skin termed the areola. The areola contains sebaceous glands that aid in the lubrication of the nipple.

1.2 Connective Tissue Stroma

The connective tissue stroma surrounds the mammary glands and act as a supporting structure. It has both fibrous and fatty components. The suspensory ligaments of Cooper are formed by the condensation of the fibrous stroma. These ligaments have two main functions: (a) they attach the breast to the dermis and underlying pectoral fascia, and, (b) they separate the secretory lobules of the breast (Fig. 1.3). The space between the mammary glands and the deep fascia is the retro-mammary space (i.e., loose connective tissue plane, allowing free movement). The mammary gland's main bulk is filled with variable amounts of fat, though the nipple and the areola are devoid of fat.

Quadrants of the Breast The breast is arbitrarily divided into four quadrants as depicted in Fig. 1.4.

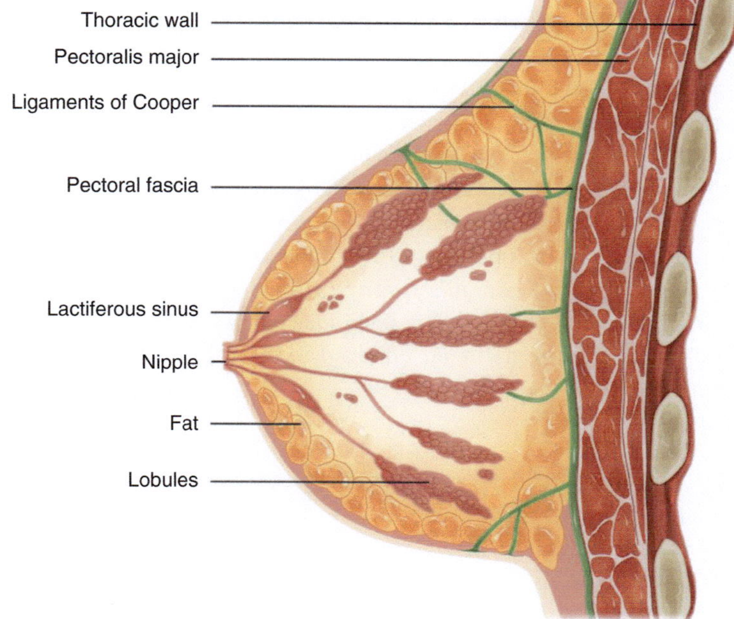

Fig. 1.3 Structure and relation of the breast

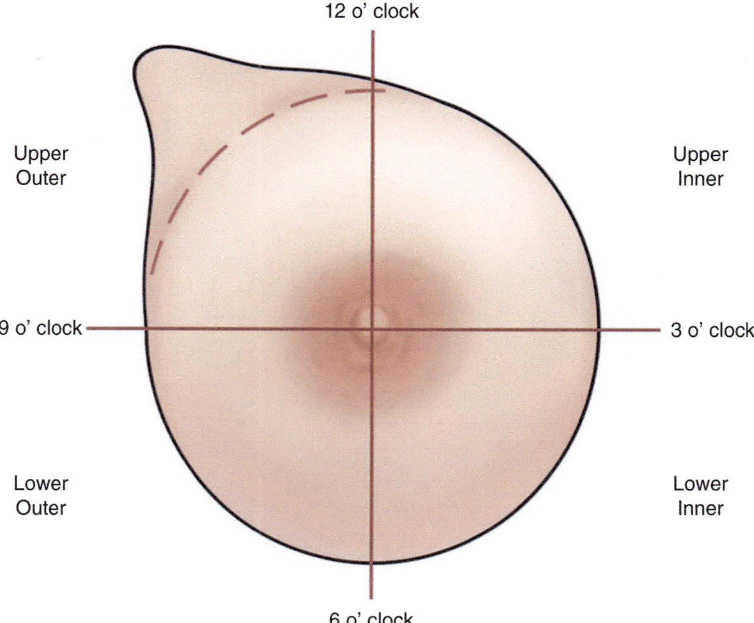

Fig. 1.4 Quadrants of the breast

1.3 Clinical Application

Majority of cancers develop in the upper outer quadrant as there is a large amount of glandular tissue here. A tongue of breast tissue often extends into the axilla, and this forms the axillary tail of Spence.

1.4 Axillary Tail of the Breast

The breast tissue that extends into the axilla forms the axillary tail of Spence [2]. This tissue pierces the deep fascia and extends into the axilla up to the level of the third rib. It is the smaller part of the breast that runs along the inferior lateral edge of the pectoralis major toward the axillary fossa (Fig. 1.5). The axillary tail hypertrophies during lactational period, and a malignant lump here can be mistaken for an enlarged axillary lymph node.

1.5 Vasculature of the Breast

The medial aspect of the breast gets its arterial supply from the internal thoracic artery (also known as internal mammary artery)—a branch of the subclavian artery (Fig. 1.6).

The lateral part of the breast receives blood from four vessels:

Lateral thoracic and thoraco-acromial branches—originate from the axillary artery.

Lateral mammary branches—originate from the posterior intercostal arteries. They supply the lateral aspect of the breast in the second, third, and fourth intercostal spaces.

Mammary branch originating from the anterior intercostal artery.

The veins of the breast correspond with the arteries and drain into the axillary and internal thoracic veins. These veins form an anastomotic circle around the nipple, which divides into superficial and deep sets.

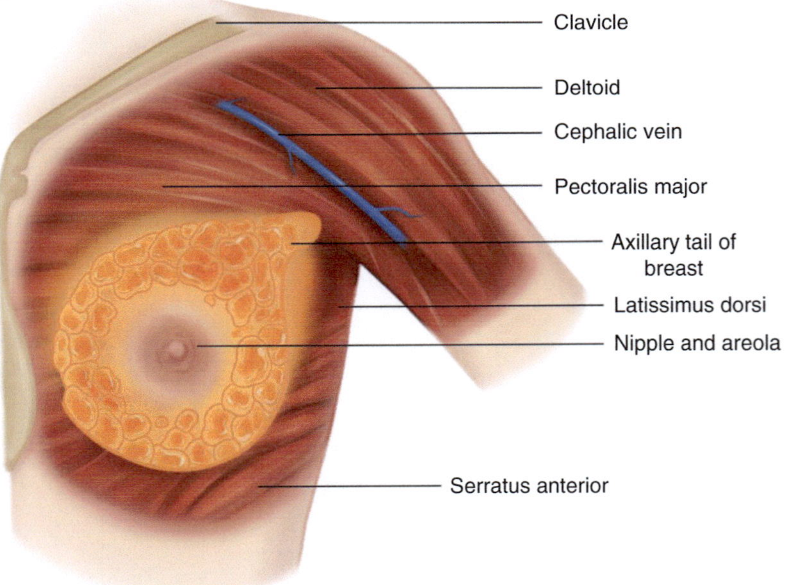

Fig. 1.5 Axillary tail of breast

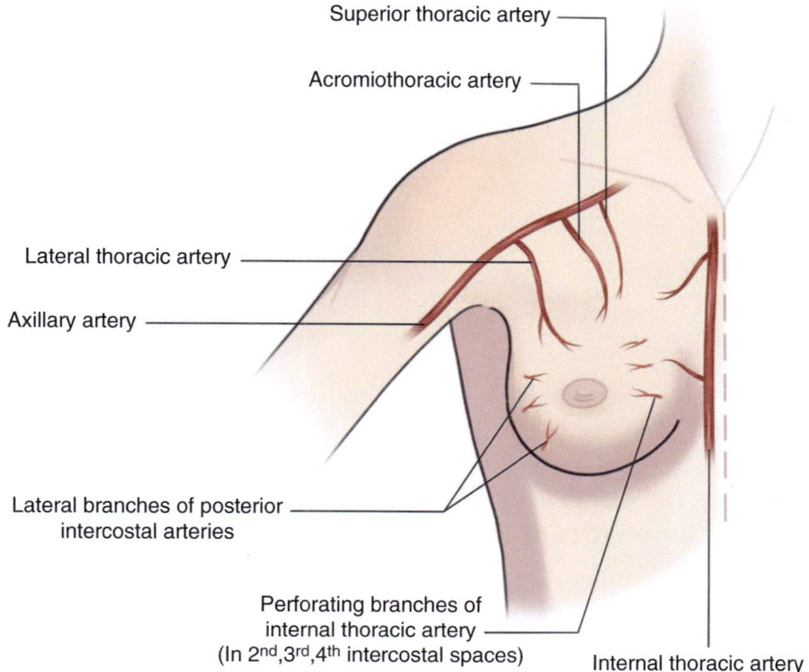

Fig. 1.6 Arterial supply of breast

- Superficial veins drain into the internal thoracic and superficial veins of the lower neck.
- Deep veins drain into internal thoracic, axillary, and posterior intercostal veins.

Clinical Importance Carcinoma of the breast may spread through deep veins (especially through the posterior intercostal veins) into the Batson's vertebral plexus of veins that drain the vertebral bodies. These are valveless veins, allowing a bidirectional flow of blood and communicate with the internal vertebral plexus of veins. Thus, a breast carcinoma can metastasize to the vertebral column and, in turn, to the spinal cord. It can also lead to the collapse of the vertebral bodies, compressing the spinal cord, and thus resulting in paraparesis or paraplegia.

1.6 Nerve Supply of the Breast

The nerve supply to the breast is by the anterior and lateral cutaneous branches of the fourth to sixth intercostal nerves. These nerves are composed of both sensory and autonomic nerve fibers (the autonomic fibers regulate smooth muscle and blood vessel tone).

Clinical Importance Long Thoracic Nerve is derived from ventral rami of C5–C7 and supplies serratus anterior superficially. The function of this muscle is to hold the upper limb to the thoracic wall. Damage to this nerve can occur during mastectomy, resulting in a "winged scapula" (Fig. 1.7).

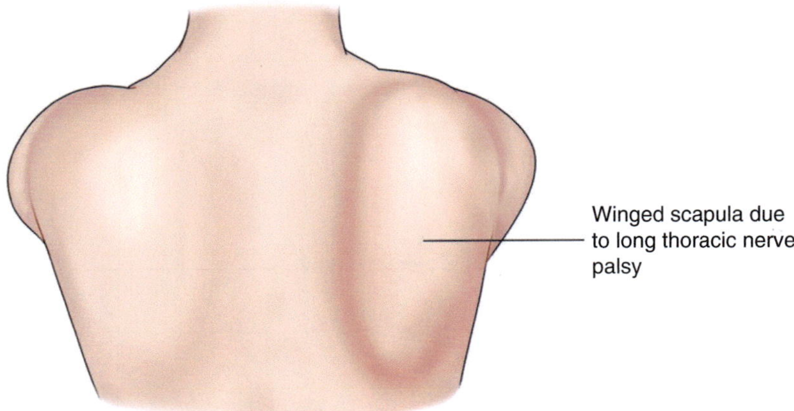

Fig. 1.7 Winged capsula

1.7 Lymphatics of the Breast

Lymphatic drainage of breast starts from the breast lobules and flows into a subareolar plexus, called Sappey's plexus. From this plexus, lymphatic drainage takes place through three main pathways that run parallel to the venous tributaries. Lymphatics from the left breast terminate in the thoracic duct and the left subclavian vein, and those from the right breast drain into the right subclavian vein.

1.8 Axillary or Lateral Pathway

This is the dominant pathway (receives >75% of lymph from breasts). This drains lateral aspect of the breast either directly or via Sappey's plexus to the axillary nodes. This pathway either runs along the inferior border of pectoralis major to reach the pectoral group of lymph nodes or pass directly to the subscapular group.

1.9 Internal Mammary Pathway

This pathway starts from both the medial and lateral quadrants of the breast. This passes through the intercostal spaces and pectoralis major into parasternal/internal mammary lymph nodes. Connections may cross the midline and hence, lymphatic metastasis can spread to the contralateral breast.

1.10 Retromammary Pathway

This comes from the deeper portion of the breast and drains to the sub-clavicular plexus. Other pathways open up when usual channels are blocked in disease. Lymph may pass to the contra-lateral breast, cervical nodes, peritoneal cavity, and liver through the diaphragm or through the rectus sheath.

1.11 Lymphatic Drainage of the Breast

The lymphatics from the breast drain to a series of nodes:

Lateral drainage is via five groups of axillary nodes: Pectoral (anterior) nodes, Subscapular (posterior) nodes, Humeral (lateral) nodes, Central nodes, and Apical nodes (Fig. 1.8).

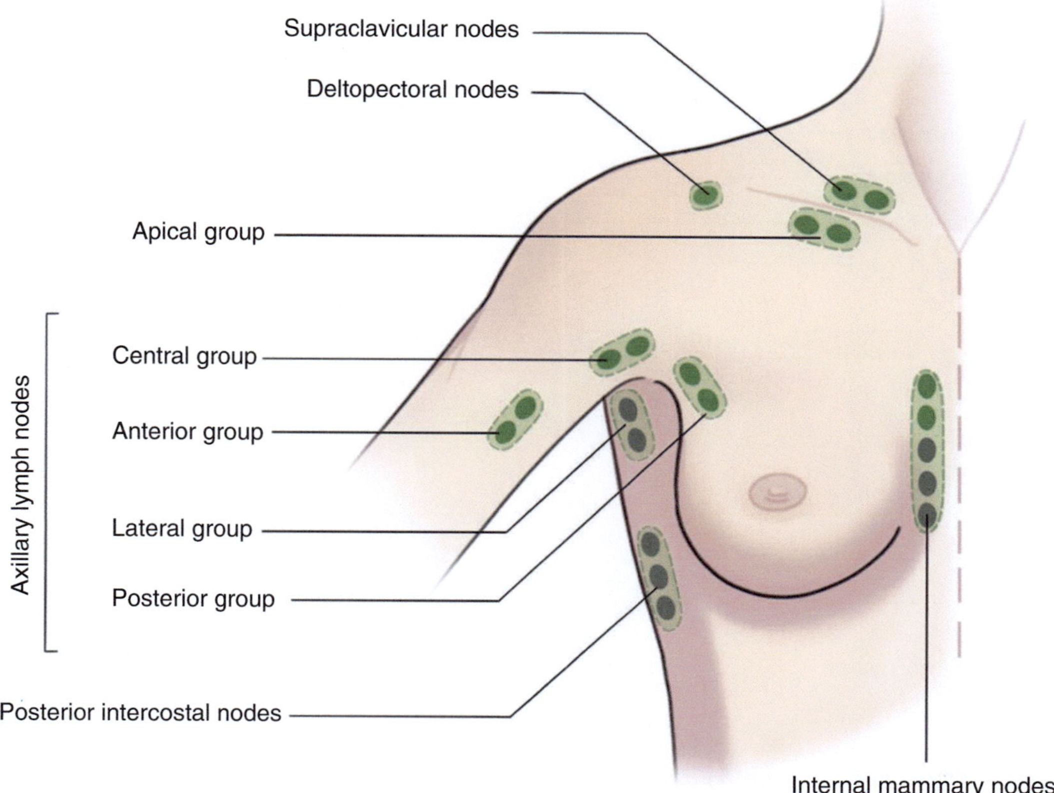

Fig. 1.8 Lymphatic drainage of breast

Superior drainage is via one group of interpectoral (Rotter's) nodes.

Medial drainage is via one group of parasternal nodes.

Clinical Importance As carcinoma breast metastasizes through the lymphatics, the surgeons need to have complete knowledge of the lymphatic drainage of the mammary gland; this will allow the appropriate removal of lymph nodes during a radical mastectomy. Typical spread is superiorly/laterally to the axillary lymph nodes. More than 75% of drainage occurs via the axillary lymph nodes. The remaining drainage is medially to the parasternal nodes. Unilateral lymphatic blockage may occur. Lymph (with cancer cells) can then drain to the opposite side.

1.12 Contents of the Axilla (Fig. 1.9)

- Axillary sheath (axillary artery and brachial plexus)
- Axillary vein and lymphatics (outside sheath)
- Fat and connective tissue
- Cutaneous nerves

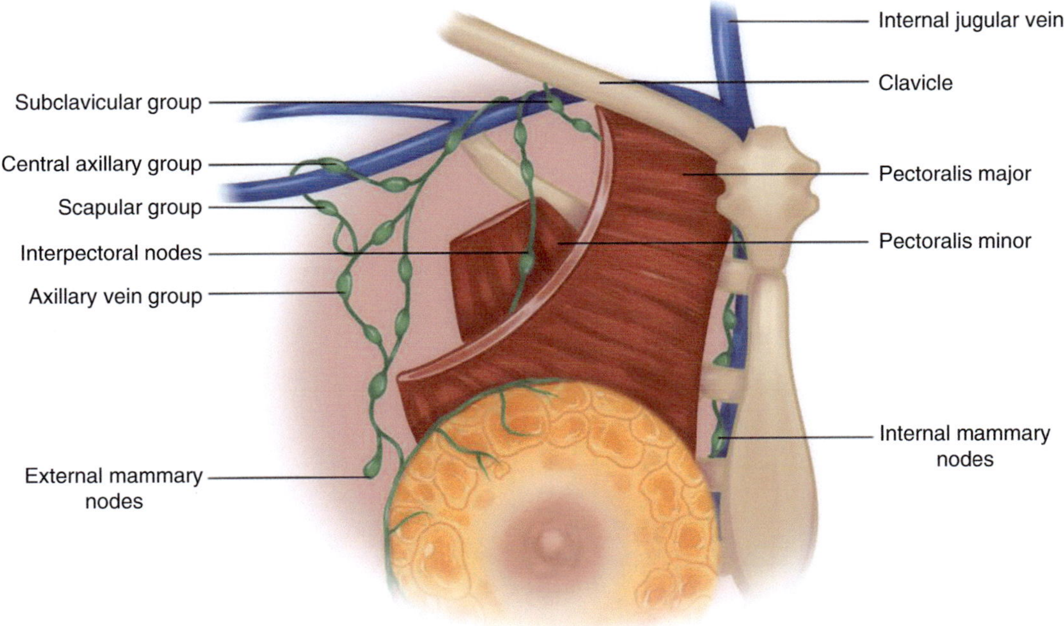

Fig. 1.9 Axillary contents

1.13 Clinical Notes on Axillary Lymph Node Dissections

Three levels of lymph nodes are described in relation to the pectoralis minor muscle.

- **Level I**–below (lateral to) pectoralis minor
- **Level II**–deep to pectoralis minor
- **Level III**–above (medial to) pectoralis minor

Radical mastectomy, as described by Halstead, involved removal of axillary lymph nodes up to level III. The current technique of modified radical mastectomy involves axillary dissection only up to level II lymph nodes.

1.14 Surgical Approach to the Axilla

The axilla is approached surgically through the axillary skin, and then, the clavipectoral fascia is divided for the excision of the axillary lymph nodes, as part of the staging and treatment of breast cancer. During axillary dissection, the intercostobrachial, long thoracic, and thoracodorsal nerves are at risk and need to be safeguarded, unless they are found adherent to involved nodes. The thoracodorsal artery is accompanied by the nerve of the same name and its preservation ensures adequate blood supply to latissimus dorsi, which is used in breast reconstruction. The axillary vein must be taken care of, when dividing its subscapular tributaries.

1.15 Early Breast Cancer

This may manifest as a painless lump or may be incidentally recognized on a screening mammogram. The patient may or may not have enlarged axillary nodes. A thorough physical examination of both breasts and axillae and the supraclavicular regions should be done. The most common site of origin of malignancy is the ducts and therefore, the most common pathology is infiltrating ductal carcinoma. Infiltrating ductal carcinoma involves the lactiferous ducts, causing retraction of the nipple.

1.16 Locally Advanced Breast Cancer (LABC)

Tumors may grow through the retromammary space and subsequently invade the deep fascia and pectoralis major muscle. This leads to fixation of the malignant breast lesion to the chest wall. Chest wall, with regard to carcinoma breast staging, includes the serratus anterior, intercostal muscles and the ribs. The tumor may also infiltrate and shorten the suspensory (Cooper's) ligaments. This, in turn, leads to irregular dimpling of skin and tethering. Involvement and blockage of the subdermal lymphatics results in peau d'orange appearance of the skin over the breast.

Surgery is the treatment of choice for malignant lesions of the breast, ranging from lumpectomy to radical mastectomy. The following are the boundaries that are followed while doing a mastectomy: clavicle forms the superior boundary; the inferior boundary is formed by the inframammary fold (above the rectus sheath); sternum forms the medial boundary of dissection and the anterior border of the latissimus dorsi forms the lateral boundary.

Knowledge of the anatomy of the breast will help in planning the surgery, especially oncoplastic breast surgery. Knowledge of lymphatic drainage of the mammary gland is essential for surgeons, in order to treat the axillary metastatic nodes effectively. Addressing the axilla in patients with breast cancer is very essential as involvement of axillary nodes is an important prognostic factor. This has led to recent advances like sentinel lymph node biopsy and thereby, avoiding axillary dissection in certain groups of patients with carcinoma breast.

References

1. Khan YS, Sajjad H. Anatomy, thorax, mammary gland. Treasure Island, FL: StatPearls; 2021. https://www.ncbi.nlm.nih.gov/books/NBK547666/
2. Sinnatamby CS. Upper limb. In: Last's anatomy. 12th ed. Amsterdam: Elsevier; 2011. pp. 50–8.

2 Radiological Anatomy

Harini Gnanavel

Abstract

Breasts are essentially modified exocrine glands responsible for lactation. Understanding the breast anatomy is important to recognize the disease processes that may occur within the breast. The key anatomical structures in the breast include skin, fat, fascial layers, Cooper ligaments, fibroglandular tissue, lymphatics, and neurovascular structures, all positioned over the chest wall. In women, fibroglandular tissue volumes vary with age, with many women having a predominance of fat within the breasts after menopause. Radiological appearance of normal breast structures varies between each imaging modality and is crucial for radiologists to have knowledge of the imaging anatomy to determine radiological–pathological concordance or discordance after a breast biopsy, to understand imaging correlates, and to plan interventional procedures.

Keywords

Breast anatomy · Imaging anatomy · Lesion localization

2.1 Introduction

A basic knowledge of breast anatomy is required to understand its pathologies and imaging features. Breast is composed of glandular tissue, fibrous tissue, fatty tissue, Cooper's ligaments, and ducts, which form the parenchyma of mammary gland (Fig. 2.1). Each lactiferous duct drains into the nipple independently [1].

H. Gnanavel (✉)
Department of Radiology, Sri Ramachandra Institute of Higher Education and Research, Chennai, India
e-mail: harini@sriramachandra.edu.in

B. Dev, L. D. Joseph (eds.), *Holistic Approach to Breast Disease*,
https://doi.org/10.1007/978-981-99-0035-0_2

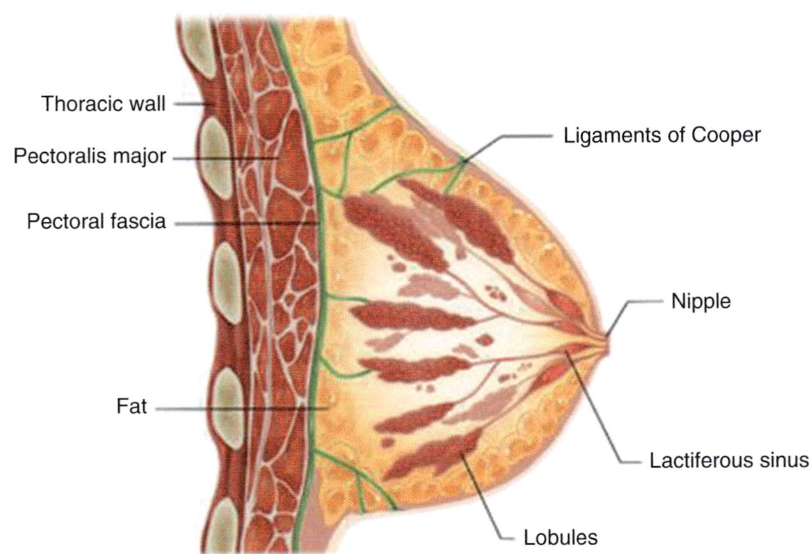

Fig. 2.1 Gross anatomy of breast

2.2 Mammogram

Mammogram is a basic, gold standard radiographic imaging modality used for breast imaging in women above age of 40 years. It uses low dose of X-rays and helps in detecting breast pathologies in early stages with good sensitivity and specificity [1].

Equipment Digital revolution has also pervaded into the field of mammography and has led to the discovery of specialized method of acquiring the breast images, namely, full field digital mammogram and digital tomosynthesis, practiced in most of the places now.

Imaging Anatomy Various structures in breast are identified in mammogram (Figs. 2.2 and 2.3).

Skin: appears as thin hyperdense layer.

Subcutaneous plane: is seen as thin hypodense layer.

Nipple and areola: appear as well-defined hyperdensity.

Intramammary fat: is seen as uniform hypodensity with fat attenuation.

Ducts and fibroglandular tissue: cannot be differentiated by their radio-opacities, since they attenuate X-rays as soft tissue elements. But due to the presence of intramammary fat in most breasts, the soft tissue elements are seen separately [2].

Coopers ligament: is seen as thin dense lines interspersed in the fibroglandular tissue.

Pectoralis muscle: appears as hyperdense band in posterior aspect.

Axillary lymph node: is seen as oval hyperdense structure in axilla.

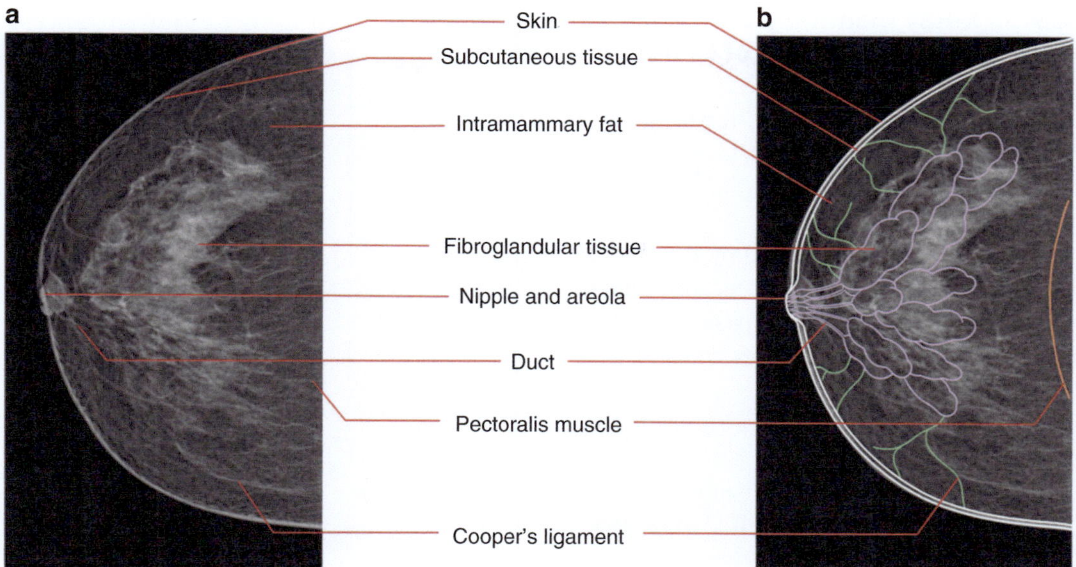

Fig. 2.2 (**a**) X-ray mammogram CC view demonstrating normal anatomy of breast. (**b**) Schematic presentation showing mammographic anatomy in CC view

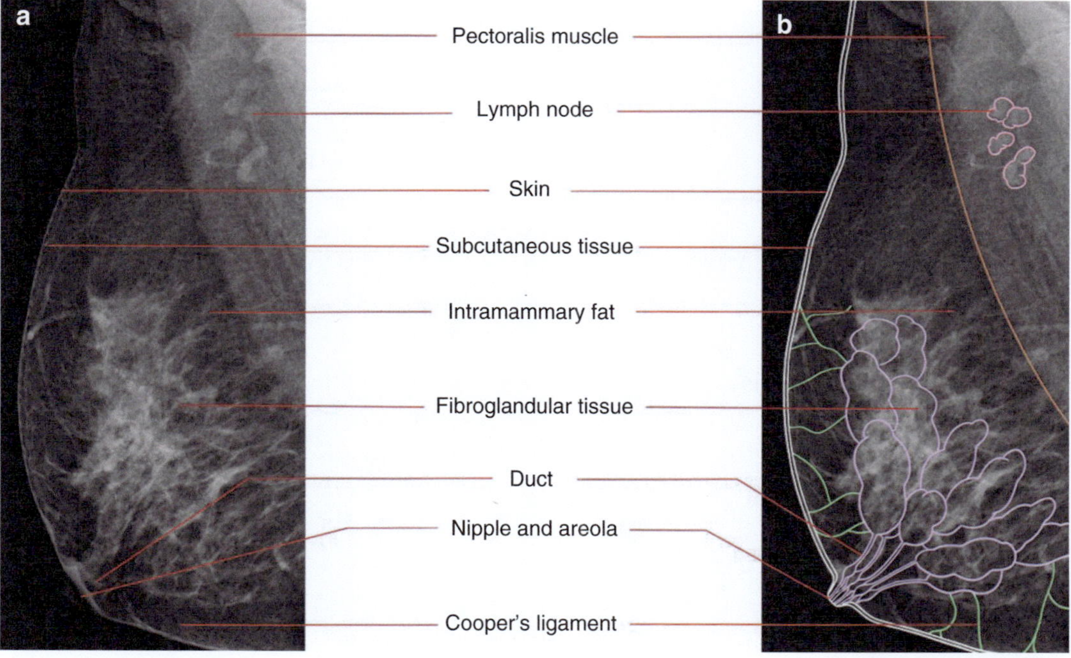

Fig. 2.3 (**a**) X-ray mammogram MLO views demonstrating normal anatomy of breast. (**b**) Schematic representation showing mammographic anatomy in MLO view

2.3 X-Ray Mammogram Views and Localization of Lesion

The routinely taken view for X-ray mammogram includes Cranio Caudal (CC) view and Medio Lateral Oblique (MLO) view. (For detailed technique, refer Chap. 4).

The lesion can be localized by the quadrants (upper, lower, inner, outer), the location (anterior, middle, posterior), and clock position (1–12) as mentioned below (Figs. 2.4, 2.5, and 2.6).

> **Highlight**
>
> Clock face location is first inferred from the CC position with the MLO view used predominantly to determine whether the mass is in upper (above the nipple) or lower (below the nipple) quadrant of breast.

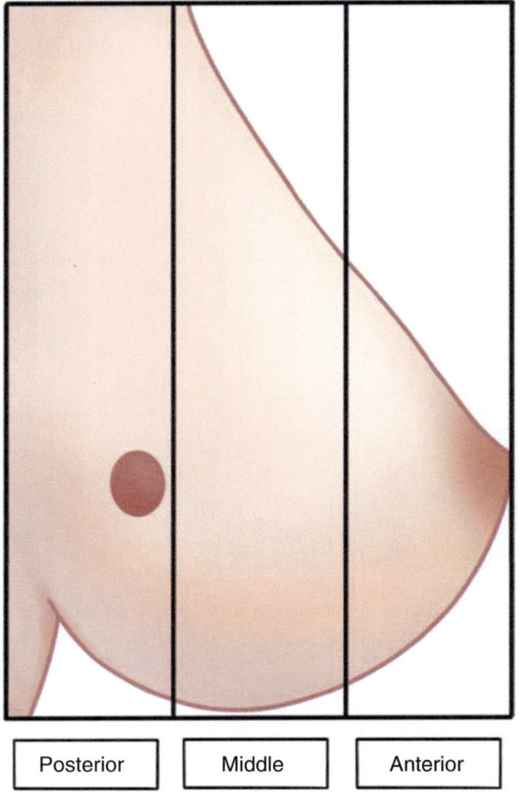

Fig. 2.5 Line diagram representing location of lesions in breast as anterior, middle and posterior

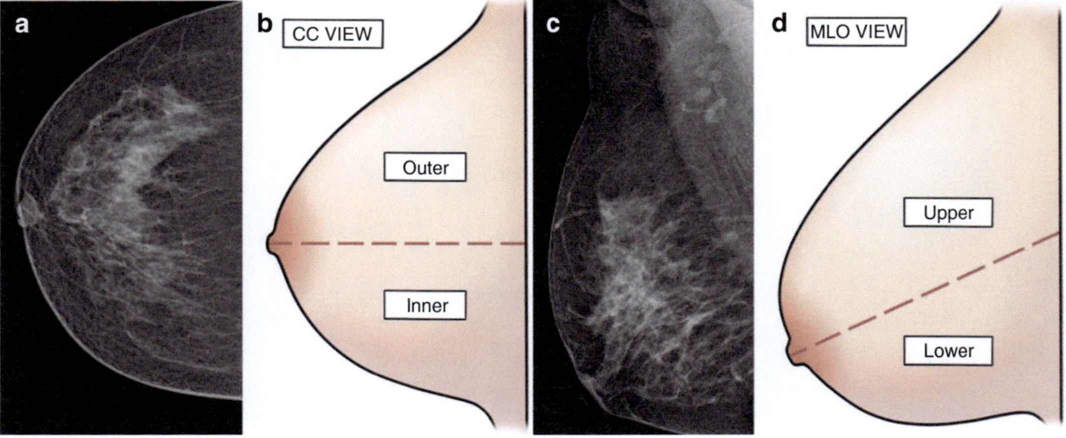

Fig. 2.4 (**a**, **b**) X-ray mammogram and line diagram in CC view demonstrating quadrants of breast. (**c**, **d**) X-ray mammogram and line diagram in MLO view demonstrating quadrants of breast

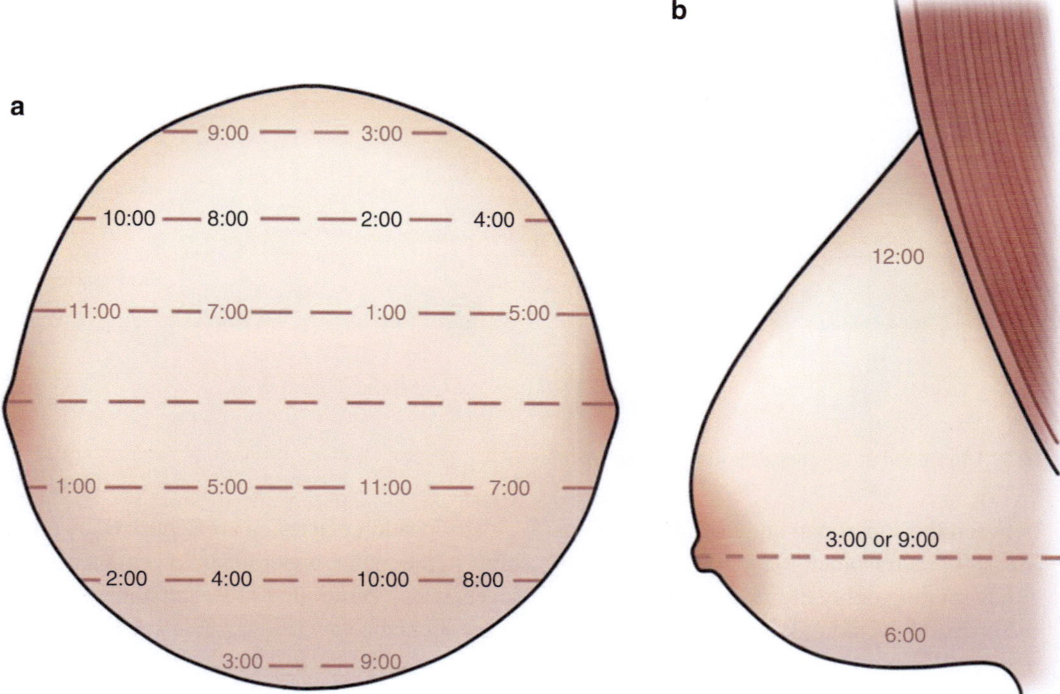

Fig. 2.6 (**a**, **b**) Line diagram in CC view and MLO view demonstrating clock face location

2.4 Ultrasound of Breast

Depending on the volume of fat interspersed within the glandular tissue of the breast, the imaging pattern on ultrasound varies.

Equipment Ultrasound of breast is done with a high-resolution ultrasound machine using high-frequency linear probe of 5–12 MHz

Imaging Anatomy Ultrasound (USG) anatomy of breast can be explained by dividing it into three zones, each zone containing specific structures (Fig. 2.7)

2.4.1 Premammary Zone

Skin—appears as a thin hyperechoic layer
Subcutaneous fat—seen as a hypoechoic layer
Superficial fascia—occasionally seen as another thin echogenic line below the skin

2.4.2 Intramammary Zone

It is composed of interspersed fat and glandular tissue that appears hypoechoic and echogenic, respectively.

2.4.3 Retromammary Zone

Fat—appears as a hypoechoic layer above the pectoralis muscles.
Pectoralis muscle—displays as a typical fibrillar pattern.
Ribs—present posterior to the pectoralis muscle and show posterior acoustic shadowing.
Ducts—Ducts are seen as tubular, branching anechoic structures, these are larger under the areola and become progressively small toward the periphery of the breast. Normal duct measures less than or equal to 2 mm.
Cooper's ligaments—Provide framework for the breast parenchyma. This ligament runs

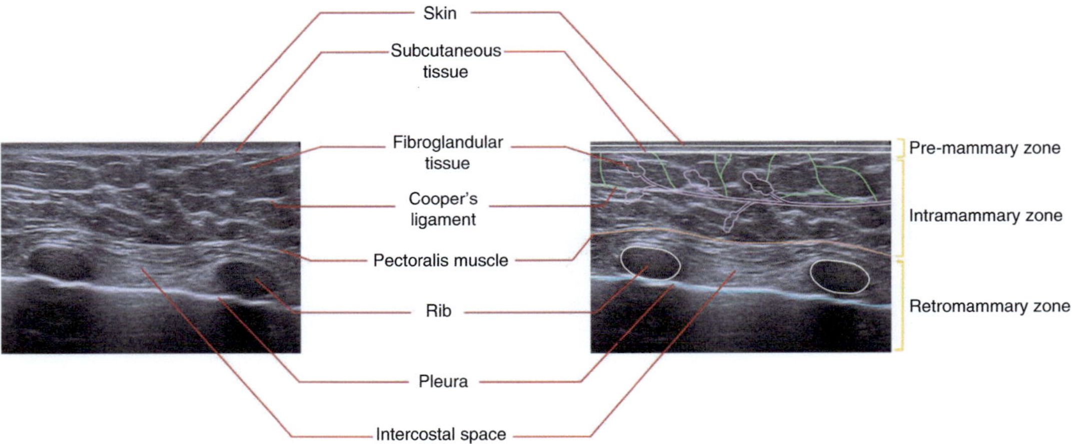

Fig. 2.7 Ultrasound of the breast showing normal anatomy

between the superficial and deep fascia of the breast. On ultrasound, it appears as echogenic bands running obliquely from the posterior of the breast to the skin [3].

2.5 Ultrasound Views and Localization of Lesion

Breast is analyzed in three planes—radial, longitudinal, and transverse (For detailed technique, refer Chap. 4).

The location of a lesion is categorized by quadrants (upper outer, upper inner, lower outer, lower inner), clock position (1–12), and zones (1, 2, 3) as mentioned below (Figs. 2.8, 2.9, and 2.10).

> **Highlight**
>
> After scanning the breast in three planes on a ultrasound, the location of the lesion should be reported with its quadrant, clock position, and zone position for reproducibility.

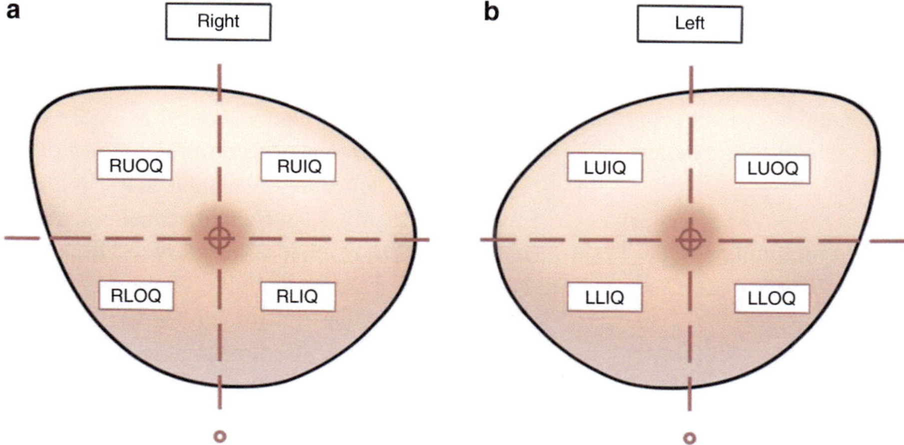

Fig. 2.8 (**a**, **b**) Line diagram showing demarcation of quadrants on breast ultrasound

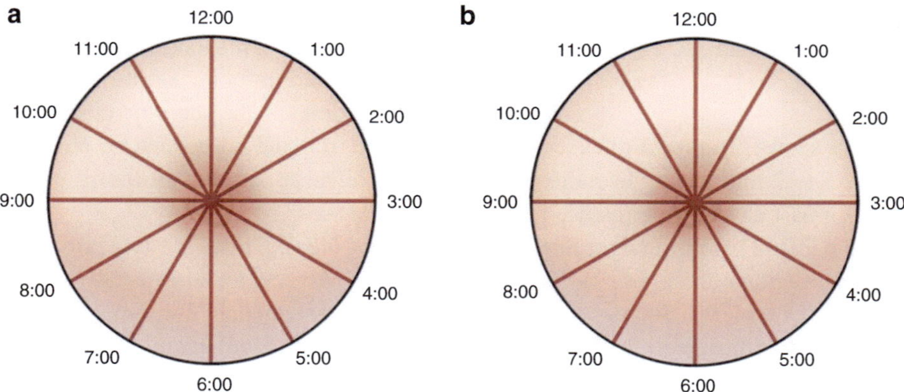

Fig. 2.9 (**a**, **b**) Line diagram showing clock position on ultrasound of breast

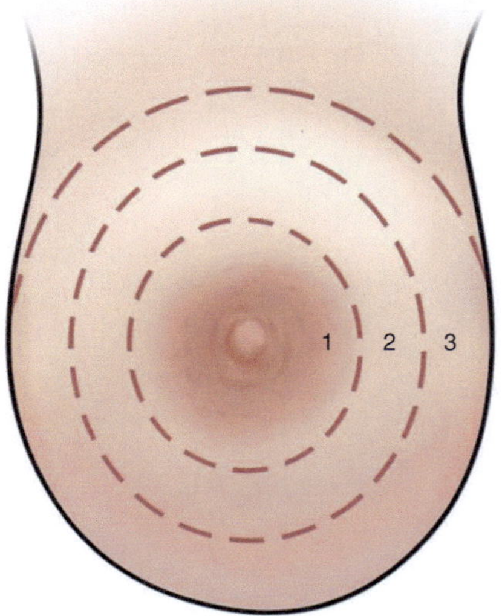

Fig. 2.10 Line diagram showing demarcation of breast into three zones

2.6 MR Mammogram

In Magnetic Resonance Imaging (MRI), both breasts are examined at the same time using a multichannel phase-array breast coil in prone position.

Equipment A minimum of 1.5 Tesla machine and dedicated breast coil is required for imaging.

Imaging Anatomy On MRI, each structure of the breast is seen as different intensity in individual sequence and does not remain consistent as in X-ray or ultrasound of breast. These specific sequences make normal breast components like fibroglandular tissue, fat, muscles and varied pathologies like hemorrhage, edema, etc., more vivid on MRI (Fig. 2.11).

Skin: The skin shows a uniform thickness ranging from 0.5 to 2 mm along the entire perimeter of the breast and is hyperintense in most of the sequences. There is a slight thickening in the areolar region normally.

Areola-Nipple Complex: Shows significant enhancement after the injection of the IV contrast owing to its intense vascularization, although this has no pathological significance.

Lactiferous Ducts: Appear as linear T2 high signal intensities converging toward the nipple. When studying the ducts, it is preferable to do highly T2-weighted sequences, such as Short Tau Inversion Recovery (STIR), and the multiphase study, with pre- and postcontrast subtraction images, in order to rule out the presence of intraductal lesions.

Fibroglandular Tissue: Appears as low signal intensity on T1 and T2 sequences.

Adipose Tissue: Follows the fat signal.

Cooper's Ligaments: These appear as low signal intensity in all sequences as they traverse the adipose tissue.

Muscle Plane: This consists of the pectoralis major and minor muscle, identified as an extension on the anterior costal wall, separated from the fibroglandular plane. It appears hypointense in the precontrast T1 and T2 sequences.

Lymph Nodes: These are typically oval shaped with fatty center and usually show intense enhancement on IV contrast owing to their significant vascularization [4].

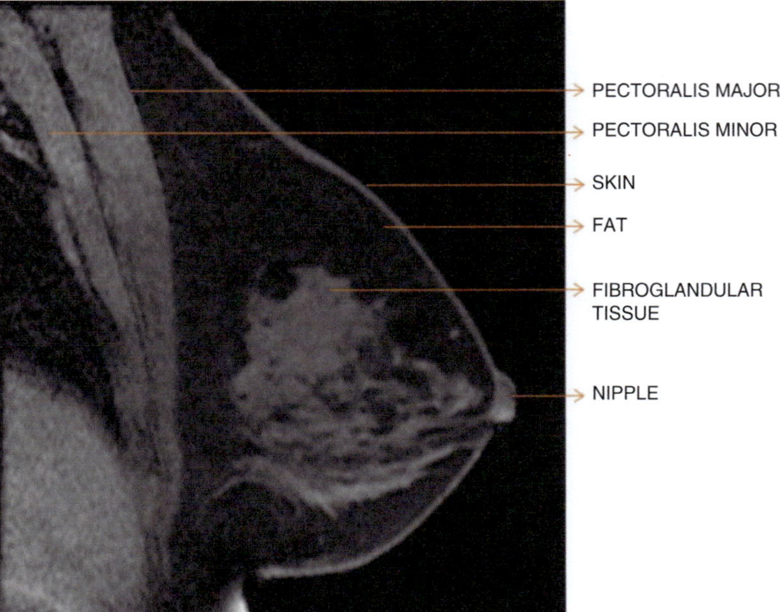

Fig. 2.11 MRI mammogram in sagittal plane showing normal anatomy

2.7 MRI Mammographic Views and Localization of Lesion

The breast is assessed in axial and sagittal planes routinely. Coronal planes are preferred by a few radiologists.

Localization of the lesion is determined by assessing whether the mass is in upper (above the nipple) or lower (below the nipple) quadrant of breast on a sagittal plane. On an axial plane, it can be categorized as inner (medial) and outer (lateral) quadrants. The coronal plane gives the clock position of the lesion as in X-ray/Ultrasound (Fig. 2.12).

Highlight

The vascularization of the breast can be clearly identified in the dynamic MRI sequence by depicting the path of the lateral thoracic vessels and the internal thoracic vessels with their branches.

- Contrast-enhanced MRI should preferably be done between 7 and14 days of menstrual cycle in a regular 28 day cycle. When the background enhancement of the normal breast tissue is low; the abnormalities are better picked up [5].
- In case of irregular menstrual cycle or history of hysterectomy before 50 years of age, the need for blood sampling with serum progesterone might be required to determine the optimal time for MRI [6].

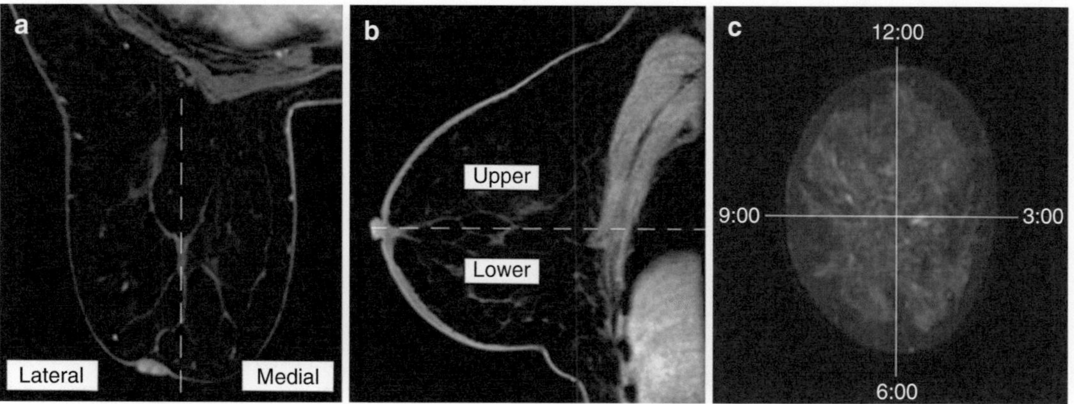

Fig. 2.12 (a–c) MRI showing the localization of lesion on various imaging planes—axial, sagittal and coronal

2.8 References

1. Reeves RA, Kaufman T. Mammography. Treasure Island, FL: StatPearls; 2020. https://www.ncbi.nlm.nih.gov/books/NBK559310/
2. De Benedetto D, Abdulcadir D, Giannotti E, Nori J, Vanzi E, Capaccioli L. Radiological anatomy of the breast. Ital J Anat Embryol. 2016;121:20–36.
3. Geddes DT. Ultrasound imaging of the lactating breast: methodology and application. Int Breastfeed J. 2009;4(1):1–7.
4. Carmona MS, Vega MC, Alfageme M, Fontanilla T, Pastrana M, Gonzalez C. Mammography. In: US and MRI: review of normal anatomy and variants. Vienna: European Congress of Radiology-ECR; 2017.
5. Dhillon GS, Bell N, Ginat DT, Levit A, Destounis S, O'Connell A. Breast MR imaging: what the radiologist needs to know. J Clin Imaging Sci. 2011;1:48.
6. Mann RM, Balleyguier C, Baltzer PA, Bick U, Colin C, Cornford E, Evans A, Fallenberg E, Forrai G, Fuchsjäger MH, Gilbert FJ. Breast MRI: EUSOBI recommendations for women's information. Eur Radiol. 2015;25(12):3669–78.

3 Breast Histology

Archana B

Abstract

Histologically, the mammary gland is composed of the glandular and connective tissue components. Glandular component comprises of a ductal-lobular system lined by two layers of cells: the inner epithelial and outer myoepithelial, which have distinct ultrastructural and immunohistochemical features. The terminal duct lobular unit (TDLU) is the basic functional unit of the breast. The histology of breast tissue varies actively with age, menstrual cycle, and hormonal influences, thus exhibiting a wide range of appearances.

Keywords

Gland · Myoepithelium · Terminal duct lobular unit · Hormone

3.1 The Inactive Mammary Gland

The mammary gland is a functional gland, the histologic structure of which varies with physiological changes. The suspensory ligaments of Cooper connect the glandular component to the overlying skin. The skin shows a pigmented circular area called the areola with a central projection, the nipple. The nipple is lined by pigmented stratified squamous epithelium (that extends into the duct), is supported by fibrous tissue containing smooth muscle, and contains numerous sebaceous glands. The epidermis of nipple and areola has a basal pigmented layer containing melanin pigment and contains clear cells representative of clear keratinocytes or toker cells. The areola has numerous nerve endings.

Each breast is composed of 15–20 lobes within which are numerous lobules containing terminal duct lobular units (TDLU), the basic functional

A. B (✉)
Department of Pathology, Sri Ramachandra Medical College, Chennai, India
e-mail: archanab@sriramachandra.edu.in

B. Dev, L. D. Joseph (eds.), *Holistic Approach to Breast Disease*,
https://doi.org/10.1007/978-981-99-0035-0_3

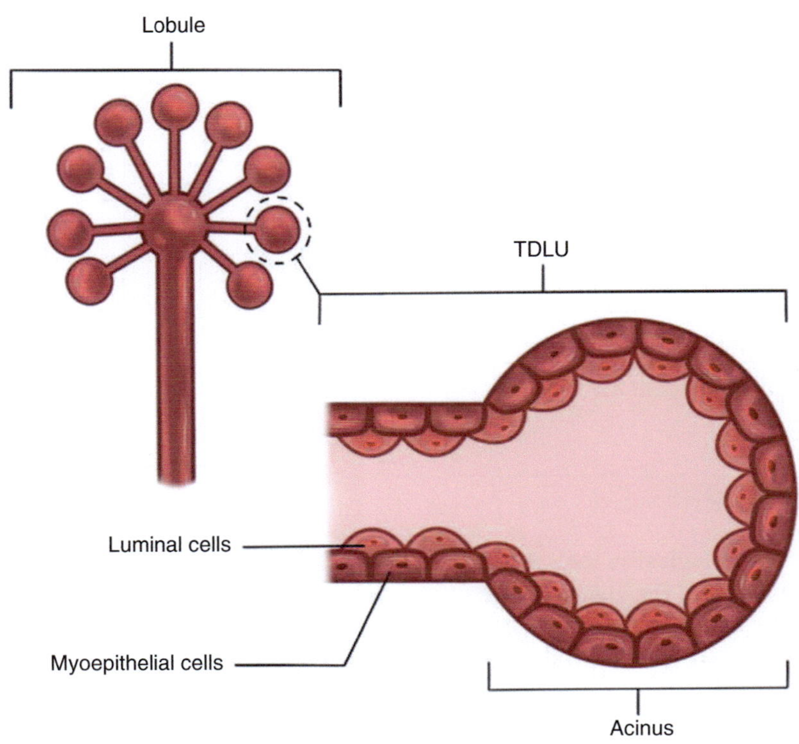

Fig. 3.1 Diagrammatic representation of TDLU

unit of the breast [1] (Fig. 3.1). Each lobe drains into lactiferous duct, which opens at the nipple. A fusiform dilatation known as lactiferous sinus is present just beneath the nipple.

3.2 Glandular Component

The glandular tissue comprises of the lobes and ducts. The interlobular ducts, intralobular ducts and alveoli (also known as acinus during pregnancy/lactation) are lined by two layers of cells, which are the inner luminal epithelial cells and the outer basal myoepithelial cells (Fig. 3.2). While the smaller ducts are lined by columnar epithelium, the larger ones are lined by pseudostratified columnar epithelium. Luminal epithelial cells express low-molecular-weight cytokeratins like 7, 8, 18, 19 and myoepithelial cells express high-molecular-weight keratins like 5, 6, 14, 17 along with other markers like p63, CD10, and S100 [2]. It is postulated that both epithelial and myoepithelial lineages arise from a common committed stem cell that expresses CK5 [3].

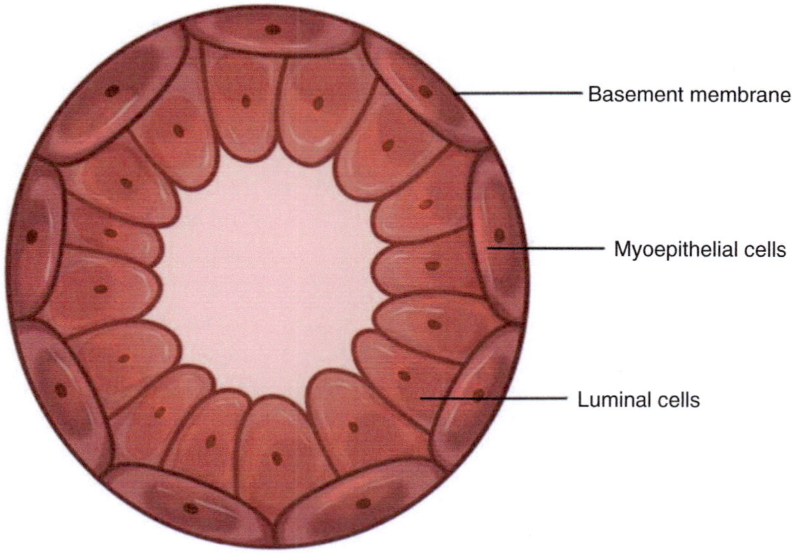

Fig. 3.2 Diagrammatic representation of the lining of the ducts

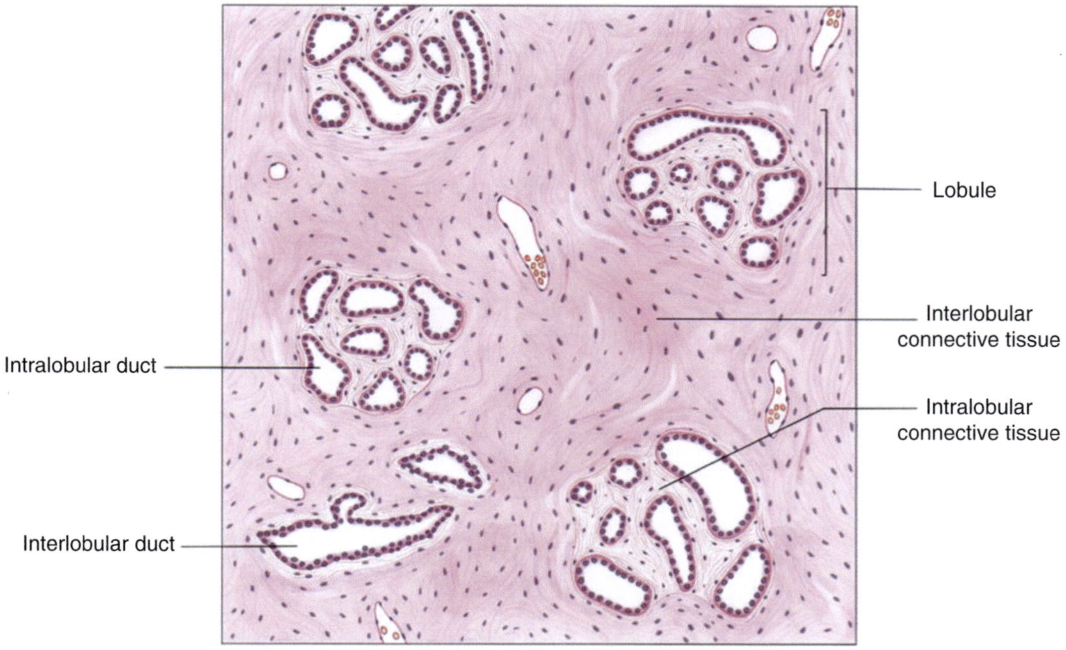

Fig. 3.3 Diagrammatic representation of the connective tissue components

3.3 Connective Tissue Component

The connective tissue component is made of intralobular and interlobular connective tissues. The intralobular connective tissue is loose, and is composed of fibroblasts, lymphocytes, plasma cells, and eosinophils. The interlobular connective tissue is denser, more collagenous containing blood vessels and adipocytes (Fig. 3.3).

3.4 Variations During Physiological Conditions

Some variations occur in the breast parenchyma during physiological conditions. Between puberty and pregnancy, the breast tissue consists of connective tissue and fat, which widely separates the glandular elements (Fig. 3.4). Alveoli may be few or absent during this period.

During pregnancy, there is a marked proliferation and branching of ducts. Alveoli increase in number and become secretory [4] (Fig. 3.5). Intralobular, interlobular ducts and lactiferous ducts also contain secretory material. Intralobular connective tissue decreases, while interlobular connective tissue increases because of increase in glandular elements. These changes appear in response to hormones such as estrogen and progesterone. The cells lining the glands bear receptors for these hormones.

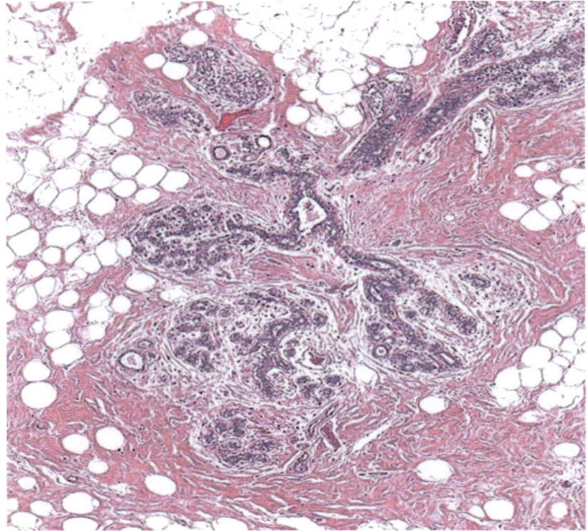

Fig. 3.4 Breast tissue from a woman of reproductive age showing terminal duct lobular unit surrounded by relatively dense fibrous interlobular and adipose tissue (H&E)

During lactation, under the influence of prolactin, the glandular elements become much more prominent. Hypertrophy of the alveoli occurs, which also demonstrates irregular branching. The interlobular connective tissue is reduced. The active alveoli are lined by enlarged epithelial cells that have a hobnail appearance with flattened myoepithelial cells. The alveoli are filled with eosinophilic material containing vacuoles of fat droplets (Fig. 3.6). Inactive alveoli have empty lumen lined by taller epithelium. Oxytocin causes contraction of the myoepithelial cells around the alveoli and excretory ducts, resulting in milk ejection. Glands are apocrine in nature; portion of the apical part of the alveoli are shed along with the secretions.

In the postpregnancy phase, the glandular tissue returns to the resting state. Atrophy of the glandular tissue, hyalinized stroma with increase

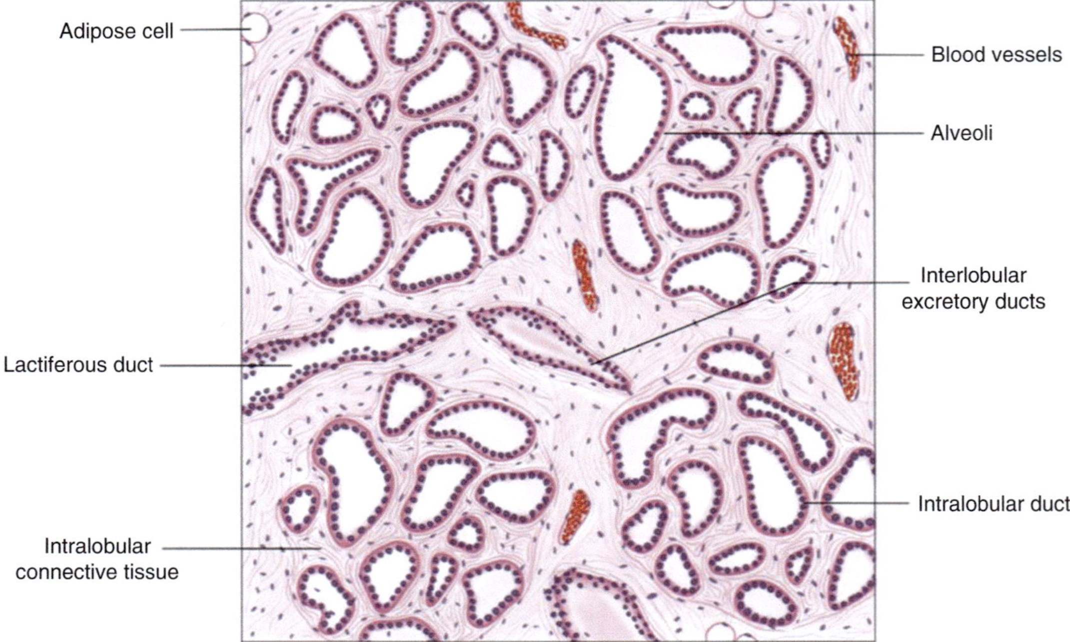

Fig. 3.5 Diagrammatic representation of the histology during pregnancy showing increase in number of alveoli and dilated alveoli

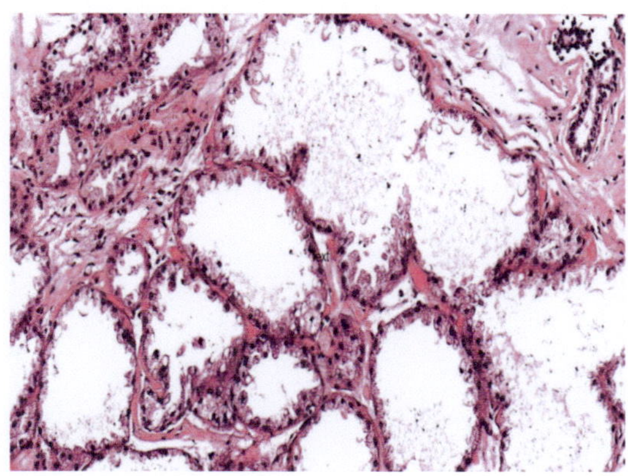

Fig. 3.6 Alveoli in lactation showing epithelial cells that are cuboidal to columnar with cytoplasmic vacuoles and apical snouts (H&E)

in fat is noted after menopause. Decrease in estrogen and progesterone results in these involutory changes.

Thus, breast is a dynamic tissue demonstrating a plethora of histomorphologic differences due to physiological variations.

References

1. Young B, Woodford P, O'Dowd G. Wheater's functional histology E-book: a text and colour atlas. Philadelphia: Elsevier Health Sciences; 2013.
2. Moriya T, Kozuka Y, Kanomata N, Tse GM, Tan PH. The role of immunohistochemistry in the differential diagnosis of breast lesions. Pathology. 2009;41(1):68–76.
3. Boecker W, Buerger H. Evidence of progenitor cells of glandular and myoepithelial cell lineages in the human adult female breast epithelium: a new progenitor (adult stem) cell concept. Cell Prolif. 2003;36:73–84.
4. Eroschenko VP, Di Fiore MS. DiFiore's atlas of histology with functional correlations. Philadelphia: Lippincott; 2013.

Part II

Clinical Approach to Breast Disease

4 Clinical Features of Breast Disease

Ramya Ramakrishnan

Abstract

The most common cause of clinical breast symptoms in a woman is a benign breast disease; breast cancer is the cause in only 3–6% of cases. The common symptoms of benign breast disease are breast pain, lump, or nipple discharge. Women with breast cancer can present with either a breast lump, nonlump breast symptoms like nipple retraction, skin changes, contour changes or with nonbreast metastatic or general symptoms. As breast cancer is the most common cancer in women, any patient with symptoms of breast disease should undergo a thorough triple assessment in order to make a correct diagnosis and initiate the appropriate treatment.

Keywords

Benign breast disease · Breast pain · Breast lump · Nipple discharge · Breast cancer · Triple assessment

R. Ramakrishnan (✉)
Sri Ramachandra Institute of Higher Education & Research (Deemed University), Chennai, India
e-mail: ramya.r@sriramachandra.edu.in

Data from the western countries reveal that around 3% of women's consultations with their general practitioners (GPs) are about breast symptoms [1]. Breast cancer is the most common form of cancer in women, occurring in approximately one in eight women at some time during their lives. For this reason, breast symptoms cause a lot of anxiety in patients and therefore, these patients should be thoroughly examined and investigated to arrive at the correct diagnosis. The majority of the patients presenting with symptoms related to the breast do not have breast cancer. Breast cancer is detected in only 3–6% of women with clinical symptoms, and in most cases, the cause of the symptoms is benign. Benign breast changes are more common in women of child-bearing age, peaking between the ages of 30 and 50, whereas the incidence of breast cancer peaks during the postmenopausal period.

4.1 Symptoms and Signs of Benign Breast Disease

4.1.1 Mastalgia

The terminology mastalgia is used to indicate pain related to the mammary gland. It is also referred to as mastodynia. Mastalgia can be classified into two broad categories such as cyclical and noncyclical.

B. Dev, L. D. Joseph (eds.), *Holistic Approach to Breast Disease*,
https://doi.org/10.1007/978-981-99-0035-0_4

The prevalence of breast pain in clinical populations has been reported to range from 41% to 69% [2]. The prevalence of breast pain in the general population is around 52%. Two-thirds (66%) of sufferers reported cyclic breast pain, which is comparable with previous clinical findings, with symptoms most commonly occurring in the week before menstruation [3]. Surveys have revealed that more than 50% of all women report significant breast pain, which impairs their everyday and sexual life in around 40% of cases. In two-thirds of cases, the pain is cyclical and is worst around the perimenstrual period. Cyclic mastalgia manifests at around 30 years of age; noncyclic mastalgia occurs usually later, at a mean age of 41. What causes mastalgia is unknown. As cyclical mastalgia improves during pregnancy and lactation or, when women attain menopause, we can assume that this is because of the response of the breast and pain pathway to the hormonal changes occurring during these phases. In a woman with noncyclic mastalgia, inflammatory, neoplastic, and vascular pathology need to be ruled out. Differential diagnoses to be considered are chest pain of extramammary origin such as intercostal neuralgia and pain due to cardiac causes. In patients with no underlying pathology, spontaneous remission of mastalgia occurs within a few months to up to 3 years.

4.1.2 Mastitis

When a patient complains of swelling of the breast associated with severe pain and fever, one should suspect mastitis—either lactational (puerperal) or nonlactational. Nonpuerperal mastitis refers to all forms of mastitis occurring other than during the lactation period. The most common ones are bacterial mastitis (59%), nonbacterial mastitis (25%), and other special forms of nonpuerperal mastitis (14%) [4].

Puerperal mastitis usually occurs during the first 3 months after delivery. Its incidence all over the world has been reported at 2–50%, and in selective subsets of the population, a higher incidence has been observed.

The symptoms of puerperal mastitis, as defined by the World Health Organization (WHO), are

- Pain
- Local redness, warmth, and swelling of the breast
- Fever and aching limbs
- General feeling of illness

Nonpuerperal mastitis includes all forms of periductal mastitis, granulomatous mastitis, and mastitis due to iatrogenic causes like surgery or radiotherapy. Breast cancer should be excluded in older patients with mastitis, by a thorough triple assessment. Periductal mastitis is an inflammatory condition of the subareolar ducts and has a prevalence of 5–9% in nonbreastfeeding women [5]. It often occurs in overweight women with macromastia and a history of chronic smoking. The clinical manifestations of periductal mastitis are peri-areolar signs of inflammation (redness, swelling, warmth). Abscess and fistula formation occur due to secondary bacterial infection.

Granulomatous mastitis is an inflammatory breast disease of young women in the childbearing age. The etiology of this rare disease is unknown. Patients commonly present with a painful palpable mass, often with redness and swelling. This may be associated with skin retraction. The symptoms and the features on imaging mimic that of a diffuse breast cancer. In some cases, abscess formation can be visualized on breast ultrasonography. Diagnosis is confirmed by performing a percutaneous core biopsy.

4.1.3 Lump in the Breast

The second most common presenting complaint in a patient with benign breast disease is a lump in the breast. With an incidence of 25%, fibroadenoma is the most common benign tumor of the breast; peak onset is between 15 and 35 years of age [6]. In terms of etiology and pathogenesis, a hormonally triggered mechanism is likely, as suggested by early onset during the premeno-

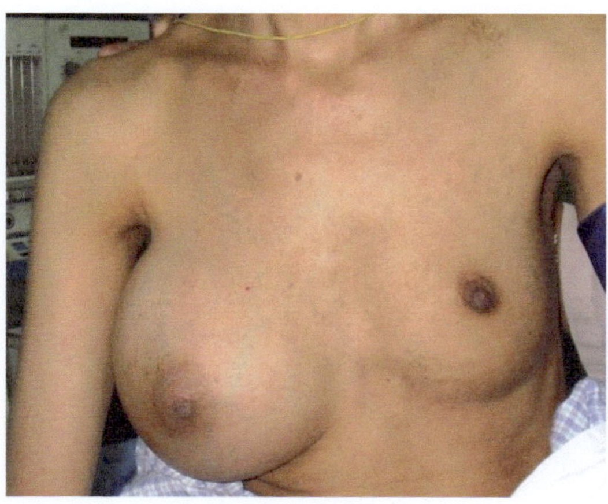

Fig. 4.1 Giant Fibroadenoma of the right breast

pausal period, growth during pregnancy or estrogen therapy, and regression during menopause. A classic clinical characteristic is a palpable mass measuring up to 5 cm (Fig. 4.1). These lumps are usually painless. If there is sudden increase in the size of the lump with associated pain, one should suspect a cyst that has suddenly become big, either by itself or due to hemorrhage into the cyst [7].

4.1.4 Nipple Discharge

Any nipple discharge that is spontaneous and unilateral is considered as pathological. The most common cause is intraductal papilloma (50% of cases). Duct ectasia is the pathology in 2–35% of cases, and in 5–15% of cases, breast carcinoma is the cause [8].

Nipple discharge that is spontaneous, unilateral, from a single duct, and bloody is significant. Greenish/brownish discharge indicates fibrocystic disease. Purulent discharge indicates infection.

Galactorrhoea indicates a milky nipple discharge, which is often bilateral. This could be due to physiological conditions like puberty and pregnancy or medication induced by drugs like dopamine antagonists such as tricyclic antidepressants or Selective Serotonin Reuptake Inhibitors (SSRIs). Other drugs that cause milky nipple discharge are methyl-dopamine, clonidine, verapamil, cimetidine, ranitidine, oestrogens, and oral contraceptive pills. Endocrine causes of galactorrhoea are hypo- or hyperthyroidism or renal failure. A prolactinoma of the pituitary gland should be suspected in any patient with a serum prolactin concentration of >200 ng/ml. The patient should be referred for a consultation with an endocrinologist and should get an MRI of the brain done to visualize the tumor. If the prolactin concentration is normal and the nipple discharge is not spontaneous, no further investigations are needed [9].

4.2 Clinical Presentation of Breast Malignancy

4.2.1 Symptoms of Breast Cancer

Many early breast carcinomas are asymptomatic. Most patients present due to an abnormal mammogram in those parts of the world where there are well-organized breast cancer screening programs. Breast lump is the most common symptom, in about 83% of all women [10]. Other commonly reported presenting symptoms are nipple abnormalities (7%), breast pain (6%), and breast skin abnormalities (2%).

Broadly, the symptoms of breast cancer can be divided into three categories:

1. Breast lump
2. Nonlump breast symptoms
3. Nonbreast symptoms

4.2.1.1 Breast Lump

Breast lump is the most common symptom at presentation, especially in developing countries that do not have a dedicated screening program. Patients usually present with a painless mass. Pain or discomfort is not usually a symptom of breast cancer; only 5% of patients with a malignant mass present with breast pain [11].

4.2.1.2 Nonlump Breast Symptoms

If the patient has not noticed a lump, then symptoms indicating the possible presence of breast cancer may include the following:

- Change in breast size or shape (contour abnormalities)
- Skin dimpling or skin changes (e.g., thickening, swelling, redness, rash, or ulceration) (Figs. 4.2 and 4.3)
- Nipple abnormalities like recent nipple retraction, skin change, ulceration or spontaneous, unilateral bloody discharge. Nipple ulceration is classically seen in Paget's disease (Fig. 4.4). Recent nipple retraction indicates the possibility of an infiltrating ductal carcinoma being the cause for the retraction (Fig. 4.5)

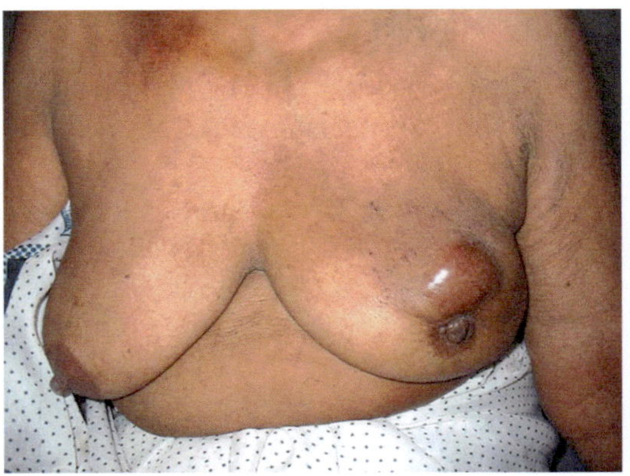

Fig. 4.2 Left breast lump with overlying skin redness along with nipple retraction

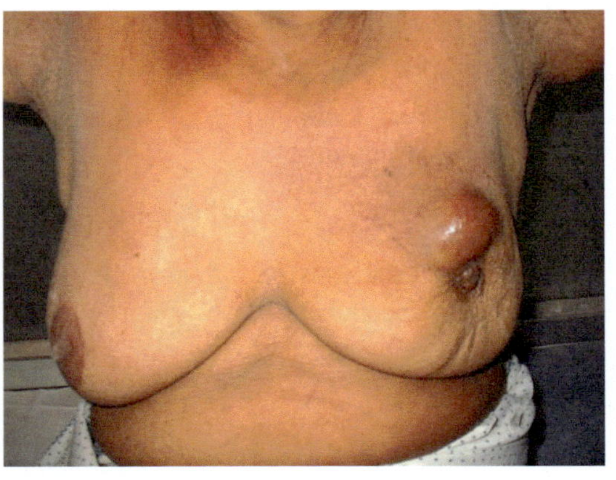

Fig. 4.3 Skin dimpling on raising the arms above the head

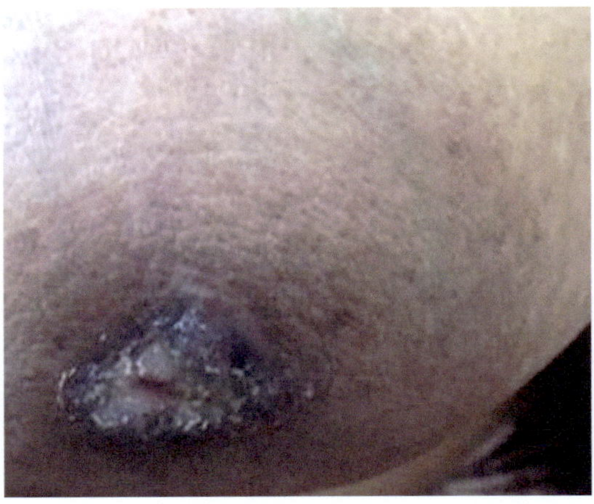

Fig. 4.4 Paget's disease of the nipple with ulceration of the nipple

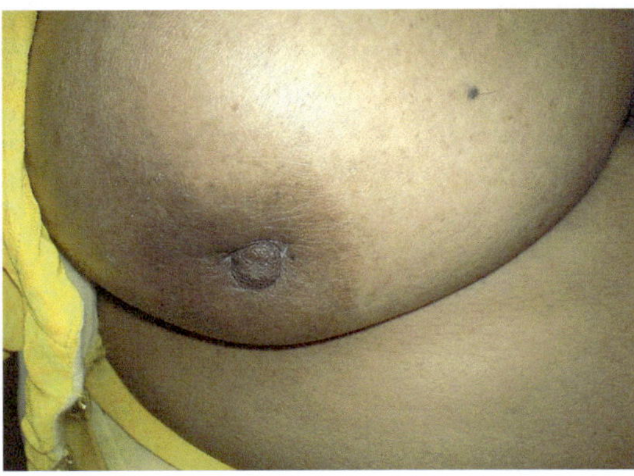

Fig. 4.5 Nipple retraction

4.2.1.3 Nonbreast Symptoms

This may be those relating to regional or distant metastases or general symptoms.

Regional Metastases may present in the form of axillary pain, axillary swelling, arm edema, or a neck swelling (supraclavicular lymph node enlargement) [12].

Symptoms of systemic metastatic spread may be any of the following:

Bone pain, backache
Breathlessness, dry cough
Abdominal pain/distension
Jaundice

Altered cognitive function
Headache, vomiting
New-onset seizures
Rarely, symptoms of hypercalcemia like excessive thirst/micturition, lethargy, irritability, depression nausea, constipation, muscle aches, easy fatiguability, etc., may be present.

4.2.2 General Nonspecific Symptoms

These may be in the form of musculoskeletal pain, fatigue, weakness, or rarely weight loss.

4.2.2.1 History

Once the patient presents with symptoms suggestive of malignancy, a detailed menstrual, obstetric, family, personal and treatment history should be obtained from her.

Menstrual History

The age of menarche and menopause should be ascertained from the patient. An early menarche (<11 years of age) and a late menopause (>55 years of age) poses a higher risk to develop breast cancer due to the excessive and continuous exposure to estrogen. It is also important to know the menopausal status of the patient—whether she is premenopausal or postmenopausal. This will determine the type of adjuvant hormonal therapy to be given in case the tumor is positive for hormonal receptors.

Obstetric History

Childbirth and breast feeding are protective to the mother from breast cancer. This is explained by the fact that pregnancy and lactational amenorrhoea reduces the estrogen stimulus on the breast and thereby reduces the chance of cancer. Nulliparous women are at a higher risk for developing breast cancer. For parous women, age of the woman at first childbirth is also important. Age greater than 30 years is an independent risk factor for the development of breast cancer.

Family History

History of malignancy in the patient's first- and second-degree relatives should be asked for. Breast, ovarian, endometrial, colorectal, gastric, pancreatic, and prostatic cancers can occur in these family members.

Personal History

Details about the patient's diet (whether it is of the low fiber western type of diet), obesity, and consumption of alcohol should be obtained, as these factors contribute to the rising incidence of breast cancer [13].

Treatment History

Long-term hormone replacement therapy (HRT) and treatment with ionizing radiation for some other disease (e.g., Hodgkin's lymphoma) are two important aspects of the treatment history that should be ascertained. Both these are risk factors for developing breast cancer. Previous history of breast biopsy with a pathological diagnosis of atypical ductal hyperplasia places the woman at a higher risk for developing cancer. History of prior treatment for cancer in the opposite breast should also be obtained.

4.2.3 Physical Examination

The examination must include an assessment of the breasts with the patient sitting up with arms by the side and then raised, in order to detect early changes in breast contour and skin dimpling/tethering. Then the patient should be examined with arms raised above her head and then while leaning forward and finally with arms pressing down on her hips (Figs. 4.6 and 4.7).

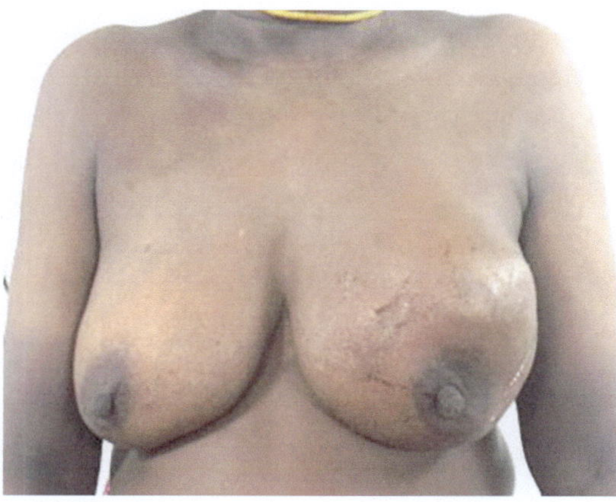

Fig. 4.6 Large breast lump in the upper outer and lower quadrants of the left breast

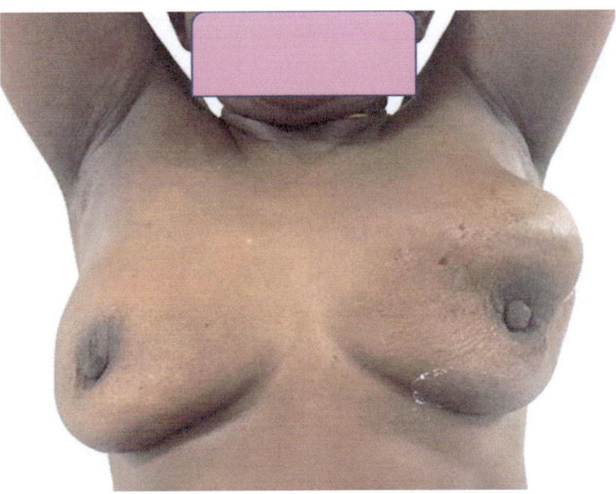

Fig. 4.7 Accentuated appearance of the large breast lump with Nipple retraction on raising the arms above the head

The following findings should raise concern:

Lump or contour change
Skin tethering
Nipple inversion
Dilated veins
Ulceration
Mammary Paget disease
Edema or peau d'orange

Next, the patient is made to lie in a semirecumbent position and the breasts are palpated with the palmar surface of the examiner's fingers to make out any discrete lump.

The following features about the palpable lump should raise concern:

Hardness
Irregularity
Focal nodularity
Asymmetry with the other breast
Fixation to skin or muscle (assess fixation to muscle by moving the lump in the line of the pectoral muscle fibers with the patient pressing her hands down on her hips).

The examination is completed on assessment of the axillae and supraclavicular fossae, chest and sites of skeletal pain, followed by an abdominal and neurologic examination. The clinical examination findings are substantiated by imaging, and a confirmed diagnosis is obtained by an appropriate core needle biopsy and pathological examination.

References

1. Stachs A, Stubert J, Reimer T, Hartmann S. Benign breast disease in women. Dtsch Arztebl Int. 2019;116:565–74. https://doi.org/10.3238/arztebl.2019.0565.
2. Smith RL, Pruthi S, Fitzpatrick LA. Evaluation and management of breast pain. Mayo Clin Proc. 2004;79:353–72.
3. Scurr J, Hedger W, Morris P, Brown N. The prevalence, severity, and impact of breast pain in the general population. Breast J. 2014;20(5):508–13. https://doi.org/10.1111/tbj.12305.
4. Spencer JP. Management of mastitis in breastfeeding women. Am Fam Physician. 2008;78(6):727–32.
5. Boakes E, Woods A, Johnson N, Kadoglou N. Breast infection: a review of diagnosis and management practices. Eur J Breast Health. 2018;14:136–43. https://doi.org/10.5152/ejbh.2018.3871.
6. El-Wakeel H, Umpleby HC. Systematic review of fibroadenoma as a risk factor for breast cancer. Breast. 2003;12:302–7.
7. Brennan M, Houssami N, French J. Management of benign breast conditions. Part 2–Breast lumps and lesions. Aust Fam Physician. 2005;34(4):253–5.
8. Dupont SC, Boughey JC, Jimenez RE, et al. Frequency of diagnosis of cancer or high-risk lesion at operation for pathologic nipple discharge. Surgery. 2015;158:988–94.
9. Verhelst J, Abs R. Hyperprolactinemia: pathophysiology and management. Treat Endocrinol. 2003;2:23–32.
10. Koo MM, Von Wagner C, Abel GA, McPhail S, Rubin GP, Lyratzopoulos G. Typical and atypical presenting symptoms of breast cancer and their associations with diagnostic intervals: evidence from a national audit of cancer diagnosis. Cancer Epidemiol. 2017;48:140–6. https://doi.org/10.1016/j.canep.2017.04.010.
11. Joe BN. Clinical features, diagnosis, and staging of newly diagnosed breast cancer. 2022. https://www.uptodate.com/contents/clinical-features-diagnosis-and-staging-of-newly-diagnosed-breast-cancer. Accessed 28 Jan 2022.
12. Chalasani P. Breast cancer clinical presentation. 2022. https://emedicine.medscape.com/article/1947145-clinical. Accessed 28 Jan 2022.
13. McTiernan A. Behavioral risk factors in breast cancer: can risk be modified? Oncologist. 2003;8(4):326–34.

Part III

Radiological Approach to Breast Disease

5 Diagnostic Imaging Investigations: Techniques

Sheila Elangovan, Bhawna Dev, and Veenashankari Padmanabhan

Abstract

Radiological imaging of breast tissues includes mammogram, Ultrasound Breast, and dynamic contrast-enhanced MRI of both breasts. Mammography is used both as a diagnostic tool in symptomatic patients and as a screening tool in asymptomatic patients who are at risk due to strong family history of breast carcinoma. This aids detection of carcinoma at a much early stage, wherein, the treatment strategy is much more effective.

Keywords

Mammogram · USG breast · MRI breast · Patient positioning · Dedicated MR coil

S. Elangovan (✉)
Faculty of Allied Health Sciences, Department of Radiology & Imaging Sciences, Sri Ramachandra Institute of Higher Education and Research, Chennai, India
e-mail: sheila@sriramachandra.edu.in

B. Dev
Department of Radiology, Sri Ramachandra Institute of Higher Education and Research, Chennai, India
e-mail: bhawnadev@sriramachandra.edu.in

V. Padmanabhan
Fellow in Breast Imaging and Intervention, Department of Radiology, Sri Ramachandra Institute of Higher Education and Research, Chennai, India

5.1 Imaging

Mammography aids in early detection of breast pathologies even before women experience symptoms such as pain, lump, skin dimpling, or nipple discharge. Successful interpretation of mammographic images requires optimal image quality free from patient-related artifacts, technique-related artifacts, and processing-related artifacts [1].

Adequate level of training, experience, effective communication with the patient, and interaction with the radiologist can improve sensitivity, specificity, and lesion detection with reduced recall rate [2].

5.2 When to Get a Mammogram Done?

It is ideal to get a mammogram done within the first 10 days of menstruation, since the breast tissues are less tender, reduce patient discomfort, and also to avoid irradiating an unknown fetus [3].

Technologists must explain the mammogram procedure and reassure apprehensive patients to overcome anxiety. Patient must be educated not to use talcum powder, deodorant on the day of mammogram as these can mimic calcifications. Breast and axilla is cleaned before the procedure, and it must be ensured that jewelry and clothing

B. Dev, L. D. Joseph (eds.), *Holistic Approach to Breast Disease*,
https://doi.org/10.1007/978-981-99-0035-0_5

in the region of examination are removed prior to mammogram.

5.3 Positioning Protocol

Technologists should develop ideal positioning techniques that yield good-quality images successful for radiologist's interpretation. Minimal modification of positioning method is necessary based on patient's body habitus. Standard positioning techniques must be reviewed periodically to analyze the percentage of redos and supplementary projections. Validation of developed positioning protocol is necessary prior to implementation.

5.4 Breast Compression

Breast compression is an important aspect in mammogram though it causes pain and discomfort to the patient. Compression of breast tissue is achieved by means of radio-translucent paddles (Fig. 5.1). Breast compression aids uniform film density (homogenous breast thickness), increases geometric unsharpness, and also results in lesser radiation dose, since the breast tissue to be penetrated is reduced.

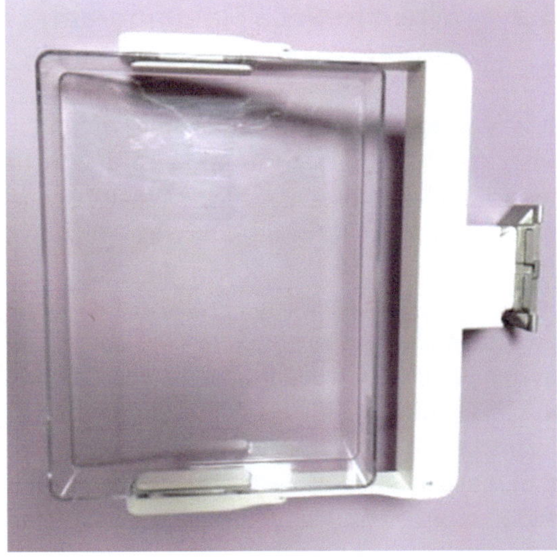

Fig. 5.1 Translucent breast compression paddle

5.5 Working Principle

The patient's breast is positioned on the mammography table and a small burst of X-rays passes through the breast onto the detector. The detector can be either a photographic film plate or a solid-state detector. The latent image captured on the photographic film plate is processed in darkroom on daylight dry view systems, whereas in solid-state detector, the electrical signals are transmitted to a computer to form a digital image.

5.6 Mammographic Projections

Cranio-caudal (CC) and mediolateral oblique (MLO) views are the standard mammographic projections. Ideally positioned CC and MLO views should image the entire breast tissue. Supplementary projections such as true lateral, spot magnification, spot compression, and cleavage views are to be taken as and when indicated.

5.6.1 Cranio-Caudal (CC) Projection

Optimal CC image demonstrates the nipple in profile, inframammary angle, lateral and medial aspect of the breast, central part of the retroglandular fat tissue, and the pectoral muscle on the posterior edge of the breast (Fig. 5.2).

Prerequisite for successful positioning:

- Cassette holder/detector in horizontal position (nil tube angulation).
- Direction of the X-ray beam must be perpendicular to the floor.
- The technologist stands at 90° to the patient on the opposite side of the breast being imaged.
- Technologist ensures that the patient's shoulder of the side being examined is relaxed to include upper-outer quadrant breast tissue and also to avoid skinfolds.

5.6.1.1 Positioning of CC View

Appropriate compression paddle and bucky/detector is to be used. The technologist stands on

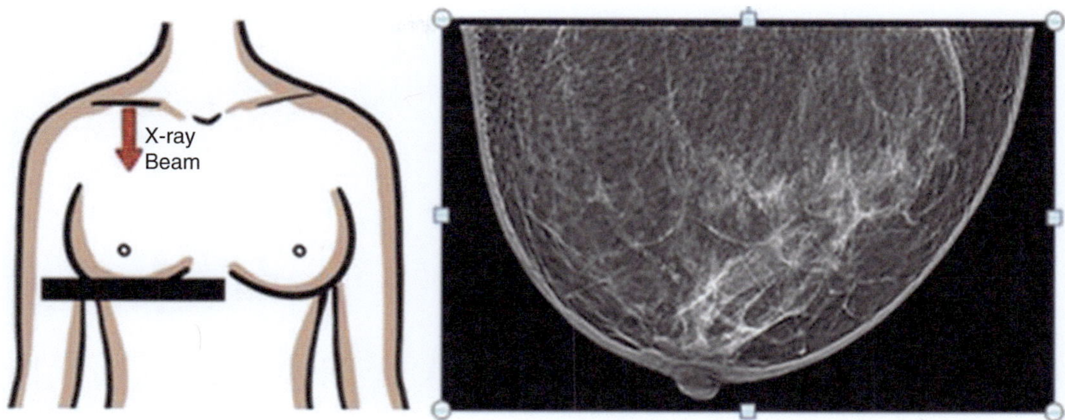

Fig. 5.2 Detector position, direction of X-ray beam, and corresponding CC image

the opposite side of the breast being imaged. Height of the detector is adjusted according to the patient such that the edge of the cassette holder is at the level of the elevated inframammary fold and the posterior nipple line (PNL) is parallel to the cassette holder. The breast is lifted up by the technologist's right hand pulling the breast forward. Both the medial and lateral portions of the breast are included, while the technologist's other hand moves the shoulder out of field of view. Skin folds, if any, are flattened. It is always better to include the cleavage portion of the opposite breast on the CC view (Fig. 5.2). Gradual compression is to be given manually, while the technologist prepositions and positions the breast keeping the nipple in profile. Compression force needs to be steady and strong.

5.6.2 Mediolateral Oblique (MLO) Projection

Optimal MLO view demonstrates the entire breast tissue, nipple in profile, pectoral muscle extending up to below the nipple line and inframammary angle [1].

Prerequisite for successful positioning;

- The cassette holder/detector is vertical, and the direction of X-ray beam is horizontal.
- The X-ray tube angle varies for each patient between 45° and 75° based on patient's height and size of the breast.
- Edge of the cassette holder/detector is parallel to the patient's pectoral muscle when the shoulders are at the same level and the upper arm is horizontal.
- Technologist stands on the side opposite to the breast being imaged.

5.6.2.1 Positioning of MLO View

Appropriate compression paddle is used. The patient stands facing the mammogram machine, turning her body slightly away from the breast to be imaged such that her feet are approximately 45° to the supporting edge of the cassette holder/detector. Technologist stands on the side opposite to the breast being imaged and places her right hand flat against the patient's upper abdomen just below the breast to be imaged. The other hand reaches the patient's back to enable inclusion of maximum breast tissue. The hand under the breast slides upward, holding the breast from below. This helps elevation of the breast and pulls the pectoral muscle away from the chest wall [4]. It is important to include the inframammary fold. The patient is moved toward the detector, upper arm is lifted, and rotated internally. Patient's upper body is flexed forward for better body contact with the detector. This movement enables viewing maximum soft tissue of the axilla, axillary tail, and posterolateral aspect of the breast attached to the chest. Edge of the detector is placed high in the axilla. Technologist's hand, which is placed on the patient's upper arm, moves to the top of the shoulder, slouching it, and patient

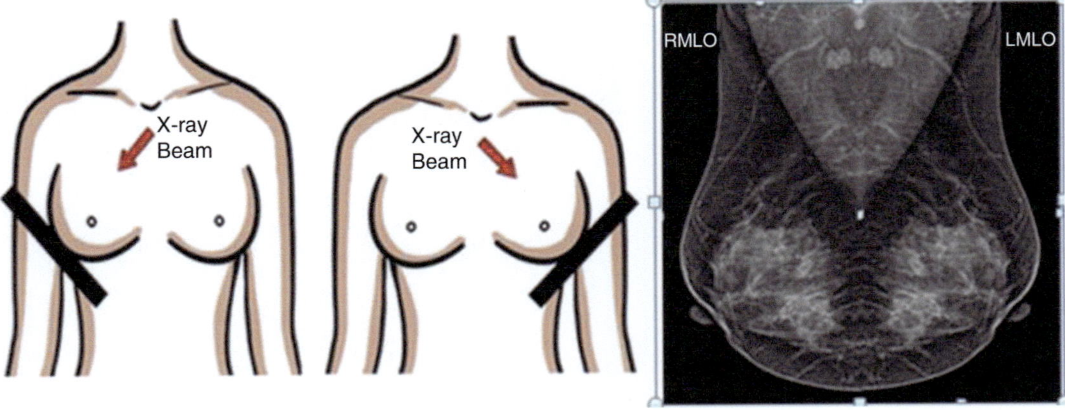

Fig. 5.3 Detector position for both breasts, direction of X-ray beam, corresponding MLO image

holds the handle bar with elbow flexed. The patient is slowly turned toward the detector, and the breast is pulled up (medially) and away (anteriorly) from the chest wall. Gradual compression using foot switch is applied while the technologist's hand slides toward the nipple, eliminating skin folds. Abdominal fold is pulled down to open the inframammary fold. Patient's face is turned to one side to avoid nose, chin, ear, or shoulder inside the field of view. It must be ensured that the patient's sternal angle and image receptor are parallel to each other, so that maximum breast tissue is compressed effectively. Other breast is to be pulled by patient using his/her contralateral hand throughout the study. Patient is asked not to move until the entire study is complete/compression paddle is released (Fig. 5.3).

5.7 Supplementary Mammographic Procedures

Few of the breast abnormalities involving the extreme medial or lateral aspect of the breast can be missed out as CC and MLO views do not image the entire breast tissues [5]. Supplementary projections provide additional information necessary to confirm an abnormality or to rule out a suspicious finding seen on only one of the standard views and not seen on the corresponding standard projection. Skilled radiologist reviews the standard view and suggests an appropriate supplementary view to confirm abnormalities/perceived abnormalities.

5.7.1 Lateral View

A true lateral view is taken with the X-ray tube rotated to 90°. Lateral view can be either lateromedial (LM) or mediolateral (ML) with the tube rotation either lateral or medial to the breast, respectively. This view helps to triangulate lesions and helps determine the trajectory in breast biopsies. This view demonstrates majority of the breast tissue, pectoral muscles, nipple in profile, and inframammary angle.

5.7.1.1 Positioning of Lateral View

Patient stands facing the mammogram equipment, and the X-ray tube is rotated by 90°. For lateromedial projection, the image receptor/detector is centered on the midsternal line (Fig. 5.4) and the width of the image receptor presses/pushes the contralateral breast [6]. This ensures deep medial breast tissue is included in the image. For mediolateral projection, detector is placed on the lateral aspect of the breast (Fig. 5.4). Patient's neck is extended with chin resting on top of image receptor. Patient's elbow is flexed to relax pectoralis muscle, while the arm is gently raised out of the field of view. Compression is applied gradually rotating the breast until it is in true lateral position. Abdominal tissue is pulled down to open the inframammary fold.

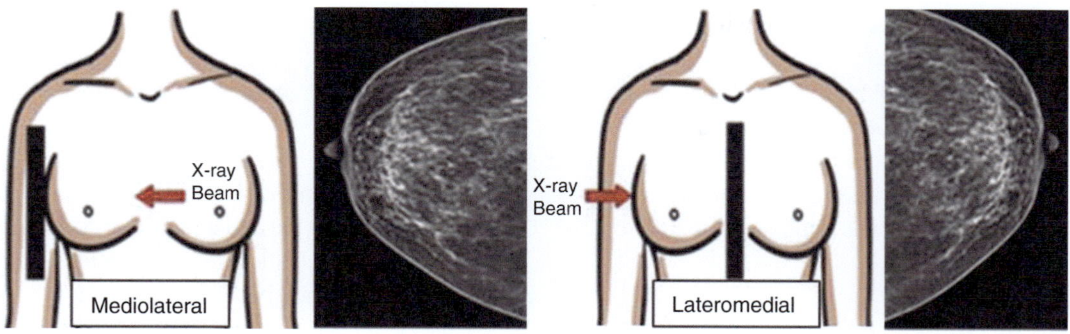

Fig. 5.4 Detector position, direction of X-ray beam, and corresponding lateral images

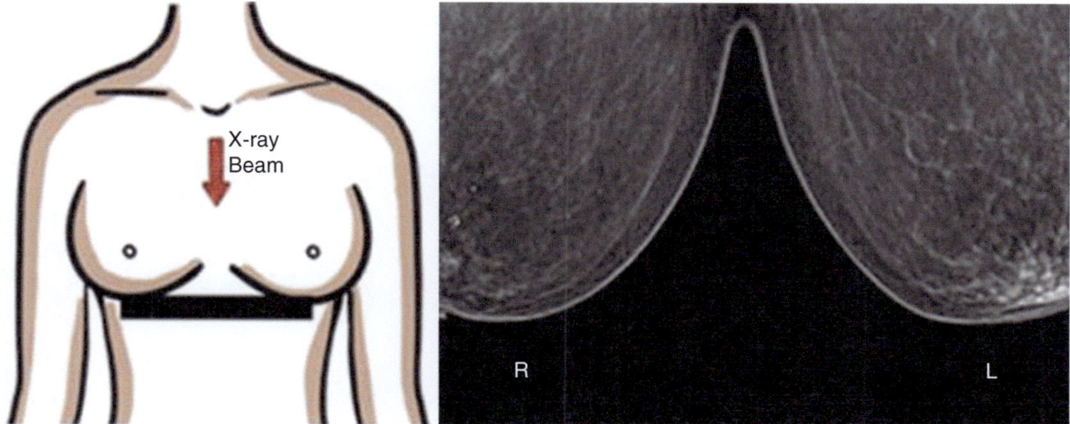

Fig. 5.5 Detector position, direction of X-ray beam, and corresponding cleavage view

5.7.2 Cleavage View

Purpose of cleavage view is to visualize the extreme medial portions of both breasts. Cleavage view helps visualize deep lesions in the postero-medial aspect of the breasts (valley between both breasts). Radiologists insist for a cleavage view when a finding is observed in the medial quadrant but not seen on the cranio-caudal view. This is because some of the breast tissue being imaged gets pulled out of the field of view during compression. Manual exposure is done if the cleavage is centered, and automatic exposure control (AEC) is a better option if the cleavage is off-centered [4].

5.7.2.1 Positioning of Cleavage View

Patient stands facing the machine in close proximity to the horizontal image receptor/detector. Technologist stands behind the patient and elevates inframammary folds of both breasts using his/her hands, on either side of the detector table. The medial portions of both breasts are placed on the detector and compression is applied gradually. Side markers are placed on the lateral aspect of both breasts (Fig. 5.5).

5.7.3 Exaggerated Cranio-Caudal View (XCCL)

Purpose of this view is to better visualize lateral or medial portion of the breast particularly posterolateral breast tissue.

5.7.3.1 Positioning of XCCL

Positioning for this view is similar to that of cranio-caudal view. Inframammary fold is elevated and patient's upper trunk is slightly rotated medially to include entire lateral aspect of the breast into the FOV (Fig. 5.6). Tube angulation is modified by 5° based on patient's body habitus to avoid shoulder joint. Compression is applied gradually and exposure is similar to that of cranio-caudal view is done.

5.7.4 Rolled View

Purpose of this view is to confirm the presence of an abnormality seen on only one standard view by separating superimposed breast tissues. Rolled views are of two types, namely, "Rolled medially" for a lesion located superiorly and "Rolled laterally" for a lesion located inferiorly. Subareolar, central, medial, and posteromedial breast tissues are visualized better on rolled views (Fig. 5.7).

5.7.4.1 Positioning of Rolled View

Patient stands facing the horizontal cassette holder/detector, and the technologist stands on the opposite side of the breast being imaged. She places one hand on the superior aspect of the breast and the other hand on the inferior aspect of the breast. In rolled lateral view, the technologist rolls the superior aspect of the breast laterally and the inferior aspect medially and in rolled medial view, the superior aspect of the breast is rolled medially and the inferior aspect is rolled laterally (Fig. 5.6).

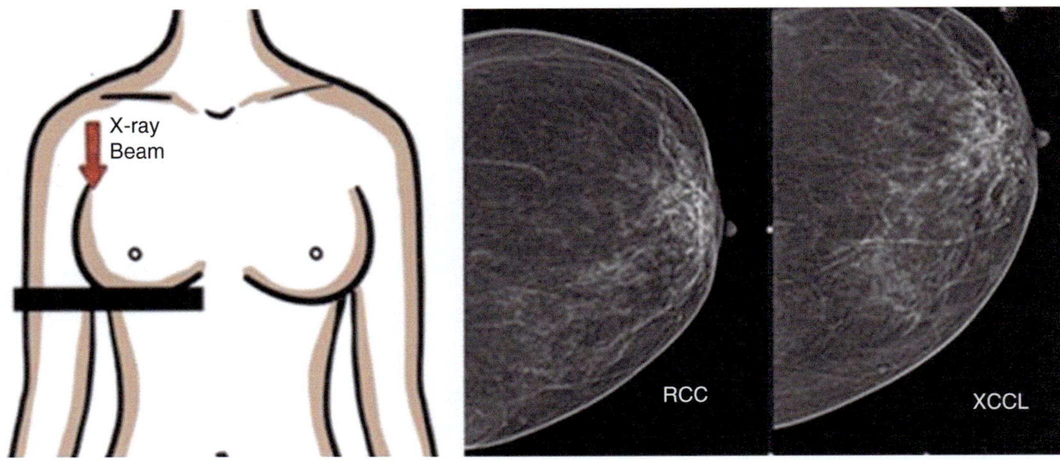

Fig. 5.6 Detector position, direction of X-ray beam, corresponding CC, and exaggerated lateral image

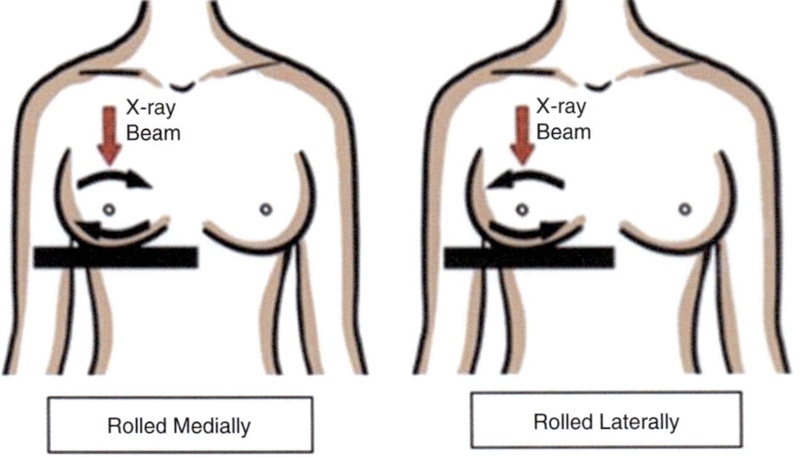

Fig. 5.7 Detector position, direction of X-ray beam with breast tissue rolled medially and laterally

Labeling of rolled views is of utmost importance for image interpretation. Rolled lateral view is labeled Cranio-caudal RL (CC rolled laterally) and rolled medial view is labeled Cranio-caudal RM (CC rolled medially).

5.7.5 Magnification View

Purpose of this view is to assess microcalcifications, their extension, suspicious lesions and also to delineate the borders of a suspicious mass. Magnification is achieved using a magnification device. The breast is positioned on the device closer to the X-ray source, which increases the distance between breast and cassette holder/detector. Area of interest is reduced with increased magnification and spatial resolution. One of the most important applications of magnification technique is specimen mammography (Fig. 5.8).

5.7.6 Spot Compression View

Purpose of this view is to eliminate pseudomass, evaluate focal asymmetry, architectural distortion, and depict margins of a mass. Spot compression is achieved by applying compression to a small defined region of breast tissue by means of a small compression paddle (Fig. 5.9). This compression is much more effective and breast tissue is spread more evenly. An important aspect of positioning technique is that the technologist must ensure rolling of breast and to avoid tube rotation.

5.7.7 Tangential View

Purpose of this view is to demonstrate superficial interdermal lesions, calcifications and palpable masses on dense glandular breasts. Tangential view is imaged within the subdermal layer by avoiding the skin. A palpable mass or suspicious lesion is imaged within the subdermal layer avoiding the skin and free from overlapping structures. A BB marker is placed on the exact site of the lesion/palpable mass, and an imaginary line is drawn between the BB marker and nipple. Mammographic tube is angled tangential to the BB marker (Fig. 5.10), and the resultant images show increased contrast and lesion details.

5.7.8 Axillary Tail View

Purpose is to demonstrate the axillary tail in its entirety. The mammographic tube is rotated parallel to the patient by 60–80° based on the patient's body habitus. Patient is turned to bring the axillary tail portion in contact with the detector. Patient's elbow is flexed, and the hand is made to rest on the handle bar of the machine. Technologist pulls the axillary portion outward

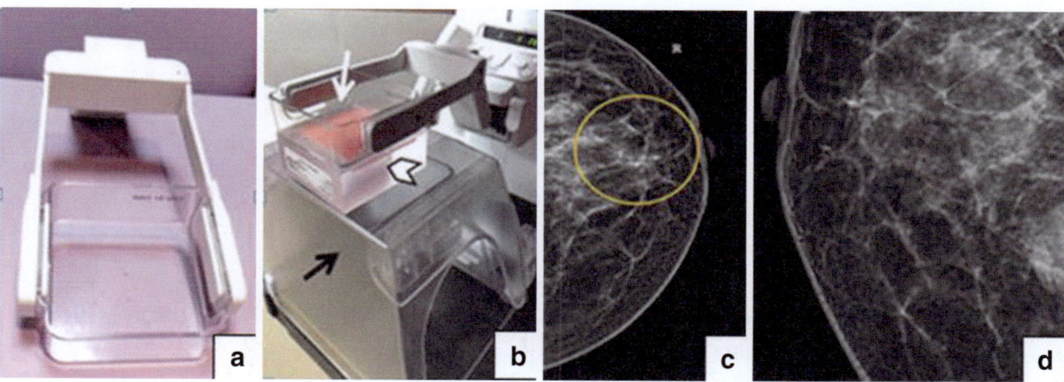

Fig. 5.8 (**a**) Magnification compression paddle, (**b**) compression paddle (white arrow), magnification device (black arrow), phantom (white arrow head), (**c**) craniocaudal image with a suspicious foci (**d**) magnified image

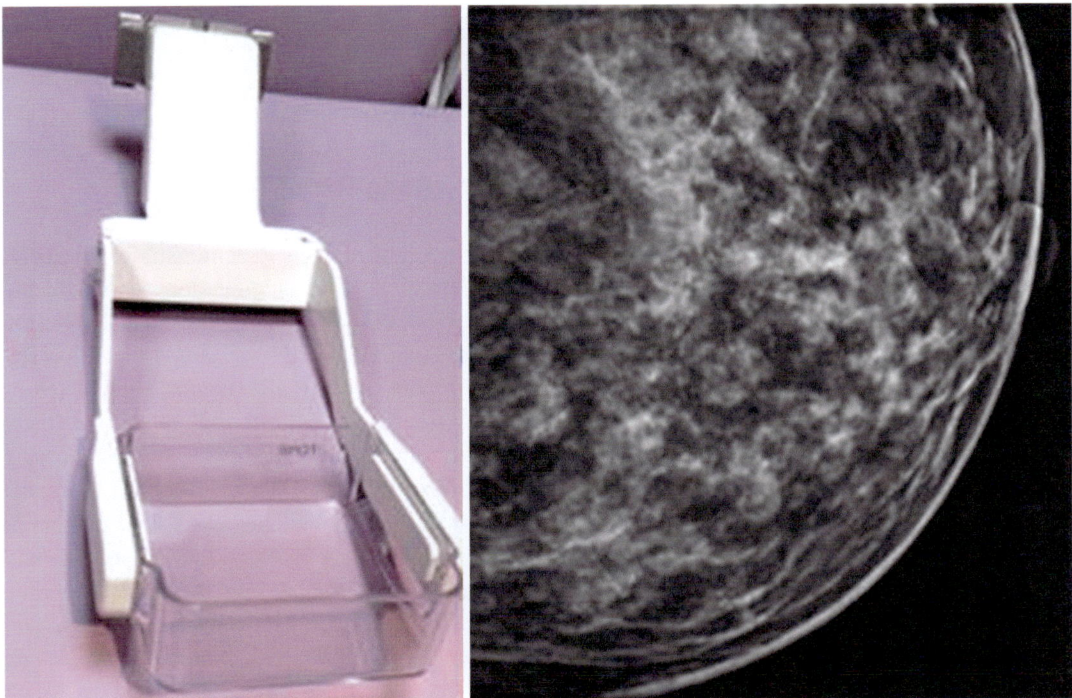

Fig. 5.9 Spot compression paddle and spot compressed image

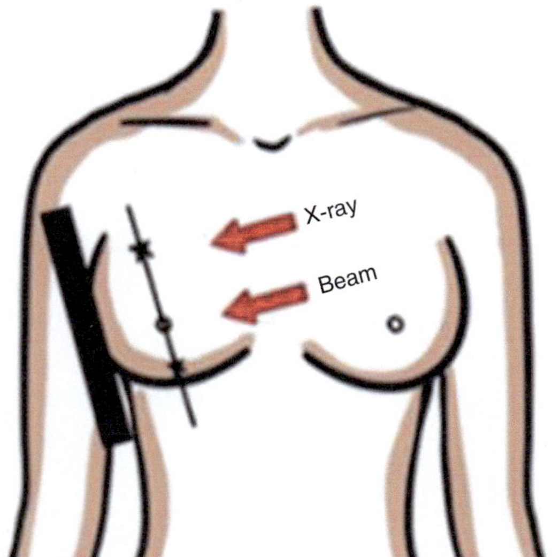

Fig. 5.10 BB marker, detector position, and direction of X-ray beam

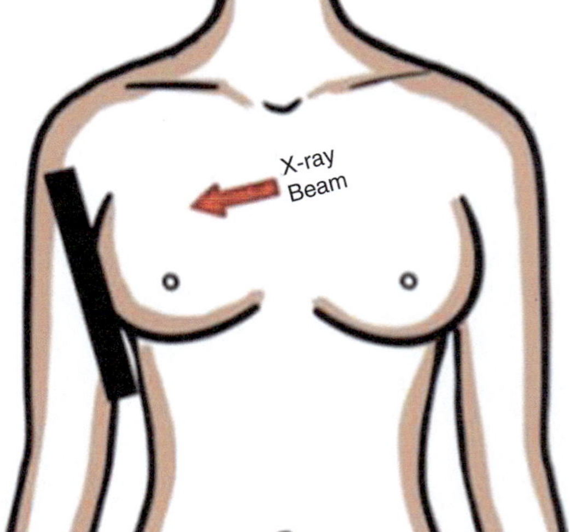

Fig. 5.11 Detector position and direction of X-ray beam

and away from the chest wall ("out and away") and holds it in place on the detector while compression is applied gradually. This view demonstrates the breast tissue high in the axilla without superimposition of pectoral muscle (Fig. 5.11).

5.8 Implant Mammography

Purpose of this view is to image breast tissues with implant in situ and with implant displaced. In the former view, mammography is performed by applying breast compression normally without displacing the breast implant (Fig. 5.12) and in the later view, mammography is performed by displacing the implant (pushing the implant posteriorly and superiorly), pulling the breast tissue forward (anteriorly), and applying compression to the breast free from superimposition of implant.

5.9 Posterior Nipple Line (PNL)

Posterior nipple line on a mediolateral oblique (MLO) view refers to a line drawn from the nipple posteriorly and perpendicular toward the pectoral muscle and on a cranio-caudal (CC) view, it refers to a line drawn from the nipple perpendicular to the posterior edge (Fig. 5.13).

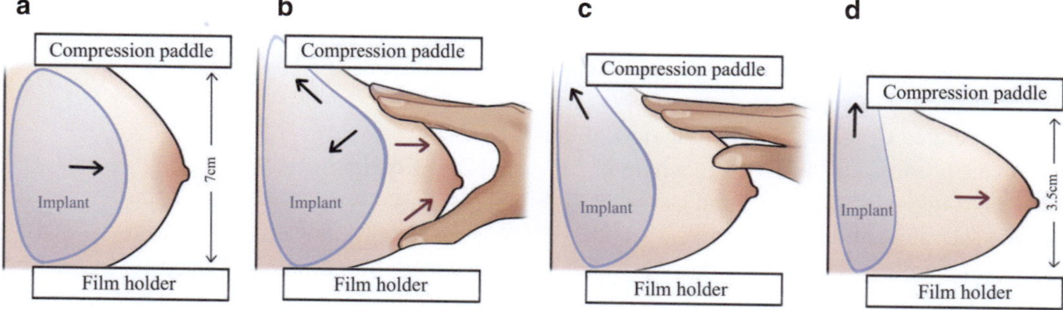

Fig. 5.12 Schematic representation of mammography in patients with breast implants (**a**) normal positioning without implant displacement and (**b–d**) implant being displaced posteriorly, superiorly and breast compression free from superimposition of implant respectively

Fig. 5.13 PNL measurement on CC and MLO views

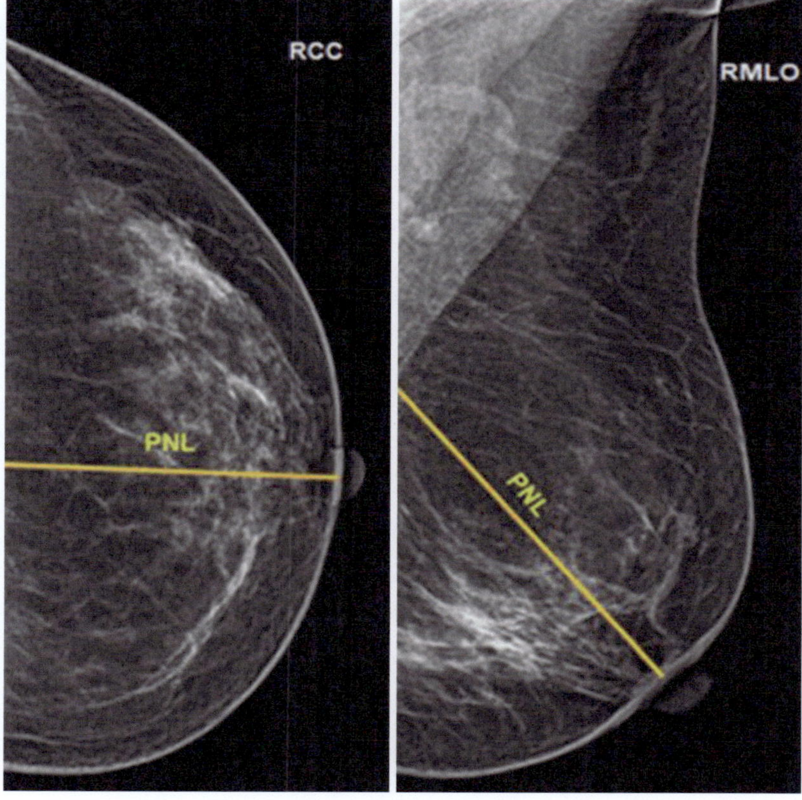

On an ideally positioned mammogram, the difference in the PNL measurements on a CC and MLO views should be less than 1 cm.

5.10 Labeling and Side Markers

An ideal mammographic image must include appropriate annotations and labeling. According to ACR guidelines, on a standard Cranio-caudal view, right (R) and left (L) side markers are to be placed on the lateral aspect of each breast. For example, Right CC view is annotated as RCC on the lateral aspect of right breast.

Exaggerated Cranio-caudal lateral view of the left breast is annotated as LXCCL, where in "X" denotes exaggerated technique and last letter "L" denotes lateral position.

5.11 Artifacts

Artifacts in mammography significantly degrade image quality, cause technical difficulties for technologist, and pose challenges in image interpretation for radiologist. Adequate knowledge about the cause, manifestation, and remedial measures are mandatory for each mammogram technologist.

Mammographic artifacts are either equipment-related, technique-related, processing-related, or patient-based artifacts. Regular calibration and maintenance of equipment is highly recommended to prevent equipment-related artifacts. Periodical training and education of technologists can reduce technique-related artifacts. Appropriate counseling and ideal patient preparation can minimize patient related artifacts.

5.12 Ultrasound Breast

Ultrasonography (US) is complementary to both mammography and magnetic resonance (MR) imaging of the breast.

Imaging dense breast parenchyma with X-ray poses challenges and requires ultrasound as an additional modality. Due to this reason, ultrasound and magnetic resonance imaging (MRI) are being used as part of supplementary breast screening procedures.

Ultrasound breast is the primary imaging modality for younger women less than 30 years of age.

The sensitivity for breast cancer detection using both mammography and ultrasound increases to 97.3%, with the false-positive rate of ultrasound measured as 2.4%.

5.12.1 Equipment

When scanning the breast, a linear 12–5-MHz transducer is commonly used (Fig. 5.14a). However, in small-breasted women (with breast thickness, 3 cm) or when performing targeted US to evaluate a superficial lesion, a linear 5–17 MHz transducer may be used. Such high-frequency transducers provide superb spatial and soft-tissue resolution, permitting substantially improved differentiation of subtle shades of gray, margin resolution, and lesion conspicuity in the background of normal breast tissue (Fig. 5.14b). The only drawback is decreased penetration due to the attenuation of ultrasound beam, making visualization of deep posterior tissue difficult.

During the initial US survey of the region of interest in the breast, the depth should be set so that the pectoralis muscle is visualized along the posterior margin of the field of view. Initial gain settings should be adjusted so that fat at all levels is displayed as a midlevel gray.

Time gain compensation (TGC), which adjusts image brightness at different depths from the skin to compensate for attenuation of the ultrasound beam, may be set manually or automatically during real-time scanning or even during postprocessing of the image.

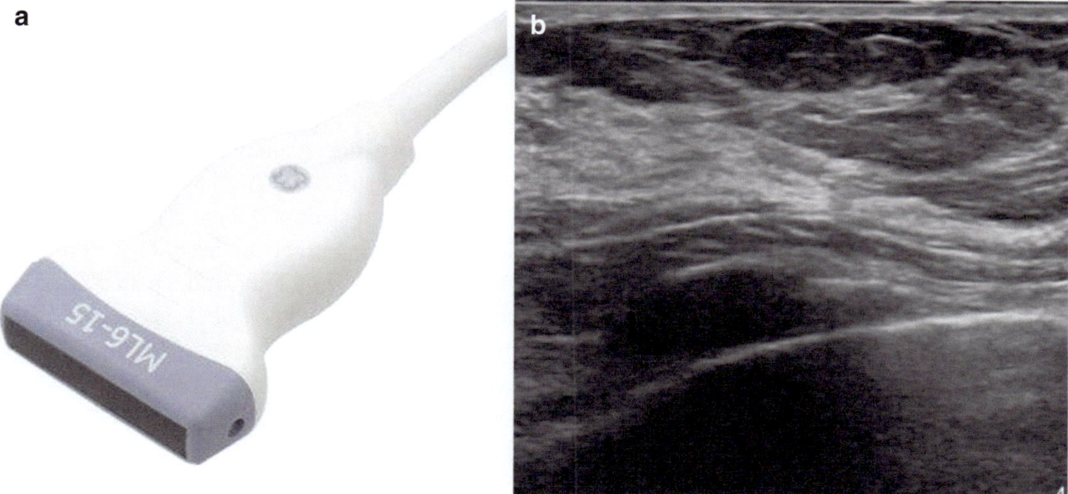

Fig. 5.14 (**a**) High-frequency linear transducer 6–15 MHz. (**b**) Ultrasound of breast showing different shades of grey separating different structures within the area scanned

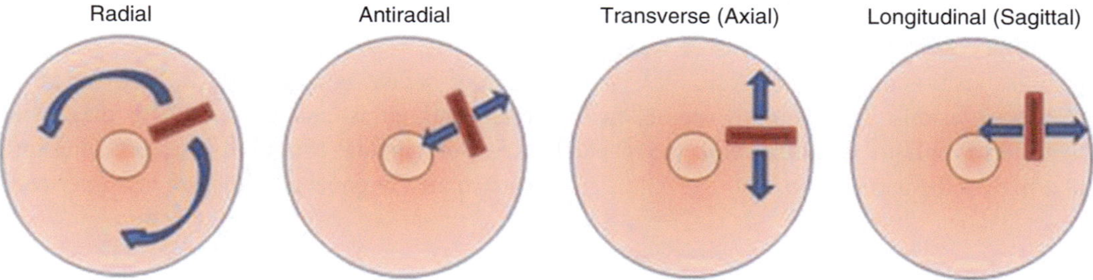

Fig. 5.15 Radial, antiradial, transverse, and longitudinal approach of performing ultrasound on breasts

5.12.2 Preparation

Breast ultrasound is a noninvasive procedure with none or very little special preparation required. Patient is encouraged to wear loose clothing to be able to undress the upper half of the torso before the examination.

5.12.3 Technique

Initial breast imaging of the patient should include a full clinical breast self-examination (BSE) to assess and validate all palpable masses, either identified by the patient or by the physician. Following BSE, a bilateral breast ultrasound is performed with a sequential sweeping of the breast surface.

The breast is assessed in the four main quadrants, namely, outer upper, outer inner, lower outer, and lower inner quadrants. Any lesions identified during the examination should be marked as a breast 'o clock position for future follow-up sessions.

The most common imaging technique used is a radial, antiradial, longitudinal, or transverse sweep of the entire breast Fig. 5.15, extending to the axillary space, parasternal, and clavicular surfaces.

The retro-areolar space should also be evaluated systematically; the dense tissue causes posterior acoustic shadowing, limiting its visibility. This anatomical limitation can be overcome by either angling the probe upward toward the retroareolar ducts or using a gel standoff pad with decreased focal zone and altering the time gain compensation controls, visualizing the soft tissue posterior to the dense nipple tissue.

5.12.4 Patient Position While Scanning

The optimal protocol for performing breast US requires the patient to lie in the supine position with the chest undressed and with arms flexed above the head to flatten the breast and in the oblique position for scanning the lateral part of the breast and, when needed, axilla.

Medial lesions: The patient is supine, with the ipsilateral arm over patient's head Fig. 5.16a.

Lateral lesions: The patient lies with the ipsilateral arm over the patient's head. The degree of obliquity depends on the breast size, pendulousness, and the location of the lesion within the breast Fig. 5.16b. In a large breast, a complete decubitus position might be the best.

Superior lesions: The patient is supine, opposite posterior oblique or sitting, with the ipsilateral arm over the patient's head.

Inferior lesions: The patient is supine, and the breast can be held superiorly.

Varying degree of pressure is used to flatten the breast parenchyma as well as bring the conical surface of the glandular tissue into a more orthogonal plane.

Given the real-time dynamic nature of ultrasound imaging, and the tendency of the breast to change its shape with gravity, the patient position should be optimized to the examination. This may be done several times to allow the acquisition of high-quality, reproducible images. Different positions are especially useful in large breasts. Inadequate positioning may cause portions of the breast to become inaccessible, the breast to fall over the transducer, or the lesions to appear displaced on follow-up examinations.

5.13 MRI of both Breasts

MRI of breasts is an adjunct to X-ray mammogram and ultrasound of breasts in diagnosing breast carcinoma. It is used as a screening tool, particularly in patients with high and intermedi-

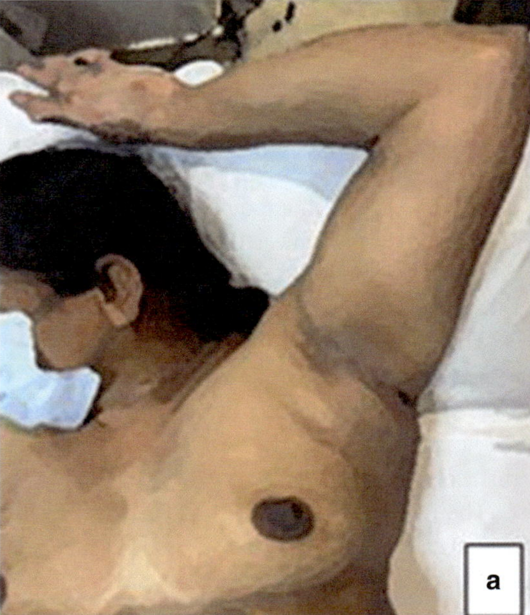

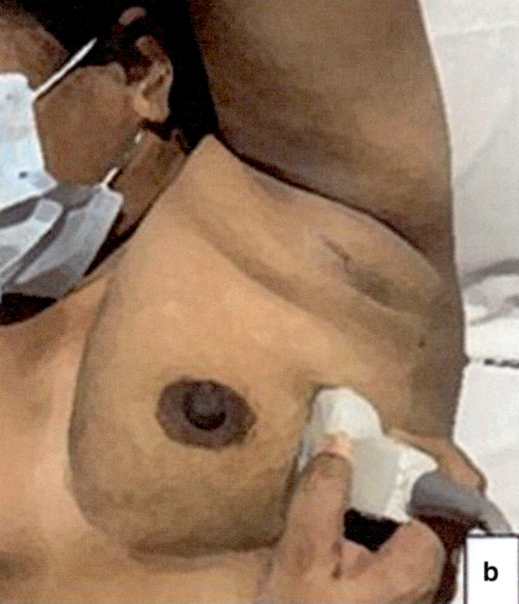

Fig. 5.16 (**a**) Patient position while scanning, (**b**) Slightly oblique (10–15°) position of the patient for clear visibility of the lateral quadrants

ate risk of breast carcinoma. MRI of breasts with its inherent soft tissue contrast yields images with excellent spatial resolution. When performed with administration of gadolinium-based contrast agent, it aids better detection of breast carcinoma. In comparison to X-ray mammogram and ultrasound of breasts, MRI provides morphological, physiological, and also functional information at the molecular level. Unlike X-ray mammogram, breast density is not a limitation for breast MRI.

MRI perfusion performed by multiphase dynamic acquisition following intravenous administration of GBCA is highly sensitive in providing information on contrast kinetics and single voxel MR Spectroscopy.

5.13.1 MR Safety Screening

Patient screening by means of a detector and questionnaire needs to be completed to rule out absolute and relative contraindications. Hormonal status (LMP/menopause/follicular phase or luteal phase, lactating history etc.), past surgical history, HRT status, family history of carcinoma, and radiotherapy/chemotherapy status are to be checked.

5.13.2 Procedure

The linchpin of MR of both breasts is appropriate coil selection and patient positioning.

Prerequisites of appropriate patient positioning are

- Entire breast tissue coverage
- Absence of skin folds
- Homogenous fat suppression

A dedicated breast coil with parallel imaging capabilities (Fig. 5.17a) is imperative for optimal imaging and successful image interpretation. It significantly improves the diagnostic sensitivity. Homogenous fat suppression is a unique advantage of employing dedicated breast coil for imaging. Positioning the patient and patient's comfort is an important attribute that addresses several artifacts. Patient's comfort throughout the examination yields conspicuous images free from movement-related artifacts. In open coil system, coils are designed with two apertures side by side for accommodating the breasts within (Fig. 5.17b). Patient lies prone on her abdomen with the breasts enveloped within the right and left apertures. The arms are placed by the sides with patient's head placed on a prime headset to enhance patient's comfort. An opening on the lateral aspect of each aperture enables the technologist to adjust the position of the breast and avoid skin folds (Fig. 5.17c) Providing foam pads and wedges below the abdomen facilitates better slouching of both shoulders, pulling the breast as far as possible from the chest wall so that entire breast tissue is encompassed within the coil with downward erection of nipple in the center. Immobilizing the breast minimizes motion artifacts that have a significant impact on subtraction sequences. Technologist ensures breast is immobilized by adjusting the side frames on the lateral aspect of the coil (Fig. 5.17d). Care is taken to avoid too much compression or flattening on the

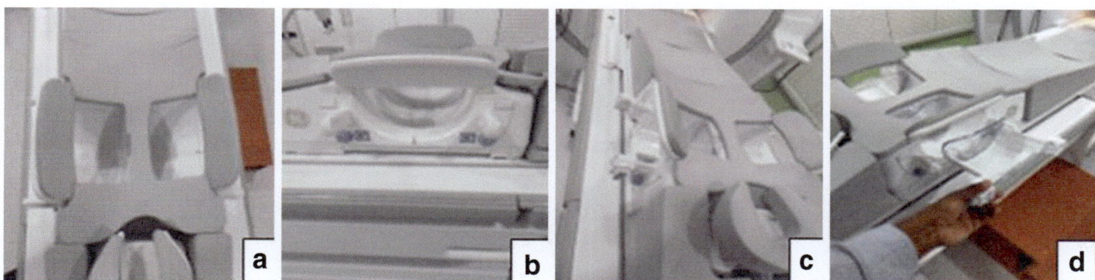

Fig. 5.17 (**a–d**) MR Breast coil from different angles

lateral aspect that might otherwise mimic deformed breast shape.

Thus, in each imaging modality (mammogram, USG breast, MRI breast), positioning of the patient is of utmost importance for reaching an adequate diagnosis.

References

1. Kopans DB. Mammography positioning in Kopans. In: Daniel B, editor. Breast imaging. 3rd ed. Philadelphia: Lippincott; 2007. p. 281–322.
2. Louise M, Henderson LM, Benefield T, Bowling JM, Durham DD, Marsh MW, Schvoeder BF, Yankarkas BC. Do mammographic technologists affect radiologists' interpretation performance? AJR. 2015;204(4):903–8. https://doi.org/10.2214/AJR.14.12903.
3. White E, Velantgas P, Margaret T, Mandolson CD, Lehman JG, Elmore PP, Yasui Y, Taplin SH. Variation in mammographic breast density by time in menstrual cycle among women aged 40–49yrs. J Natl Cancer Inst. 1998;90(12):906–10. https://doi.org/10.1093/jnci/90.12.906.
4. Tabar L, Parsons W, Vedin B, Petersen A. Mammographic positioning techniques.
5. Kelly J. Supplementary mammographic projection. National Health Science; 2015. https://doi.org/10.1007/978-3-319-04831-4-24.
6. Miller LC. Mammography positioning: basic and advanced. SBI Breast Imaging Symposium. 2016.

BI-RADS: An Overview

6

Priya K. Palanisamy, Bhawna Dev, and M. C. Sheela

Abstract

The American Collage of Radiology (ACR) structured a reporting system Breast Imaging Reporting and Data System (BI-RADS) with an aim of establishing consistency between the reports worldwide which enhances a clear communication between the radiologists and breast physicians. BI-RADS provides a standard lexicon of descriptors, reporting template, assessment categories depending on the imaging findings and recommendations for each category. In this chapter, we have briefly highlighted the revisions made to BI-RADS in the fifth edition by comparing with its forerunners.

Keywords

BI-RADS lexicon · ACR · Mammogram · Ultrasound · MRI

Breast Imaging Reporting and Data System is a standardized system of reporting breast pathologies seen on mammogram, ultrasound (USG), and Magnetic resonance imaging (MRI). Before the advent of the BI-RADS lexicon, the mammography and MRI breast reports were ambiguous, which, in turn, made the clinical management difficult for the referring physicians.

The American College of Radiology (ACR) in 1993 formulated the first edition of the BI-RADS lexicon system with the aim of standardizing the mammography reporting format. The lexicon descriptors enable the radiologists to communicate with the consulting physicians clearly and consistently by providing a uniform reporting structure that predicts the benign and malignant findings and provides recommendations regarding the final assessment, specific management protocol, and outcome monitoring. BI-RADS also helps in eliminating the ambiguity in the report and allows automated data collection.

Multiple revisions to the BI-RADS system have been made since 1993, with addition of imaging atlas with example of each descriptor in 1998, introduction of USG and MRI standardization in 2003. **Currently, the Fifth edition of the ACR BI-RADS system is being widely followed since Feb 2014** [1]. The final standardized report should be concise and organized using the following structure according to the ACR BI-RADS guidelines:

P. K. Palanisamy (✉)
Maidstone and Tunbirdge Wells NHS Trust, Kent, UK
e-mail: p.palanisamy@nhs.net

B. Dev · M. C. Sheela
Department of Radiology, Sri Ramachandra Institute of Higher Education and Research, Chennai, India
e-mail: bhawnadev@sriramachandra.edu.in; sheelamc@sriramachandra.edu.in

B. Dev, L. D. Joseph (eds.), *Holistic Approach to Breast Disease*,
https://doi.org/10.1007/978-981-99-0035-0_6

1. Indication for examination
2. Succinct descriptors of the overall breast Composition
3. Clear description of any important Findings
4. Comparison of previous examination(s), if deemed appropriate by the interpreting physician
5. Assessment
6. Management

6.1 A Brief Review on Revisions in the Fifth Edition BI-RADS: Mammography Lexicon Updates [2, 3]

The recent fifth edition of ACR Breast Imaging Reporting and Data System (BI-RADS) lexicon was published in February 2014 [1]. Since the Fourth edition of BI-RADS (published in 2003) was in practice for more than 10 years, many radiologists have difficulties in learning the changes made in the Fifth edition. In this segment, we briefly describe the updates made in the Mammography, USG, and MRI sections of the lexicon. These updates were built on clarifying previous term with aim of risk stratification.

The mammography lexicon has been changed from previous edition by eliminating and/or consolidating the descriptors along with few new additions. These changes are summarized in the Table 6.1.

Table 6.1 Summary of changes within mammography between BI-RADS fourth and fifth edition

Modified Descriptors	4th Edition	5th Edition changes
Breast composition	**Previously described in percentages** (a) Almost entirely fatty (less than 25% fibroglandular tissue) (b) Scattered fibroglandular densities (25–50%) (c) Heterogeneously dense (50–75%) (d) Extremely dense (more than 75%)	**Percentages have been removed** (a) The breast almost entirely fatty (b) There are scattered areas of fibroglandular densities (c) The breasts are heterogeneously dense, this may obscure small masses (d) The breasts are extremely dense, which lowers the sensitivity of mammography
A. Masses	**Shape**: Lobular **Density**: Fat containing radiolucent	Lobular is removed in fifth edition Omitted radiolucent
B. Calcification:		
1. Typically benign	**1. Typically benign:** • Eggshell or rim calcification • Lucent centered calcification	Combined egg-shell and lucent centered calcification into rim calcification
2. Suspicious morphology	2. **Intermediate morphology, suspicious calcification** • Amorphous or indistinct • Coarse heterogenous	Combined intermediate, suspicious calcifications and high probability of malignancy into suspicious calcifications
	3. **High probability of malignancy** • Fine pleomorphic • Fine linear or fine linear branching	
Distribution	Diffuse/scattered Grouped/clustered	Omitted "scattered" Omitted "clustered"

Table 6.1 (continued)

Modified Descriptors	4th Edition	5th Edition changes
C. Architectural distortion	**No changes**	
D. Asymmetries	Was included under **D. Special cases:** 1. Asymmetric tubular structure/solitary dilated duct 2. Intramammary nodes 3. Global asymmetry 4. Focal asymmetry	Added separate section for asymmetry **D. Asymmetries** 1. Asymmetry 2. Global asymmetry 3. Focal asymmetry 4. Developing asymmetry (**NEW**) Given under separate category: **E. Intramammary lymph nodes** **F. Skin lesions** **G. Solitary dilated ducts** Omitted asymmetric tubular structure
H. Associated findings	1. Skin retraction 2. Nipple retraction 3. Skin thickening 4. Trabecular thickening 5. Skin lesions 6. Axillary adenopathy 7. Architectural distortion 8. Calcifications	Omitted "skin lesions" 1. Skin retraction 2. Nipple retraction 3. Skin thickening 4. Trabecular thickening 5. Axillary adenopathy 6. Architectural distortion 7. Calcifications
I. Location of lesion	1. Location 2. Depth	**Added new findings** 1. Laterality 2. Quadrant and clock phase 3. Depth 4. Distance from skin

6.2 Use of Radio-Opaque Markers

In the fifth edition of BI-RADS, the use of radio-opaque markers explains about the application of markers for skin, palpable lesions and recommends including what the marker represents as an image annotation or as a descriptor to be added in the final report.

6.3 Revisions in BI-RADS Assessment Category

Clarifications in view of usage of BI-RADS 3 lesions have been given in the fifth edition, specifically in the context of screening detected abnormalities, **BI-RADS 3 should be reserved for lesions that has been fully evaluated in diagnostic settings.** Similarly BI-RADS Category 4 and 5 should also be reserved until after the completion of the diagnostic workup of the lesion.

6.4 Ultrasound Lexicon Updates [2, 3]

Includes addition of new subsection called "general considerations" and few changes in the US lexicon to improve the consistency across all modalities and addition of new modalities like Elastography in breast imaging. The complete list of changes is listed in Table 6.2.

Table 6.2 Summary of changes within US between BI-RADS fourth and fifth edition

Modified descriptors	4th edition	5th edition changes
General considerations	**N. S**	A. Breast anatomy B. Image quality C. Labeling and measurement D. Documentation
Composition	Described as background echotexture	Renamed as tissue composition
Masses	Lesion boundary: • Abrupt interface • Echogenic halo Posterior acoustic features: • No posterior features • Enhancement • Shadowing • Combined pattern	Removed lesion boundary category Renamed as posterior features: • No posterior features • Enhancement • Shadowing • Combined pattern
Calcifications	Macrocalcifications Microcalcifications: • Microcalcification in a mass • Out of a mass	Removed macro-/microdistinction and combined as calcifications • Calcification inside a mass • Calcification outside a mass • Intraductal calcification **(NEW)**
Surrounding tissue attributed now found under associated features	Surrounding tissue: • Architectural distortion • Duct changes • Edema • Skin thickening • Skin retraction	Renamed as associated features: • Architectural distortion • Duct changes • Edema • Skin thickening • Skin retraction • Vascularity: (a) Absent (b) Internal vascularity (c) Vessels in rim
Vascularity	Was a separate section • Present or absent • Present immediately adjacent to the lesion • Diffusely increased vascularity seen in the surrounding tissue	Omitted dedicated "Vascularity" section and included in "Associated Features" section
Elasticity assessment	**N. S**	Included under associated features Elasticity assessment: • Soft • Intermediate • Hard
Special cases and vascular abnormality	**N. S**	Special cases: • Simple cysts • Postsurgical fluid collection • Fat necrosis Vascular abnormalities: • Arteriovenous malformations/ Pseudoaneurysms • Mondor disease

N. S: Not Specified
N. A: Not Applicable

6.5 MRI Lexicon Updates [2, 3]

The fifth edition has included new additions like amount of fibro-glandular tissue, degree of background parenchymal enhancement, and consolidated few terms in masses and nonmass enhancement section of fourth edition. Also, the "Associated Findings" section has been expanded with new descriptors and descriptors about Implants have been added in the fifth edition as described in Table 6.3.

Table 6.3 Summary of changes within MRI between BI-RADS fourth and fifth edition

Modified descriptors	4th edition	5th edition changes
Breast composition	N. S	Amount of fibro glandular tissue A. Almost entirely fatty B. Scattered C. Heterogeneously dense D. Extremely dense
Background parenchymal enhancement	N. S	Level: A. Minimal B. Mild C. Moderate D. Marked Symmetric/asymmetric
Focus	–	Changed definition of focus: A tiny dot of enhancement that does not represent a space occupying lesion or mass and does not clearly show a mass on precontrast images.
Mass		Omitted "lobulated"
• Shape	• Round • Oval • Lobulated • Irregular	• Round • Oval • Irregular
• Margins	• Smooth • Irregular • Spiculated	• Circumscribed • Not circumscribed: – Irregular – Spiculated
• Internal enhancement	• Homogenous • Heterogenous • Rim • Dark internal septation • Enhancing internal septation • Central enhancement	Omitted "enhancing internal Septations" and "central enhancement"
Non mass enhancement	Modified sections Distribution: Ductal Internal enhancement: • Stippled/punctate • Dendritic/reticular	Removed Removed and replaced with "clumped enhancement"
New findings category	N. S	Includes • Intramammary lymph node • Skin lesions
Associated features		
New terms	N. S	• Skin invasion: Direct invasion, inflammatory cancer • Axillary adenopathy • Chest wall invasion • Architectural distortion

(continued)

Table 6.3 (continued)

Modified descriptors	4th edition	5th edition changes
Renamed terms	Nipple retraction/ inversion	Renamed as "nipple retraction"
Removed terms	N. A	• Precontrast high duct signal • Edema • Lymphadenopathy • Hematoma-blood • Abnormal signal void • Cyst
Fat containing lesions	N. S	Newly added (a) Lymph node: • Normal • Abnormal (b) Fat necrosis (c) Hamartoma (d) Postoperative seroma/ hematoma with fat
Kinetic curve assessment	Initial phase: • Slow • Medium • Rapid	Replaced "rapid "as" fast" Initial phase • Slow • Medium • Fast
Implants		
1. Implant Material and Type	N. S	**A. Material:** Silicone/saline/other material **B. Lumen type** **C. Intact/ruptured**
2. Implant location	N. S	Retro glandular/retro pectoral
3. Implant focal bulge	N. S	Abnormal implant contour/focal bulge
4. Intracapsular implant findings	N. S	**Intracapsular silicone findings** Radial folds, subcapsular line Keyhole sign, linguine sign
5. Extracapsular findings	N. S	**Extracapsular silicone in** A. Breast B. Lymph nodes
6. Others	N. S	• **Implant water droplets** • **Peri-implant fluid**

N. S: Not Specified
N. A: Not Applicable

6.6 BI-RADS Assessment Categories and Management Recommendations [1]

The most important change in the BI-RADS-fifth edition is the subdivision of the Category 4 into A, B, and C for Mammography and USG (not for MRI) based on the level of suspicion for malignancy as described in Table 6.4 and the addition of management recommendations as detailed in Fig. 6.1.

BI-RADS 0: Almost always used for screening situation. Under some circumstances used in diagnostic mammography report, If US equipment or the personnel not available or the patient is unwilling/unable to complete the diagnostic examination. Additional imaging includes—spot compression ± magnification, special mammography views and USG. **Other BI-RADS 1& 2**: can includes Intra mammary Lymph node, Vascular calcification, architectural distortion due to surgery—may be excluded from the report and in that case, the Final assessment is considered as BI-RADS 1 (Normal). **BI-RADS 3**: Not an indeterminate category to be used when in case of unsure findings whether to give BI-RADS-2 (Benign) or BI-RADS-4 (Suspicious). But reserved for the ones that have specific imaging findings known to have >0% to <2% likelihood of malignancy (1) and not expected to change over the period of follow-up.

Table 6.4 Concordance between BI-RADS category and Likelihood of Malignancy

Categories	Final assessment	Likelihood of cancer
Category 0	**Mammography:** Incomplete: needs additional imaging evaluation and/or prior mammogram for comparison **USG and MRI:** Incomplete: needs additional imaging evaluation	N/A
Category 1	Negative	Essentially 0% likelihood of malignancy
Category 2	Benign findings (calcified fibroadenoma, skin calcifications, metallic clips, fat containing oil cysts/lipoma/galactocele) and others	Essentially 0% likelihood of malignancy
Category 3	Probably benign	> 0% but <2% likelihood of malignancy
Category 4	Suspicious for malignancy **4A: Low suspicion** for malignancy. **4B: Moderate suspicion for malignancy** **4C: High suspicion f**or malignancy	> 2–<10% likelihood of malignancy >10–<50% likelihood of malignancy >50–<95% likelihood of malignancy
Category 5	Highly suggestive of malignancy	> 95% likelihood of malignancy
Category 6	Known biopsy proven *(presurgical)*	N/A

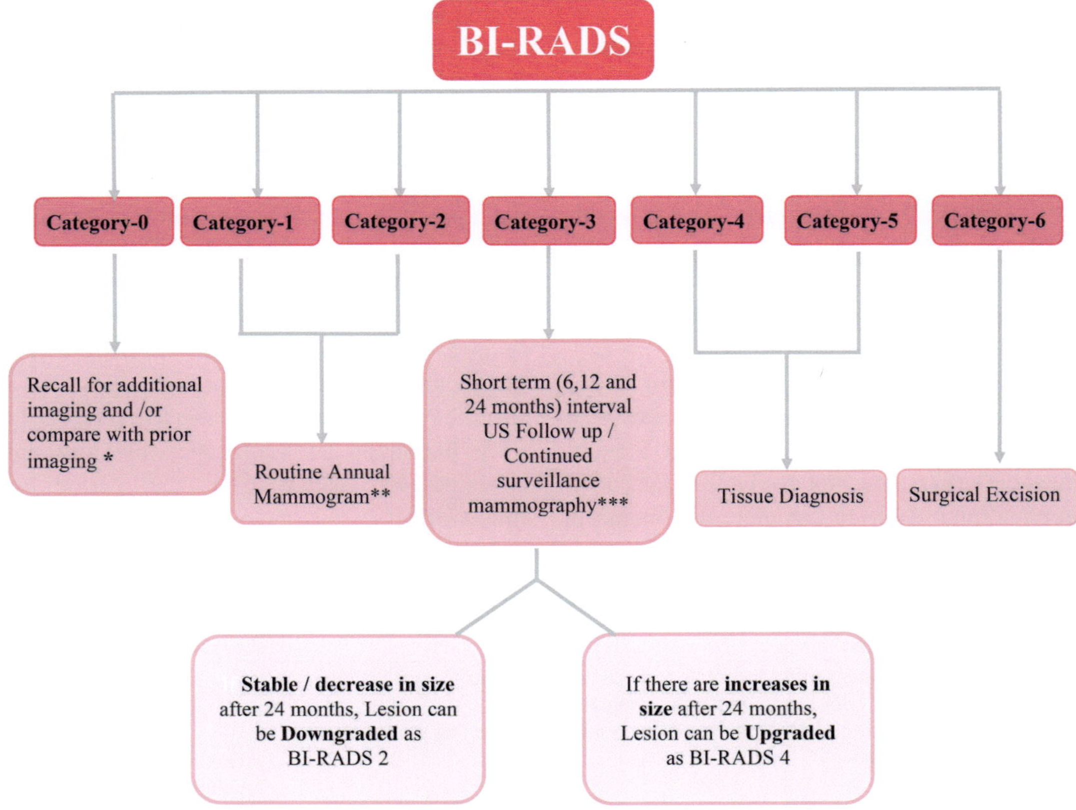

Fig. 6.1 Assessment category and management recommendations [1]

References

1. D'Orsi CJ, Sickles EA, Mendelson EB, Morris EA, et al. ACR BI-RADS® atlas, breast imaging reporting and data system. Reston, VA: American College of Radiology; 2013.
2. Rao AA, Feneis J, Lalonde C, Ojeda-Fournier H. A pictorial review of changes in the BI-RADS fifth edition. Radiographics. 2016;36(3):623–39.
3. Spak DA, Plaxco JS, Santiago L, Dryden MJ, Dogan BE. BI-RADS® fifth edition: a summary of changes. Diagn Interv Imaging. 2017;98(3):179–90.

Screening Recommendations

7

Priya K. Palanisamy, Bhawna Dev, and Harini Gnanavel

Abstract

Breast cancer screening is defined as the evaluation of a population of asymptomatic women (healthy pre- and postmenopausal women), who have no overt signs or symptoms of breast cancer, aimed to detect unsuspected cancer earlier in its growth, which would not be diagnosed without the application of a screening test. There are a wide variety of screening programs practiced across the world: the most popularly used are the screening mammograms. Though there are some significant merits of screening mammograms like early diagnosis and early treatment, which in turn reduces the mortality and morbidity rate, many claim that there are a few disadvantages to screening programs with mammography, like false positivity, high cost, and risk of ionizing radiation. In this chapter, we aim to give a brief review of the advantage, discuss if these disadvantages are justifiable, and, most importantly, the various recent screening recommendations proposed and followed across the world.

Keywords

Screening program · Screening recommendation · Breast cancer · Screening mammograms

7.1 Introduction and Background

According to recent statistics in 2020, breast cancer is the most common cancer among women worldwide with over two million women diagnosed each year [1]. The prime reason for the increase in the mortality secondary to breast cancer prior to the implementation of the national screening program even in many of the developed countries like European Union and Americas is the advanced nature of these cancers at the time of diagnosis. These cancers were picked up clinically by palpation and often the outcome of such tumors was bad, as most of them had systemic spread at the time of diagnosis (advanced stage). Therefore, the main goal of a screening program is to diagnose breast cancer when they are small and impalpable and to detect in situ carcinomas, which are usually clinically impalpable.

The interval between the imaging/mammographic detectability and the clinical presentation

P. K. Palanisamy (✉)
Department of Radiology, Maidstone and Tunbridge Wells NHS Trust, Kent, UK
e-mail: p.palanisamy@nhs.net

B. Dev · H. Gnanavel
Department of Radiology, Sri Ramachandra Institute of Higher Education and Research, Chennai, India
e-mail: bhawnadev@sriramachandra.edu.in; harini@sriramachandra.edu.in

B. Dev, L. D. Joseph (eds.), *Holistic Approach to Breast Disease*,
https://doi.org/10.1007/978-981-99-0035-0_7

of breast cancer is variable and depends on the tumor biology and the patient's age. This interval is called the **sojourn time**, and this is when the cancer needs to be diagnosed to reduce the mortality rate. The screening interval also depends on this and should usually be less than the sojourn time so that the interval cancer rate is less in the screening program.

Various randomized control and observational studies around the world indicate that a well-structured regular screening mammogram can reduce the mortality due to breast cancer considerably. In a well-known randomized control trial **"Swedish two county trial" by Tabar et al.**, they compared a total of 77,080 women of age 49–74 years randomly clustered into two groups of women, those who were invited for screening mammograms in 33-month interval and those who were not invited. There was a reduction of 30% in the mortality rate among women who were invited for screening than those who weren't [2]. In the same trial, there was a significant reduction of 40% in the mortality rate among women who attended these screening mammograms to those who did not make it [2, 3].

7.2 The Efficacy of a Screening Test

There is no absolute definition of Efficacy. In general, a new technique is believed to be an efficient screening tool if the stage at which the disease is detected is reduced than previous methods and ultimately results in reductions in the mortality from the disease or reduces the need for dangerous or harsh treatment. Furthermore, the degree of benefit must be balanced against the human risks and as well as the economic costs.

7.3 Mammography as a Screening Modality

Mammography is the most widely accepted and used screening tool across the world due to its ability to detect small invasive cancers and in situ carcinomas, which are usually asymptomatic. Screening mammograms are recommended to have two-view mammograms of both breasts with adequate exposure for accurate and standardized reporting. Recently, the use of digital mammography as a screening modality in comparison to the aboriginal film-screen mammograms is increasing. This can be attributed to the fact that digital mammography is beneficial in imaging dense breasts with low radiation in contrast to the conventional full field screen-film mammogram. However, several studies have found little or few differences between conventional and digital mammography [4]. Digital mammography still is the preferred modality especially in screening settings as it has the added advantage of image storage and transmission, which helps in making a comparison of mammograms. Computer-Aided Detection (CAD) using computer software can increase the sensitivity of screening mammogram but at the same time reduces the specificity and increases the number of visits post screening.

7.4 Advantages of Screening Mammography

In a study by Fletcher et al., a meta-analysis of all randomized control trials, which tested the efficiency of screening mammograms, they have concluded that there is a significant reduction of about 25–30% in breast cancer mortality due to screening mammogram among 50–69-year age group women and lower yet significant number among 40–49-year age group [4].

Decrease in morbidity is secondary to the diagnosis of cancer at an early stage and as they are diagnosed at a much earlier stage, they can be treated with breast conservation surgery without the need for chemotherapy [5]: better 5-year survival rate of 99% in the localized stage, 84% in regional disease, and 23% in metastatic disease. However, there are several debates and squabbles around the world as to when should screening commence in a screening program, how often should we do screening mammograms, and when should we stop.

7.5 Mammographic Screening: Various Recommendations

Worldwide the recommendations for screening mammograms defer and we have briefly discussed the updates made below with a summary in Table 7.1.

7.5.1 In Developed Nations

The U.S Preventative Services and Task Force (USPSTF) recently updated their 2009 recommendation as biennial screening mammograms starting at 50 years of age till 74 years [6]. This decision was based on their convincing evidence that there was a significant reduction in the absolute mortality rate of breast cancer among women in age group 50–74 years rather than 40–49 years. They also stated that women aged 40–49 years with high-risk factors like first-degree relatives (siblings, parent, or a child) diagnosed with invasive/in situ breast cancer may benefit with screening mammograms rather than average-risk women <50 years. They also insisted that this recommendation should be an individualized one with the patient making a well-informed decision. The USPSTF also recommends that no screening mammogram is needed for women of <40 years of age and also concluded that there are no benefits in performing screening mammograms for women >74 years of age [6]. This recommendation against the screening mammograms for the woman in their 40s stirred up lot of controversies in the US radiological arena. The American Society of Breast imaging, American Cancer Society (ACS) along with breast imaging commission of the American College of Radiology (ACR) recommend annual screening mammograms for women at average risk starting from 40 years [7]. For the woman with genetic mutations in BRCA 1/BRCA 2 genes or those with first-degree relative who are BRCA positive, an annual screening mammogram is recommended at the age of 30 years and the same applies to the woman with sisters or mothers having premenopausal breast cancer or having >20% lifetime risk of breast cancer based on family history [7]. Women with a history of mantle or chest radiation for Hodgkin's lymphoma should have a yearly screening mammogram starting from 8 years post irradiation but not less than 25 years of age. At last, they also recommend that women with history of lobular/ductal in situ carcinoma, atypical ductal hyperplasia, invasive breast, or ovarian cancers should undergo annual screening mammograms irrespective of the age of diagnosis [7].

In the United Kingdom, the National Health Service Breast Screening Programme (NHS BSP), which was started in 1989 and implemented throughout the country by 1995, recom-

Table 7.1 Summary of worldwide screening mammogram program recommendations by different organizations of developed countries

Organization	Screening modality	Age group recommendation	Recommended interval	High-risk group recommendation
USPSTF	Mammogram	50–74 years	Annually	40–49 years annual mammogram. Supplemented with MRI in dense breast
ACS	Mammogram	Same as USPTF		
ACOG	Mammogram	40–75 years	Annually	–
CTPHC	Mammogram	50–74 years	Annually	40–49 years, individual decision
UK	Mammogram	50–74 years	3 years once	MRI screening alone if <40 years of age and MRI + mammogram if >40 years of age annually
CCA	Mammogram	50–74 years	Biennial	–
Russia	Mamo	Starting 40 years	Biennial	–

ACOG American College of Obstetricians and Gynaecologists, *ACS* American Cancer Society, *CCA* Cancer Council of Australia, *CTPHC* Canadian Taskforce on Preventative Health Care, *MRI* magnetic resonance imaging, *USG* ultrasonography, *USPSTF* United States Preventive Services Task Force

mends 3 yearly screening mammograms starting from 50 years of age [8]. Many updates have been made to the program for the past 20 years and the current program development includes extending the invitation to 70 years of age after evaluation through research [9] There are further extensions to the program currently with an additional screen between 47–50 years and 70–74 years [9], which was suspended during the pandemic era and resumed recently. The current NHS BSP also offers MRI screening for women at high genetic risk of breast cancer [9].

Many European countries follow the International Agency for Research on Cancer (IARC) recommendation, which is updated recently in 2015 and promotes screening mammograms every 2–3 years from 50 years of age [10].

The Canadian Task Force on Preventive Health Care (CTFPHC) recommended screening mammograms from 50 to 74 years of age and concluded the mortality rate associated with screening mammograms is not significant between the age of 40 and 74 years. Moreover, they stated that potential harmful effects like overdiagnosis and extra biopsies were greater secondary to screening mammograms in younger women [11].

The Cancer Council of Australia (CCA) also recommends biennial screening mammograms between the age group of 50 and74 years. However, women aged 40–49 years and older than 74 years can have screening mammogram if they wish but will not be invited by invitation letter [12].

Russia recommends screening mammograms at 40 years at a 2-year interval with two view mammograms [13]. Countries like China and South Africa at present do not have any nationwide breast cancer screening program. The Cancer Association of South Africa revealed that the risk of breast cancer in an African woman is 1 in 33 [14]. In 2005, China started a screening program by performing screening mammograms and ultrasounds for 100,000 women but stopped it due to significant false-positive results in their study and inadequate funding [15].

7.5.2 In Developing Nations

In the past, low- and middle-income countries (LMICs) have reportedly lower incidence of breast cancer compared to the Americas and European countries. Recently, in the past two decades, there has been a notable increase in the incidence and mortality from breast cancer among low- and middle-income countries [16]. In a worldwide study (GLOBOCAN) conducted by Ferlay J. et al., they predicted that about 45% of the breast cancer incidence burden and 55% of breast-cancer-related deaths worldwide would be contributed by low and middle resource countries [17]. Even though the rise in the mortality rate of women dying of breast cancer is more/less equal to pregnancy-related deaths in LMIC, more resources and fundings are focused on maternal health. Most of the women in LMIC present to the clinic at tragically late stage for diagnosis and treatment. This is mainly due to the lack of awareness about breast cancer and its symptoms, and stigmas and inappropriate attitude toward the self-breast examination. Compounding this problem is the concerning fact that most of these LMICs don't have prevention of breast cancer by screening/early diagnosis in their public health agenda. In LMIC countries like India, there is only a limited data available about the true incidence of breast cancer nationwide and the available data are mostly from small geographic areas, which are extrapolated to larger areas, as there are no dependable cancer registries as in the developed Americas and Europe.

Implementation of population level program for screening/early detection of breast cancer, along with the use of ways to improve awareness among women regarding breast cancer, should be the overall agenda of LMIC going forward. The use of ultrasound as a screening tool could be a cost-effective alternative in these countries.

7.6 Quality Assurance in Screening Program

A screening program should be avouched by good-quality imaging being available population wide. Having a standardized quality assurance recommendation for a screening program would avoid any harm caused due to the program to the population, by reducing and avoiding unnecessary workup of benign conditions, which in turn causes anxiety to the patient, inappropriate economic cost, and justification of using ionizing radiation. The U.S. congress charged Federal Drug Administration (FDA) in developing and implementing Mammogram Quality Standards Act (MQSA). The main aim of this act was to establish minimum national quality standards for mammography facilities that undergo periodic certification by accredited bodies to ensure safe and reliable screening images [18].

In the UK, since 1989, we have multiple documents promoting standard guidelines for screening program, which includes quality standards further divided into core radiological, general radiological, and quality standards for screen reading. There are also standards for working practice for breast radiologists, surgeons, mammographers, and nurses. Detailed discussion about the NHS BSP is beyond the scope this chapter and could be referred in the NHS BSP website [9]. Similarly, the European guidelines for screening program quality assurance (QA) demand the need for QA for all screening units and robustly recommended that all staff should have specialist training and hold professional qualifications to interpret and report screening mammograms.

7.7 Claims About the Potential Drawbacks of Screening Mammography Program

There have been multiple articles published recently in the lay press and medical journals about the potentially harmful effects of mammographic screening programs. The concerns that are raging against screening mammograms are increasing false positives, overdiagnosis, overtreatment, missed cancers, and radiation exposure. **Daniel B Kopans**, in his recently published open letter to the panels that are deciding guidelines for breast cancer screening, has tried to elucidate such misinformation that is propagating in the media and recent medical literature [19]. He has described in this letter that these allegations are due to various factors like the panels taking into consideration articles, which have not passed peer reviews, excluding experts in these panels for making guidelines and most importantly pointing out that the reviews and media claiming that there is only minimal or nil benefit in reducing the mortality rate from screening have all been flawed as they have ignored the "**length bias sampling.**" He stated that a delay of 5 or more years is expected to see a decline in breast cancer mortality secondary to screening and 2.2 years are far short to see the impact of screening [19].

(a) *False Positives*: These are reported to be suspicious on screening and proven to be benign on further assessment. But the usage of the word "False positive" in screening program is misleading. These should be called "**screening recalls**," which require few further imaging and biopsies occasionally. The recall rates from screening are 10% and less, which is comparable to that of cervical cancer screening with a pap smear. Only 1–2% of women get biopsies from screening and about 40–60% of these screening biopsies are cancerous, which is still a high yield than biopsies from symptomatic lumps [20].

(b) *Overdiagnosis*:

This refers to conditions like in situ carcinoma and atypical hyperplasia, which, if left untreated, would have disappeared on their own or not have turned into cancers. This claim made in an article published in the New England Journal of Medicine (NEJM) in which the authors guessed that about 70,000 women who were diagnosed to have cancer in 2008 would have regressed or disappeared on their own if not detected in screening mammogram [21]. Later these authors confronted that they were their "best guesses" and couldn't support their theory as there were no data.

(c) *Lack of immediate benefit*:

The reduction in the mortality rate of breast cancer due to screening is not a short-term effect but rather a delayed benefit, which could be evident after 5–7 years. This is a misunderstanding among analyst due to length bias [22].

(d) *Missed Cancers*:

Mammograms do have their own limitations and unfortunately, false negativity is a significant one. The sensitivity of the mammogram depends mainly on the density of the breasts. In these scenarios, usage of additional imaging modalities like the whole breast USG and MRI could aid in reducing the number of missed cancers in the screening program. Also studying the imaging characteristics of these notorious missed cancers in mammograms will help the radiologist to improve their sensitivity and is a good learning exercise. In the UK, one of the QA that we must decrease the number of missed cancers is by recommending double reading every screening mammogram by two qualified breast specialist radiologists/radiographers [10].

(e) *Radiation Exposure*:

The carcinogenic effect of ionizing radiation and the incidence of radiation-induced breast cancer from repeated screening mammograms over a period is a topic of scientific speculation. In a recent study by Ernest KJ et al. [23] in 2016, they concluded the ratio of induced incidence rate over baseline incidence rate in western European countries is 1.6% in women who don't have a genetic predisposition and stated that a ratio less than 0.7% could be excluded. This serves the need to consider risk-to-benefit ratio and encourages the individual to make an informed decision. Women who are at an increased risk of DNA damage should have careful consideration of screening mammograms and may benefit from other nonionizing radiation involving modalities like USG and MRI.

7.8 Nonmammographic Screening Methods for Breast Cancer

(a) **Breast Self-Examination (BSE)**: It is the examination of breasts by women themselves preferably once every month during the sixth to tenth day of their menstrual cycle to reduce the interference by fibroadenomas and fibrocystic changes.

Advantage: Noninvasive and inexpensive technique. No radiation is involved, so better tolerated over time. These can be taught to women and, in turn, makes them self-aware of breast health.

Disadvantage: several controlled studies on BSE as screening method declared that there is no convincing evidence in the reduction of breast cancer mortality rate. The Cochrane meta-analysis in China and Russia showed no advantage in women who performed monthly BSE over women who didn't [24].

Recommendation: USPSTF supports that all women should be aware of their breast changes; however, it did not update its recommendation on teaching women on about BSE. ACOG and American Medical Association recommend monthly BSE. In the UK, NHS BSP promotes and recommends women to do monthly BSE even in high-risk patients [10].

(b) **Clinical Breast Examination (CBE)**: It includes detailed personal and family history, through clinical examination by inspection and palpation of both breasts and axilla by a breast clinician.

Advantage: Detects masses and skin, nipple changes that could potentially be missed in imaging. Helps to differentiate benign from malignant lesions, stage the disease, and plan surgical treatment.

Disadvantage: There are no studies to evaluate the efficacy of CBE alone worldwide.

Recommendation: In 2009, USPSTF recommended that there is no added advantage of CBE. And in Feb 2016, USPSTF did not update its recommendation on CBE. Similarly, ACS guidelines in 2015 did not recommend CBE as well [6].

(c) **Digital Breast Tomosynthesis (DBT)**: Cross-sectional imaging of breast tissue with conventional X-ray tubes that are three-dimensionally reconstructed.

Advantage: Beneficial in dense breasts. Better localization, assessment of shape, size, and multifocality. Minimizes the need for additional imaging.

Disadvantage: prolonged acquisition time and relatively more radiation exposure.

Recommendation: USPSTF stated that there is insufficient data about the merits and demerits of DBT as a primary screening modality and continuous research on this worldwide before DBT can be recommended as a primary screening modality [6]. For now, DBT is widely used as an adjuvant modality in screening recall assessment clinics.

(d) **Whole Breast Ultrasound**: High-frequency sound waves (13 MHz) for imaging breast tissue. The sensitivity of USG in women with negative screening mammogram is 80–83% and 86–90% specificity [25]. Automated Breast UltraSound (ABUS) has been recently approved by FDA as a first-line screening tool among <30 years of age [25].

Advantage: Beneficial in dense breasts compared to mammogram; no radiation involved, so no risk of screening-induced breast cancer; and can be used in young and pregnant/lactational women. Easy availability, patient friendly, and cost-effectiveness.

Disadvantage: Microcalcifications cannot be usually visualized in USS, which could be the only early presentation of invasive cancer or ductal carcinoma in situ (DCIS). Lack of spatial resolution. Time consuming to do a whole breast ultrasound of both breasts under screening setting, limiting the number of scans that can be done by radiologists.

Recommendation: USG is not approved by FDA or any other organization as a single modality for screening breast cancer. It is widely used as an adjuvant tool with screening mammograms in dense breast and sometimes with MRI in high-risk patients.

(e) **Breast MRI**: Three-dimensional imaging of both breasts using radio waves and magnetic fields. Has sensitivity of 77–100% and specificity of 78–89% [26].

Advantage: can image both breasts entirely in all planes, no radiation, and good spatial resolution. Accurate sizing, multifocality, and staging, in detecting occult and residual malignancies. High negative predictive value than mammography/USG. Excellent in BRCA 1/2-positive patients and in women with breast implants.

Disadvantage: less availability, high cost, usage of contrast agents, and limitations like contraindicated in patients with pacemaker/non-MRI-compatible metal prosthesis and patients who cannot lie prone due to kyphoscoliosis.

Recommendation: In the updated USPSTF recommendation in 2016, it is stated that MRI can only be added as a supplement to screening mammography in dense breast and BRCA1/2-positive patients (high-risk patients). The ACS and ACOG recommends MRI as a supplement to mammography only in women with >20% risk for breast cancer and in BRCA-mutation-positive patients and not in average-risk population [27].

7.9 High-Risk Breast Cancer Screening [10]

Includes six categories:

(a) Women with a genetic predisposition—BRCA 1-/BRCA 2-positive mutation
(b) Women with a first-degree relative having premenopausal breast cancer
(c) Women with a previous prolonged history of mantle/chest irradiation
(d) Women with a lifetime risk of 20–25% and above in the risk screening tool
(e) Women with other genetic conditions like Li Fraumeni, Cowden syndrome, etc.
(f) Women with a previous history of invasive cancer

Moderately high risk:

1. Women with an average lifetime risk of 5–20%
2. Women with dense breast
3. Women with previous precancerous/carcinoma in situ like Ductal/Lobular carcinoma in situ (DCIS/LCIS) and atypical ductal and lobular hyperplasia (ADH, ALH)

Most of the worldwide recommendation for the average-risk women for screening is annual screening mammograms starting from the age of 40 years and for higher-risk women annual mammography or annual MRI should be started as early as 30 years of age [28].

7.10 Conclusion

Screening mammography till date is proven to be the gold standard screening modality in reducing the breast cancer mortality rate as seen in various Randomized Control Trial (RCT). However, these data and observations are based on the developed nations who have standardized screening program and quality assurance. In the Low- and Middle-Income Countries (LMICs) like India, to control the increase in the incidence and mortality rate due to breast cancer will require country wide implementation of a screening program. Until then various cost-effective alternatives like self-breast examination, awareness about breast health and risk factors, efforts in demystifying the old maid myths, clinical examination, and whole breast USG could be an effective propaganda.

References

1. Cancer Tomorrow. International agency for research on cancer. http://gco.iarc.fr/tomorrow/graphicisotype?type=0&population=900&mode=population&sex=2&cancer=39&age_group=value& apc male=0&apc_female=0. Accessed 5 Jan 2020.
2. Tabár L, Fagerberg CJG, Gad A, et al. Reduction in mortality from breast cancer after mass screening with mammography: randomized trial from the breast cancer screening working group of the Swedish national board of health and welfare. Lancet. 1985;1:829–32.
3. Tabar L, Fagerberg G, Chen HH, et al. Efficacy of breast cancer screening by age. New results from the Swedish two-county trial. Cancer. 1995;75:2507–17.
4. Fletcher SW, Elmore JG. Clinical practice: mammographic screening for breast cancer. N Engl J Med. 2003;348:1672–80.
5. Barth RJ Jr, Gibson GR, Carney PA, Mott LA, Becher RD, Poplack SP. Detection of breast cancer on screening mammography allows patients to be treated with less-toxic therapy. AJR Am J Roentgenol. 2005;184:324–9.
6. US Preventive Services Task Force. Screening for breast cancer: U.S. preventive services task force recommendation statement. Ann Intern Med. 2009;1519(10):716–26. W-236.
7. Lee CH, Dershaw DD, Kopans D, Evans P, Monsees B, Monticciolo D, et al. Breast cancer screening with imaging: recommendations from the society of breast imaging and the ACR on the use of mammography, breast MRI, breast ultrasound, and other technologies for the detection of clinically occult breast cancer. J Am Coll Radiol. 2010;7:18–27.
8. Forrest P. Department of Health and Social Security. Breast cancer screening, report to the Health Ministers of England, Wales, Scotland, and Northern Ireland. London, UK: Her Majesty's Stationery Office; 1986.
9. Patnick J. NHS Cancer Screening Programmes. NHS Breast Screening Programme Annual Review 2010, Overcoming Barriers. Sheffield, UK; 2010.
10. Giordano L, von Karsa L, Tomatis M, Majek O, de Wolf C, Lancucki L, Eunice Working Group, et al. Mammographic screening programmes in Europe: organization, coverage and participation. J Med Screen. 2012;19(Suppl 1):72–82.
11. Miller AB, Wall C, Baines CJ, Sun P, To T, Narod SA. Twenty-five-year follow-up for breast cancer incidence and mortality of the Canadian National Breast Screening Study: randomized screening trial. BMJ. 2014;348:366.
12. Australian Government, Australian Institute of Health, and Welfare (AIHW). Breast Screen Australia monitoring report 2010–2011. Cancer Series No. 77. Canberra: AIHW; 2013.
13. Zakharova N, Duffy SW, Mackay J, Kotlyarov E. The introduction of a breast cancer screening programme in a region with a population at medium risk for developing breast cancer: Khanty-Mansiysky autonomous OkrugUgra (Russian Federation). Ecancermedicalscience. 2011;5:195.
14. Apffelstaedt J. Reflections on the USPSTF breast screening recommendations from a South African perspective. S Afr J Gynaecol Oncol. 2010;2:13–4.
15. Wang F, Zhi-Gang Y. Current status of breast cancer prevention in China Department of Breast Surgery. Chron Dis Transl Med. 2015;1:2–8.
16. Porter PL. Global trends in breast cancer incidence and mortality. Salud Publica Mex. 2009;51(Suppl 2):S141–6.

17. Ferlay J, Bray F, Pisani P, GLOBOCAN, et al. Cancer incidence, mortality and prevalence worldwide. In: IARC cancer-base No 5, Version 2.0. Lyon: IARC; 2002. http://www-dep.iarc.fr/globocan/database.htm.
18. FDA. Mammography quality standards act of 1992. Mammography facilities requirement for accrediting bodies, and quality standards and certifying requirements: interim rules (21 CFR 900). 1993;58:57558–57572.
19. Kopans DB. An open letter to panels that are deciding guidelines for breast cancer screening. Breast Cancer Res Treat. 2015;151(1):19–25. https://doi.org/10.1007/s10549-015-3373-8.
20. Spivey GH, Perry BW, Clark VA. Predicting the risk of cancer at the time of breast biopsy. Am Surg. 1982;48(7):326–32.
21. Bleyer A, Welch HG. Effect of three decades of screening mammography on breast-cancer incidence. N Engl J Med. 2012;367(21):1998–2005.
22. Kopans DB. Screening for breast cancer and mortality reduction among women 40–49 years of age. Cancer. 1994;74(1 Suppl):311–22.
23. Pauwels EKJ, Foray N, Bourguignon MH. Breast cancer induced by X-ray mammography screening? A review based on recent understanding of low-dose radiobiology. Med Princ Pract. 2016;25(2):101–9. https://doi.org/10.1159/000442442.
24. Kösters JP, Gøtzsche PC. Regular self-examination or clinical examination for early detection of breast cancer. Cochrane Database Syst Rev. 2008;2003(3):CD003373.
25. Berg WA, Bandos AI, Mendelson EB, Lehrer D, Jong RA, Pisano ED. Ultrasound as the primary screening test for breast cancer: analysis from ACRIN 6666. J Natl Cancer Inst. 2015;108(4):djv367.
26. Melnikow J, Fenton JJ, Whitlock EP, Miglioretti DL, Weyrich MS, Thompson JH, et al. Supplemental screening for breast cancer in women with dense breasts: a systematic review for the U.S. Preventive Service Task Force. 2016;164(4):268–78.
27. American College of Obstetricians and Gynaecologists. Response of the American College of Obstetricians and Gynaecologists to new breast cancer screening recommendations from the U.S. Preventive Services Task Force; 2010.
28. Ren W, Chen M, Qiao Y, Zhao F. Global guidelines for breast cancer screening: a systematic review. Breast. 2022;64:85–99. https://doi.org/10.1016/j.breast.2022.04.003.

Reporting Template: Mammogram, USG, MRI

8

Priya K. Palanisamy, Bhawna Dev, and M. C. Sheela

Abstract

In this chapter, we have formulated reporting templates for Mammogram, USG, and MRI based on the reporting atlas provided by the American College of Radiology (ACR) in the fifth Edition of BI-RADS. The goal is to establish uniformity, reduce ambiguity in the reporting style, and to improve the communication between the breast radiologist and the clinician worldwide.

Keywords

BI-RADS · Reporting template · Mammogram USG · MRI

P. K. Palanisamy (✉)
Maidstone and Tunbridge Wells NHS Trust, Kent, UK
e-mail: p.palanisamy@nhs.net

B. Dev · M. C. Sheela
Department of Radiology, Sri Ramachandra Institute of Higher Education and Research, Chennai, India
e-mail: bhawnadev@sriramachandra.edu.in; sheelamc@sriramachandra.edu.in

8.1 Reporting Template for Mammogram [1]

The mammogram report should be concise and organized in the following structure

1.	Indication for the examination
2.	Overall breast composition
3.	Findings: Mass description
4.	Findings on correlation with USG
5.	Comparison with previous studies
6.	Final assessment/impression
7.	Management recommendation

1. **Indication for the examination**: One of the following indications should be mentioned.
   (a) Screening Mammogram of an asymptomatic woman.
   (b) Post **Left/Right** mastectomy, on Surveillance screening.
   (c) Evaluation of the screening detected lesion/Clinical finding (Mention the side, location, and specific finding).
   (d) Follow-up study (either of a benign BI-RADS-3 finding/Malignancy post conservation surgery).
2. **Overall Breast Composition**: These are categorized as **a, b, c, and d** so as to avoid confusion with the numbered BI-RADS final assessment categories.
   (a) The breasts are almost **entirely fatty**.
   (b) There are **scattered areas** of Fibroglandular densities.

B. Dev, L. D. Joseph (eds.), *Holistic Approach to Breast Disease*,
https://doi.org/10.1007/978-981-99-0035-0_8

 (c) **Heterogeneously dense** breast parenchyma, which may obscure small masses on mammography.
 (d) **Extremely dense** breast parenchyma, which lowers the sensitivity of Mammography.
3. **Findings: Mammogram**: Clear descriptions of important abnormal findings must be described using BI-RADS Mammogram Lexicon (Refer Chap. 6).

> Note: The findings of both breasts can be given separately in the order of clinical relevance.

Abnormality: Mass/Suspicious calcification/Architectural distortion/Asymmetry

 (a) **Mass**: Shape, Margin, Density, Associated features (calcifications)
 (b) **Calcification**: Morphology—typically benign/Suspicious morphology (describe the shape of calcification), Distribution
 (c) **Architectural distortion**:
 (d) **Asymmetries**: **Focal/global/developing**
   - Location
   - Associated calcifications
   - Associated features
 (e) **Intramammary Lymph node** (rarely important)
 (f) **Skin lesion** Location
 (g) **Solitary dilated duct**: (rarely present)

> Note: if there are no important abnormal findings in the mammogram, the following clause can be added to the report—"There are no suspicious masses, architectural distortion, or calcifications in the bilateral breasts in X-ray mammography."

4. **Findings on correlation USG**: A composite report, if USG done on the same day
5. **Comparison**: A statement indicating that the current examination has been compared to previous study (most recent study with specific date)/no comparison has been made should be mentioned as—**Prior study/studies in/No prior studies are available.**
6. **Final Assessment/Impression**: The report should conclude with
 (a) Statement about the breast composition
 (b) A concise summary of pertinent Mammography and ultrasound findings with a final assessment using **BI-RADS categories 0–6** and the phrases associated with them.

> Note: When correlation USG is done on the same day, the final assessment category and management recommendation should be given based on the combined findings.

7. **Management Recommendation**: the BI-RADS assessment categories are designed to be concordant with management recommendation (Refer Chap. 6) to enhance sound medical practice.

   BI-RADS 0: usually given for screening examinations when additional imaging evaluation is recommended. In such cases, a recall (category 0) assessment should include specific suggestions for the next course of action (spot-compression magnification views, US, etc.).

   For example: "**Further recommendation will be based on the ultrasound findings/prior examination.**"

   When the prior examination report becomes available, an addendum should be added to the initial assessment and a Final revised assessment category and management recommendation should be given in the report within 30 days.

> Note: **Category 0** should never be given in a diagnostic mammography finding, which requires further evaluation with MRI. Rather in such cases final assessment category should be provided in the report by the breast radiologist before the MRI is performed.

BI-RADS 1 & 2: Negative or benign examination, recommendation can be as "Screening Mammogram after a year to establish baseline parenchymal stability."

BI-RADS 3: Probably benign masses**, should be** recommended for initial short-term (6 months) followed by long-term (12–24 months) follow-up for probably benign lesions and the recall period should be mentioned in the report.

BI-RADS 4 & 5: In case of suspicious findings,

(a) Biopsy is advised, mention the modality preferred for biopsy of the suspicious finding (USG-guided/stereotactic biopsy using Mammogram/MRI)
or
(b) Bilateral Dynamic Contrast-Enhanced MRI (DCEMRI) breasts to evaluate the extent of the disease if clinically not contraindicated and BCS (breast conservation surgery) is being considered.

8.2 Report Template for USG [2]

1.	Indication for the examination
2.	Technique of examination
3.	Overall breast composition
4.	Findings: Mass description
5.	Comparison with previous studies
6.	Final assessment/impression
7.	Management

1. **Indication**: Initial imaging technique of choice in young women <35 years, lactating and Pregnant women.
   (a) Evaluation of the Clinical finding (Mention the side, location, and specific finding).
   (b) Follow-up study (either of a benign BI-RADS-3 finding/Malignancy post conservation surgery).
   (c) Postmastectomy screening.
2. **Technique of Examination**: real-time USG with color Doppler, Sheer wave elastography, Automated 3D scanner.
3. **Overall Breast Composition**: **(Only in Screening USG)**
   (a) Homogenous background echotexture —Fat.
   (b) Homogenous background echotexture —Fibroglandular.
   (c) Heterogenous background echotexture.
4. **Findings**: Descriptions using US BI-RADS lexicon, and the findings of both breasts can be given separately in the order of clinical relevance.
   (a) **Mass**:
      - Shape.
      - Size—in 3 dimensions (largest horizontal × vertical × orthogonal).
      - Morphology—shape and margins.
      - Location—In clock face, distance from the nipple.
      - Associated effect on surrounding tissues.
      - Associated features.

> NOTE: in case of multiple simple/complicated cysts in either breasts, no need to mention each cyst separately in the report. The largest in each breast will suffice

5. **Comparison**: Prior study/studies in/No prior studies are available.
6. **Final Assessment**: The report should conclude with a concise summary of pertinent US findings with final BI-RADS US categories 0–6 and the phrases associated with them.
7. **Management**: Clear recommendations should be made as to the next course of action.

In case if Biopsy/FNAC is recommended, the type of imaging (stereotactic, US, or MRI guidance) should be mentioned in the report.

8.3 Reporting Template for MRI [3]

The reporting system should be concise and organized in the following structure

1.	Indication for the examination
2.	Technique of examination
3.	Comparison with previous studies
4.	Overall breast composition
5.	Findings: mass description
6.	Final assessment/impression
7.	Management

1. **Indication**: description of the patient's clinical history, including
   (a) Reason for performing the exam (e.g., screening, follow-up of a probably benign lesion or Breast cancer post neoadjuvant chemotherapy, staging or problem solving, Evaluation of breast implant)
   (b) Clinical abnormalities, including size, location, and duration
   - Palpable finding
   - Nipple discharge
   - Other pertinent clinical findings or history

   (c) Previous biopsies
   - Biopsy type
   - Biopsy location
   - Benign or malignant pathology (cytology or histology)

   (d) Hormonal status if applicable
   - Pre- or postmenopausal
   - Menstrual cycle phase (second week or other) or last menstrual period
   - Peripartum
   - Exogenous hormone therapy, tamoxifen, aromatase inhibitors
2. **Technique**: Following should be described in this section:
   (a) Right, left, or both breasts
   (b) Location of markers and their significance (clips, scar)
   (c) Weighting: T1 weighted, T2 weighted, Fat saturation, Scan orientation and plane, Other pertinent pulse sequence features
   (d) Contrast dose: Name of contrast agent, Dosage (mmol/kg) and volume, Injection type: bolus or infusion, Timing (relationship of bolus injection to scan start time and scan length)
   (e) Postprocessing techniques: MPR/MIP, Time/signal intensity curves, Subtraction and Other techniques
3. Comparison: includes
   (a) Previous MRI—date of examination
   (b) Other imaging studies (mammogram, US, nuclear medicine examination, others) and date of examination
4. **Overall Breast Composition**: This includes the following features in an MRI:
   (a) Amount of Fibroglandular Tissue (FGT):
   (b) Background Parenchymal enhancement: Level and Symmetric/asymmetric
   (c) Implant: if present, should include composition (silicone, saline, or others) and number of lumen (single or multiple)
5. **Findings**: the BI-RADS MRI lexicon descriptors are used (Refer Chap. 6) and findings of both breasts can be given separately in the order of clinical relevance.

   In case of describing the **Location** of the abnormality—Should include
   (a) Right or left breast
   (b) Breast quadrant and clock-face position (or central, retro-areolar, and axillary tail descriptors)
   (c) Distance from nipple, skin, or chest wall in centimeters (if applicable)
6. **Final Assessment**: The report should conclude with a concise summary of the pertinent MRI findings with a final BI-RADS MRI categories 0–6 and the phrases associated with them.

Note: An incomplete assessment (category 0) is used when full diagnostic imaging has not been performed and should be given only when additional imaging or clinical evaluation is recommended to establish the benignity of a finding (e.g., a possible intramammary lymph node or fat necrosis at MRI may require additional mammography and/or US examination)

7. **Management Recommendation**: Clear recommendations should be made as to the next course of action.

   In case of Category 0, a specific suggestion for the next course of action should be given (physical examination, diagnostic mammography, targeted diagnostic US, etc.).

References

1. D'Orsi CJ, Sickles EA, Mendelson EB, Morris EA, et al. ACR BI-RADS® atlas, breast imaging reporting and data system. Reston, VA: American College of Radiology; 2013.
2. Mendelson EB, Böhm-Vélez M, Berg WA, et al. ACR BI-RADS® ultrasound. In: ACR BI-RADS® atlas, breast imaging reporting and data system. Reston, VA: American College of Radiology; 2013.
3. Morris EA, Comstock CE, Lee CH, et al. ACR BI-RADS® magnetic resonance imaging. In: ACR BI-RADS® atlas, breast imaging reporting and data system. Reston, VA: American College of Radiology; 2013.

9 Approach to Architectural Distortion and Asymmetry

M. C. Sheela, Bhawna Dev, Harini Gnanavel, and Leena Dennis Joseph

Abstract

Breasts are generally symmetric with a similar distribution of density and architecture. Asymmetry of breast tissue is an area with increased density compared to the contralateral breast. It is essential to rule out underlying malignancy in such asymmetric densities. Architectural distortion refers to distortion of normal parenchyma, which necessitates differentiating from a malignant mass causing architectural distortion.

Keywords

Asymmetry · Architectural distortion · Radial scar · Developing asymmetry · Sclerosing adenosis

M. C. Sheela (✉) · B. Dev · H. Gnanavel
Department of Radiology, Sri Ramachandra Institute of Higher Education and Research, Chennai, India
e-mail: sheelamc@sriramachandra.edu.in; bhawnadev@sriramachandra.edu.in

L. D. Joseph
Department of Pathology, Sri Ramachandra Institute of Higher Education and Research, Chennai, India

9.1 Asymmetry of Breast

Breasts are generally symmetric with a similar distribution of density and architecture. The term *asymmetric breast tissue* refers to a greater volume or density of breast tissue in one breast than in the corresponding area in the contralateral breast. Asymmetric breast tissue is seen in approximately 3% of mammograms [1]. Most commonly, the asymmetric breast tissue is due to summation of normal overlying tissues, normal variation, postoperative change, or hormone replacement therapy. The important concern of the asymmetry in a breast is a developing mass or underlying cancer.

The ***ACR BI-RADS fifth edition*** has divided asymmetry into four groups:

1. Asymmetry
2. Global asymmetry
3. Focal asymmetry
4. Developing asymmetry

9.1.1 Asymmetry

It is an area of fibroglandular tissue visible on *only one mammographic projection*, caused by *the superimposition of normal breast tissue* (Fig. 9.1). It lacks convex border and occupies less than a quadrant of the breast [2]. It is found in 3.3% of screening mammograms. In approxi-

B. Dev, L. D. Joseph (eds.), *Holistic Approach to Breast Disease*,
https://doi.org/10.1007/978-981-99-0035-0_9

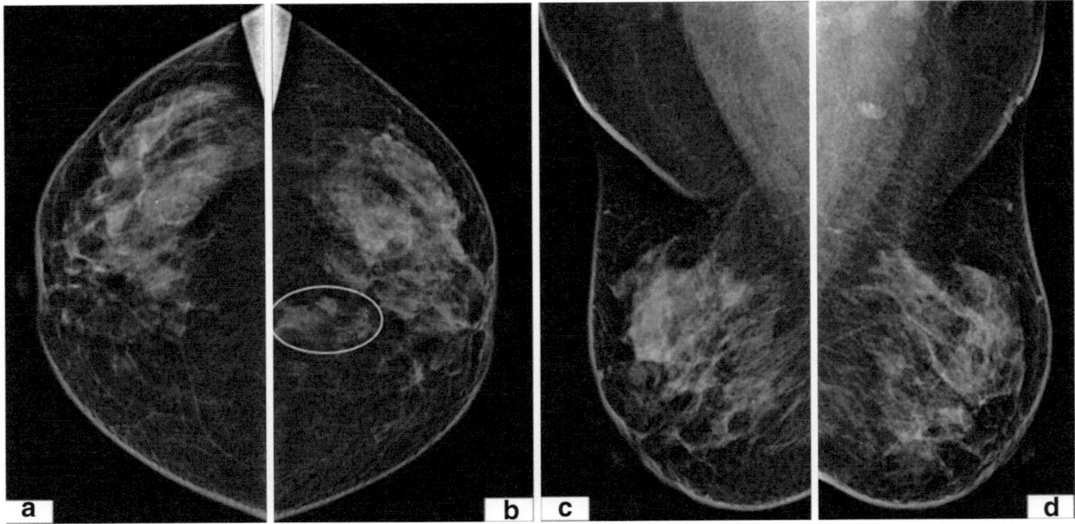

Fig. 9.1 CC view (**a**) right and (**b**) left breast, MLO view (**c**) right and (**d**) left breast. (**b**) Asymmetric glandular tissue (circled) noted in the central region of left breast, seen only on CC view

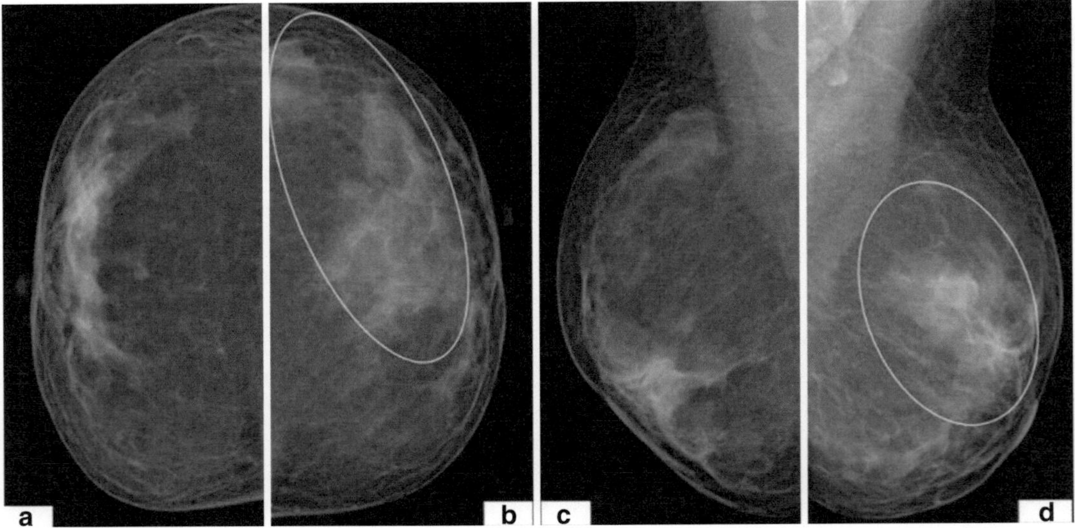

Fig. 9.2 CC view (**a**) right and (**b**) left breast, MLO view (**c**) right and (**d**) left breast. Asymmetric glandular tissue noted (circled in **b** and **d**) in the upper outer quadrant and central region of left breast, noted in both projections, occupying more than a quadrant

mately 82.7%, it is caused by benign superimposition of breast tissue—summation artifact—and hence generally not reproducible in other projections. The overall likelihood of it being malignant in screening mammogram is 1.8% [3]. In screening mammography, approximately 10.3% of persistent asymmetries have been reported to be malignant [3].

9.1.2 Global Asymmetry

It consists of asymmetry *seen in two views, in at least one-quarter of the breast (>1 quadrant)* without any associated mass, suspicious calcifications, or architectural distortions (Fig. 9.2). It is usually seen in approximately 3% of mammograms [1]. It is generally a normal variant; however, if there is a corresponding palpable abnormality, it is significant and requires further evaluation.

9.1.3 Focal Asymmetry

Focal asymmetry, in comparison to asymmetry, is *a lesion seen in at least two different mammographic projections that has concave outward margins* and may appear interspersed with fat in contrast to mass (Fig. 9.3). It occupies a volume *of less than one quadrant* of the breast and is of more concern. It is seen in 0.87% of screening mammograms with approximately 0.67% of likelihood of malignancy [3].

If a focal asymmetry develops in a patient undergoing hormone replacement therapy, repeat mammography after discontinuation of therapy may demonstrate resolution of the finding. If the density does not resolve, a biopsy is indicated. A developing asymmetry that becomes less evident but persists after discontinuation of hormone replacement therapy could hypothetically represent estrogen-sensitive breast cancer [2].

9.1.3.1 Alarming Signs of Focal Asymmetry

- If the asymmetry is palpable
- Associated with architectural distortion (Fig. 9.4)

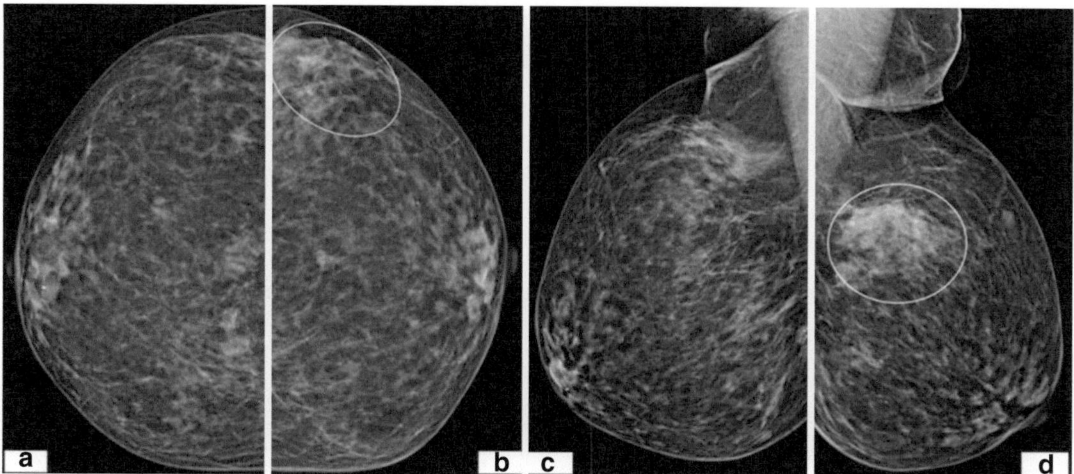

Fig. 9.3 CC view (**a**) right and (**b**) left breast, MLO view (**c**) right and (**d**) left breast. Focal asymmetric glandular tissue noted (circled in **b** and **d**), noted in both projections—upper outer quadrant of left breast, occupying less than a quadrant

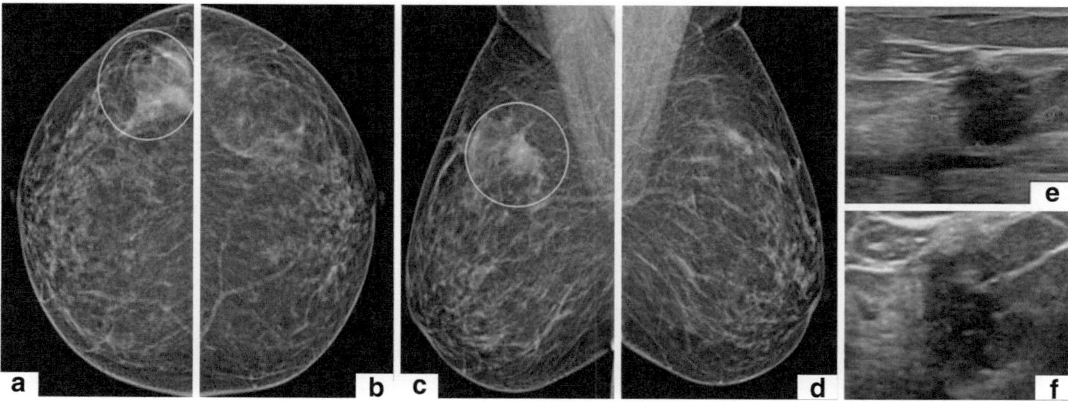

Fig. 9.4 CC view (**a**) right and (**b**) left breast, MLO view (**c**) right and (**d**) left breast. Focal asymmetric glandular tissue noted in the upper outer quadrant of right breast, noted in both views, and occupies less than a quadrant (circled in **a** and **c**). The lesion was palpable and on ultrasound revealed irregular spiculated hypoechoic mass (**e**) and USG-guided tru-cut biopsy (**f**) revealed an invasive ductal carcinoma

- Along with suspicious microcalcifications
- Suspicious axillary adenopathy

Note If the focal asymmetry without any alarming features is stable over 2–3 years, the BI RADS category can be downgraded from BI RADS 3 to BI RADS 2 [3].

9.1.4 Developing Asymmetry

A developing asymmetry is a focal asymmetry that is new or more conspicuous over time (Fig. 9.5). It is an uncommon mammographic finding, reported in less than 1% of cases, but this *carries a 12.8% risk of malignancy when seen at screening mammography and a 26.7% risk of malignancy when it persists at diagnostic mammography* [4].

A developing asymmetry that cannot be accounted for by differences in imaging technique and positioning, hormone replacement therapy, surgery, trauma, or infection at the site should raise suspicion of malignancy.

9.1.4.1 Developing Asymmetry: Points to Ponder [5]

1. It is important to *compare* the current study with previous studies performed at least 2 years earlier, if available, because an area of increasing density may not be apparent over a shorter follow-up period [6].
2. The finding of developing asymmetry on mammography should be evaluated with additional imaging to identify possible malignancy. The initial evaluation usually involves diagnostic mammographic views, including 90° lateral (for lesions seen only on MLO) [7], shallow oblique, and rolled views (for lesions seen only on CC views) and spot-compression (with or without magnification) views. Digital breast tomosynthesis, if available, gives better clarification than 2D imaging, obliviating the need for additional views mentioned earlier.

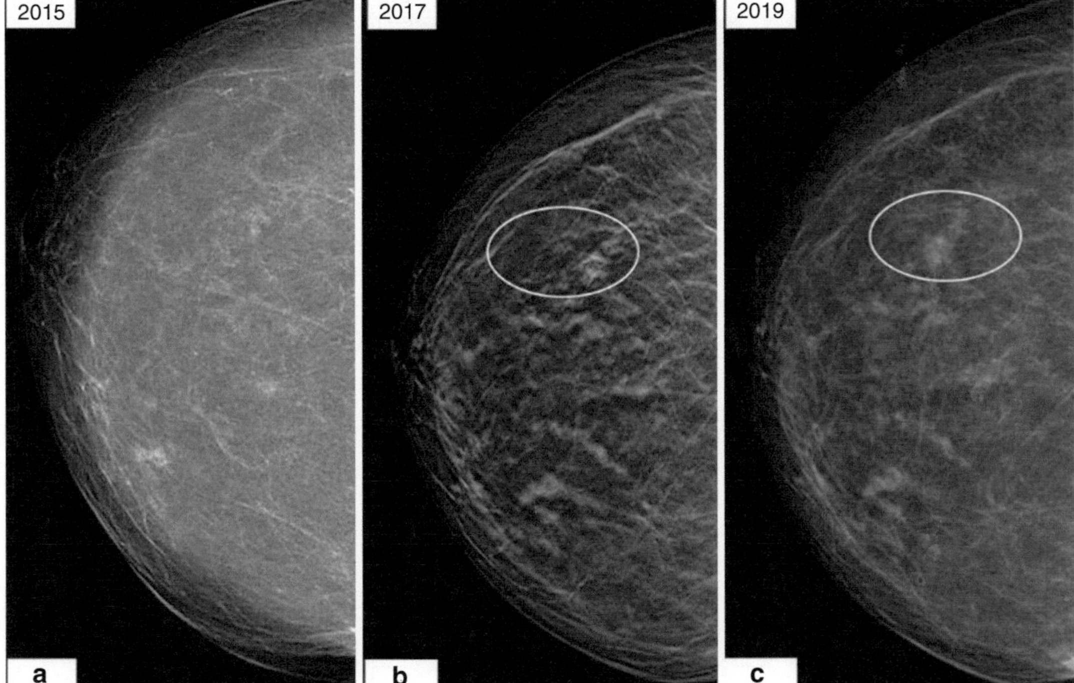

Fig. 9.5 Serial CC views (**a**–**c**) of right breast done during the period 2015–2019. Focal developing asymmetry is noted in the outer quadrant of right breast (circled in **b** and **c**). Stereotactic biopsy revealed ductal carcinoma in situ

3. Ultrasound correlation may help to categorize the developing asymmetry as either definitely benign or suspicious lesion. Also it may aid to plan image-guided biopsy if warranted.
4. MRI has no established role in the evaluation of breast asymmetry.
5. It is essential to have biopsy correlation even if a developing asymmetry is nonpalpable or have no ultrasound correlate.
6. Cancer manifesting as developing asymmetry can be of any histologic type, including DCIS.

Youk et al. [8] have suggested a very practical approach to assess asymmetry.

In our institute, we follow the following algorithm (Flow Chart 9.1).

9.2 Differentiation of Asymmetry Versus Masses

- Asymmetries have different border contours than true masses and lack the conspicuity of masses
- Asymmetry appears *similar to other discrete areas of fibroglandular tissue*, except they are unilateral, that is, no mirror image correlate in the contralateral breast
- *Asymmetry demonstrate concave outward border* and is usually interspersed with fat, whereas *mass demonstrates convex outward borders* and appears denser in the center than at the periphery (Fig. 9.12)

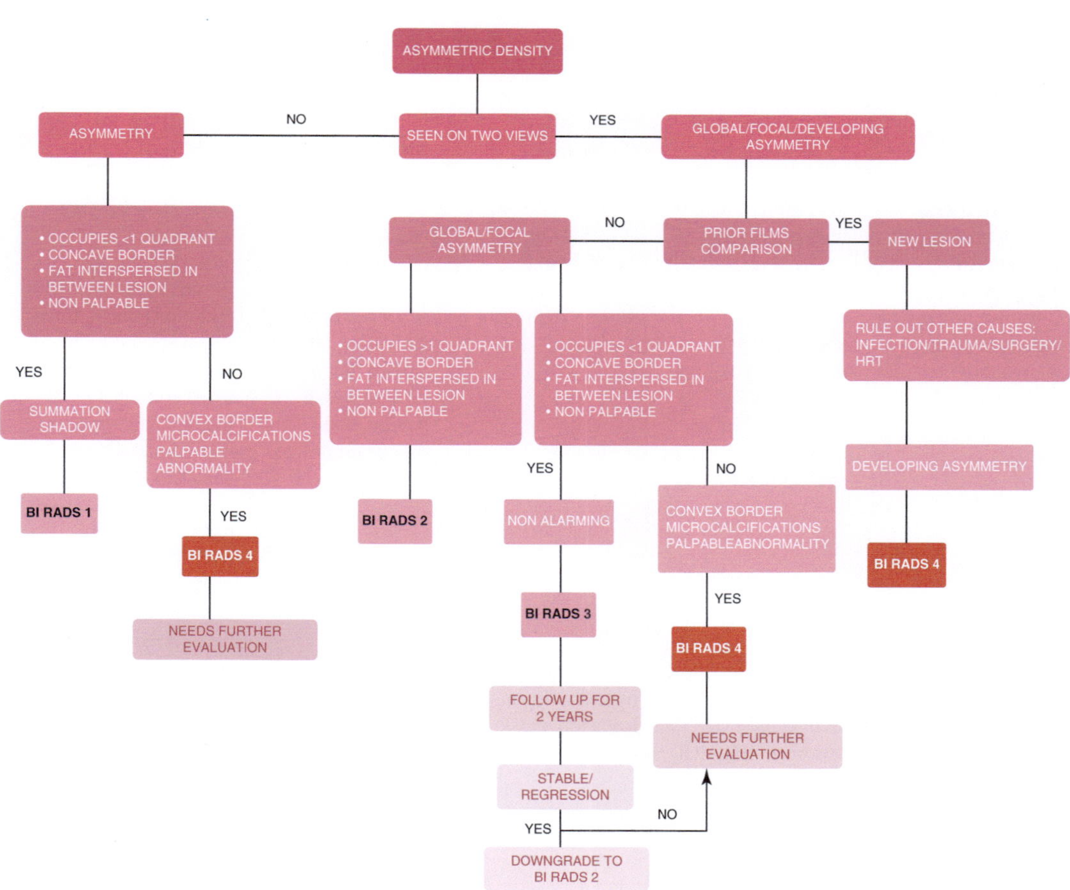

Flow Chart 9.1 A practical approach to asymmetry

To summarize, the asymmetry can be assigned with different BI-RADS category as in Table 9.1.

Table 9.1 Types of asymmetry and the corresponding BI RADS category

Type of asymmetry	BI RADS category
Asymmetry at screening—overlapping tissues	BI-RADS 1
Nonpalpable global asymmetry or stable focal asymmetry	BI-RADS 2
Baseline nonpalpable focal asymmetry	BI-RADS 3
Palpable focal asymmetry or nonpalpable with suspicious features **Developing asymmetry**	BI-RADS 4

9.3 Architectural Distortion

Architectural distortion is the third most common mammographic appearance of nonpalpable breast cancer, representing nearly 6% of abnormalities detected on screening mammography [1].

Architectural distortion is defined by the Breast Imaging Reporting and Data System (BI-RADS) system as an appearance in which "**the normal architecture of the breast is distorted with no definite mass visible**. This includes spiculations radiating from a point and focal retraction or distortion at the edge of the parenchyma. Architectural distortion can also be an associated finding along with a malignant mass."

There are various causes of architectural distortion. Few common etiologies and their imaging findings are enlisted in Table 9.2.

Table 9.2 Common etiologies presenting with asymmetry and imaging findings

Etiology	Mammography	Ultrasound	MRI	Pathology
Benign causes 1. **Radial scar** (<1 cm and around 40% develop malignancy) **Complex sclerosing lesions** (>1 cm; malignant potential unknown)	Focal architectural distortion, typically with radiolucent centre (Fig. 9.6) and spiculated margins; sometimes associated with microcalcifications "*BLACK STAR*" as referred by Tabar et al.	Commonly seen as a hypoechoic mass (Fig. 9.7) or parenchymal distortion that mimics malignancy	The morphologic features and contrast enhancement patterns of radial scars and complex sclerosing lesions cannot reliably differentiate a benign from malignant process	Radial scar and complex sclerosing lesions are characterized by fibroelastotic core with entrapped ducts. It may be associated with atypical and typical usual epithelial hyperplasia, adenosis, papillomatosis, sometimes may even be associated with ductal carcinoma in situ (DCIS) or even invasive carcinoma within or adjacent to areas of radial scar
2. **Sclerosing adenosis**	Microcalcifications, mass, focal architectural distortion (Fig. 9.8) It can coexist with both invasive and in situ cancers	A circumscribed, hypoechoic, or isoechoic mass	No specific MRI findings to differentiate from malignancy	Sclerosing adenosis shows an increase in the glandular elements along with stromal fibrosis and sclerosis that distorts and compresses the glands. Lobular architecture is maintained at low power with rounded and well-defined nodules. This may be associated with microcalcification or even fibrocystic changes

Table 9.2 (continued)

Etiology	Mammography	Ultrasound	MRI	Pathology
3. **Fat necrosis**	Usually either oval radiolucent oil cysts with thin capsules or thickening and deformity of the skin and subcutaneous tissue (Fig. 9.9) If the fibrotic component predominates, then may present as a spiculated lesions with skin thickening and retraction	Usually cystic or solid with mixed internal echotexture May appear as spiculated lesion with no significant internal vascularity	When spiculated or distorted, fat necrosis can be differentiated from malignancy on MRI as it *typically follows the signal intensity of fat on all sequences*	Fat necrosis shows disruption of the fat, admixed with lipid-laden macrophages, chronic inflammation and foreign body giant cell reaction. Hemosiderin-laden macrophages may also be seen
4. **Postprocedural changes**	Parenchymal scar with focal architectural distortion, swirling pattern after mammoplasty (Fig. 9.10) (Usually decrease by 35% by 2 years)	Frank distortion after breast biopsy/lumpectomy can reveal an irregular hypoechoic mass with posterior shadowing and no significant internal vascularity	Distortion with no significant enhancement on postcontrast scans *Any enhancement in the surgical bed on MRI that persists for 18 months or more after surgery is concerning for recurrence*	Following a lumpectomy or any other procedure, there can be areas of fat necrosis or inflammation, which can be seen in the breast parenchyma
5. **Rare benign lesions** [9] A. **Breast fibromatosis** B. **Granular cell tumor** [9] (Painless mobile masses, usually the upper inner quadrant)	Spiculated mass without microcalcification On mammography, this entity may have various appearances, ranging from an ill-defined and spiculated mass with architectural distortion (Fig. 9.11) to a round and well-circumscribed mass, usually without microcalcifications	Irregular hypoechoic mass with posterior acoustic shadowing, indistinguishable from malignancy The ultrasound appearance is similarly varied, manifesting as poorly circumscribed or well-circumscribed with posterior shadowing	Isointense mass on unenhanced T1-weighted images, heterogeneously, low- to high-intensity mass on fat-suppressed T2-weighted images, and heterogeneous gradual enhancement on dynamic MRI No specific MRI findings	Fibromatosis is characterized by the presence of long intersecting fascicles of bland spindle cells with indistinct borders, hyperchromatic nuclei, with occasional nucleoli and eosinophilic cytoplasm. The background stroma has thickened collagen, resembling keloid. Lymphoid aggregates may be seen at the periphery Granular cell tumor is composed of infiltrating sheets or cords of polygonal bland cells with well-defined cell borders, abundant eosinophilic granular cytoplasm, and round to oval nuclei with prominent nucleoli. The stroma in the background is collagenous

(continued)

Table 9.2 (continued)

Etiology	Mammography	Ultrasound	MRI	Pathology
6. **Malignant causes** A. **DCIS** B. **Invasive ductal and lobular carcinoma**	Pleomorphic, linear/branching microcalcifications with focal architectural distortion Mass with radiating spicules from *the central mass* (Fig. 9.12) (**Note:** Lobular carcinoma may have subtle finding as the tumor spreads in single file pattern, i.e., permeation without much displacement of the adjacent tissue)	Hypoechoic masses and microcalcifications Irregular spiculated hypoechoic mass with or without posterior features	Typically shows clumped linear or ductal nonmass-like enhancement An enhancing mass with plateau or washout kinetics can be seen	DCIS is classified on architectural growth pattern, mainly based on the arrangement of ductal cells whether in a cribriform, papillary, micropapillary, flat, solid, or comedo type of DCIS The nuclear grade may be low grade, intermediate or high grade. Myoepithelial cell layer surrounding duct spaces containing DCIS is intact, but may be attenuated especially in high grade DCIS. Associated stromal reaction (chronic inflammatory infiltrate, fibrosis/sclerosis) may be prominent in areas surrounding DCIS, especially in high grade DCIS and does not indicate invasion

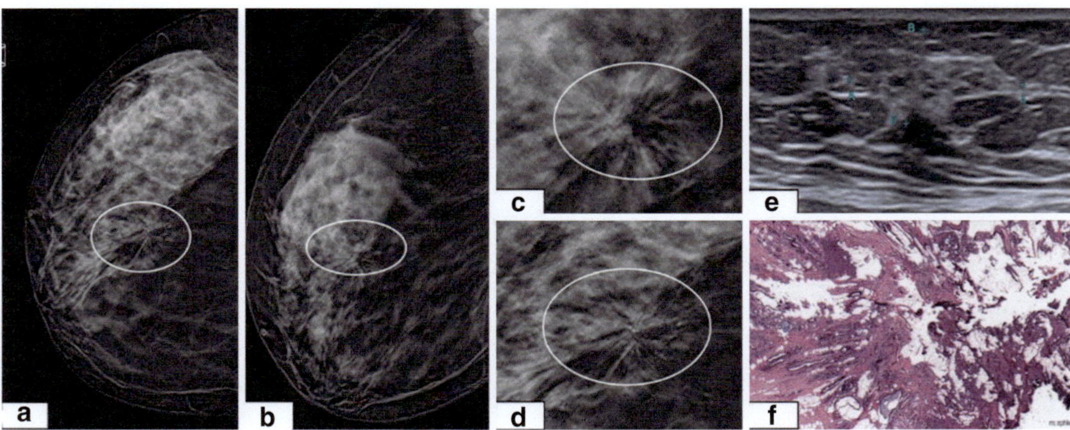

Fig. 9.6 Radial scar. (**a**, **b**) CC and MLO views of right breast. A focal architectural distortion with central radiolucency in upper outer quadrant (circled in **a** and **b**). (**c**, **d**) Magnified image of architectural distortion (circled in **c** and **d**). (**e**) Ultrasound shows a focal irregular heterechoic lesion. (**f**) Photomicrograph showing a central fibroelastotic stromal core with radiating ducts and lobules of varying degrees of proliferative and cystic changes (H&E×40)

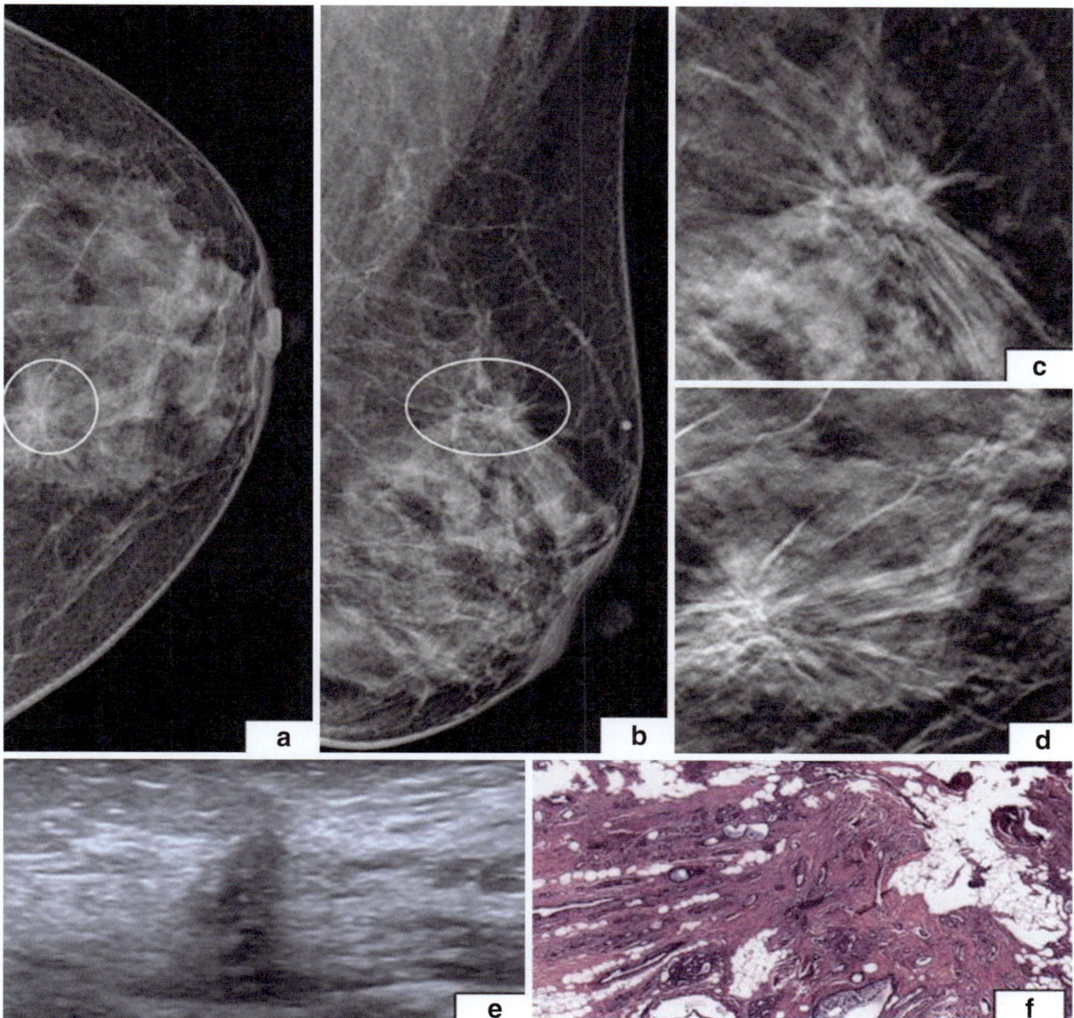

Fig. 9.7 Radial scar. (**a**, **b**) CC and MLO views of left breast— A focal architectural distortion with central radiolucency and peripheral radiating spicules in upper outer quadrant (circled in **a** and **b**). (**c**, **d**) Magnified image of architectural distortion. (**e**) Ultrasound shows a focal irregular hypoechoic lesion. (**f**) Photomicrograph showing a central fibroelastotic stromal core with radiating ducts and lobules of varying degrees of proliferative and cystic changes (H&E×100)

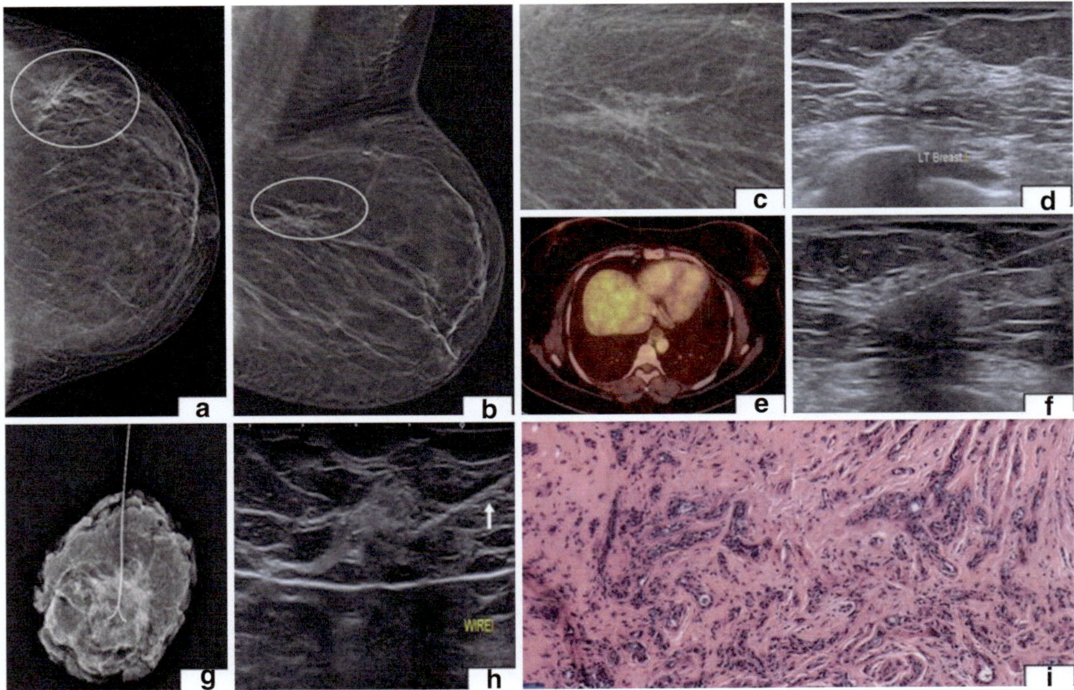

Fig. 9.8 Sclerosing adenosis (Known case of carcinoma of right breast). (**a**, **b**) CC and MLO views of left breast—A focal architectural distortion with radiating spicules in upper outer quadrant (circled in **a** and **b**). (**c**) Magnified image of architectural distortion. (**d**) Ultrasound shows a focal irregular isoechoic lesion. (**e**) PET CT shows increased uptake in the lesion. (**f**) USG-guided wire localization. (**g**, **h**) Specimen radiograph of the excisional biopsy revealing architectural distortion and wire in situ. (**i**) Photomicrograph showing increased and compressed glands, surrounded by stromal fibrosis (H&E×200)

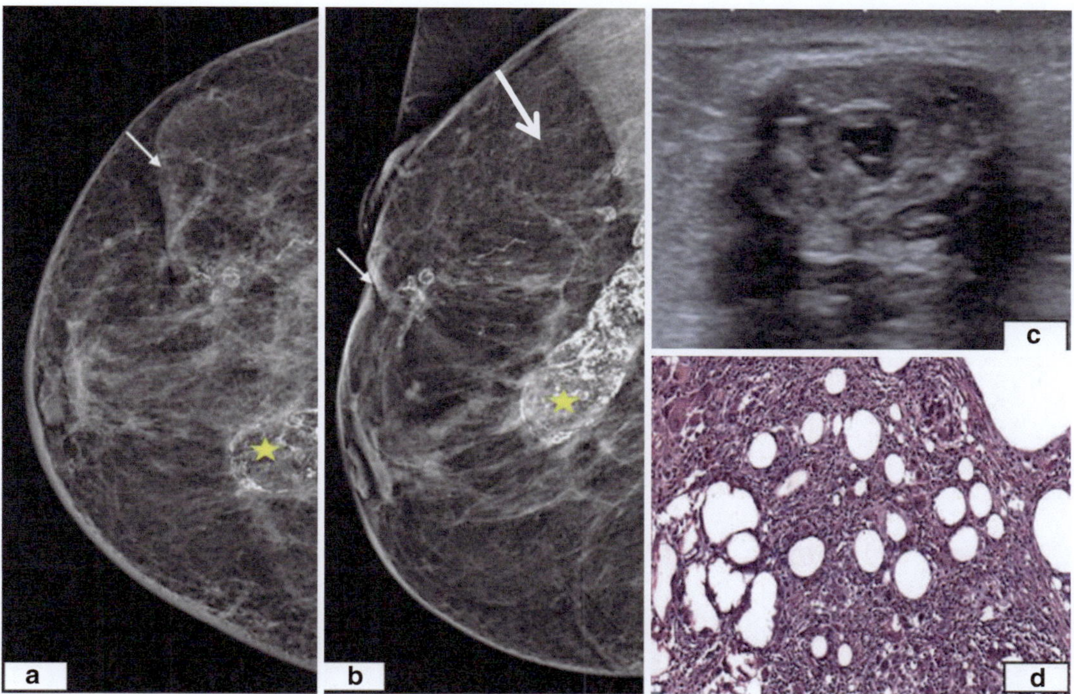

Fig. 9.9 Fat necrosis. (**a**, **b**) CC and MLO view of right breast—Architectural distortion noted in the upper outer quadrant (arrow) due to prior breast conservation surgery. Dystrophic calcification noted in the upper inner quadrant (star). (**c**) Ultrasound revealed irregular heteroechoic mass. (**d**) Photomicrograph showing necrotic adipose tissue with foamy histiocytes, chronic inflammatory cells, and multinucleated giant cells (H&E×200)

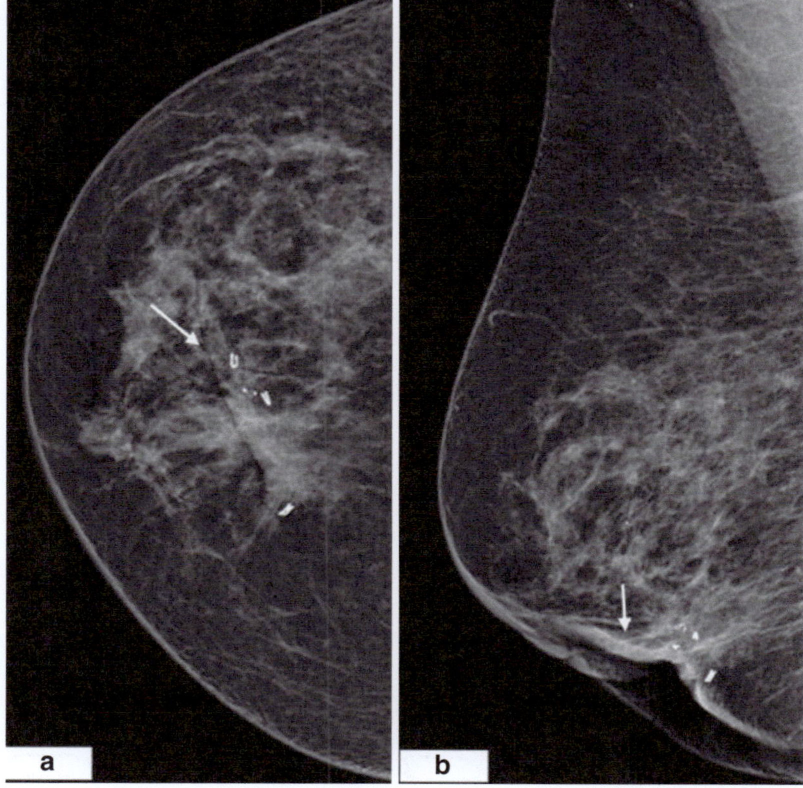

Fig. 9.10 Postoperative breast: (**a**, **b**) CC and MLO view of right breast—Architectural distortion (arrow) is seen involving the lower inner and central regions with few surgical staples adjacent to it

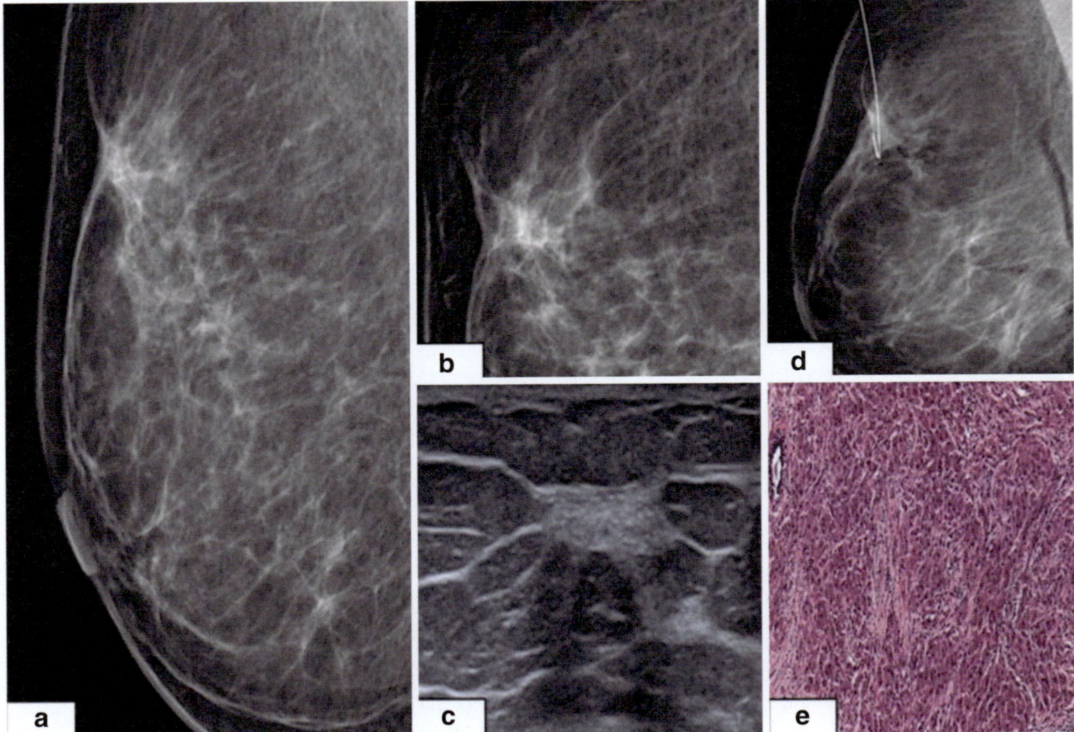

Fig. 9.11 Granular cell tumor. (**a**) MLO view of right breast shows focal architectural distortion with retraction of the overlying skin in the upper quadrant. (**b**) spot compression reveals persistence of the distortion. (**c**) Ultrasound reveals focal heteroechoic lesion. (**d**) Wire localization of the lesion done. (**e**) Photomicrograph showing infiltrating sheets of polygonal bland cells with well-defined cell borders, abundant eosinophilic granular cytoplasm, and round/oval nuclei with prominent nucleoli (H&E×200)

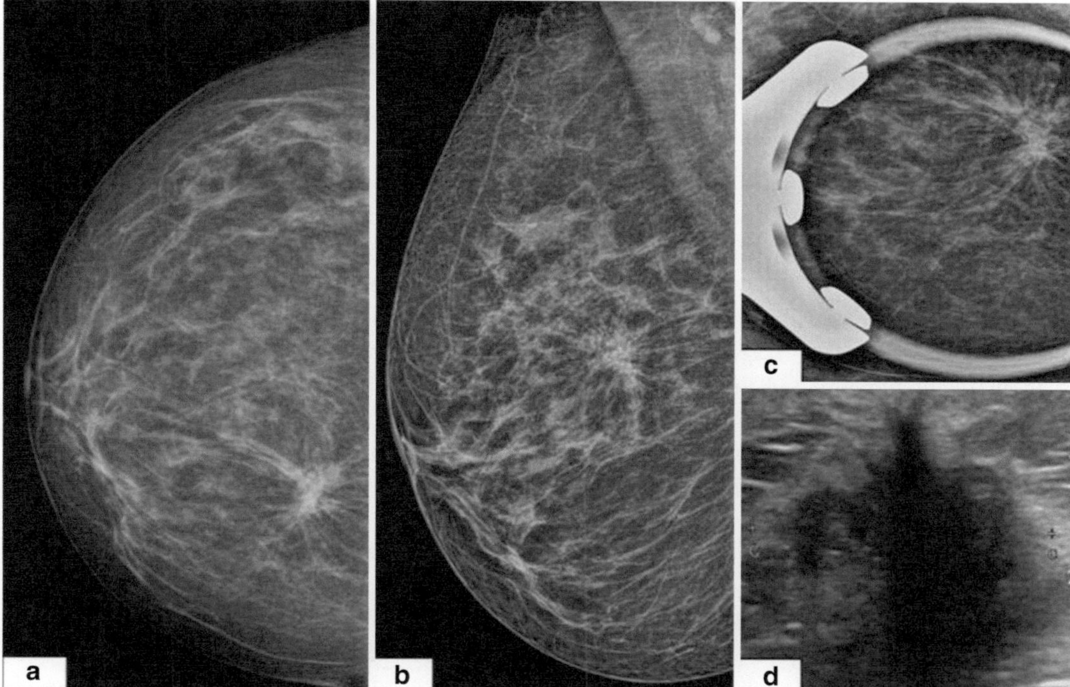

Fig. 9.12 Infiltrating Ductal Carcinoma. (**a**, **b**) CC and MLO view of the right breast reveals a focal spiculated mass with peripheral architectural distortion (**c**) Magnified image reveals central mass in contrary to radiolucent center as seen in radial scar. (**d**) USG reveals an irregular spiculated mass, favoring malignancy

9.4 Conventional 2D Mammography vs. Digital Breast Tomosynthesis

At conventional 2D screening mammography, 12–45% of missed breast cancers are retrospectively noted to be areas of architectural distortion. Invasive ductal and lobular carcinomas and ductal carcinoma in situ may manifest as architectural distortion [10].

Digital breast tomosynthesis can better demonstrate architectural distortion compared with 2D mammography, especially in dense tissue. Invasive lobular carcinoma, with its characteristic single-file growth that often permeates rather than displaces normal structures, can manifest with subtle findings at mammography and may be mammographically occult at 2D imaging.

In a study by Partyka et al. [11], it is found that architectural distortion was identified more readily with tomosynthesis than with 2D mammography, with 73% of identified distortions seen at tomosynthesis only, and 21% of those 2D-occult distortions yielding a cancer diagnosis.

9.5 Role of Ultrasound

Targeted Ultrasound identifies a sonographic correlate of distorted parenchyma or a mass. If the correlation is vague, a skin marker can be placed over the ultrasound finding, and additional mammographic views can be obtained to confirm a match.

Post-biopsy mammographic imaging of the biopsy marker is of value to confirm the accurate correlation of the lesions seen at tomosynthesis and ultrasound.

If the correlate is convincing, USG-guided biopsy can be performed for histopathological correlation.

9.6 Role of MRI

Indicated in the absence of no correlate found on ultrasound and the lesion is visible on only one view in mammography (when the stereotactic biopsy is not feasible).

MRI may reveal a corresponding suspicious enhancing area from where MRI-guided biopsy can be attempted.

9.7 Indeterminate Lesions

Management is primarily dependent on the patient's risk assessment status in a 2D detected subtle architectural distortion. Few studies [11] suggest that if no ultrasound correlate is found, the lesion is probably benign—BI-RADS 3 and short-term follow-up. Some studies recommend a biopsy correlation, as a significant percentage turned out to be malignant lesions [12]. Hence, it is preferable to do the biopsy in high-risk cases.

If a tomosynthesis-detected questionable subtle architectural distortion has no US or MR imaging correlate, the following options may be considered at the radiologist's discretion: tomosynthesis-guided needle localization, tomosynthesis-guided stereotactic biopsy, or short-interval follow-up tomosynthesis [10].

9.8 Suggested Algorithm to Interpret Architectural Distortion

1. Identify the architectural distortion in both the views.
2. Rule out any occult mass associated with architectural distortion.
3. Review Digital Breast Tomosynthesis images if available.
4. Compare with prior imaging and review clinical history for any prior interventions in breast like postbiopsy/lumpectomy/mammoplasty.
5. If the Architectural distortion is seen only on one view, for example, only CC or MLO, or in limited sequences in DBT, use cross-localization bar to localize in the other breast.
6. If still seen in only one view, use any other marker adjacent to it viz., cyst/calcification.
7. Use additional spot compression images for better analysis.

   NOTE: *If the lesion is convincing in the 2D image and disappears in spot (spot away), still it warrants biopsy correlation* [10].
8. Find an ultrasound correlate and characterize the lesion.
9. If there are no ultrasound correlates and the lesion is seen on the only view, MRI is warranted.
10. If there is no US/MR correlate, the lesion is probably a benign finding (BI-RADS 3). However, in high-risk patients, an image-guided biopsy is warranted.

9.9 BI RADS Category

If the architectural distortion is convincingly alarming, BI-RADS 4 is assigned, followed by image-guided biopsy as most of the lesions are nonpalpable.

9.10 Image-Guided Biopsy

1. If USG correlate is found, USG-guided core needle biopsy or Vacuum-assisted biopsy is the ideal technique.
2. If mammography is the only modality in which the lesion is seen, either stereotactic biopsy or wire localization can be performed for excision biopsy.
3. If lesion visibility is better on MRI with no ultrasound or mammography correlate, MRI-guided biopsy is suggested.

References

1. Kopans DB, Swann CA, White G, McCarthy KA, Hall DA, Belmonte SJ, Gallagher W. Asymmetric breast tissue. Radiology. 1989;171(3):639–43.
2. D'Orsi CJ, Sickles EA, Mendelson EB, Morris EA. ACR BI-RADS® atlas. Breast imaging reporting and data System. Reston, VA: American College of Radiology; 2013. p. 5.
3. Sickles EA. Findings at mammographic screening on only one standard projection: outcomes analysis. Radiology. 1998;208(2):471–5.
4. Rao AA, Feneis J, Lalonde C, Ojeda-Fournier H. A pictorial review of changes in the BI-RADS fifth edition. Radiographics. 2016;36(3):623–39.
5. Leung JWT, Sickles EA. Developing asymmetry identified on mammography: correlation with imaging outcome and pathologic findings. Am J Roentgenol. 2007;188(3):667–75.
6. Kopans DB. Suspicious lesions and lesions with a high probability of malignancy. In: McAllister L, editor. Breast imaging. 3rd ed. Philadelphia, PA: Lippincott; 2007. p. 513–53.
7. Samardar P, de Paredes ES, Grimes MM, Wilson JD. Focal asymmetric densities seen at mammography: US and pathologic correlation. Radiographics. 2002;22(1):19–33.
8. Youk JH, Kim E-K, Ko KH, Kim MJ. Asymmetric mammographic findings based on the fourth edition of BI-RADS: types, evaluation, and management. Radiographics. 2009;29(1):e33.
9. Gaur S, Dialani V, Slanetz PJ, Eisenberg RL. Architectural distortion of the breast. Am J Roentgenol. 2013;201(5):W662–70.
10. Durand MA, Wang S, Hooley RJ, Raghu M, Philpotts LE. Tomosynthesis-detected architectural distortion: management algorithm with radiologic-pathologic correlation. Radiographics. 2016;36(2):311–21.
11. Partyka L, Lourenco AP, Mainiero MB. Detection of mammographically occult architectural distortion on digital breast tomosynthesis screening: initial clinical experience. Am J Roentgenol. 2014;203(1):216–22.
12. Freer PE, Niell B, Rafferty EA. Preoperative tomosynthesis-guided needle localization of mammographically and sonographically occult breast lesions. Radiology. 2015;275(2):377–83.

Approach to Calcifications

10

Harini Gnanavel, Bhawna Dev,
Leena Dennis Joseph,
Anupama Chandrasekharan,
and Priya K. Palanisamy

Abstract

Breast calcifications are seen frequently in day-to-day practice on mammogram. Their frequency increases with age of the patient. Calcifications can be seen within a lesion or present as an isolated finding with no clinically palpable lump. Calcium deposition occurs within ducts, acini, stroma, or vessels in the form of calcium oxalate and calcium phosphate. Calcium oxalate is mostly seen in benign conditions and calcium phosphate is more commonly associated with malignant etiology. Calcium phosphate is more easily recognized on histopathology than calcium oxalate. X-ray mammogram remains the gold standard in detecting calcification till date. Ultrasound detects larger calcifications; however, it does not help in characterization of morphology. BI-RADS fifth edition classifies calcification according to morphology and distribution. These two categories are subdivided into benign and malignant according to the descriptors.

Keywords

Breast calcification · X-ray mammogram · Ultrasound · Benign · Malignant calcification

H. Gnanavel (✉) · B. Dev · A. Chandrasekharan
Department of Radiology, Sri Ramachandra Institute of Higher Education and Research, Chennai, India
e-mail: harini@sriramachandra.edu.in; bhawnadev@sriramachandra.edu.in

L. D. Joseph
Department of Pathology, Sri Ramachandra Institute of Higher Education and Research, Chennai, India
e-mail: leenadennisj@sriramachandra.edu.in

P. K. Palanisamy
Maidstone and Tunbridge Wells NHS Trust, Kent, UK

10.1 Introduction

Breast calcifications are encountered in our routine practice on mammography and their frequency increases with the age of the patient. While the majority of microcalcifications are benign, some specific grouped patterns can be caused by malignant disease or high-risk lesions. These can present as a nonpalpable lesion or as an isolated finding as in Ductal Carcinoma In Situ (DCIS). Some of these calcifications are not only seen in pure DCIS, but also correspond to the intraductal portion of infiltrating carcinomas [1].

10.2 Pathophysiology

The mechanism of calcium deposition, though not clearly understood, is proposed to be due to an active cellular process, or an effect of cellular degeneration. Calcium deposition occurs within

B. Dev, L. D. Joseph (eds.), *Holistic Approach to Breast Disease*,
https://doi.org/10.1007/978-981-99-0035-0_10

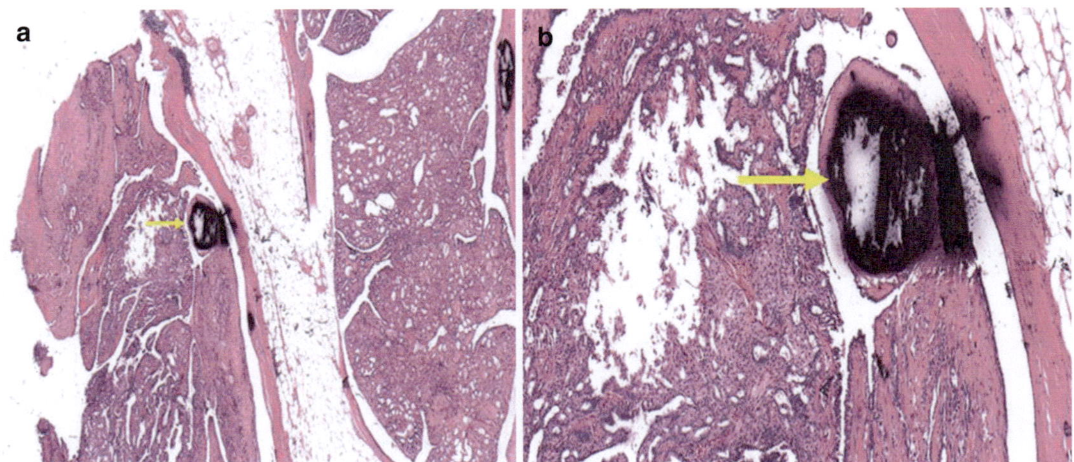

Fig. 10.1 (**a**) Photomicrograph showing intraductal papilloma with calcification (yellow arrow) seen as basophilic material (H&E×100) (**b**) Benign intraductal papilloma with calcification (yellow arrow) (H&E×200)

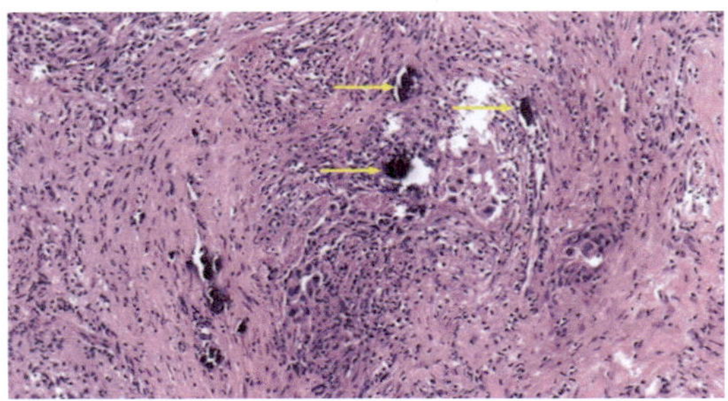

Fig. 10.2 Photomicrograph showing invasive mammary carcinoma with calcification (yellow arrows) (H&E×200)

ductal system, breast acini, stroma, or vessels in the form of calcium oxalate and calcium phosphate.

10.3 Histopathology

Calcium oxalate crystals are produced by apocrine cells of the breast and are colorless. On routine histopathology, these crystals are not seen. However, they can be seen under polarized microscope They are mainly seen in relation to benign cystic changes and sometimes seen in association with breast cancer. Calcium phosphate is more easily recognized on histopathology. It stains purple with haematoxylin and eosin (Figs. 10.1 and 10.2). Calcium phosphate is usually seen in the form of calcium hydroxyapatite. It is more commonly associated with malignant lesions than calcium oxalate [2]. Calcium phosphate microcalcifications are associated with benign and malignant disease and are seen as blue/purple psammoma-like structures. Histochemical stains like Von Kossa stain can demonstrate the calcifications.

10.4 Imaging

Presently, digital mammography is the first-line imaging modality of choice for evaluating and characterizing the calcifications.

The majority of calcifications are not visible on ultrasound (US), and it only detects large ones or those that are associated with masses or cysts. Although it is demonstrated as echogenic foci, it is not possible to adequately characterize them by US [1].

In general, features that suggest benign calcification on mammogram are [2]

- Multiple similar groups of calcification in more than one quadrant in one or both breasts
- Uniformity of the individual flecks of calcification
- Lack of interval change

Features that require further evaluation/suggest suspicious calcification include [2]

- Pleomorphic calcification (variability in shape, size, and density)
- Linear and branching forms
- Segmental distribution within a lobe of the breast
- Interval change

Note
It is must to take a spot magnification view to read the morphology of calcifications.

10.5 BI-RADS Fifth Edition Mammographic Descriptors of Calcifications

Calcification is categorized according to distribution and morphology (Fig. 10.3)

10.5.1 Distribution Descriptors

It refers to the arrangement of the calcifications in the breast (Fig. 10.4) and suggests the probability of malignancy.

1. *Diffuse distribution*: Calcifications are randomly distributed (Fig. 10.5) within the breast and are almost always benign [1].
2. *Regional distribution*: Calcifications in an extensive area, greater than 2 cm in their largest dimension and involving more than one quadrant (Fig. 10.6).The risk of malignancy is low; however, the morphology should be considered for final BI-RADS assessment [1].
3. *Grouped distribution*: Few calcifications (lower limit of 5 calcifications) are found in a small area of tissue (lower limit of 1 cm and upper limit of 2 cm) (Fig. 10.7). They require further evaluation with magnified views and should be seen as grouped calcifications in both projections to consider them as such [1]. This can be seen in benign or malignant conditions. If the group is a loose group (<10/cm^2), it is more likely to represent a benign condition, whereas a compact group (>20/cm^2) is more likely to be due to malignant disease [3] (term cluster is replaced by group in ACR BI-RADS fifth edition).
4. *Linear distribution*: Calcifications are arranged in a linear path (Fig. 10.8) and can show branching pattern, suggesting calcium deposits within a duct. Vascular or thick linear calcifications may present in this distribution; however, they have a characteristically benign morphology. The probability of malignancy is described approximately 60% [1].
5. *Segmental distribution*: This distribution pattern suggests deposition of calcium in the ducts and its branches, following the anatomical shape of a breast lobe, that is, triangular shape, with the tip of calcifications directed toward the nipple (Fig. 10.9). It can occur in benign pathology, such as secretory calcifications, or in extensive or multifocal cancer. A probability of malignancy is described as about 62% [1].

10.5.2 Morphology Descriptors

This refers to the morphology of calcifications within the breast tissue. It is divided into typically benign and suspicious calcifications. Typically benign calcifications often do not require magnification views or warrant increased monitoring. Suspicious calcifications require magnification for characterization and histological evaluation in the majority of cases [1].

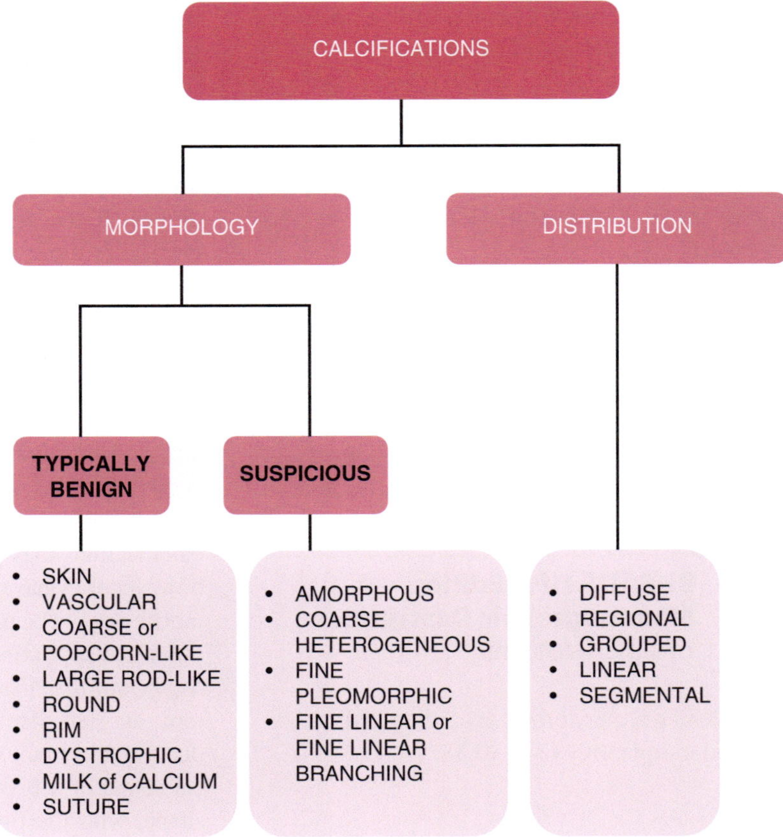

Fig. 10.3 Flow chart showing classification of calcification

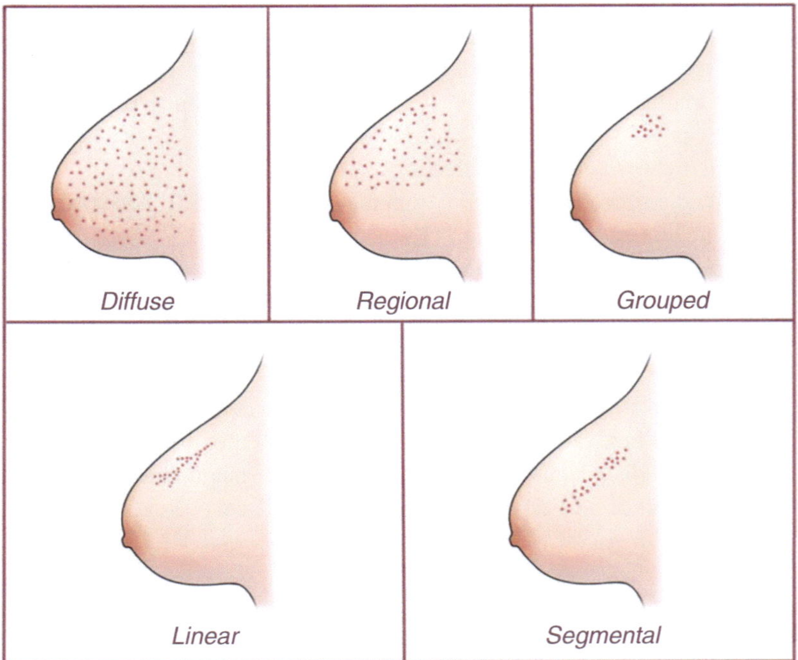

Fig. 10.4 Illustration of distribution of calcification

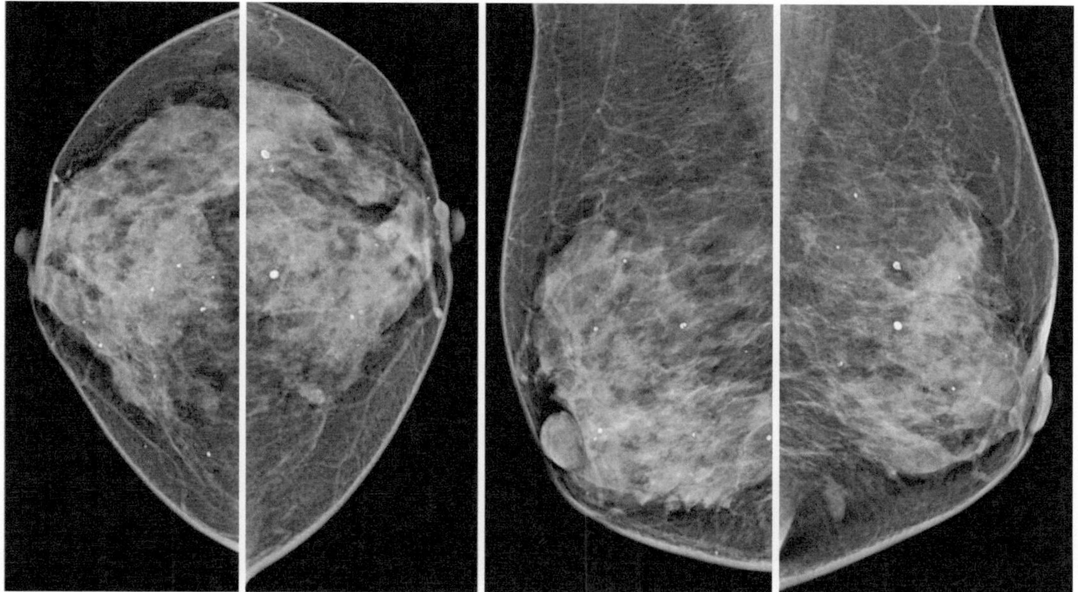

Fig. 10.5 X-ray mammogram of both breasts showing calcification in a diffuse distribution

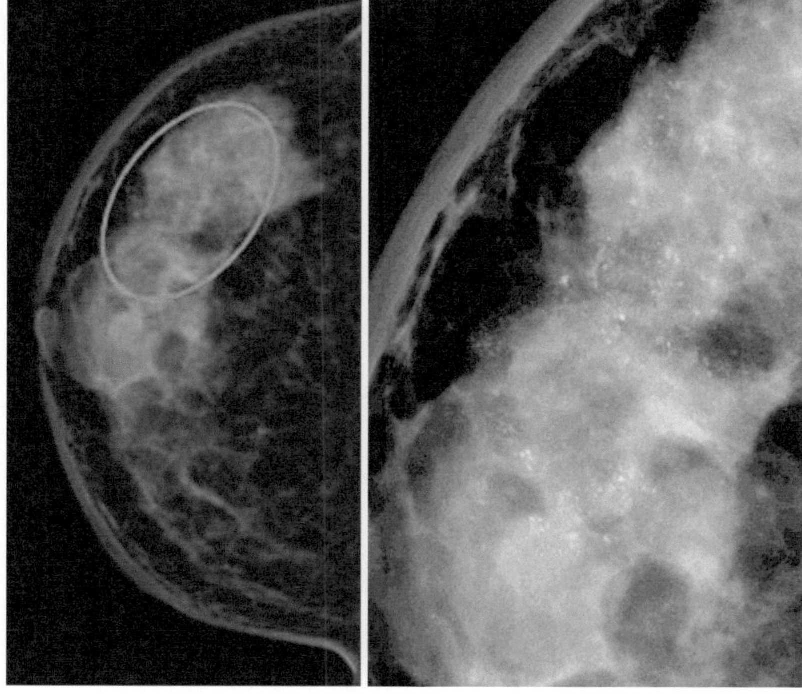

Fig. 10.6 X-ray mammogram showing calcification in a regional distribution

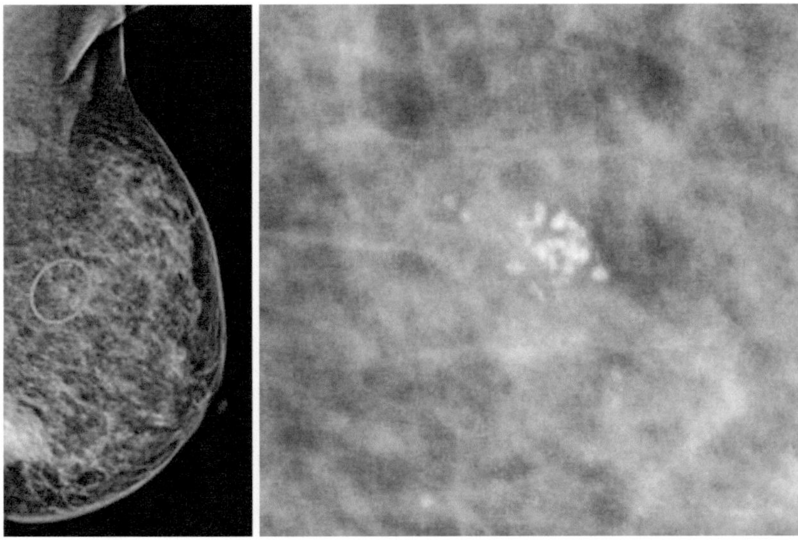

Fig. 10.7 X-ray mammogram showing group calcification

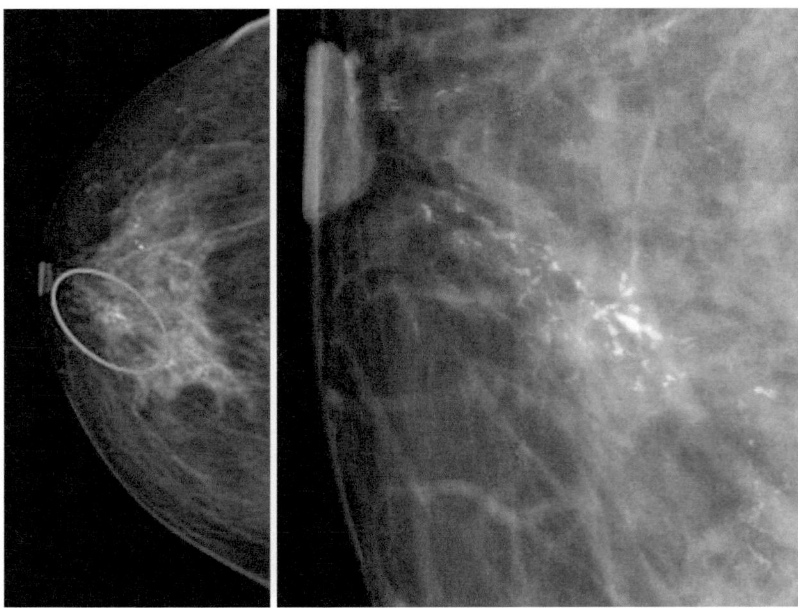

Fig. 10.8 X-ray mammogram showing calcification in a linear distribution

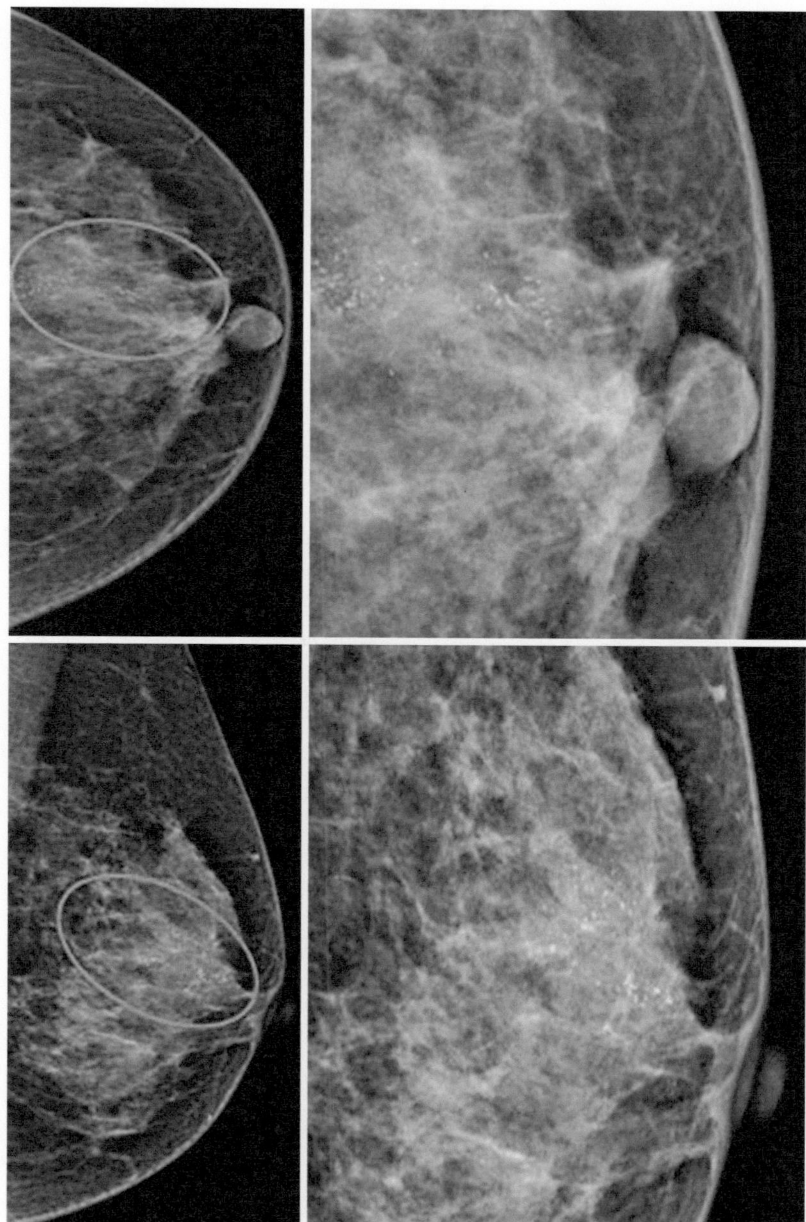

Fig. 10.9 X-ray mammogram showing calcification in a segmental distribution, tip of calcifications pointing to the nipple

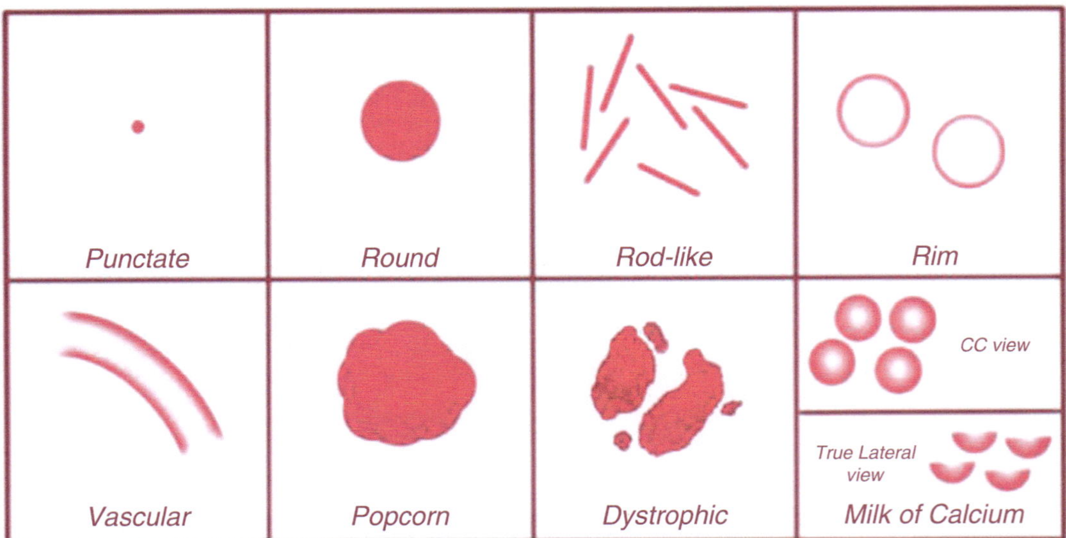

Fig. 10.10 Illustration of benign morphology calcification

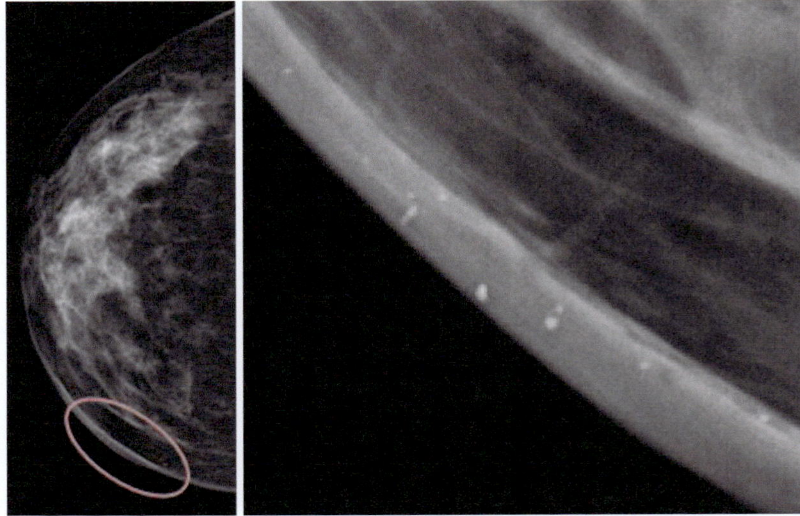

Fig. 10.11 X-ray mammogram showing skin calcification

10.6 Benign Calcifications [1]

10.6.1 Pictorial Representation of Typically Benign Calcifications (Fig. 10.10)

1. *Skin calcifications*: They correspond to small calcifications of the sebaceous gland, usually associated with inflammatory processes such as chronic folliculitis. They are usually multiple and pathognomonic. Their morphology is polygonal, sometimes round (Fig. 10.11), with radiolucent center. They measure between 1 and 2 mm. A useful sign in these cases is the "tattoo" sign, where the group of calcifications does not change its arrangement in the different projections, which confirms their superficial location.
2. *Vascular calcifications*: These are calcific deposits in the walls of the mammary arteries. They are usually bilateral and seen as parallel paths or "railroad tracks" and may be continuous or discontinuous (Fig. 10.12).

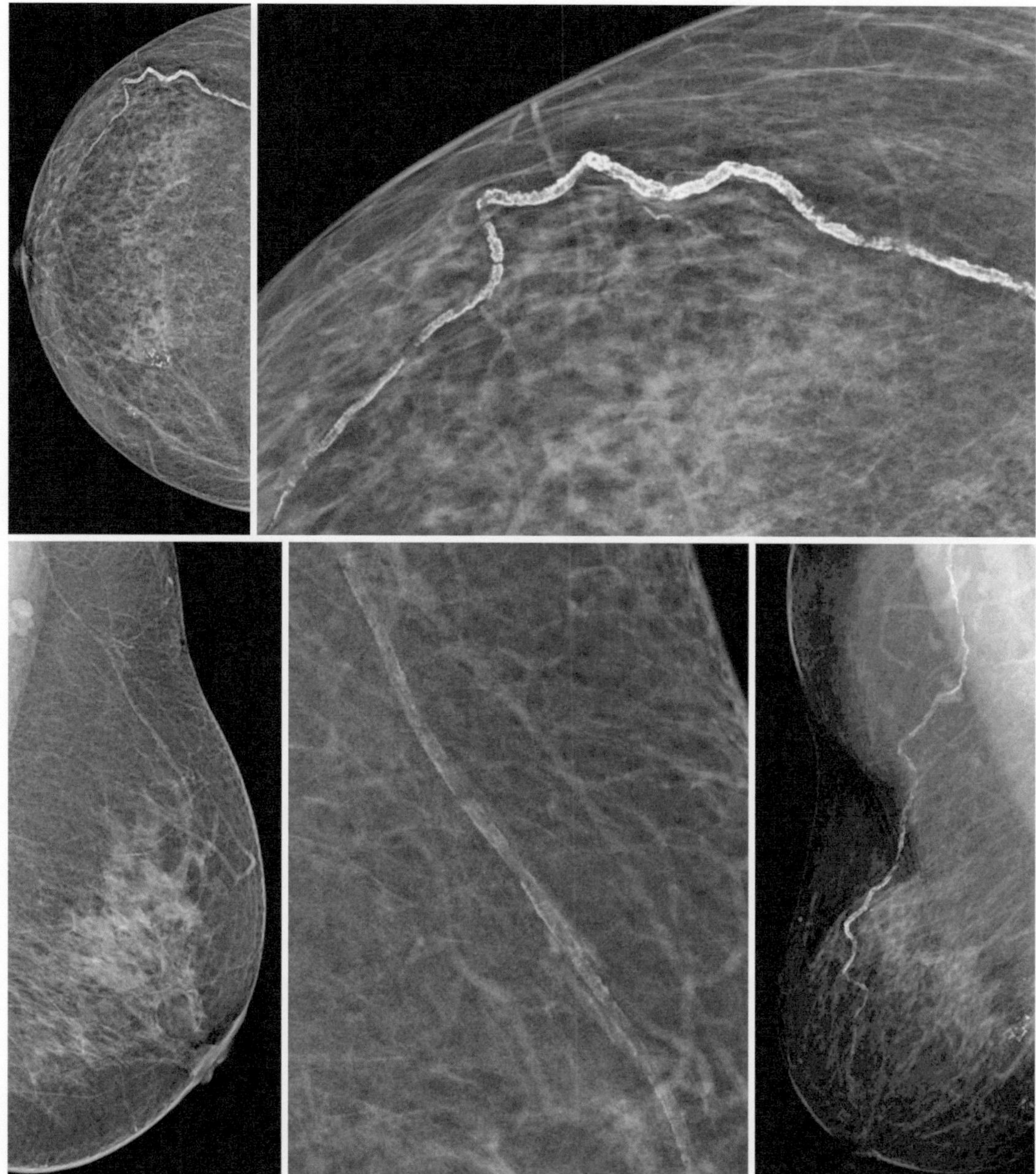

Fig. 10.12 X-ray mammogram showing vascular calcifications

3. *Coarse or popcorn-like calcifications*: These are dense, thick, larger than 2–3 mm, which over time tend to coalesce (Fig. 10.13), suggestive of fibroadenomas in involution. The initiation of calcification takes place at the periphery of the nodule.
4. *Large rod-like calcifications*: They correspond to calcifications located in the ducts, associated with ductal ectasia, secretory disease, or plasma cell mastitis. These are commonly seen in sixth decade. They are linear with smooth and regular edges with a bilateral distribution (Fig. 10.14)—unlike suspicious linear calcifications.
5. *Round calcifications*: These are round calcifications of various sizes and have their origin at

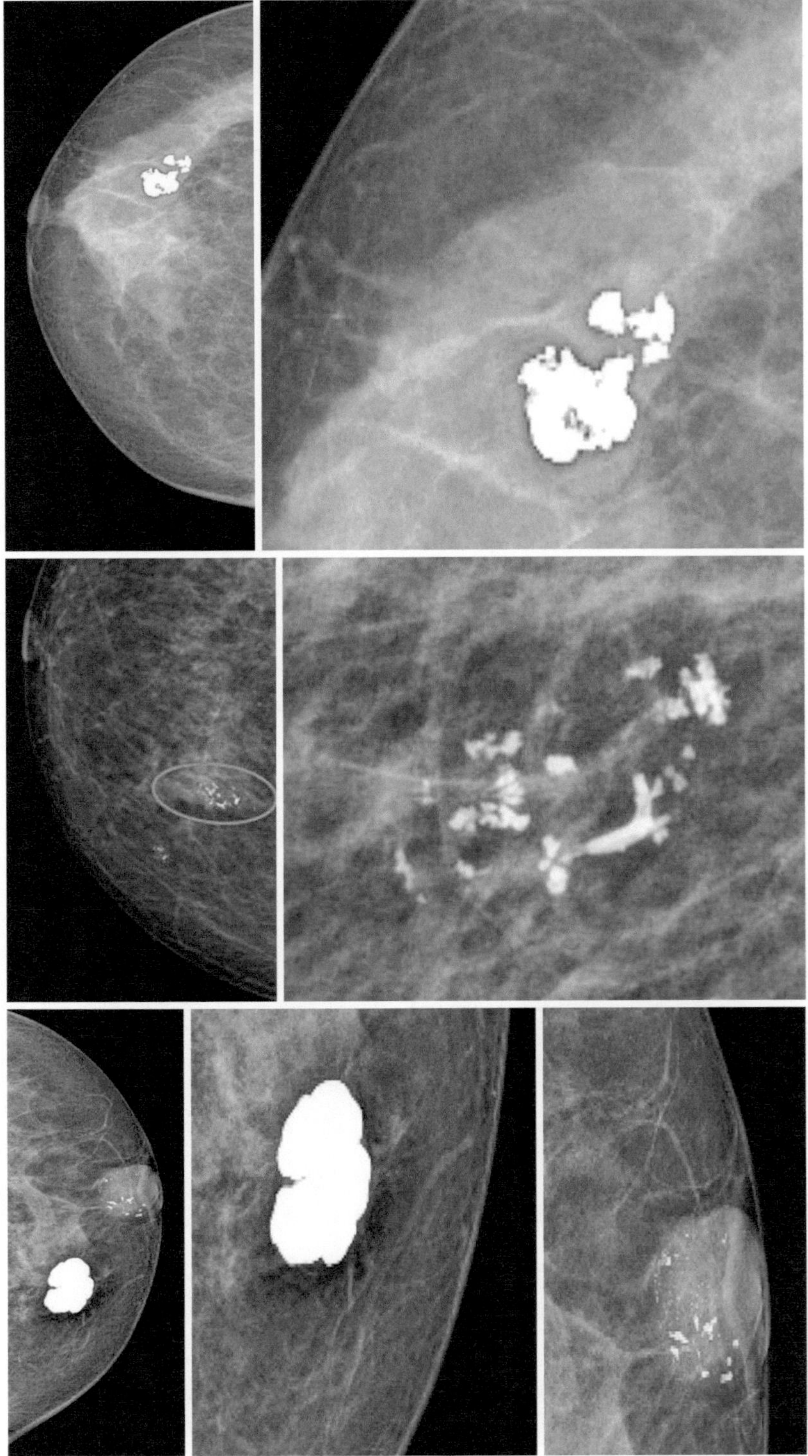

Fig. 10.13 X-ray mammogram showing various presentation of benign coarse/popcorn-like calcification

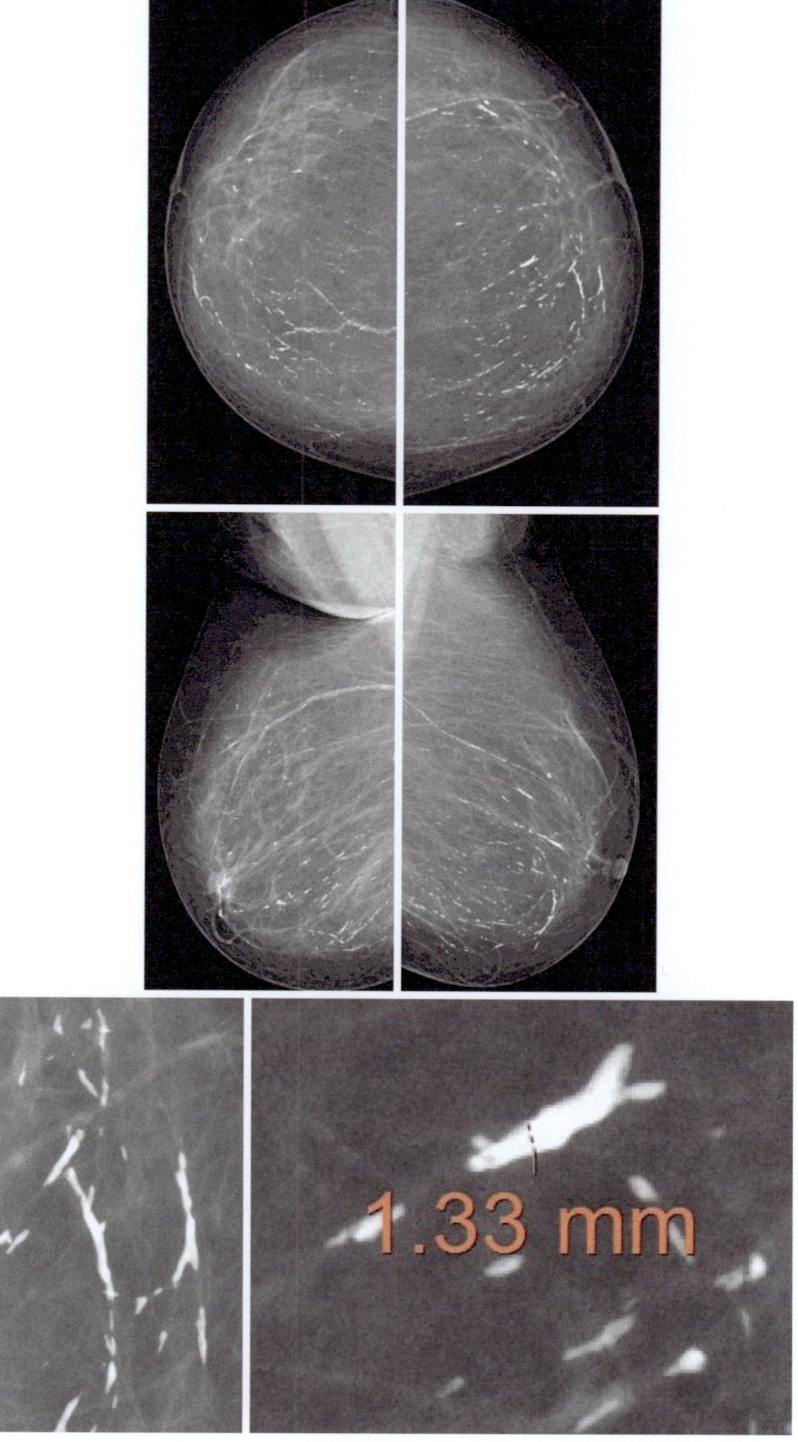

Fig. 10.14 X-ray mammogram showing rod-like calcification. The last image depicts the diameter of the calcification, which is larger in comparison to malignant calcification

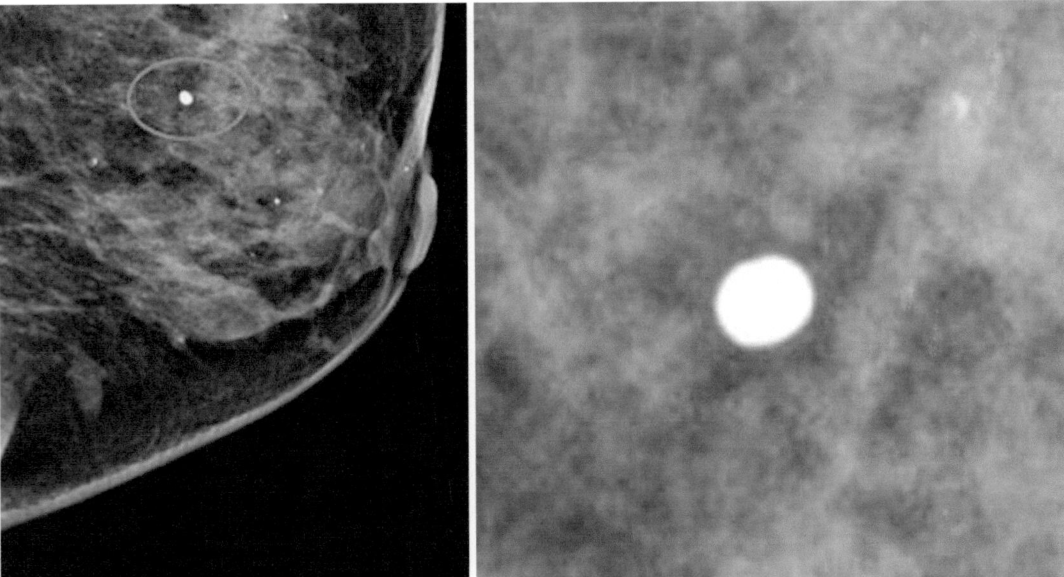

Fig. 10.15 X-ray mammogram showing round calcification

the acinar or lobular level. They appear punctate when they are smaller than 0.5 mm (Fig. 10.15). These are seen commonly in over 40 -year-old patients. When they are grouped, they deserve short-term monitoring, 6-month follow-up, and comparison with previous examinations. If the group is of recent appearance, more numerous than in previous controls or of linear or segmental distribution or adjacent to a known cancer, it is advisable to perform a histological study (term punctate and round are combined as single term "round" in ACR BI-RADS fifth edition).

6. *Rim calcifications*: These are peripheral thin rim of calcification around simple cysts or cystic lesions containing fat. They may be associated with a history of trauma or surgery. Radiologically, it appears as round or oval lesion with radiolucent center with peripheral thin rim of calcification (Fig. 10.16).
7. *Dystrophic calcifications*: These correspond to areas of fat necrosis in response to a trauma like surgery, radiotherapy, etc. to the breast tissue. Hence, relevant clinical history is important for the diagnosis. Dystrophic calcifications usually occur adjacent to the surgical scar, usually 3–5 years after surgery. They are usually greater than 1 mm, thick, rough, irregular calcifications (Fig. 10.17), which tend to coalesce, sometimes becoming very large and palpable. The presence of radiolucent areas, which indicate the existence of fat, is important for diagnosis.
8. *Milk of calcium calcifications*: These correspond to small particles of calcium oxalate settling within saccular dilatations of the TDLU (macro- or microcysts). It is noted in the peri- and postmenopausal women, usually located in the central and posterior regions of the breast, bilaterally. These calcifications are less evident in routine craniocaudal and oblique projection. True lateral projection is mandate for the typical—teacup appearance (Fig. 10.18), observed as a crescent with upper concavity. Milk of calcium calcifications shows change of morphology in the different projections.
9. *Suture calcifications*: These represent calcium deposited in the suture material. They are linear or tubular calcifications (Fig. 10.19) that may represent knots. These calcifications are common in patients who have undergone radiotherapy possibly because the damage induced by radiation alters the healing and delays the reabsorption of catgut, providing a matrix for calcium deposit.

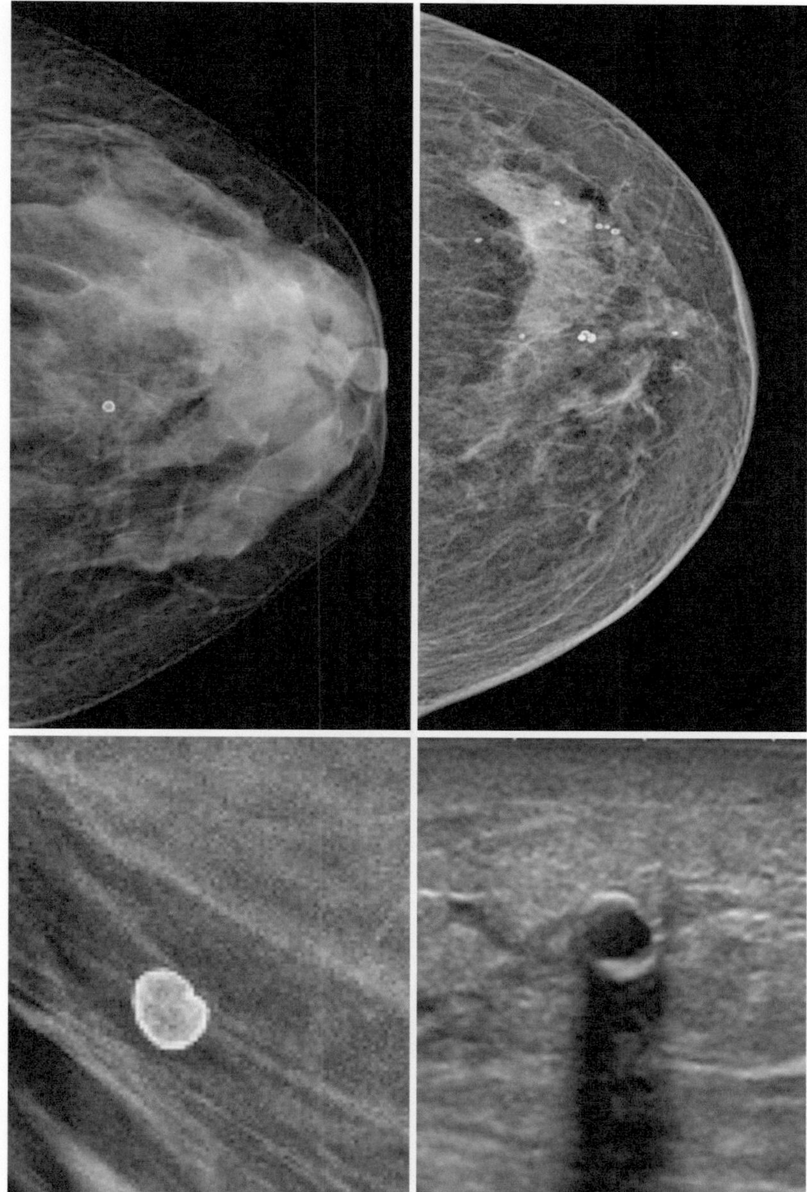

Fig. 10.16 X-ray mammogram showing rim calcification. The fourth image is an ultrasound showing rim calcification

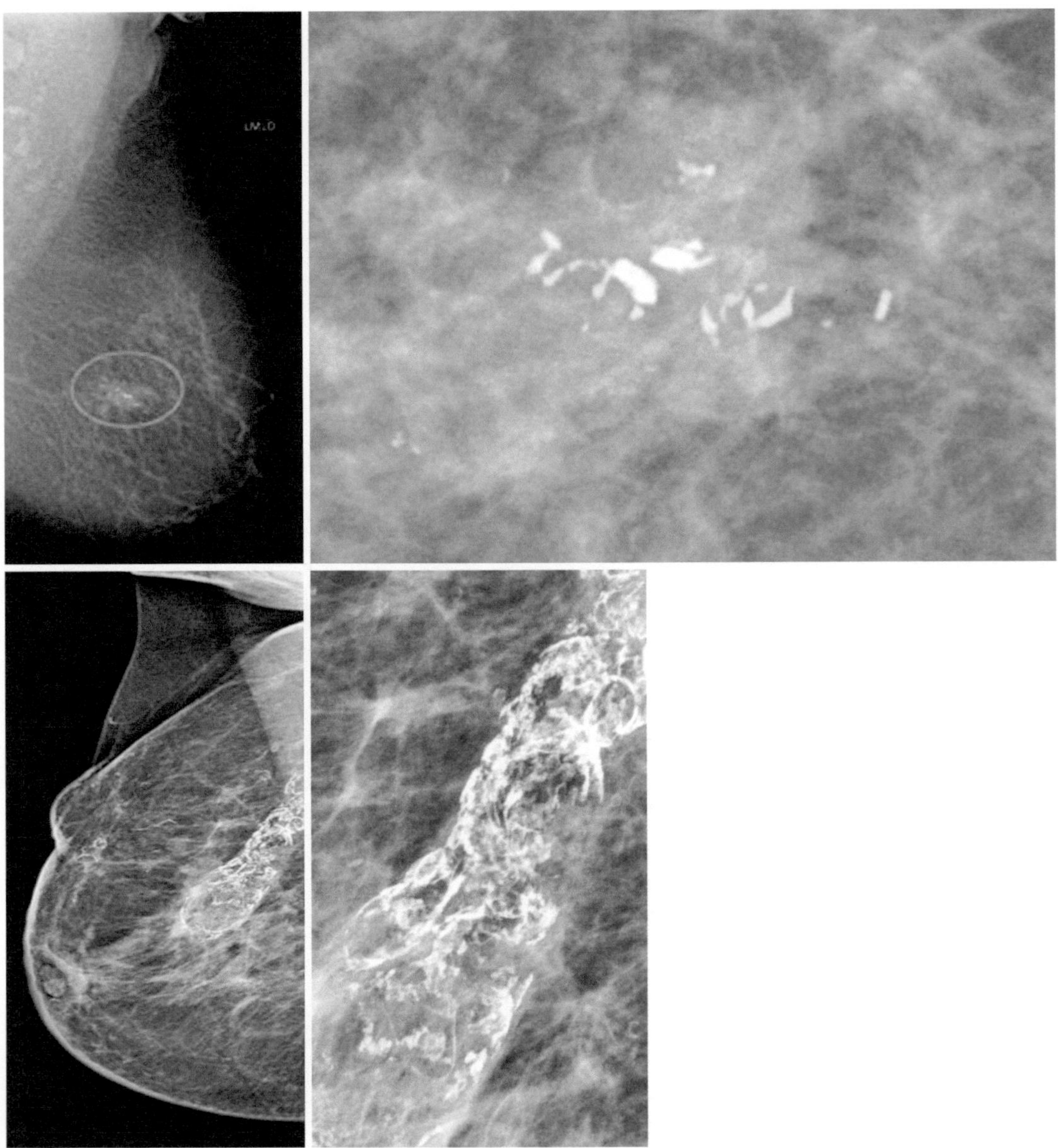

Fig. 10.17 X-ray mammogram showing various presentation of dystrophic calcification

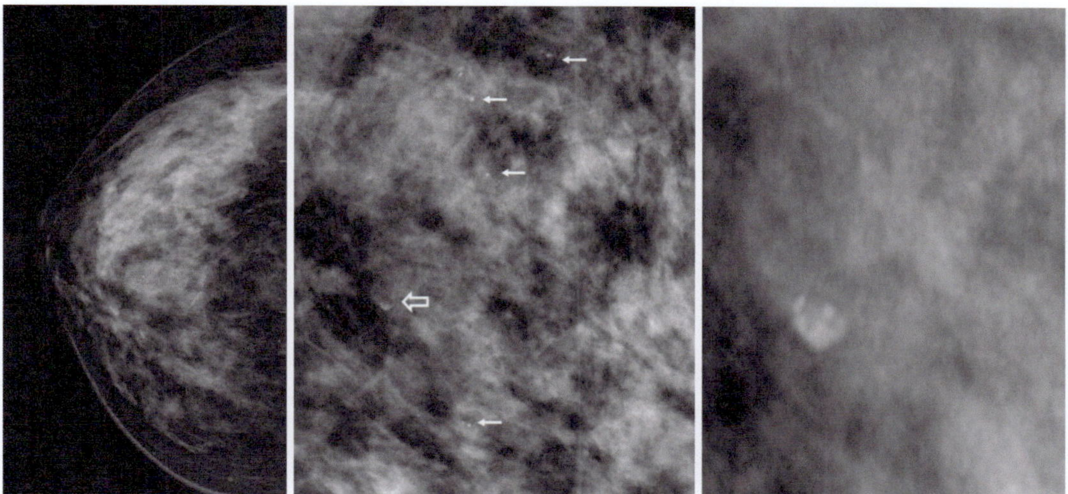

Fig. 10.18 X-ray mammogram showing milk of calcium calcification and tea-in-cup appearance on true lateral view

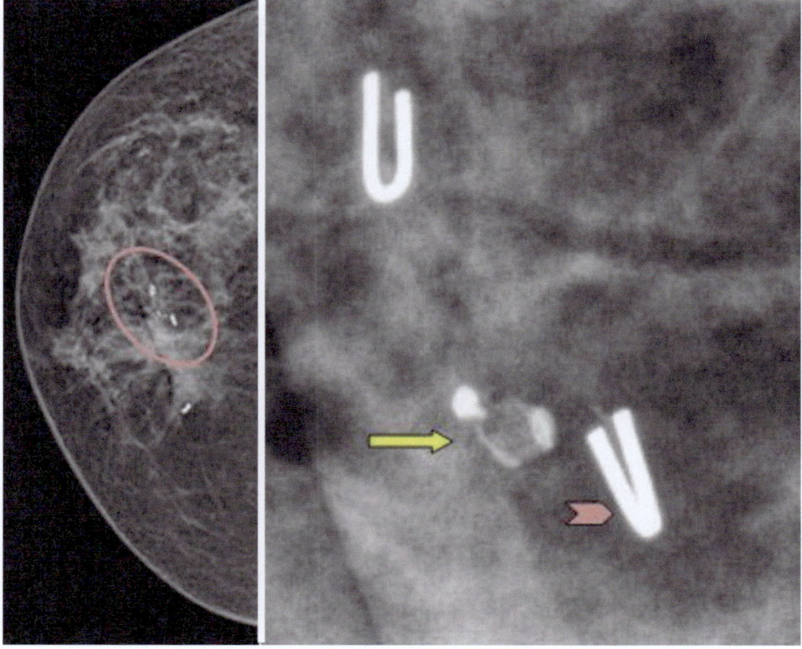

Fig. 10.19 X-ray mammogram showing suture calcification (yellow arrow) and surgical clip (pink arrow head)

Fig. 10.20 Illustration of suspicious morphology of breast calcifications

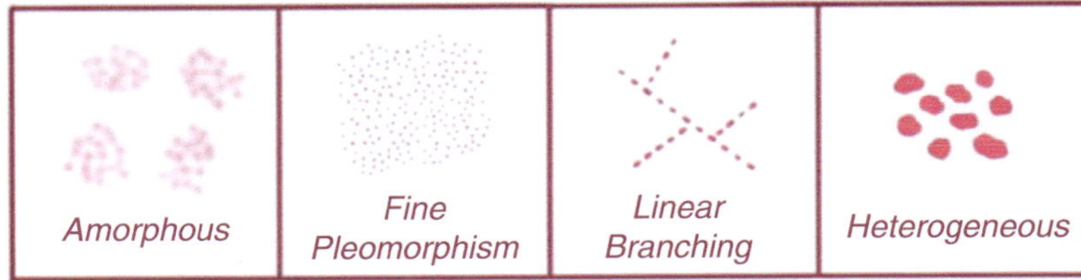

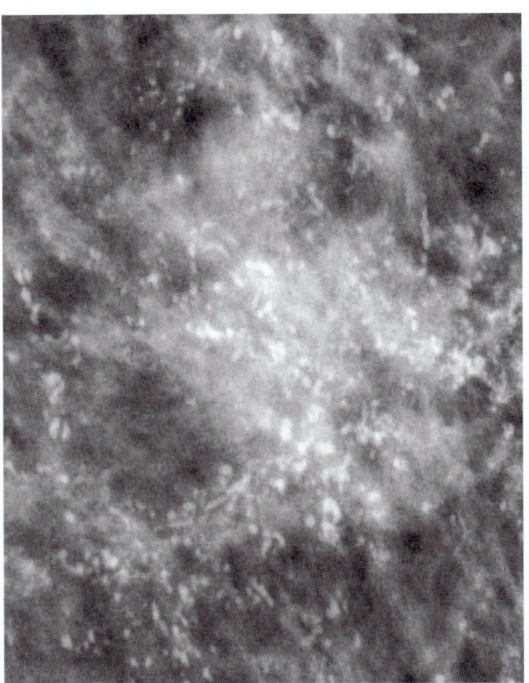

Fig. 10.21 X-ray mammogram showing coarse heterogeneous calcification

10.7 Suspicious Calcification [1]

10.7.1 Pictorial Representation of Suspicious Calcifications (Fig. 10.20)

1. *Coarse heterogeneous calcifications*: They are irregular and defined calcifications (Fig. 10.21), which tend to coalesce. Measuring more than 0.5 mm, that is, more than the pleomorphic calcifications but less than the dystrophic calcifications. These may be located in the breast stroma or ducts.
2. *Amorphous calcifications*: They correspond to small calcifications (less than 0.1 mm) that are not possible to count nor determine the shape, hence the name "amorphous" (shapeless) (Fig. 10.22). It gives the appearance of "powder," "cloud," or "cotton." To categorize them as amorphous, these calcifications should not decant in the strictly lateral projections, as in that case they would correspond to milk of calcium calcifications.
3. *Fine pleomorphic calcifications*: They correspond to calcifications of different shapes and sizes, angled, heterogeneous, with a size between 0.5 and 1 mm, smaller than the coarse heterogeneous like a crushed stone appearance (Fig. 10.23).
4. *Fine linear or branched calcifications*: These correspond to small calcifications, less than 0.5 mm, thin, linear, usually discontinuous and with irregular edges (Fig. 10.24), which originate in calcified necrotic debris within a duct compromised by carcinoma, that is, they present calcium molds in an irregular duct. They may branch in different directions forming "letters" (L, V, Y, X). The probability of malignancy is high in these calcifications.

10.7.2 Miscellaneous

Artifacts: Breast calcifications may be simulated by artifacts, including radiopaque material on the skin such as antiperspirants, deodorants, powders, surgical clips (Fig. 10.25), many of which contain metals such as aluminum, magnesium, iodine, or zinc oxide [4].

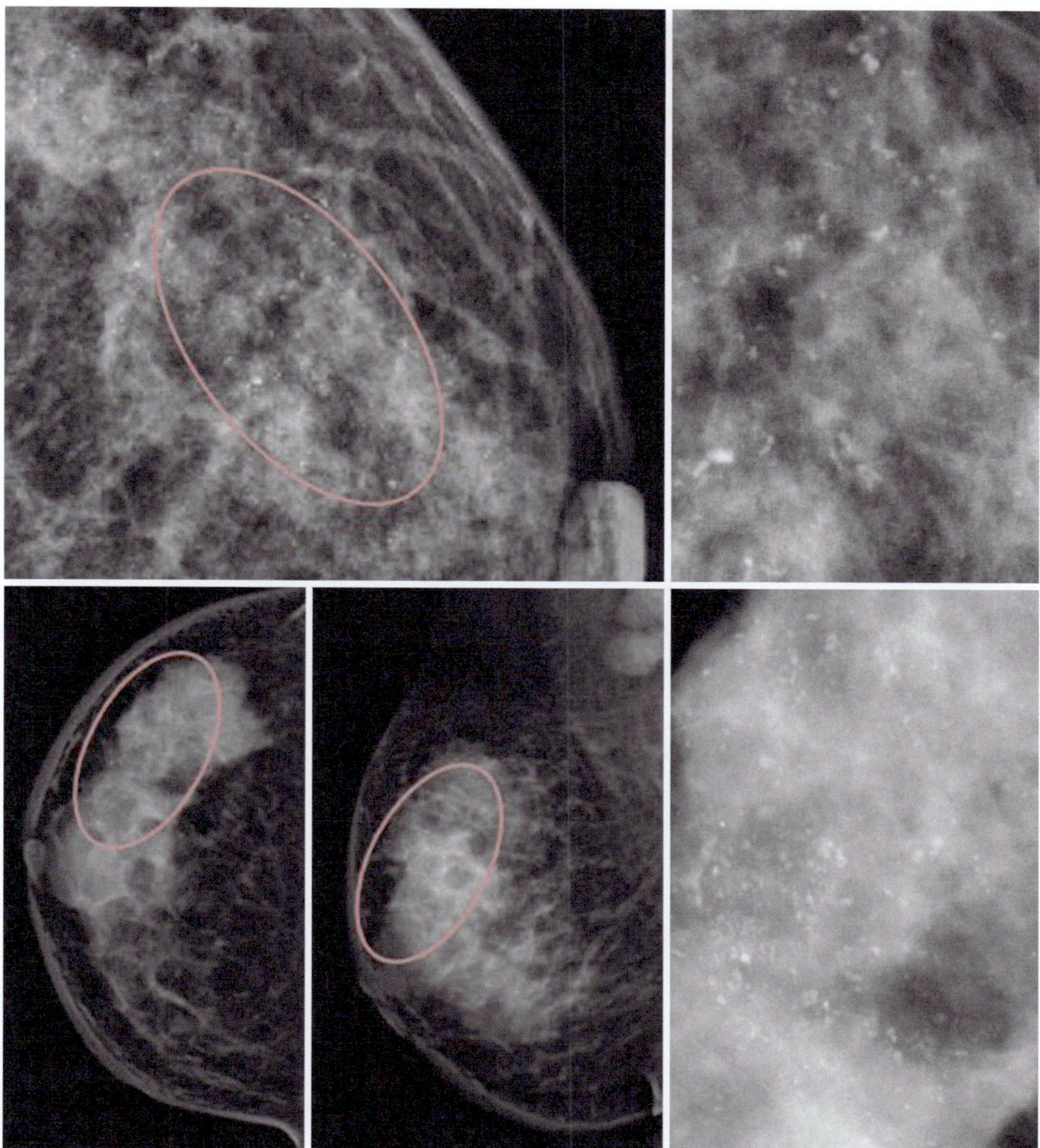

Fig. 10.22 X-ray mammogram showing amorphous calcification

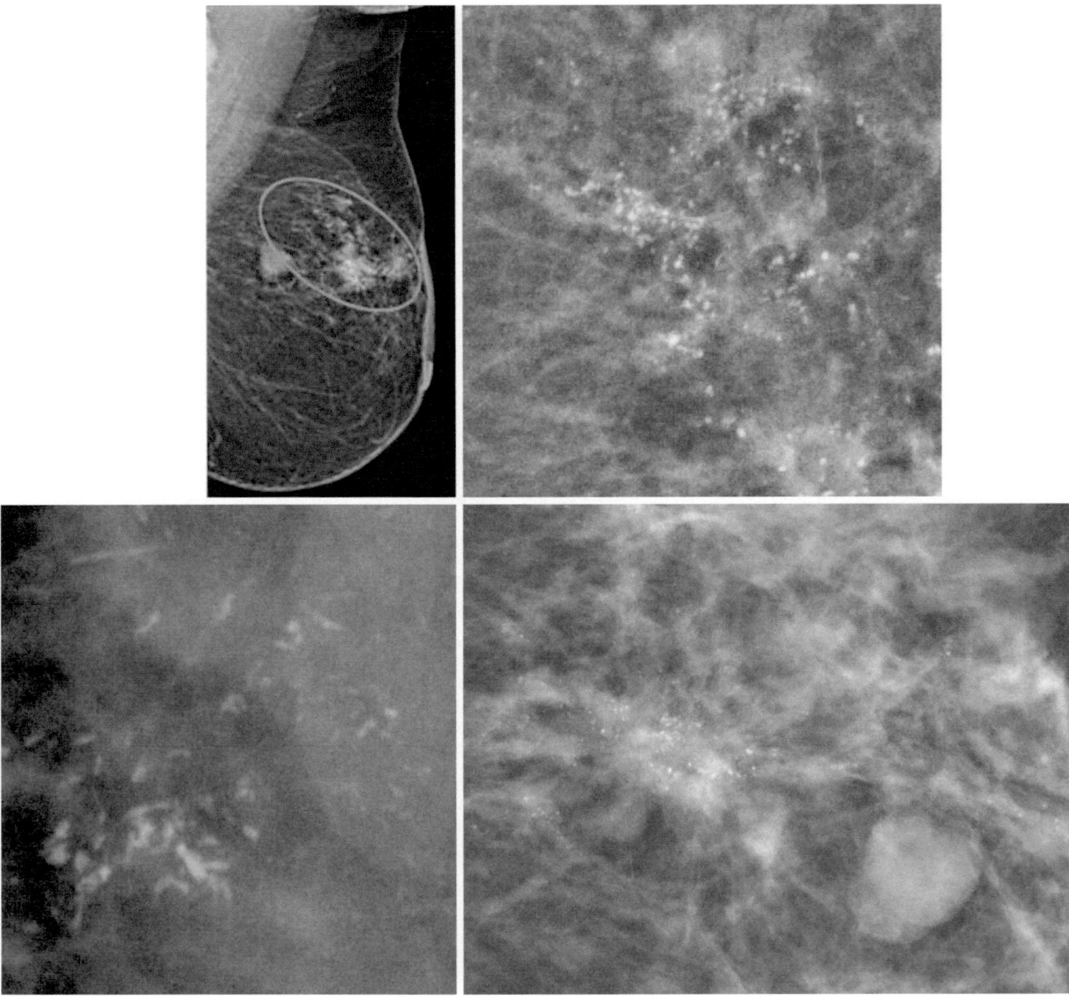

Fig. 10.23 X-ray mammogram showing pleomorphic calcification

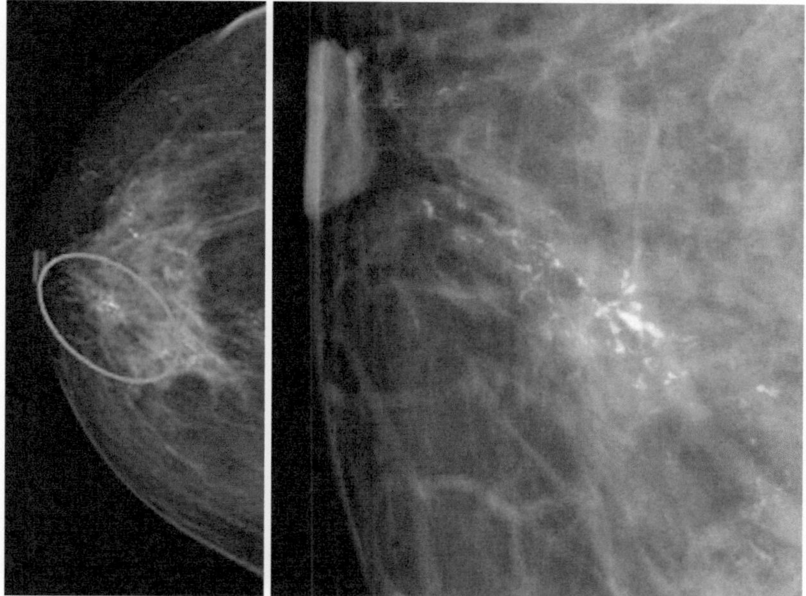

Fig. 10.24 X-ray mammogram showing fine linear or branched calcifications

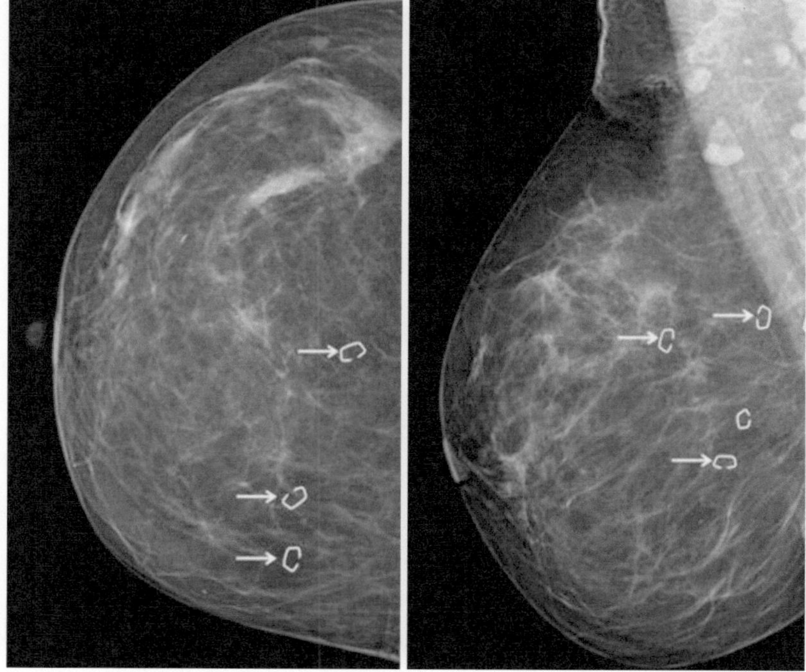

Fig. 10.25 X-ray mammogram showing surgical clips—artifact

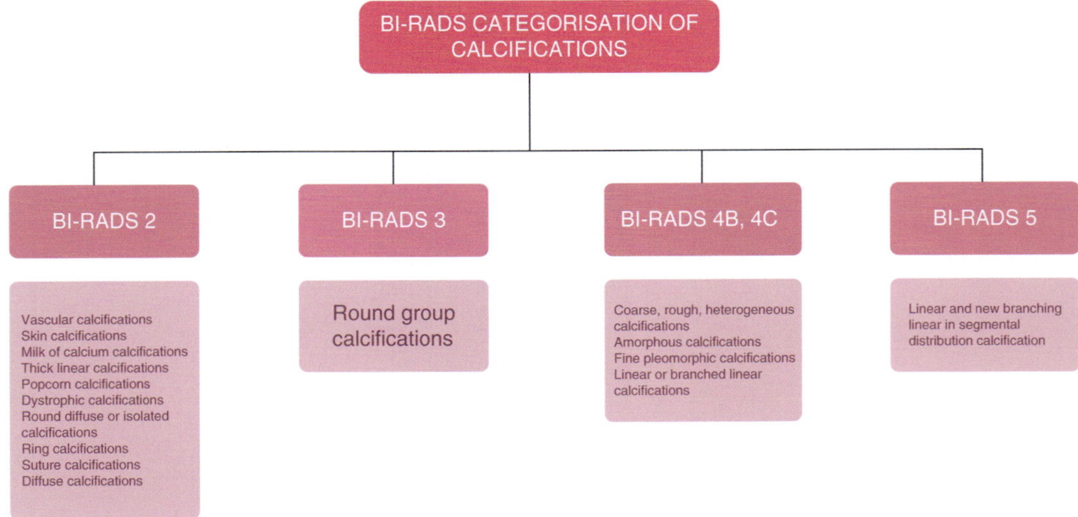

Fig. 10.26 Flow chart showing categorization of calcification according to BI-RADS

Note

The stability of breast calcifications should be ideally assessed with previous imaging wherever possible, to evaluate any change in the number of calcifications, morphology, and associated findings.

Spot magnification views should be done in suspicious calcifications to define the morphology better.

Various calcifications are described with their distribution and morphology and each are given a separate BI-RADS categorization (Fig. 10.26).

10.8 BI-RADS Fifth Edition Ultrasound Descriptors of Calcifications [5]

The revised classification has 3 descriptive terms (Fig. 10.27)

- Calcifications in a mass
- Calcification outside a mass
- Intraductal calcification

(The terms micro- and macrocalcification are omitted)

10.8.1 Intervention

Nonoperative diagnosis by image-guided sample is essential in cases of suspicious calcifications.

In an ideal situation, suspicious calcifications should be sampled by using vacuum-assisted biopsy (VAB) under stereotactic guidance. VAB needles range from 7 to 12 G and can be used to remove tissue volumes equivalent to the weight of a surgical specimen. It also allows multiple samples to be collected with a single percutaneous introduction. However, due to its availability and cost, it is not being used much.

Stereotactic biopsy, using a 14 G needle (Fig. 10.28), is the widely and commonly done procedure for suspicious calcifications due to VAB not being easily available. A 14-G needle sample may be confidently used to establish diagnosis [2].

When appropriate, vacuum-assisted biopsy can be performed using ultrasound. Successful identification of calcification on ultrasound relies on accurate localization of the cluster in the cor-

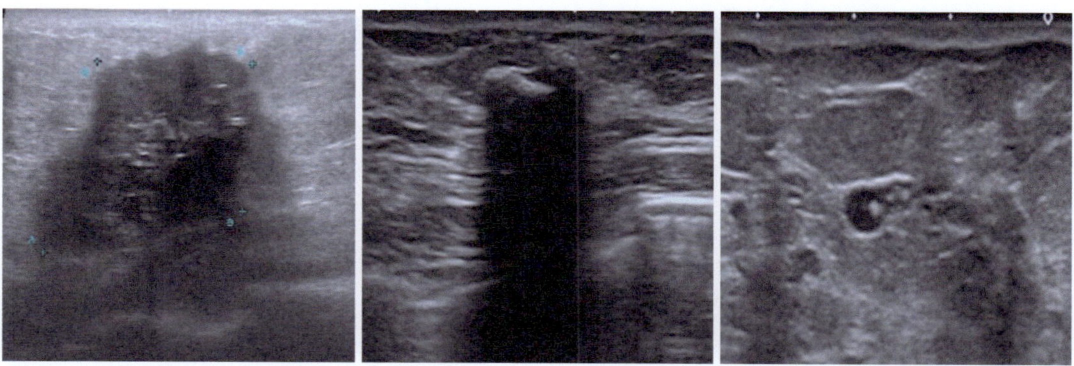

Fig. 10.27 Ultrasound images showing calcification in a mass, calcification outside a mass, and intraductal calcification

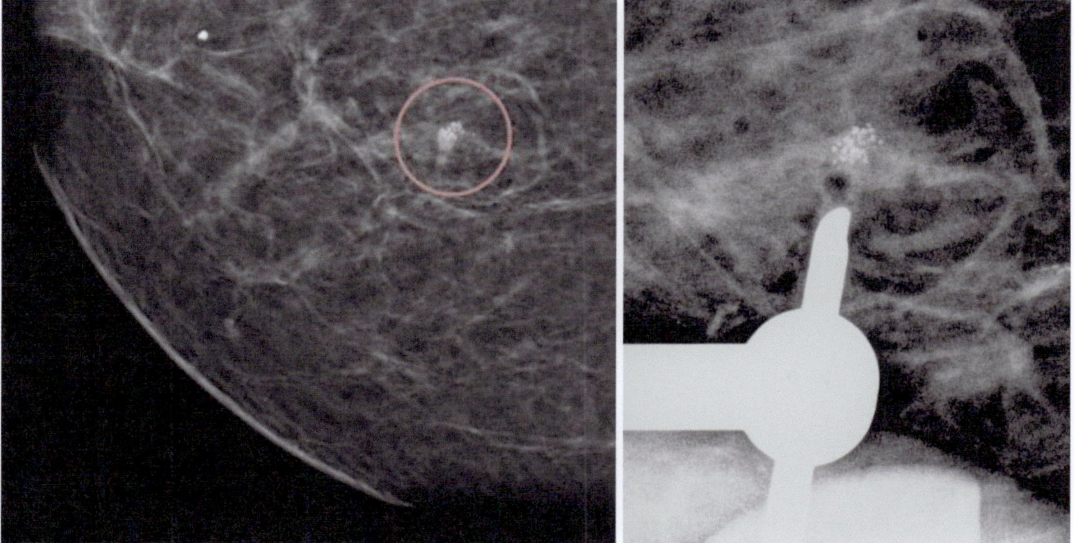

Fig. 10.28 Images showing stereotactic-guided biopsy of grouped calcification

rect quadrant, distance from the nipple, and depth below the skin surface. Immediate specimen radiography is essential to assess the adequacy of the specimen [2].

Note

At least five flecks of calcification should be seen or flecks in three separate cores to ensure that the sample is representative. It is important to ensure that calcification seen on specimen radiography correlates to the size and morphology of the calcification on mammography [2].

10.9 BI-RADS Category

When multiple masses/calcifications are encountered, each mass/calcification is given a separate BI-RADS according to the morphology and distribution and suggested HPE correlation.

References

1. Hernández PL, Estrada TT, Pizarro AL, Cisternas ML. Breast calcifications: description and classification according to BI-RADS 5th edition. Rev Chil Radiol. 2016;22(2):80–91.
2. Wilkinson L, Thomas V, Sharma N. Microcalcification on mammography: approaches to interpretation and biopsy. Br J Radiol. 2017;90(1069):20160594.
3. Nalawade YV. Evaluation of breast calcifications. Indian J Radiol Imaging. 2009;19(4):282–6.
4. Demetri-Lewis A, Slanetz PJ, Eisenberg RL. Breast calcifications: the focal group. Am J Roentgenol. 2012;198(4):W325–43.
5. Rao AA, Feneis J, Lalonde C, Ojeda-Fournier H. A pictorial review of changes in the BI-RADS fifth edition. Radiographics. 2016;36(3):623–39.

11 MRI Breast

Rupa Renganathan, S. Prema, and Suchana Kushvaha

Abstract

Magnetic Resonance Imaging (MRI) is an integral part of breast imaging services. As MRI provides both the morphological and functional information, it has the highest sensitivity and high negative predictive value in detecting invasive cancers. MRI has a role in screening of high-risk women, preoperative staging of breast cancers, assessment of response in patients undergoing neoadjuvant chemotherapy, and is used as a problem-solving tool when conventional modalities are inconclusive. It is also used for localization and biopsy of the suspicious findings detected in MRI. Because of the several advantages that MRI breast offers, it should be integrated into the management protocol of every institute offering comprehensive breast cancer care. This chapter reviews the MRI breast technique and its interpretation, various indications, MRI guided procedures, and its limitations.

R. Renganathan (✉) · S. Prema
Division of Breast and Women's Imaging, Department of Diagnostic and Interventional Radiology, Kovai Medical Center and Hospitals, Coimbatore, India
e-mail: drrupa@kmchhospitals.com

S. Kushvaha
Department of Radiology, Artemis Hospital, Gurgaon, India

Keywords

MRI breast · Sequences · Screening · Local staging · Enhancement · Implant integrity

11.1 Introduction

Ever since the first MRI breast was performed in Germany in 1986, the technology underwent rapid developments as it offered the advantage of providing functional information in addition to the morphological information to characterize the abnormality. The aim was to achieve images of both the breasts simultaneously as fast as possible without compromising on the spatial resolution. The continuous efforts have made it possible to perform ultrafast MRI acquiring isotropic 3D volumetric data sets. In clinical practice, it is often used as a problem-solving tool whenever the results of the conventional modalities are confounding. It offers several advantages over ultrasound and mammography of providing multiplanar information, functional information of the tumor, the accurate extent, and stage of the disease. It has the highest sensitivity of detecting cancers and is therefore recommended by both national comprehensive cancer network (NCCN) and American Cancer Society (ACS) as a screening tool for women who carry more than 20% lifetime risk of developing breast cancer [1, 2].

B. Dev, L. D. Joseph (eds.), *Holistic Approach to Breast Disease*,
https://doi.org/10.1007/978-981-99-0035-0_11

11.2 Technique

11.2.1 Basic Principles

The aim is to image the entire bilateral breasts simultaneously at least once within the first 2 min as the contrast flows through the blood circulation. This is because most breast cancers enhance in the first 2 min of contrast injection and the differentiation between the cancers and the normal parenchymal tissue is maximum in this time period. To achieve this, sequences with high temporal and spatial resolution are used for performing MRI Breast. This has been made possible with the advent of multichannel breast coils and parallel imaging methods such that near-isotropic volumetric acquisitions of both the breasts can be acquired within few seconds.

High spatial resolution is important as it helps one to delineate the morphology and margins of the lesion that decides the ultimate BI-RADS assessment category even if the kinetics of the lesion favor benign etiology.

11.2.2 Positioning

As for any MRI exam, triplanar scout views using body coil are obtained to ascertain the proper positioning and the adequate coverage of anatomical area of interest, in this case being both breasts, axilla, and supraclavicular fossa. Patient lies in prone position with the breasts positioned within the dedicated breast coil. Proper positioning is important to achieve homogeneous fat suppression, avoid artifacts resulting from skin folds, and to avoid missing cancers. Position is adequate if both breasts are centered with the nipple in profile. Nipple should not be pressing against the coil surface. This usually happens in case of large breasts. Help of cushions to push the patient chest off the coil may help in cases of large breasts. Arms are usually kept overhead as this is more comfortable position and avoids wrap around artifacts. However, in small built patients with small breasts, arms may be kept on sides to reduce the concavity of the breast tissue and to bring more tissue inside the coil.

11.2.3 Aquisition Planes

Images may be acquired in axial, coronal, or sagittal plane. The phase encoding direction is kept left to right or superior to inferior for axial and coronal planes, respectively, to avoid ghost artifacts from normal aortic/heart pulsations. These planes are preferred as these allow simultaneous viewing of both breasts. The near-3D postcontrast iso-volumetric acquisitions allow visualization of the images in any plane. The protocol varies with the institution and is usually performed in axial plane. However, ACR recommends obtaining both sagittal and axial images whenever MRI is being performed for evaluating implant integrity [3]. Recommended MRI parameters and sequences by the ACR committee are mentioned in Table 11.1 [3].

Table 11.1 MRI Breast protocol for performing breast MRI as per ACR recommendations

Sequence	Significance	
1. Scout images using body coil	Acts as localizer, assess for adequacy of breast position and the anatomical coverage	
2. T2w images: axial or coronal planes	Depicts edema better, lesions bright on T2w images are most often benign	
3. T1w images	Tells about the composition of breast, the morphology of the lesion	
4. Precontrast fat sat. T1w sequence	Acts as the baseline image for further subtraction and kinetic assessment Depicts high-intensity fluid, especially the biopsy changes and blood-filled ducts better	Slice thickness ≤3 mm Interslice gap: 0 mm In-plane spatial resolution: ≤1 mm
5. Minimum of two postcontrast T1w sequences	Required for kinetic assessment Two phases: Early within 2 min post contrast injection. Late phase—After 2 min post injection	

11.2.4 Diffusion Weighted Imaging

Diffusion-weighted imaging (DWI) is a rapid magnetic resonance (MR) imaging technique that measures the random movement of water molecules in tissues. The movement of water molecules is inversely related to tissue cellularity and integrity of cell membranes as well as the signal intensity in diffusion-weighted imaging. In breast, DWI along with dynamic contrast-enhanced MRI can improve the specificity in differentiating benign and malignant lesions [4], differentiate in situ from invasive disease [5], and can assess early response of cancers treated with neoadjuvant chemotherapy [5].

DWI is incorporated into standard breast imaging protocol in many of the centers but still not incorporated into the MRI Breast Imaging Reporting And Data System (BI-RADS). In order to overcome these limitations, in 2019, the European Society of Breast Radiology (EUSOBI) released a consensus statement to standardize DW MRI image acquisition and interpretation [6]. Table 11.2 shows the minimum requirements in acquisition parameters suggested by EUSOBI DWI working group [6].

Normal breast parenchyma will be hyperintense in low b value images and gets suppressed in high b value images. The reported mean Apparenr diffusion coefficient (ADC) of normal breast tissue varies over a wide range from 1.51×10^{-3} to 2.09×10^{-3} mm^2/s [5].

The lesions, which show high signal on high b value images, should be correlated with ADC maps. The lesions with true restricted diffusion exhibit low ADC values.

Cancers have increased cell density, resulting in restricted water diffusion, which leads to higher signal intensity at DWI and low ADC values. The previously reported ADC cutoff values to distinguish between benign and malignant lesions ranged from 1.1 × 10–3 to 1.6 × 10–3 mm^2/s [5].

The following lesions might be false negative on DWI: mucinous carcinoma (because of high mucin content and low cellularity), triple-negative cancers with extensive necrosis, ductal carcinoma in situ, invasive lobular carcinoma, and small cancers [5].

False-positive findings on breast DW MRI include mastitis, abscesses, hematomas, complicated cysts, intramammary lymph nodes, atypical ductal hyperplasia, intraductal papilloma, and fibroadenomas with high cellularity [5].

Table 11.2 Minimum requirements in acquisition parameters suggested by EUSOBI DWI working group [6]

Acquisition parameter	Minimum requirement	Specific remarks if any
Type of sequence	EPI based	
Orientation	Axial	
Field of view	The field of view should cover both breasts	Covering the axillary region is not mandatory
In-plane resolution	$\leq 2 \times 2$ mm^2	Acquired physical resolution, before reconstruction, and reconstructed resolution
Slice thickness	≤ 4 mm	
Number of *b* values	2	More is optional
Lowest *b* value	0 s/mm^2	In practice as close to 0 as possible, but not exceeding 50 s/mm^2
High *b* value	800 s/mm^2	
Fat saturation	Required	SPAIR is recommended
TE	Minimum possible by the system and choice of parameters	Optimize the rBW to obtain minimum TE. The reduction in SNR by increasing the rBW is usually compensated for by the shortening of TE
TR	≥ 3000 ms	
Acceleration	Parallel imaging (factor ≥ 2)	Reduces distortion, loss in SNR can be counterbalanced by increasing the number of excitations
Post-processing	Generation of ADC maps is required	Standard ADC is calculated as ADC = ln $(S_{low}/S_{high})/(b_{high} - b_{low})$ where $S_{low,high}$ are the image signal values obtained with b values $b_{low,high}$

11.2.5 Ultrafast and Abbrevtaed MRI

The groundbreaking study by Kuhl et al. [7] on the feasibility of abbreviated breast MRI showed that both the image acquisition and interpretation time could be significantly reduced without compromising the diagnostic accuracy. It consisted of a fat-saturated T1-weighted precontrast and early postcontrast with subtraction and MIP sequence. The later studies also added T2-weighted or STIR sequences, which did not influence the diagnostic accuracy but were helpful in increasing the specificity and decision to biopsy [8]. The omission of delayed postcontrast images limited the kinetic analysis. This limitation is now overcome by incorporating ultrafast imaging techniques into the abbreviated breast MRI protocols [9].

The techniques used in ultrafast sequences despite short acquisition time would still maintain high spatial resolution by using the concept of view sharing and undersampling the periphery of the k-space in addition to using parallel imaging techniques [9].

The protocol proposed by Mann et al. [10] used time-resolved angiography by view sharing and k-space undersampling. Using TWIST acquisitions, the slopes obtained allowed differentiation between benign and malignant lesions with higher accuracy with a sensitivity of 90% and specificity of 67%. Mus et al. used similar ultrafast sequences and evaluated time to enhancement (TTE) to differentiate between benign and malignant lesions with a cutoff value of 12.96 s.

The ultrafast technique using time-resolved MRI has a disadvantage of temporal blurring and inability to reconstruct in other planes. This was largely overcome by parallel imaging methods like sensitivity encoding (SENSE) and array coil spatial sensitivity encoding (ASSET).

The recently published EA1141 trial, which compared abbreviated breast MRI and DBT in screening women with dense breasts, showed that the invasive cancer detection rate of abbreviated MRI was more than twice that of DBT (11.8 per 1000 compared to 4.8 per 1000) [11].

11.3 Lesion Detection and Charecterisation

Standardized lexicons and reporting format from American College of Radiology Breast Imaging Reporting and Data System (BI-RADS) is used for reporting of breast MRI [12]. Table 11.3 shows the summary of reporting format with standard terminologies for reporting.

A standard report contains clinical indication for the scan, availability of any relevant previous studies, technical details including the sequences and amount of contrast media. Further, breast composition and amount of background parenchymal enhancement are assessed. For both the measures, higher degree is associated with higher risk of breast cancer [13]. Also, a higher amount of background parenchymal enhancement makes the interpretation difficult and is associated with a higher number of false-positive findings [14]. Multiparametric MR imaging features of a biopsy-proven left breast carcinoma are shown in Fig. 11.1.

Abnormal enhancement is identified as enhancement of higher density compared to the normal BPE on a contrast-enhanced scan. Three types of abnormal enhancement include focus, mass, and nonmass enhancement.

(a) **Focus**: A focus is a small dot of enhancement that cannot be otherwise categorized. In general, a focus is considered when the enhancing dot is less than 5 mm in size. However, when an enhancing focus irrespective of the size has an irregular shape and noncircumscribed margins, it should be termed as a mass irrespective of the size.
(b) **Mass**: A mass is a space-occupying lesion with convex outer margins. Further characterization of masses is on the basis of shape, margins, and internal enhancement pattern.

Typical malignant masses have irregular shape and margins, heterogeneous or rim enhancement pattern and show washout on dynamic postcontrast images [15]. Nonenhancing septations within a fibroadenoma will appear as dark septations in postcontrast images.

Table 11.3 Summary of reporting format with standard terminologies for reporting MRI breast according to ACR BI-RADS (1)

1. Clinical indication			
2. Technique—breast MRI sequences and postprocessing techniques, amount of contrast media			
3. Findings—descriptors			
Sequence	Descriptor	Terminologies	
T1 precontrast	Amount of fibro-glandular tissue	Almost entirely fatty; scattered; heterogeneous; extreme	
T1 90 s postcontrast SUB	Background parenchymal enhancement	Minimal; mild; moderate; marked Symmetric; asymmetric	
	Lesion	Focus; mass; nonmass enhancement	
	Focus	Focus: <5 mm of enhancement, too small to characterize	
	Mass	Shape	Round; oval; irregular
		Margin	Circumscribed; irregular; spiculated
		Internal enhancement pattern	Homogeneous; heterogeneous; rim; dark internal septations
	Nonmass enhancement	Distribution	Focal; linear; segmental; regional; multiple regions; diffuse
		Internal enhancement pattern	Homogeneous; heterogeneous; clumped; clustered ring
T1 dynamic	Kinetic curve assessment	Initial enhancement (percentage of peak signal intensity achieved at 90 s)	Slow, <50%; medium 50–100%; fast >100%
		Delayed enhancement (relative enhancement compared with peak)	Persistent >10% increase; plateau—>10% increase to >10% decrease; washout >10% decrease
T2	Signal intensity of the lesion	High; intermediate and low	
	Edema	Absent; peri-lesional; prepectoral; diffuse	
DWI	ADC (mm^3/s)	Very low, <0.9; low, 0.9–1.3; intermediate, 1.3–1.7; high, 1.7–2.1; very high, >2.1	
Nonenhancing findings: Ductal precontrast high signal, cyst, postoperative collections, posttherapy changes, nonenhancing mass, architectural distortion, signal void from clips, foreign bodies			
Associated features: Nipple retraction, nipple invasion, skin retraction, skin thickening, skin invasion, pectoralis muscle invasion, chest wall invasion, architectural distortion, axillary adenopathy			
T1 with and without FS	Fat-containing lesions	Lymph-nodes, fat necrosis, hamartoma, postoperative seroma/hematoma with fat	
4. Comparison to previous examinations			
5. Assessment			
6. Management			

(c) **Nonmass Enhancement (NME)**

Nonmass enhancement is an enhancing area that does not have convex margins and is neither a mass nor a focus. Descriptors for nonmass enhancement are distribution and internal enhancement pattern. Linear and segmental distributions of nonmass enhancement are suspicious findings, because they represent enhancement in a single duct and enhancement along a duct and its branches [16]. Among the internal enhancement patterns of non-mass enhancement, clumped and clustered ring types are suspicious [16, 17].

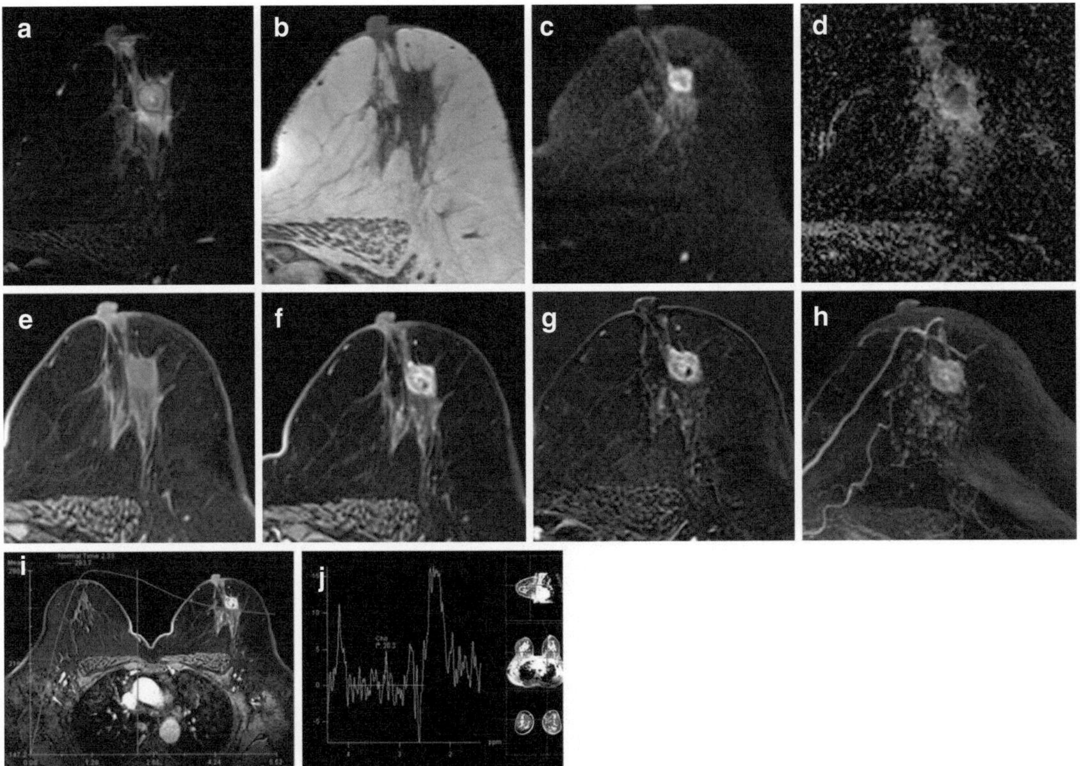

Fig. 11.1 (**a**–**j**) Multiparametric MR imaging of a patient with biopsy-proven left breast carcinoma. (**a**) T2 IR image shows an intermediate signal intensity lesion with perilesional edema. (**b**) T1 image shows that the lesion is isointense. (**c**, **d**) The lesion is hyperintense on B800 DWI images and hypointense on ADC, suggesting true restricted diffusion. (**e**–**h**) Precontrast T1 FS(E), early postcontrast T1FS(F), subtraction(G), and MIP(H) images demonstrate heterogeneous enhancement of the lesion. (**i**) Time intensity curve of the lesion demonstrates early and rapid enhancement of the lesion with washout in delayed phase. (**j**) MR single voxel spectroscopy shows choline peak within the lesion

Early and fast enhancement and washout of the lesion in dynamic contrast study suggests that the lesion is suspicious. Although findings from DWI are not included in the BI-RADS descriptors, incorporation of DWI findings improves the specificity in differentiating benign and malignant lesions.

11.4 Clinical Applications

11.4.1 Screening

Breast cancer screening recommendations are based on the individual's risk of developing breast cancer. Risk stratification of women for breast cancer is done by various risk prediction models considering the presence or absence of risk factors such as germ-line mutations, family history, and personal risk factors. Among the risk prediction models the most comprehensive one is The Tyrer-Cuzick (International Breast Cancer Intervention Study, or IBIS) model. Women are stratified into high-risk group (>20% lifetime risk of breast cancer), intermediate-risk group (15–20% lifetime risk of breast cancer), and average risk group (<15% lifetime risk of breast cancer).

MRI is recommended as a supplemental screening tool in high-risk groups by various national and international guidelines because of its highest sensitivity in cancer detection and high negative predictive value.

Screening of intermediate risk women: Intermediate-risk group includes women with 15–20% lifetime risk of breast cancer, personal history of breast cancer, dense breasts at mammography, or history of high-risk lesions at biopsy (atypical ductal hyperplasia, atypical lobular hyperplasia, or lobular carcinoma in situ). According to ACR recommendations, among the intermediate-risk group women, MRI is recommended for screening in women with personal history of breast cancer and dense breast tissue or those diagnosed before 50 years of age or personal history of high-risk lesions especially if other risk factors are present [2].

Screening of high-risk women: Women with a more than 20% lifetime risk of breast cancer, women with germ-line mutations and their untested first-degree relatives are categorized as high risk by the American Cancer Society and the American College of Radiology [2]. Annual screening MRI and mammography are recommended in this group of women. The high-risk group includes various germ-line mutations (e.g., *BRCA1*, *BRCA2*, *PALPB2*, *TP53*, *PTEN*, *CHECK2*, *CDH1*, *ATM*, and *STK11*). Annual screening MRI is also recommended for women who have undergone chest irradiation before the age of 30 years. In high-risk women, combined mammography and MRI have a greater sensitivity than mammography and ultrasound [18]. Studies have shown that in high-risk women younger than 40 years of age, there is no incremental cancer detection by mammography if a concurrent MRI is also performed [19]. Based on this evidence, it is important to reconsider mammograms when MRI is performed particularly in BRCA mutation carriers who are susceptible to the effects of radiation.

Age of screening in high-risk women: For women who are at high risk due to germ-line mutations, annual screening mammography and MRI are recommended beginning 10 years earlier than the affected relative at the time of diagnosis but not before 30 years of age [20]. MRI alone is recommended for screening for this group of women between 25 and 30 years of age. For BRCA mutation carriers, consideration of delaying mammogram until 40 years of age is recommended [20].

For women who are at high risk because of prior chest irradiation between the ages of 10 and 30, annual MRI and mammography for breast cancer screening is recommended starting 8 years after radiation therapy but not before 25 years of age [20].

11.4.2 Local Staging

The usefulness of breast MRI in local staging remains controversial as there is no strong evidence in the literature supporting detection of additional disease translating into improved outcomes.

There are various guidelines describing the indications for breast MRI in women with a new diagnosis of breast cancer and they vary widely in their recommendations. The indications for MRI breast in local staging according to various guidelines are summarized in Table 11.4 [1, 21–24].

Most studies conclude that tumor size estimation with MRI is more reliable than clinical examination, mammography, and USG. MRI is more accurate in assessing the size of the invasive lobular carcinomas, DCIS components related to invasive cancers as shown in Fig. 11.2, and pure DCIS lesions particularly high-grade lesions [4]. However, small DCIS lesions detected as mammographic calcifications may be occult at

Table 11.4 Indications for breast MRI in local staging

Indications for breast MRI—local staging
1. Invasive lobular carcinoma
2. Discrepancy in tumor size (>1 cm) in different modalities (including clinical examination)
3. High-risk women
4. Eligibility for partial breast irradiation
5. Post lumpectomy with positive margins
6. Extremely dense breast parenchyma

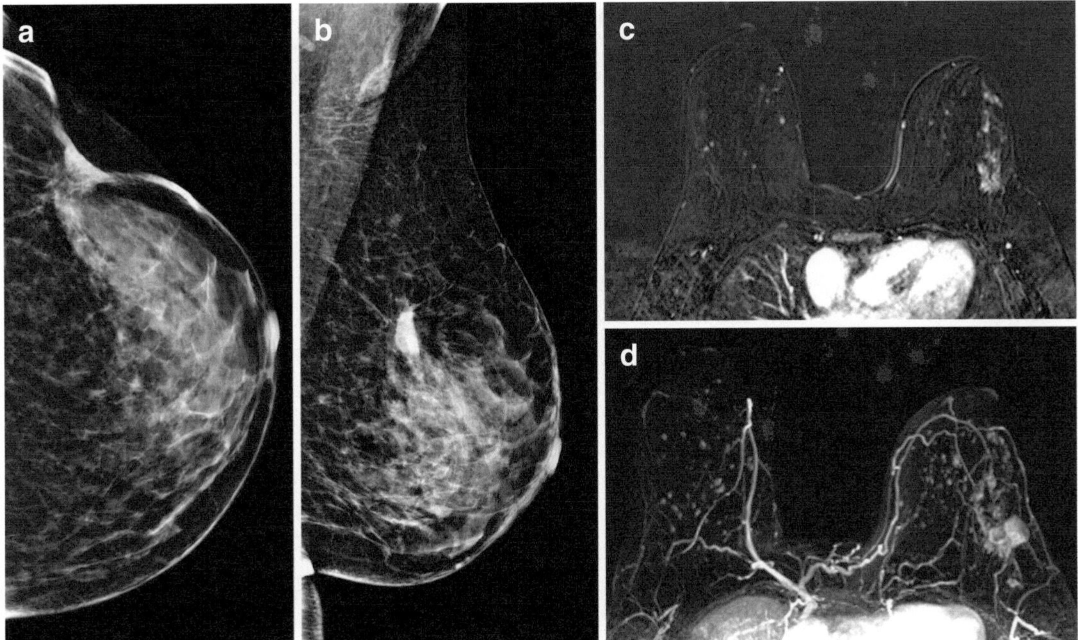

Fig. 11.2 (**a**–**d**) 58-year-old lady with left breast lump. CC and MLO image of left breast (**a**, **b**) shows extremely dense fibroglandular parenchyma and an irregular lesion with spiculated margins in upper outer quadrant of left breast with focal skin infiltration. On biopsy, it was infiltrating ductal carcinoma. Early postcontrast subtraction (**c**) and MIP (**d**) MR images show in addition to the index lesion, there is a clumped nonmass enhancement in segmental distribution anterior and inferior to the index lesion. On HPE, the nonmass enhancement was proven to be DCIS

MRI. MRI can assess the status of axillary, internal mammary and supraclavicular nodes, skin and chest wall involvement and also screen the contralateral breast. In patients with known breast cancer, MRI identifies occult contralateral cancer in 2–4% of patients (Fig. 11.3) [4].

Given the higher sensitivity of MRI, detection of mammographically occult lesions in the affected/contralateral breast is common. A meta-analysis of 50 studies [25] found that MRI detected additional disease in the same breast in 20% of women. Two-thirds (67%) of additional findings were malignant. Additional disease that impacts treatment is detected in 20% of patients out of which one-third of the conversion to mastectomy decisions were inappropriate. This highlights the importance of pathological confirmation of additional findings that impact the surgical procedure prior to treatment.

The additional lesions that need biopsy can be addressed by MR directed USG where USG identifies 57% of lesions and USG guided biopsy can be done for pathologic confirmation [26]. The findings which do not have an ultrasound correlate should be biopsied using MR guidance.

Though it is established that MRI is most sensitive in detecting additional disease, whether it translates into improvement in clinical outcome in the form of reduced re-operation rates or reduced local recurrences remains a controversy.

First randomised control trial on the breast MRI was Comparative effectiveness of MRI in Breast Cancer (COMICE) [27]. The results revealed similar reoperation rates in the groups with and without preoperative MRI.

Preoperative MRI in Breast cancer (POMB) [28] and MIPA [29] trials showed a significant reduction in re-excision rates in the MRI group (5% and 8% respectively) compared to no MRI group (15% and 14.8% respectively).

These controversial results illustrate the importance of effective utilization of informa-

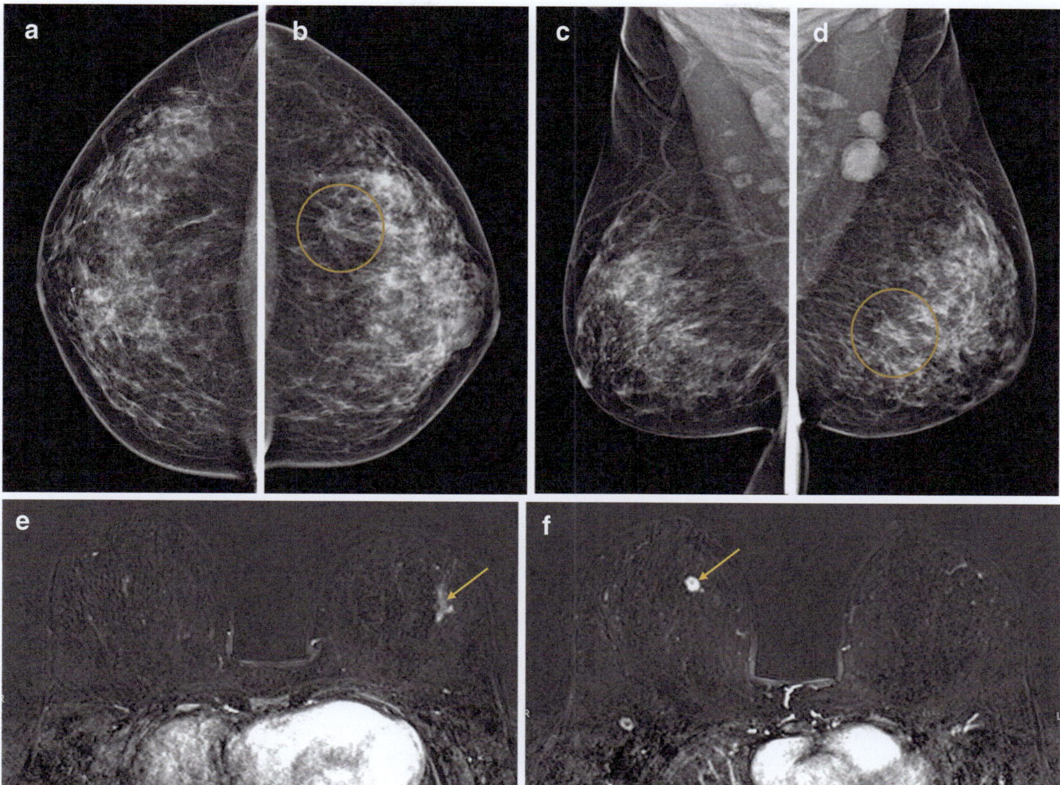

Fig. 11.3 (**a–f**) 55-year-old lady presented with left axillary lump. Mammogram of both breasts in CC and MLO views (**a–d**) shows focal asymmetry with architectural distortion in lower outer quadrant of posterior third in left breast (yellow circles) with suspicious left axillary lymphnodes. Right breast was unremarkable. Biopsy from left breast lesion was suggestive of invasive lobular carcinoma. Preoperative MRI was done for the screening of contralateral breast and to evaluate the extent of abnormality. Early postcontrast subtraction images (**e**, **f**) show heterogeneously enhancing lesion in lower outer quadrant of left breast, which was a biopsy-proven lobular carcinoma (yellow arrow in **e**) and an intensely enhancing lesion in inner central quadrant of right breast (yellow arrow in **f**). The right breast lesion was identified in second-look USG and biopsy revealed invasive lobular carcinoma

tion offered by MRI and MRI guidance in surgical planning. Effective utilization of MR offered information can be done by discussing the information in a multidisciplinary team, MR guided localization, or MRI-guided bracketing of the extent of larger tumor or DCIS.

11.4.3 Assessing Response to Neoadjuvant Chemotherapy

As the neoadjuvant chemotherapy offers several advantages over the adjuvant setting and is being offered for not only the locally advanced breast cancers but in early cancers also, it becomes imperative to assess the response to identify a nonresponder early avoiding expensive therapy and its side effects [30, 31]. Even in a patient who has responded well, imaging may play an important role in future by identifying a complete pathological response (pCR) with higher accuracy in assessing the in vivo response to chemotherapeutic drugs.

Clinical assessment of the response is subjective and is confounded by various factors like skin thickening and edema. Accurate assessment is done by comparing the pre- and posttherapy imaging and the choice of imaging modality depends on the availability of resources and the institutional protocol. ACR recommends obtaining a pretreat-

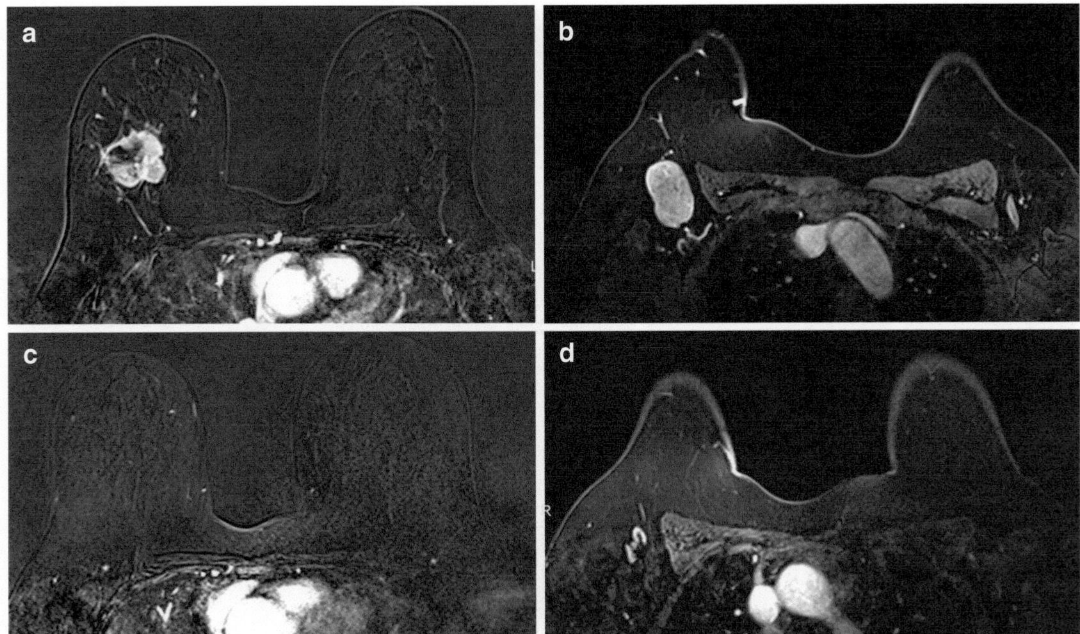

Fig. 11.4 (**a**–**d**) Postcontrast subtraction prechemotherapy (**a**) and postchemotherapy (**c**) MR images of breast showing complete resolution of irregular heterogeneously enhancing lesion in right breast (biopsy proven carcinoma, ER−, PR−, Her2−, Ki-67—62%) after chemotherapy. Postcontrast T1 FS images before (**b**) and after (**d**) chemotherapy showing complete resolution of right axillary lymph-node after chemotherapy. Findings are consistent with complete response

ment MRI owing to its highest accuracy compared to other conventional modalities, namely, ultrasound and mammography [32]. While NCCN guidelines recommend clinical breast examination and performance of imaging studies that were abnormal at the time of diagnosis [33].

Accuracy of MRI is also determined by the tumor histology and molecular subtype with the radiological complete response (rCR) being correlated well with pCR in triple-negative and her2-neu-positive tumors, while it does not correlate well in case of hormone-positive tumors [34].

MRI should be performed utilizing the same parameters and protocol every time. To identify early nonresponders, MRI is done after first 2 cycles of chemotherapy. Post NACT MRI is done prior to surgery.

Both the primary tumor, nodal disease, and the ancillary findings like skin thickening and edema are assessed. Both qualitative and quantitative parameters are assessed. Presence or absence of enhancement in early phase at the site of previous disease. Pattern of tumor response that may be categorized as concentric shrinkage in size, fragmented or stippled response, or nonmass enhancement [35]. Tumor size is assessed and compared as per the RECIST 1.1 guidelines [36]. Other measurable parameters can also be derived from multiparametric MRI study and compared. These include various perfusion parameters, ADC values on diffusion-weighted imaging, and the choline peak on proton spectroscopy. All these variables need validation from large studies for their routine application.

Although there are no standard guidelines about assessing the treatment response in breast cancer, it can be done as per the RECIST criteria [36]. The response is classified as complete response if no residual tumor is seen at the primary site with no new lesions (Fig. 11.4). Partial response, when there is reduction of >30% (Fig. 11.5), progressive disease when there are new lesions or if there is increase by >10%, stable disease if the criteria do not match for progressive disease or partial response.

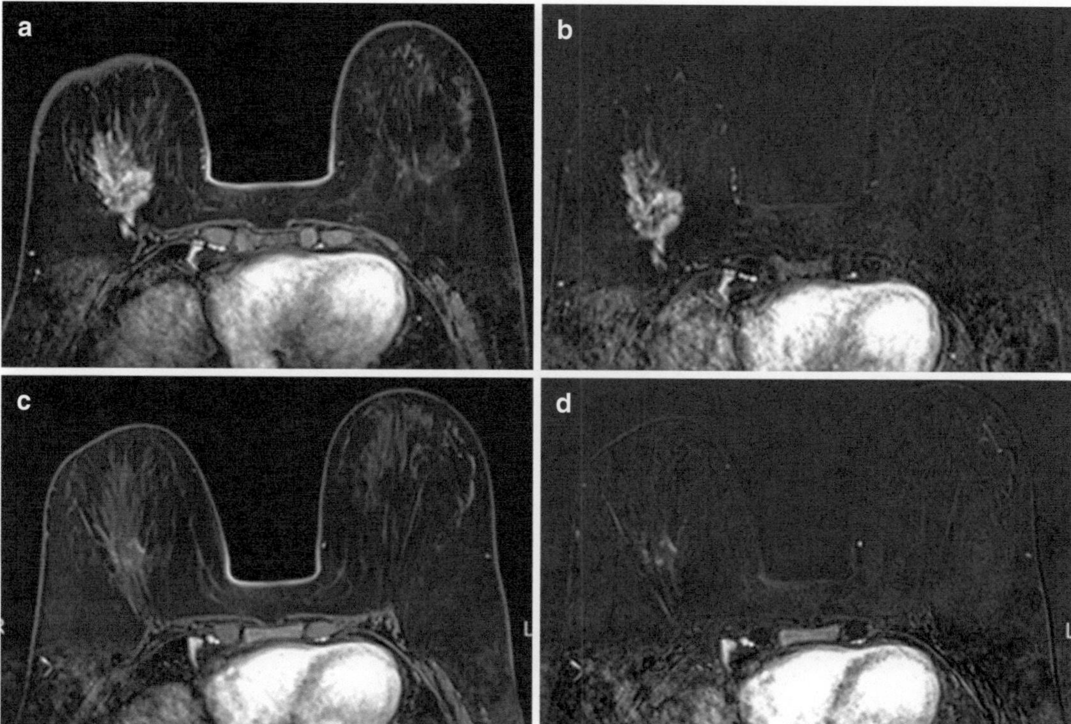

Fig. 11.5 (**a–d**) Prechemotherapy postcontrast T1 FS (**a**) and postcontrast subtraction (**b**) MR images show irregular heterogeneously enhancing lesion in right breast (biopsy-proven carcinoma, ER +, PR +, Her 2−, Ki-67: 23%). Post contrast T1 FS (**c**) and postcontrast subtraction (**d**) MR images after neoadjuvant chemotherapy shows marked reduction in size of the lesion in right breast with residual enhancement—suggestive of partial response. Partial response was confirmed on histopathology

In summary, MRI carries the highest accuracy among the imaging modalities of USG, DM, DBT for primary tumor response assessment; however, it should be borne in mind that it is still less accurate than the pathological examination. This paves way to future research for developing newer techniques and tools with 100% sensitivity and specificity when the breast surgery may be omitted in patients who achieve pCR.

11.4.4 Problem Solving

11.4.4.1 Carcinoma of Unknown Primary

When a patient presents with unilateral metastatic axillary adenopathy with a suspicion of breast primary and negative mammogram and ultrasound, modified radical mastectomy is the accepted treatment. MRI detects up to 70% of breast primary lesions, which are occult on conventional imaging modalities and facilitate breast conservation surgery as shown in Fig. 11.6 [37]. When MRI is negative in this setting, it has a high negative predictive value, and it is safe to treat the breast with radiation therapy, avoiding unnecessary mastectomies [38].

11.4.4.2 Equivocal Findings in Mammogram

MRI is helpful in further evaluating single view asymmetries and equivocal findings in tomosynthesis. When there is absence of enhancement on MRI, a biopsy can be assertively avoided as it has a high negative predictive value.

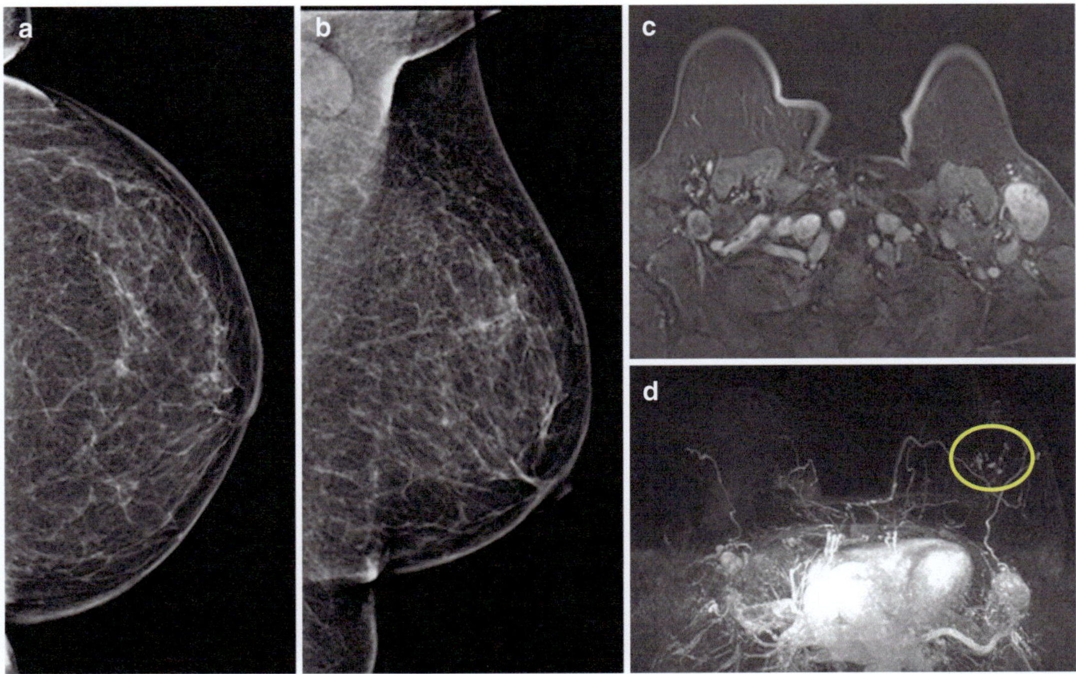

Fig. 11.6 (**a**–**d**) Mammogram of left breast in CC and MLO view (**a**, **b**) of a 50-year-old lady with left axillary lump: The left breast was unremarkable, and a suspicious left axillary lymph-node was noted. Biopsy from the node—metastatic carcinoma with probable primary from the breast. She was further evaluated with MRI. Postcontrast FS T1 MR image (**c**) showing an enlarged heterogeneously enhancing left axillary lymph-node. Early postcontrast subtraction MIP image (**d**) showing abnormal nonmass enhancement in focal distribution (yellow circle) in left breast

11.4.4.3 Pathological Nipple Discharge

If a patient presents with pathological nipple discharge, mammogram and ultrasonography are the initial modalities of evaluation. When these are negative or ultrasound could not pick up an intraductal lesion due to intraductal debris, MRI is the investigation of choice as it has high spatial resolution, high sensitivity, and high negative predictive value. MRI is more sensitive in picking up peripherally located intraductal lesions, which is helpful in planning microdochectomies as shown in Fig. 11.7. When MRI is negative in this setting, the patients can be safely followed up instead of subjecting them to surgery [39].

11.4.5 Evaluation of Breast Implants

MRI is the gold standard to detect the silicone implant ruptures especially the intracapsular ones that are often asymptomatic [40, 41]. Saline

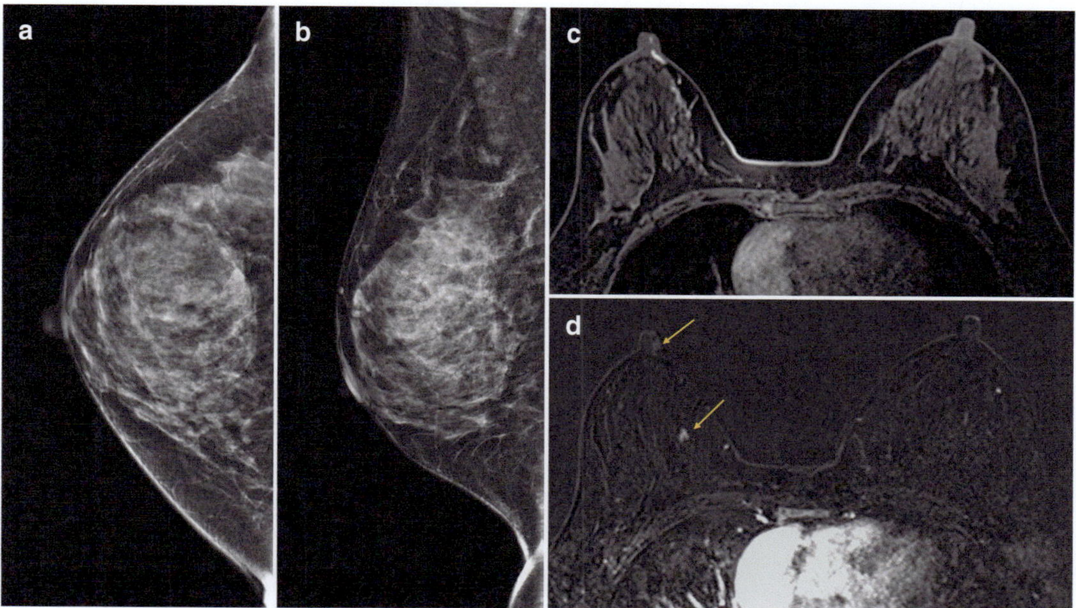

Fig. 11.7 (**a**–**d**) Right CC and MLO (**a**, **b**) images of a 44–year-old lady with right pathological nipple discharge. Mammogram was unremarkable and a supplementary USG revealed solitary dilated duct with internal debris at 3 o'clock position of right breast. She was further evaluated with MRI. T1 FS precontrast (**c**) MR image shows solitary dilated duct with hyperintense contents in inner central quadrant of right breast. Postcontrast subtraction (**d**) MR image shows two enhancing intraductal lesions (marked by yellow arrows) in inner central quadrant of right breast. On pathology, these lesions were proven to be benign intraductal papillomas

implant ruptures are easily diagnosed by the clinician and the patient herself. Mammography is diagnostic in these cases, and MRI is rarely required. An implant can be seen in either retroglandular or retropectoral location (Fig. 11.8). Silicone selective sequences are used to distinguish silicone from other water- or saline-containing structures as in double lumen implants. The pictorial diagram in Fig. 11.9 depicts the various signs of intracapsular rupture and Table 11.5 lists the various probable and definite signs. Another increasingly recognized late implant complication is breast-implant-associated anaplastic large cell lymphoma (BIA-ALCL) for which MRI is being used for staging purposes [42]. Various MRI findings that one may see include peri-implant fluid with enhancement, focal mass, and enlarged axillary lymph nodes [43]. Unlike other lymphomas where chemotherapy is the treatment of choice, breast implant removal with surgery is the treatment of choice for BIA-ALCL [44]. Other late complications that rarely need MRI include capsular retraction and herniation producing contour deformity, silicone gel bleed referring to microscopic silicone leakage with an intact implant shell [45].

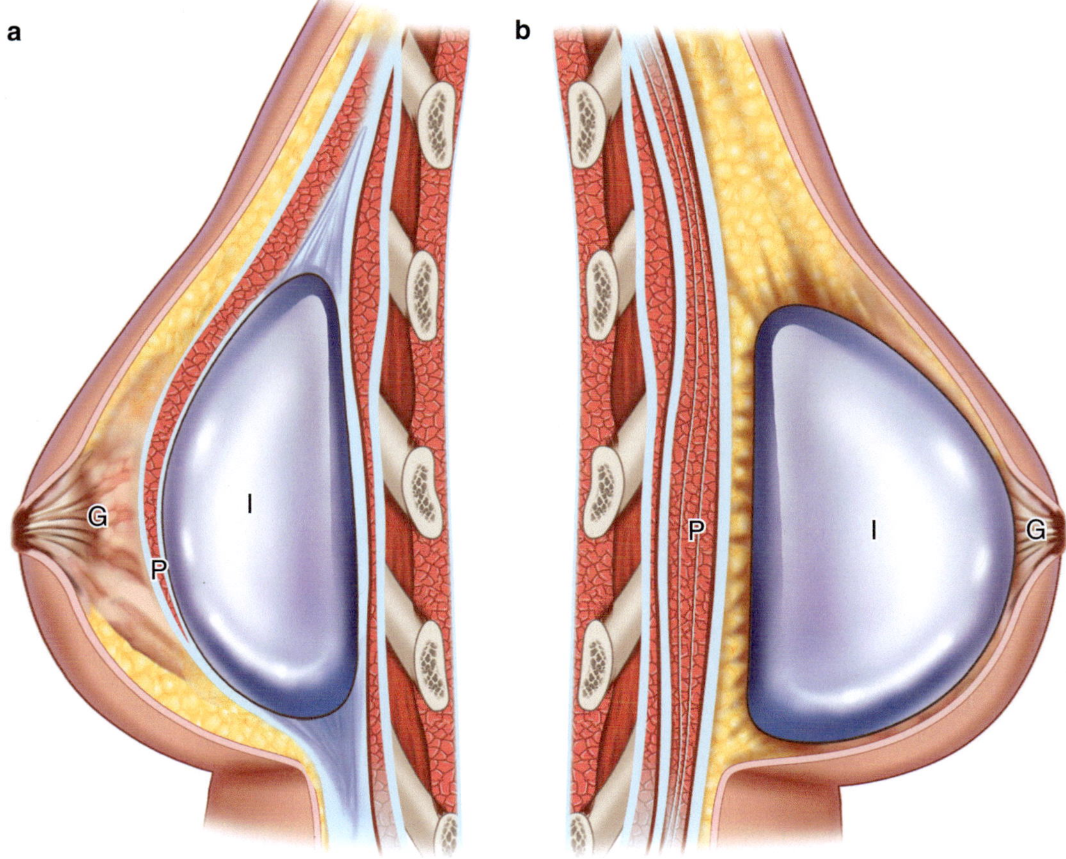

Fig. 11.8 Pictorial diagram depicting sagittal sections through breasts depicting Implants (I) in (**a**) retropectoral location beneath the pectoral muscle (p) and in (**b**) subglandular location beneath the glandular parenchyma (g)

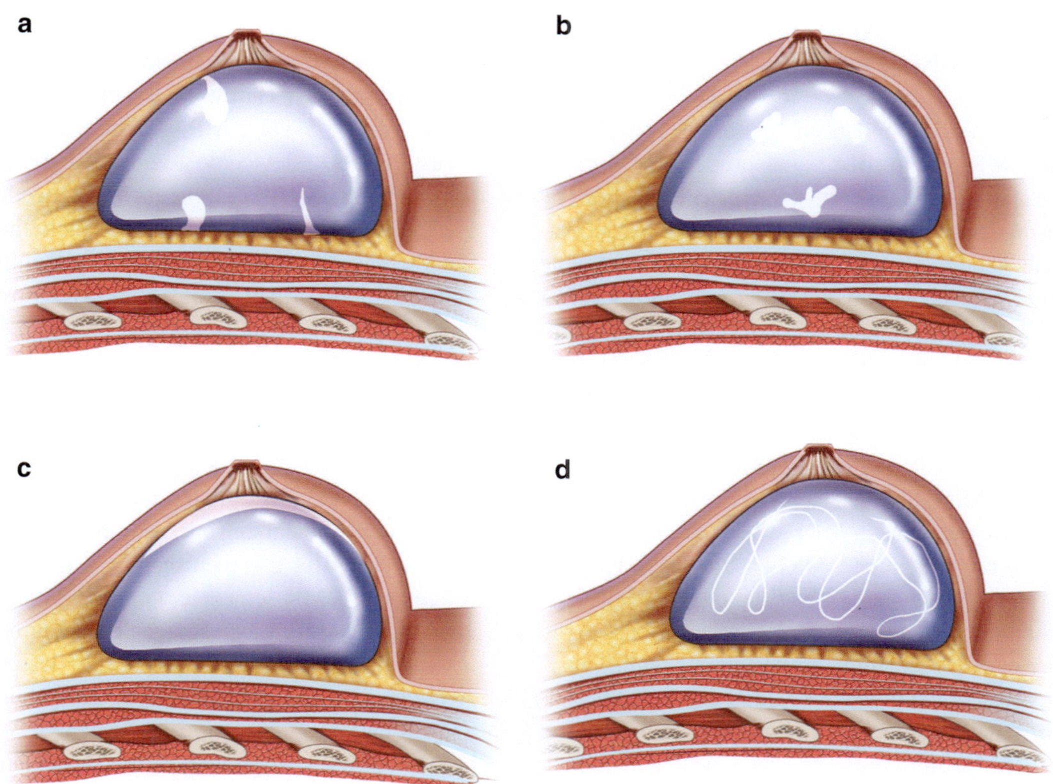

Fig. 11.9 Pictorial diagram depicting axial sections through breasts depicting different signs suggesting intracapsular rupture. (**a**) Tear drop/Noose sign and keyhole sign. (**b**) Salad oil sign. (**c**) Subcapsular lines. (**d**) Linguine sign

Table 11.5 Various MRI signs indicating intracapsular rupture of a silicone implant

Signs of intracapsular implant rupture	
Probable signs	Contour deformity Irregular margins Salad oil sign or the droplet sign Tear drop/noose/keyhole sign
Definite signs	Subcapsular lines Tram track sign Linguine sign Silicone outside the implant

11.5 Contrast Mammogrpahy VS MRI of Breast

Both contrast-enhanced mammography(CEM) and MRI exploit the same property of tumors, i.e., neo-angiogenesis, for cancer detection by using intravascular contrast agents. Contrast-enhanced mammography is emerging as a viable alternative to MRI with similar indications as that of MRI. According to previous studies, as a supplemental screening tool, CEM and MRI have similar incremental cancer detection rates of 13.1/1000 and 11.8–16.5/1000, respectively [46]. Positive predictive value of CEM (97%) is superior to MRI (85%) because of the higher number of false positives in MRI [47].

In our experience, MRI is superior to CEM in evaluating patients with pathological nipple discharge where mammography and ultrasonography are negative and clinical suspicion is high. This is because of the higher resolution of MRI in detecting small intraductal lesions such as papillomas.

The lesions close to chest wall and medial breast are difficult to image using CEM whereas they are not difficult imaging with MRI. Also, MRI provides complete nodal staging, whereas supplementary USG is needed for nodal staging when using CEM.

11.6 MRI-Guided Interventions

MR-guided interventions in breast include MRI-guided biopsy and MRI-guided wire localizations.

Indications: Lesions that are primarily detected and characterized as suspicious on contrast-enhanced MRI. The first step before considering MRI-guided intervention is reviewing the latest mammogram and performing a second-look USG to look for correlate in these modalities because it is easier to perform stereotactic or USG-guided biopsy when compared to MR-guided biopsy. According to previous studies, sonographic correlates were identifiable in up to 56% of lesions, which are primarily identified by CEMRI [48]. For the suspicious abnormalities that do not have mammographic or USG correlate, MRI-guided biopsy should be considered.

MR-guided biopsy: Hardware required for the procedure is 1.5 T/3 T MR system, dedicated breast coil, grid device/post and pillar device for compression of breast parenchyma, needle guide with fiducial, introducer set including sheath, introducer and obturator, vacuum-assisted biopsy device, and 7–11 G biopsy gun.

Procedure (Fig. 11.10): Informed consent is obtained. Patient is placed in prone position. Grid device is used to immobilize the breast with target lesion. Commonly used approaches are lateral and medial approaches. Needle guide with fiducial having gadolinium contrast is placed at C4 position of the grid for reference. T1 MR sequence with and without contrast and subtraction images are acquired in sagittal plane to localize the lesion. According to the available literature, about 8–13% of MR-guided biopsies are cancelled because of nonvisualization of the lesion during the procedure after compression [49, 50]. After visualizing the lesion, three reference points are marked, namely, the fiducial, skin surface, and the target lesion. Software automatically calculates the lesion coordinates and provides information about the site and way of placement of needle guide and depth of entry. After skin preparation and placing the obturator at the specified depth, check scan is taken. After confirming the position, vacuum-assisted biopsy is performed and a marker is always placed at the biopsy site. Immediately after the procedure, the incision site is checked for bleeding and manual compression is given to achieve hemostasis followed by postprocedure mammogram for the marker localization.

Further management is based on the biopsy report. If it is benign, follow-up with MRI is done. If it is malignant, stereotactic wire localization at the marker site and excision is performed.

MR-guided wire localization: To manage the MR detected lesions, which are at locations not amenable for biopsy such as posterior or

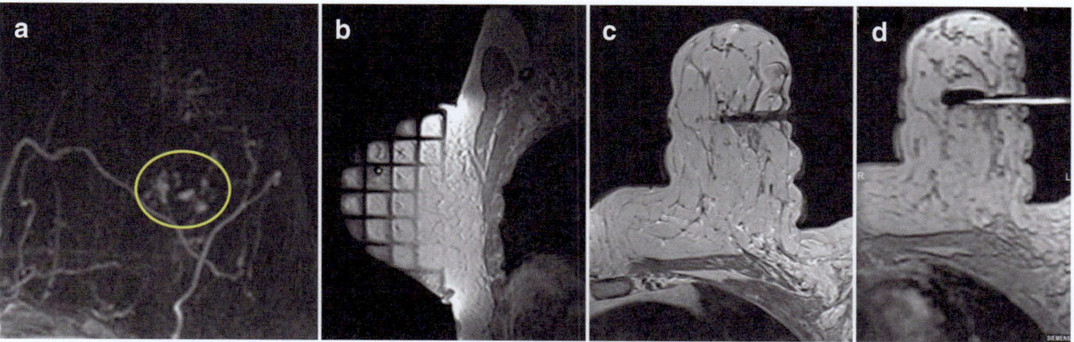

Fig. 11.10 (**a–d**) MR-guided, vacuum-assisted biopsy of left breast nonmass enhancement (yellow circle in (**a**). (**d**) Demonstrates postbiopsy cavity after sampling

superficial lesions, lesions, which are close to nipple or implant, and lesions in very thin breast, wire localization and excision is performed.

Complications: Complications are very rare following MR-guided breast interventions. The common complications include significant hematoma, infection, pneumothorax commonly in posterior lesions, marker clip displacement, and skin injury in superficial lesions.

11.7 Limitations

The limited availability and cost refrains clinicians and the radiologists from its routine use. Smaller dedicated breast centers must rely upon other MRI facilities as installing and maintaining the equipment is not a feasible option.

11.8 Conclusion

MRI breast is a powerful tool when used in an appropriate case-based setting, providing both the morphological and functional information. Owing to its highest sensitivity among the currently available imaging tools, it is recommended as a primary screening modality in high-risk women. MRI performed in a preoperative setting helps in improving overall surgical outcomes of breast conservation surgeries, reducing re-excisions, local recurrences, and avoiding unnecessary mastectomies. Likewise, when performed early during chemotherapy, it allows oncologists to stop or change the drug regime by identifying the nonresponders early. In scenarios of lesions of unknown malignant potential like architectural distortion, it can avoid biopsy and unnecessary surgery by excluding the malignancy owing to its high negative predictive value. MRI has a promising role in pathological nipple discharge and axillary nodes with suspected breast primary. Because of the several advantages that MRI breast offers, it should be integrated into the management protocol of every institute offering comprehensive breast cancer care.

References

1. National Comprehensive Cancer Network (NCCN). NCCN guidelines breast cancer screening and diagnosis, version 1. 2021. https://www.nccn.org/guidelines/guidelines-detail?category=2&id=1421
2. Monticciolo DL, Newell MS, Moy L, Niell B, Monsees B, Sickles EA. Breast cancer screening in women at higher-than-average risk. Am Coll Radiol. 2018;15(3PA):408–14.
3. American College of Radiology. ACR practice parameter for the performance of contrast-enhanced magnetic resonance imaging (MRI) of the breast. https://www.acr.org/-/media/ACR/Files/Practice-Parameters/mr-contrast-breast.pdf.
4. Mann RM, Cho N, Moy L. Breast MRI: state of the art. Radiology. 2019;292(3):520–36. https://doi.org/10.1148/radiol.2019182947.
5. Lee SH, Shin HJ, Moon WK. Diffusion-weighted magnetic resonance imaging of the breast: standardization of image acquisition and interpretation. Korean J Radiol. 2021;22(1):9–22. https://www.

acr.org/-/media/ACR/Files/Practice-Parameters/mr-contrast-breast.pdf
6. Baltzer P, Mann RM, Iima M, Sigmund EE, Clauser P, Gilbert FJ, Martincich L et al. EUSOBI International Breast Diffusion-Weighted Imaging working group. Diffusion-weighted imaging of the breast-a consensus and mission statement from the EUSOBI International Breast Diffusion-Weighted Imaging working group. Eur Radiol. 2020;30(3):1436–50. https://doi.org/10.1007/s00330-019-06510-3.
7. Kuhl C, Weigel S, Schrading S, Arand B, Bieling H, König R, et al. Prospective multicenter cohort study to refine management recommendations for women at elevated familial risk of breast cancer: the EVA trial. J Clin Oncol. 2010;28(9):1450–7. https://doi.org/10.1200/JCO.2009.23.0839.
8. Heacock L, Lewin AA, Toth HK, Moy L, Reig B. Abbreviated MR imaging for breast cancer. Radiol Clin N Am. 2020;59(1):99–111.
9. Milon A, Wahab CA, Kermarrec E, Bekhouche A, Taourel P. Breast MRI: is faster better. Am J Roentgenol. 2020;214(2):282–95.
10. Mann RM, Mus RD, van Zelst J, Geppert C, Karssemeijer N, Platel B. A novel approach to contrast-enhanced breast magnetic resonance imaging for screening: high-resolution ultrafast dynamic imaging. Investig Radiol. 2014;49(9):579–85. https://doi.org/10.1097/rli.0000000000000057.
11. Comstock CE, Gatsonis C, Newstead GM, Synder BS, Gareen IF, Bergin JT, et al. Comparison of abbreviated breast MRI vs digital breast tomosynthesis for breast cancer detection among women with dense breasts undergoing screening. JAMA. 2020;323(8):746–56. https://doi.org/10.1001/jama.2020.0572.
12. American College of Radiology. BI-RADS atlas. 5th ed. Reston, VA: American College of Radiology; 2013.
13. Dontchos BN, Rahbar H, Partridge SC, Korde LA, Lam DL, Scheel JR, et al. Are qualitative assessments of background parenchymal enhancement, amount of fibroglandular tissue on MR images, and mammographic density associated with breast cancer risk? Radiology. 2015;276(2):371–80.
14. Ray KM, Kerlikowske K, Lobach IV, Hofmann MB, Greenwood HI, Arasu VA, et al. Effect of background parenchymal enhancement on breast MR imaging interpretive performance in community-based practices. Radiology. 2018;286(3):822–9. https://doi.org/10.1148/radiol.2017170811.
15. Gity M, Arabkheradmand A, Taheri E, Shakiba M. Diagnostic investigation of breast magnetic resonance imaging in malignant and benign mass lesions. Arch Med Sci. 2018;14(5):1061–9. https://doi.org/10.5114/aoms.2016.62281.
16. Yang QX, Ji X, Feng LL, Zheng L, Zhou XQ, Wu Q, et al. Significant MRI indicators of malignancy for breast non-mass enhancement. J Xray Sci Technol. 2017;25(6):1033–44. https://doi.org/10.3233/XST-17311.
17. Lee SM, Nam KJ, Choo KS, Kim JY, Jeong DW, Kim HY, et al. Patterns of malignant non-mass enhancement on 3-T breast MRI help predict invasiveness: using the BI-RADS lexicon fifth edition. Acta Radiol. 2018;59(11):1292–9. https://doi.org/10.1177/0284185118759139.
18. Berg WA, Zhang Z, Lehrer D, Jong RA, Pisano ED, Barr RG, et al. Detection of breast cancer with addition of annual screening ultrasound or a single screening MRI to mammography in women with elevated breast cancer risk. JAMA. 2012;307(13):1394–404. https://doi.org/10.1001/jama.2012.388.
19. Phi XA, Saadatmand S, De Bock GH, Warner E, Sardenelli F, Leach MO, et al. Contribution of mammography to MRI screening in BRCA mutation carriers by BRCA status and age: individual patient data meta-analysis. Br J Cancer. 2016;114(6):631–7.
20. Expert Panel on Breast Imaging, Mainiero MB, Moy L, Baron P, Didwania AD, Diflorio RM, Green ED, et al. ACR appropriateness criteria® breast cancer screening. J Am Coll Radiol. 2017;14(11S):S383–90.
21. Sardanelli F, Boetes C, Borisch B, Decker T, Federico M, Gilbert FJ, et al. Magnetic resonance imaging of the breast: recommendations from the EUSOMA working group. Eur J Cancer. 2010;46(8):1296–316.
22. Newell MS, Giess CS, Argus AD, et al. ACR practice parameter for the performance of contrast enhanced magnetic resonance imaging (MRI) of the breast. Reston, VA: American College of Radiology; 2018.
23. The American society of breast surgeons. Consensus guideline on diagnostic and screening magnetic resonance imaging of the breast. 2017.
24. National Institute for Health and Care Excellence. Early and locally advanced breast cancer: diagnosis and management. NICE guideline [NG101]. 2018. https://www.nice.org.uk/guidance/ng101. https://www.nice.org.uk/guidance/ng101.
25. Plana MN, Carreira C, Muriel A, Chiva M, Abraira V, Ignacio J, et al. Magnetic resonance imaging in the preoperative assessment of patients with primary breast cancer: systematic review of diagnostic accuracy and meta-analysis. Eur Radiol. 2012;22(1):26–38.
26. Spick C, Baltzer PA. Diagnostic utility of second-look US for breast lesions identified at MR imaging: systematic review and meta-analysis. Radiology. 2014;273(2):401–9.
27. Turnbull L, Brown S, Harvey I, Olivier C, Drew P, Napp V, et al. Comparative effectiveness of MRI in breast cancer (COMICE) trial. Lancet. 2010;375(9714):563–71. https://doi.org/10.1016/S0140-6736(09)62070-5.
28. Gonzalez V, Sandelin K, Karlsson A, Aberg W, Lofgren L, Iliescu G, et al. Preoperative MRI of the breast (POMB) influences primary treatment in breast cancer: a prospective, randomized, multicenter study. World J Surg. 2014;38(7):1685–93.
29. Sardanelli F. Preoperative staging with MRI: did the MIPA trial solve all issues? Insights into Imaging–ECR 2018–book of abstracts. 2018; p. 106.

30. Kaufmann M, von Minckwitz G, Mamounas EP, Cameron D, Carey LA, Cristofanilli M, et al. Recommendations from an international consensus conference on the current status and future of neoadjuvant systemic therapy in primary breast cancer. Ann Surg Oncol. 2012;19(5):1508–16. https://doi.org/10.1245/s10434-011-2108-2.
31. Rastogi P, Anderson SJ, Bear HD, Geyer CE, Kahlenberg MS, Robidoux A, et al. Preoperative chemotherapy: updates of national surgical adjuvant breast and Bowel Project Protocols B-18 and B-27. J Clin Oncol. 2008;26(5):778–85.
32. Expert Panel on Breast Imaging, Slanetz PJ, Moy L, Baron P, diFlorio RM, Green ED, Heller SL, Holbrook AI, Lee SJ, Lewin AA, Lourenco AP, Niell B, Stuckey AR, Trikha S, Vincoff NS, Weinstein SP, Yepes MM, Newell MS. ACR Appropriateness Criteria® monitoring response to neoadjuvant systemic therapy for breast cancer. J Am Coll Radiol. 2017;14(11S):S462–75.
33. National Comprehensive Cancer Network Guidelines Version 6.2021 Invasive Breast Cancer. https://www.nccn.org. Accessed 20 Aug 2021.
34. Houssami N, Macaskill P, von Minckwitz G, Marinovich ML, Mamounas E. Metaanalysis of the association of breast cancer subtype and pathologic complete response to neoadjuvant chemotherapy. Eur J Cancer. 2012;48(18):3342–54.
35. Tomida K, Ishida M, Umeda T, Sakai S, Kawai Y, Mori T, et al. Magnetic resonance imaging shrinkage patterns following neoadjuvant chemotherapy for breast carcinomas with an emphasis on the radiopathological correlations. Mol Clin Oncol. 2014;2(5):783–8.
36. Scheel JR, Kim E, Partridge SC, Lehman CD, Rosen MA, Bernreuter WK, et al. ACRIN 6657 Trial Team and I-SPY Investigators Network. MRI, clinical examination, and mammography for preoperative assessment of residual disease and pathologic complete response after neoadjuvant chemotherapy for breast cancer: ACRIN 6657 trial. AJR Am J Roentgenol. 2018;210(6):1376–85.
37. Olson JA Jr, Morris EA, Van Zee KJ, Linehan DC, Borgen PI. Magnetic resonance imaging facilitates breast conservation for occult breast cancer. Ann Surg Oncol. 2000;7(6):411–5.
38. McCartan DP, Zabor EC, Morrow M, Van Zee KJ, El-Tamer MB. Oncologic outcomes after treatment for MRI occult breast cancer (pT0N+). Ann Surg Oncol. 2017;24(11):3141–7.
39. Stafford AP, Cruz LMDL, Willey SC. Workup and treatment of nipple discharge–a practical review. Ann Breast Surg. 2021;5. https://abs.amegroups.com/article/view/6921
40. Cher DJ, Conwell JA, Mandel JS. MRI for detecting silicone breast implant rupture: meta-analysis and implications. Ann Plast Surg. 2001;47(4):367–80.
41. Holmich LR, Vejborg I, Conrad C. The diagnosis of breast implant rupture: MRI findings compared with findings at explantation. Eur J Radiol. 2005;53(2):213–25.
42. Keech JA Jr, Creech BJ. Anaplastic T-cell lymphoma in proximity to a saline-filled breast implant. Plast Reconstr Surg. 1997;100(2):554–5.
43. Adrada BE, Miranda RN, Rauch GM, Arribas E, Kanagalshamanna R, Clemens MW, et al. Breast implant associated anaplastic large cell lymphoma: sensitivity, specificity, and findings of imaging studies in 44 patients. Breast Cancer Res Treat. 2014;147(1):1–14.
44. Clemens MW, Horwitz SM. NCCN consensus guidelines for the diagnosis and management of breast implant-associated anaplastic large cell lymphoma. Aesthet Surg J. 2017;37(3):285–9. https://doi.org/10.1093/asj/sjw259.
45. Yang N, Muradali D. The augmented breast: a pictorial review of the abnormal and unusual. AJR Am J Roentgenol. 2011;196(4):W451–60.
46. Covington MF. Contrast enhanced mammography implementation, performance and use for supplemental breast cancer screening. Radiol Clin N Am. 2021;59(1):113–28. https://doi.org/10.1016/j.rcl.2020.08.006.
47. Jochelson MS, Dershaw DD, Sung JS, Heerdt AS, Thornton C, Moskowitz CS, et al. Bilateral contrast-enhanced dual-energy digital mammography: feasibility and comparison with conventional digital mammography and MR imaging in women with known breast carcinoma. Radiology. 2013;266(3):743–51.
48. Meissnitzer M, Dershaw DD, Lee CH, Morris EA. Targeted ultrasound of the breast in women with abnormal MRI findings for whom biopsy has been recommended. AJR Am J Roentgenol. 2009;193(4):1025–9. https://doi.org/10.2214/AJR.09.2480.
49. Brennan SB, Sung JS, Dershaw DD, Liberman L, Morris EA. Cancellation of MR imaging-guided breast biopsy due to lesion nonvisualization: frequency and follow-up. Radiology. 2011;261(1):92–9. https://doi.org/10.1148/radiol.11100720.
50. Hefler L, Casselman J, Amaya B, Heinig A, Alberich T, Koelbl H. Follow-up of breast lesions detected by MRI not biopsied due to absent enhancement of contrast medium. Eur Radiol. 2003;13(2):344–6. https://doi.org/10.1007/s00330-002-1713-7.

Imaging-Guided Interventions

12

Bhawna Dev, Trupti Kulkarni, and M. C. Sheela

Abstract

Breast imaging plays an integral part in the triple assessment of breast disease. Image-guided intervention, both diagnostic and therapeutic, ranges from FNAC, biopsy, and localization. Image guidance helps in accurate localization of the lesion as well as in obtaining the appropriate representative area of the sample, thereby reducing misdiagnosis and eliminating need for repeat biopsies.

Keywords

USG guided biopsy · Wire localization
Marker clip placement · Magseed · VABB

12.1 Introduction

Triple assessment is the current gold standard approach to evaluate breast disease. It consists of clinical examination, imaging, and histopathology for correlation.

While mammography and sonomammography are the primary modalities employed in breast imaging and therefore intervention, other modalities such as tomosynthesis, MRI, and contrast-enhanced spectral mammography may be employed as problem-solving tools for intervention where the mass is not identified with routine imaging.

Apart from diagnostic image-guided biopsy, intervention may be used for the placement of fiducial clips or markers within cancers prior to treatment with neoadjuvant chemotherapy or primary endocrine therapy in some cases, presurgical localization of breast tumors, and as an aid to guide axillary surgery.

B. Dev (✉) · M. C. Sheela
Department of Radiology, Sri Ramachandra Institute of Higher Education and Research, Chennai, India
e-mail: bhawnadev@sriramachandra.edu.in; sheelamc@sriramachandra.edu.in

T. Kulkarni
Manchester University Hospital NHS Trust, Manchester, UK

B. Dev, L. D. Joseph (eds.), *Holistic Approach to Breast Disease*,
https://doi.org/10.1007/978-981-99-0035-0_12

12.1.1 Imaging Guided Intervention: The Basics

1. Patient selection: To confirm pathology in BI-RADS 4 and BI-RADS 5 category lesions.
   (a) Biopsy may be performed in BI-RADS 3 masses
   (b) Where patient follow-up is not assured or is difficult
   (c) In anxious patients
   (d) Where the clinical suspicion is high and/or discordant with imaging and histopathological confirmation is needed to decide if treatment is required
2. Modality selection: To choose the modality for the intended intervention in terms of feasibility and safety. This will depend on mass visualization and accessibility, availability of the imaging modality, efficiency, safety, patient comfort, and the practitioner's experience [1, 2].
3. Mass selection: If multiple masses are identified, it is mandatory to identify the mass with the most ominous features. In multiple masses, guided biopsy is indicated to rule out multifocal/multicentric disease and for treatment planning.
4. Needle selection: According to the site, size, the procedure planned viz., FNAC, biopsy, Vacuum-assisted breast biopsy (VABB)/vacuum-assisted excision (VAE).

12.2 Consent

- Informed consent is essential prior to undertaking any breast intervention procedure. Although local policies dictate whether written or electronic consent is accepted, it is imperative that the patient is explained.
  - The need for the procedure
  - The steps of the procedure (explained clearly in the language known and easily understood by the patient avoiding medical jargon, e.g., injection instead of infiltration)
  - Possible risks and complications (e.g., pain, bleeding rarely requiring surgical intervention, bruising, infection, which rarely will need antibiotics, need for repeat biopsy in case of inadequate sample, allergy to antiseptic and local anesthetic agents*, risk of damage to implant)
    **Check for allergy to local anesthetic and dressings and use an alternative if patient is allergic to a particular local anesthetic.*
  - Alternatives to the procedure if any (e.g., excision biopsy) and merits and demerits of each option
  - After-care information
  - Need for any further procedures (e.g., repeat biopsy/FNAC in case of inadequate sample)
- Although use of anticoagulants raises the risk of bleeding during breast intervention and postprocedure bruising [3, 4], it is not strictly essential to stop anticoagulation prior to all image-guided procedures. Most bleeding stops with firm pressure and image-guided biopsies on the breast can safely be performed with patients on warfarin (if INR <4) and also when patients are on Aspirin, Clopidogrel, and the newer anticoagulants (Rivaroxaban, Apixaban, etc.). Anticoagulant stoppage may be essential for procedures such as vacuum-assisted excisions and axillary core biopsies where the target lesion is deeply sited and close to blood vessels. In case there is a need to stop anti coagulants, a detailed discussion with the hematologist or other referring physician should be conducted including the need for alternative short-acting bridging (injectable) anticoagulation in some cases.
- The patient may experience pain due to breast compression in stereotactic procedures. Discomfort in ultrasound-guided procedures may occur from positioning with abduction of the arm.
- Positioning of the patient in stereo-guided procedures is decided based on location and depth of lesion and equipment available. Consideration must be given to biopsy in the lying down position for patients at risk of, or with history of, vaso-vagal attacks. In case of MR-guided biopsy, the patient has to be explained the need for lying in the prone posi-

tion and use of intravenous contrast agent, that is, gadolinium. In both stereo- and MRI-guided biopsies, it is essential the patient is placed in as comfortable a position as possible so as to avoid inadvertent movement during the procedure.
- Pneumothorax is a rare, potential complication (especially in deep-seated lesions or axillary biopsies). Proper technique makes this exceedingly rare.

12.3 Intervention Procedures

1. Fine needle aspiration
2. Biopsy
   (a) Core needle biopsy
   (b) Vacuum-assisted biopsy (VAB)
   (c) Vacuum-assisted excision (VAE)
3. Tissue marker placement
4. Localization
   (a) Wire localization
   (b) Nonwire localization—ROLL
   (c) Other nonwire localization methods
5. Therapeutic aspiration

12.3.1 FNA/FNAC

Fine needle aspiration is a simple technique, which requires local anesthesia (optional), a syringe, and needle to aspirate. Usually, a needle with a diameter of 27–18 G is used. In our institute, we preferably use 21 G or 22 G.

The sample is obtained by repeated passes through the lesion thus agitating and loosening cells with or without syringe attachment for suction. Sample collects either by capillary action or by suction (if using syringe for negative pressure creation by suction) in the needle hub. This can then be smeared on slides with or without fixation and/or sent in cytology fluid in a pot.

Sample Single or two passes through a mass are performed. Sample should be sufficient to smear on 4 slides and send in cytology fluid. Requirements differ between laboratories and pathologists' preferences should be kept in mind. Its best to discuss with pathology department to get a pulse of their preference. Some departments need sample only sent in cytology fluid.

12.3.2 Biopsy

12.3.2.1 Core Needle Biopsy

The materials needed for biopsy are antiseptic for skin, draping sheet, probe cover for the ultrasound probe (if performing the procedure under ultrasound guidance), syringe for local anesthesia (1 mL for skin and 5 mL for planned biopsy tract, although more may be needed in some patients depending on pain experienced), 11″ blade for making stab incision, biopsy gun, swabs, and container with formalin (Fig. 12.1).

Types of Biopsy Devices

Different vendors have different biopsy devices with variable needle gauges and lengths (Fig. 12.2). Irrespective of the manufacturer, the most commonly used gun is 14G (diameter) × 10 cm (Length). A study by Helbeich et al. [5] found that 14G is best suitable for biopsy and the smaller needles had significantly more tissue fragments and crush artifacts. Another study by Nath et al [6] found the quantity of specimen to be an important criterion for breast biopsies – larger needles yield wider and larger tissue samples than do smaller needles.

Automated Biopsy Guns (Figs. 12.3 and 12.4)

Automated biopsy gun is a spring-loaded automatic device. This consists of a firing stylet (fires at high speed into the target lesion) and a cutting cannula (fires rapidly following the stylet). Some devices provide the option of separately performing the two steps while also having the option of single button press for both steps to take place. The major advantage of the automated gun is the ability to cut through tough lesions and obtain good samples for diagnosis. For those devices where the two steps cannot be

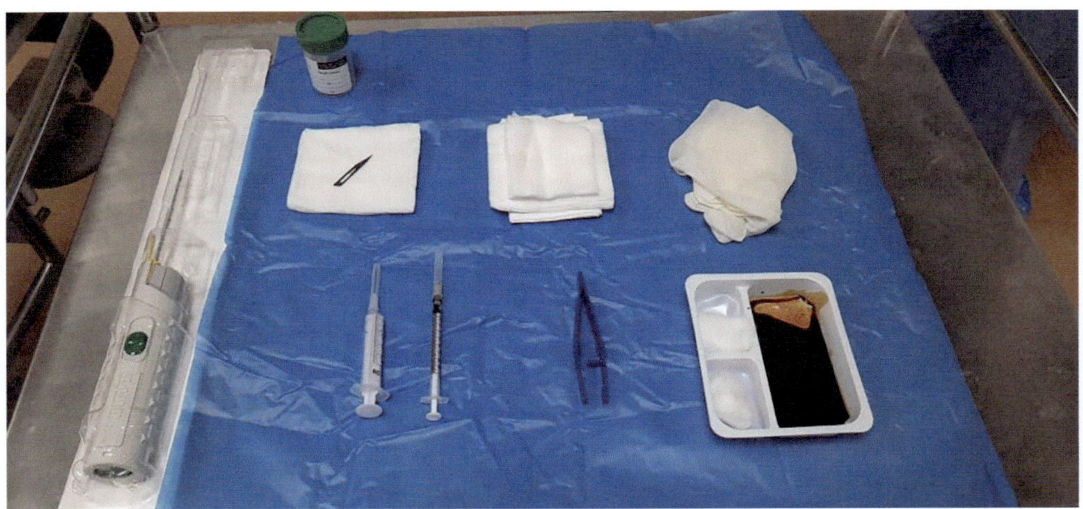

Fig. 12.1 Biopsy trolley—biopsy gun (14 G, 10 cm length, 2 cm throw) extreme left. Biopsy pot with formalin (top left). Middle row—11″ blade for incision, cotton swabs, and sterile gloves. Bottom row—1 mL syringe for skin anesthesia, 5 mL syringe (for deeper anesthesia along biopsy tract), plastic forceps to handle specimens, and a white well containing betadine solution. Some institutions also use plastic cassette for holding specimen within the formalin pot

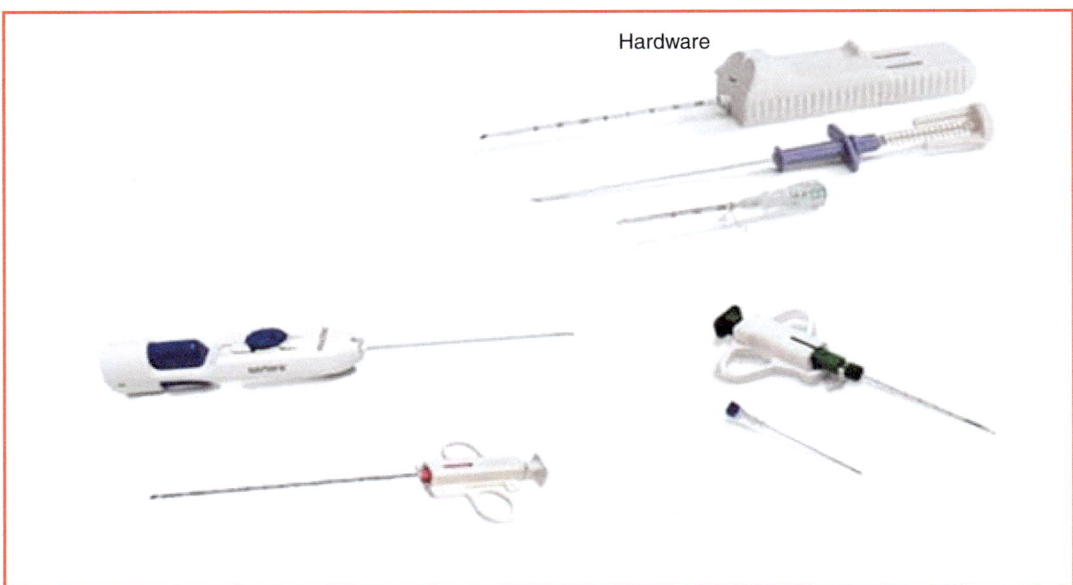

Fig. 12.2 Different types of biopsy guns

separately performed, the major disadvantage is that the course of the throw cannot always be predicted with absolute precision. Hence, it becomes crucial to ensure that sensitive structures, such as the skin, the pectoralis muscle, and large vessels, are not in the potential planned trajectory before firing such an automated device.

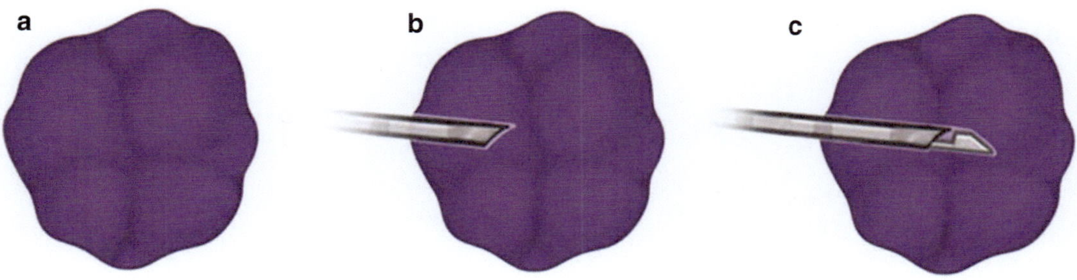

Fig. 12.3 Schematic represntation (**a**) of a mass. (**b**) Biopsy needle tip is seen at the margin of the mass (**c**) Outer cannula and cutting cannula are ejected simultaneously and seen within the mass

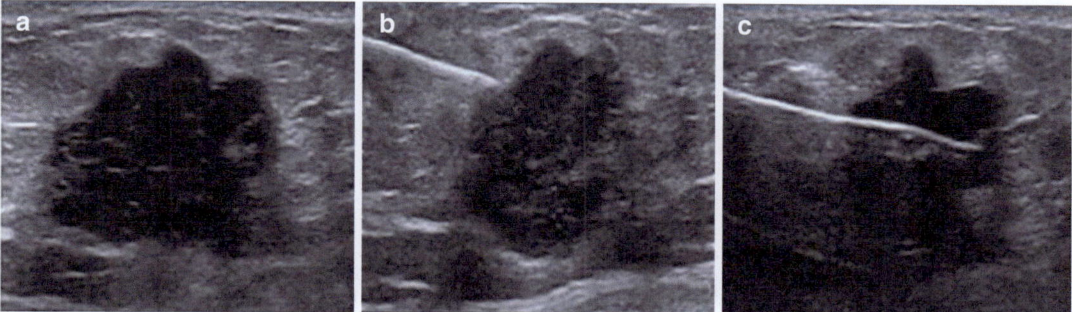

Fig. 12.4 (**a**) USG reveals irregular hypoechoic mass in right breast. (**b**) Biopsy needle tip is seen at the margin of the mass (**c**) Firing stylet and cutting cannula are simultaneously ejected into the mass

Semiautomated Biopsy Guns (Figs. 12.5 and 12.6)

A semiautomatic device is used in masses located in difficult anatomical locations where safe deployment of automatic guns is not entirely possible. In this, the inner needle containing a recessed sampling notch is fired first, followed by a hollow cutting cannula over the notched needle, shearing off the tissue. The advantage is that the stylet can be inserted independent of the cutting cannula and the open sample notch is visualized by ultrasound allowing confident verification and documentation of sample notch within the mass.

Use of Tru-Cut versus Coaxial System

- **Tru-cut core biopsy**
  In this technique, the biopsy gun is inserted under image guidance and the samples are obtained. Every time, the gun is removed with the sample core and reinserted after dislodging the core into the formalin.
- **Coaxial system** (Fig. 12.7):
  It has three parts—a guiding cannula, stylet, and biopsy needle.

In this technique, the depth of the lesion from the skin is analyzed. Using depth stop, the coaxial biopsy needle is positioned proximal to the lesion to be biopsied. Once the needle is adequately placed, the stylet is removed from the outer cannula, securing the guiding cannula within the lesion. The biopsy needle is now inserted into the guiding cannula, and the open sample notch is advanced. After confirming the position of the sample notch, biopsy is performed. The biopsy gun is withdrawn and the core dislodged into a cassette or directly into the formalin pot avoiding needle contact with the formalin. If there has been contact with formalin, this should be wiped off the biopsy gun before it is reintroduced into the guiding cannula.

The advantage of using a coaxial system is that repeated skin entry is not necessary to obtain

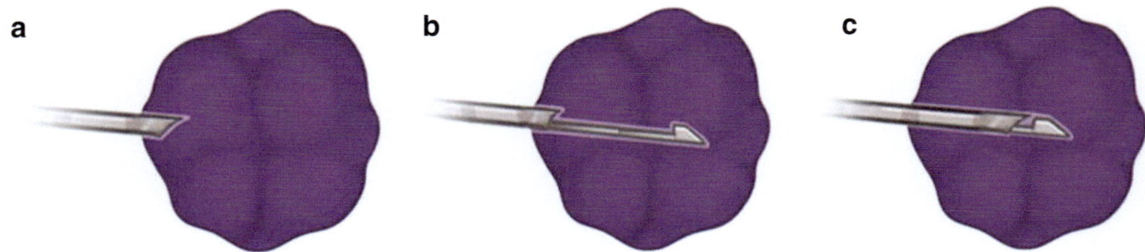

Fig. 12.5 Schematic representation showing (**a**) needle tip at the margin of the mass (**b**) on loading the biopsy needle, the recessed sample notch is seen within the mass (**c**) on firing cutting cannula is seen over the sampling notch

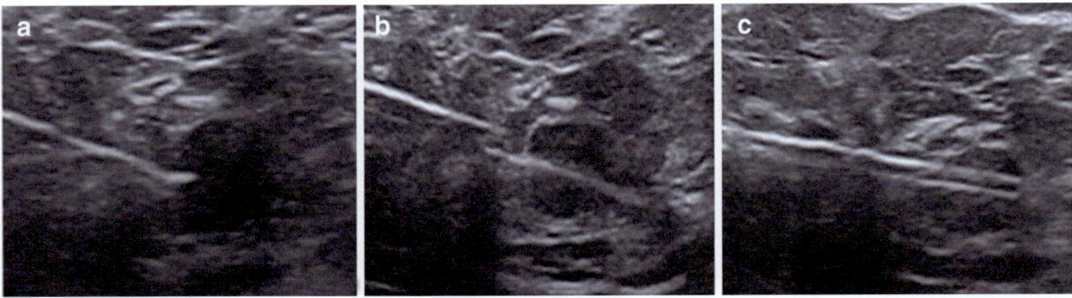

Fig. 12.6 (**a**) USG shows biopsy needle tip at the margin of mass. (**b**) On loading the gun, the recessed sampling notch is located within the mass. (**c**) Loading of the hollow cutting cannula over the notched needle

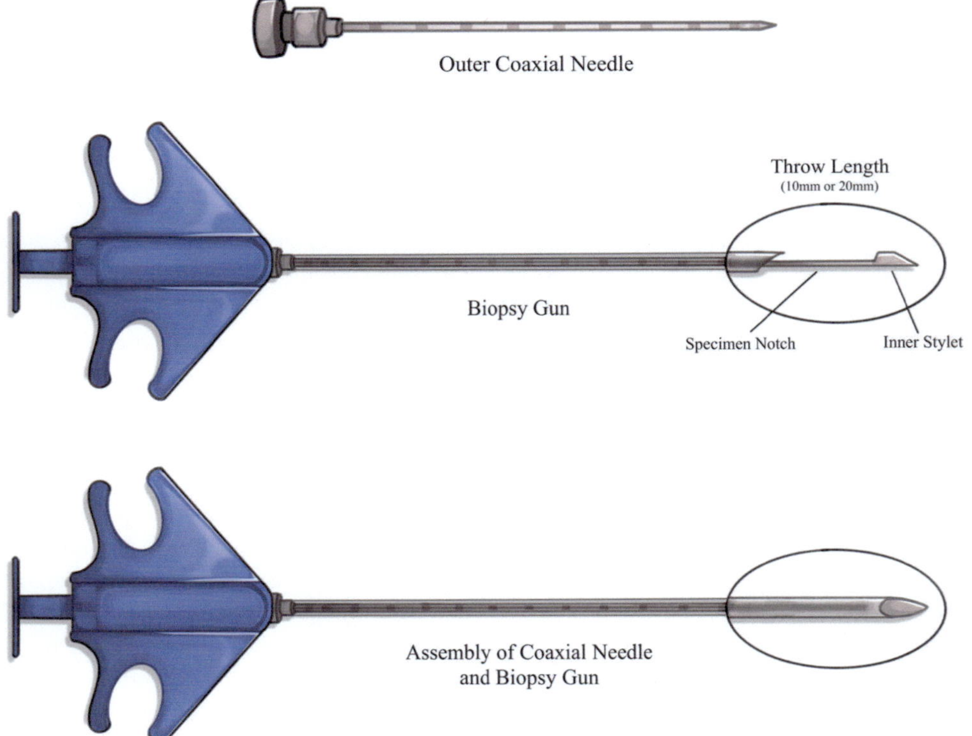

Fig. 12.7 Drawing showing parts of a coaxial biopsy needle

samples. Once the guiding cannula is placed, further sampling is through the guiding cannula. In difficult access masses, once the guiding cannula is placed, it is possible to obtain adequate samples without much additional effort. Also, a different area of the lesion can be sampled by turning the cutting edge of the biopsy needle within the cannula.

The risk of dislodgement of the cannula and assistance needed to hold the guiding cannula is one of the main disadvantages of using the coaxial system.

Sample Size

Three to four nonfragmented cores of approximately 2 cm length (that appear solid and not fatty to the naked eye or sink to the bottom of the formalin pot) obtained with 14-gauge biopsy needle are preferred [7]. Shorter length of samples may be obtained using same caliber guns with a throw of 11 mm, which is preferred for smaller lesions. A study by Lucena et al. found that even two cores are sufficient to diagnose a breast lesion [8]. Fewer cores may be obtained if there are technical difficulties (e.g., bleeding or patient fainting or withdrawing consent) encountered during biopsy.

12.3.2.2 Vacuum-Assisted Biopsy

Vacuum-Assisted Biopsy Probe/Needle consists of an outer, hollow sleeve with an aperture at its terminus (Figs. 12.8, 12.9 and 12.10). Vacuum holes are positioned opposite to the aperture designed to actively pull adjacent breast tissue within the outer sleeve of the probe when the vacuum is activated. A hollow cutter with a sharpened end is positioned within the outer sleeve. When the cutter is advanced forward, vacuum is automatically generated and breast tissue is pulled through the aperture and into the probe. The captured tissue is collected in the collection chamber automatically without needing to withdraw the probe for each sample. This occurs by withdrawing the cutter rearward within the outer sleeve of the probe, thus carrying the tissue sample back to a "knockout" pin, which pushes the captured tissue out into a specimen collection chamber.

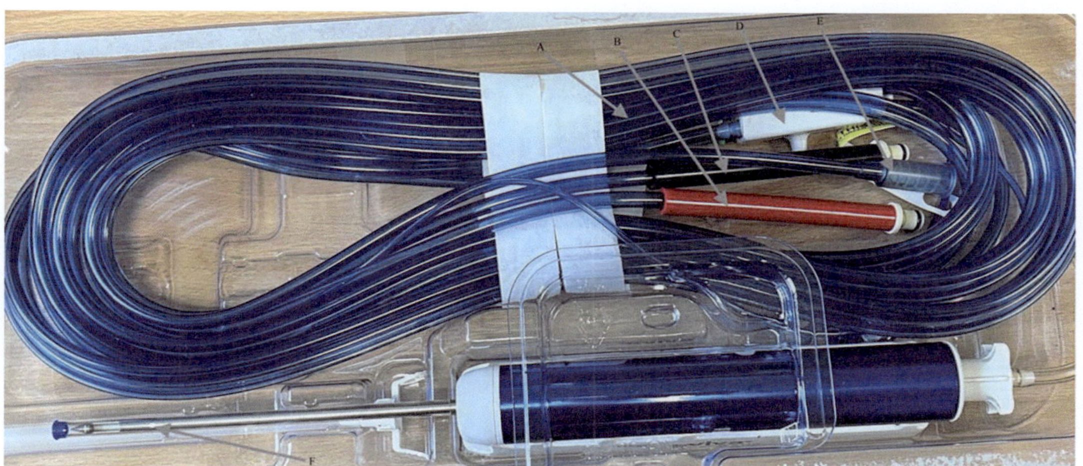

Fig. 12.8 Vacuum assisted set and accessories, labelled in picture. A—Plastic tubing, B—Red sleeve–to MRI hand piece receptacle (to be used for MRI-guided biopsies), C—Black sleeve- to non-MRI hand piece receptacle, D—Stereotactic adapter (Useful in dense breasts), E—Tube attachment to Vacuum canister, F—Needle (with notch open) connected to the blue hand piece, G—Open Cutting notch of the needle (20 mm aperture)

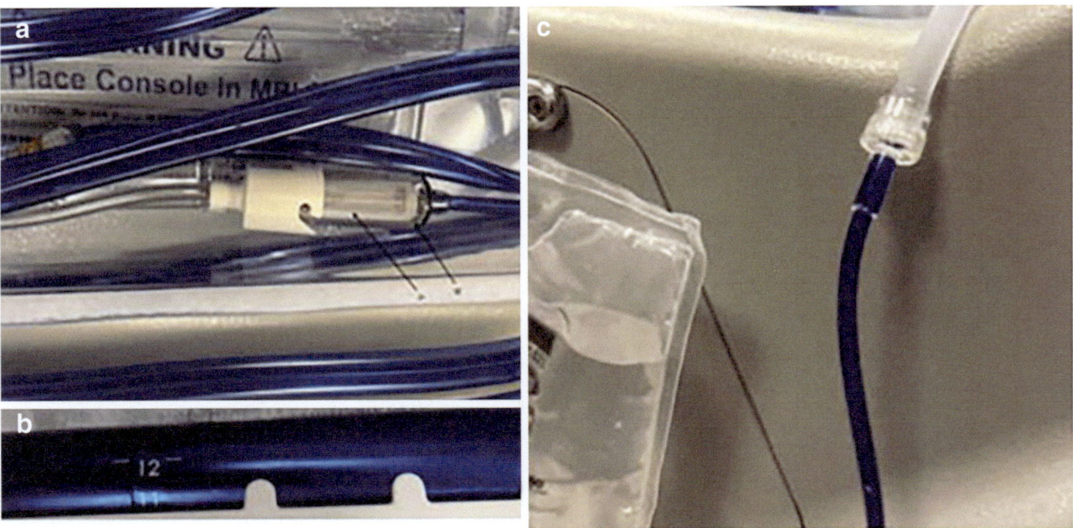

Fig. 12.9 (**a**) Parts of VAB set: A—Net filter within which specimen is captured, B—Plastic specimen chamber. (**b**) Needle base—numbers indicate clock face and can guide number of samples taken, (**c**) Saline connection for lavage

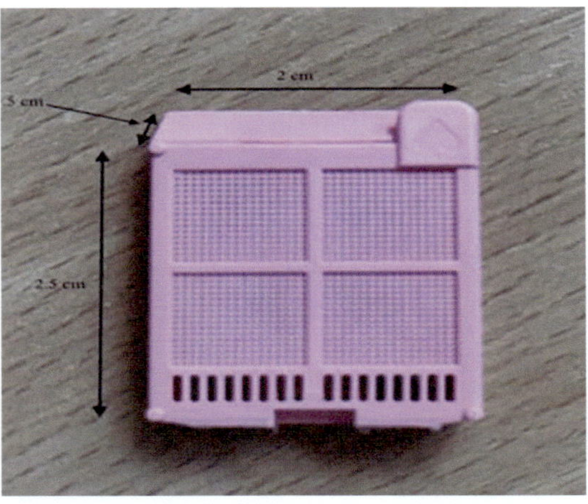

Fig. 12.10 Pink cassette for breast biopsies—this goes into the formalin pot

Vacuum biopsy probes are available in 7, 9, 10, 11, and 14 gauge sizes. The 14-gauge probe obtains approximately 40 mg of tissue per sample (compared with approximately 15 mg of tissue per sample with the automated core devices), and the 11-gauge probe obtains approximately 100 mg of tissue per sample [9].

Sample Size

The number of samples obtained depends on the needle size and whether this is being used as first line to obtain tissue for diagnosis, repeat biopsy for additional tissue with a view to upgrading the pathology or in order to excise a lesion. As a rough guide, for diagnostic purposes, 6 samples with 10/11 G needle and for upgrade purposes, 12 samples with 7–9 G needles [10] are taken.

12.3.2.3 Vacuum Assisted Breast Biopsy: Diagnostic vs. Excision [8]

If a vacuum biopsy is used for excision of a mass (used for fibroadenoma or radial scar), the needle is positioned along the deep margin of the mass, the sample notch opened, and needle position adjusted to center the mass within the opening of the sample notch. As sampling proceeds, the lesion should become visibly smaller as tissue is shaved from the inferior aspect of the lesion.

12.3.3 Tissue Marker Placement

A tissue marker can be placed following biopsy by any of the techniques mentioned above. **Indications for marker clip insertion:**

- Cancers planned to undergo neoadjuvant chemotherapy (Marker aids in checking response to various regimes of chemotherapy. It also allows for targeted wide local excision where breast conservation is planned and helps ensure excision of tumor bed in case of good response where lesion is no longer identifiable on imaging. Marker also guides pathologist to site of cancer in case of mastectomy where there has been a complete response to neoadjuvant treatment).

- Cancers in operative high-risk patients treated with first-line endocrine treatment (to check response to treatment).
- Small, impalpable, screen detected or incidentally found breast cancers (in order to localize these for surgery).
- Multiple masses with different BI-RADS biopsied (to specifically identify malignant lesions needing surgery).
- DCIS presenting as microcalcification (especially small cluster, which may be completely excised at diagnostic image-guided biopsy).
- Lesions seen only on MRI (in cases where MRI-guided biopsy is not feasible, but the lesion is amenable to clip insertion, biopsy around clip inserted can be performed using mammogram guidance).
- Marking of involved lymph nodes (especially where these may be away from the normal location in the axilla, e.g., sited extremely laterally or nodal recurrence in previously treated axilla where this would aid the clinician).
- Marking of nodes may also be indicated for certain cancer trials.

12.3.3.1 Clip Marker Types and Their Placement

Markers currently in use (Figs. 12.11 and 12.12) are titanium or stainless steel [10] which are MRI compatible. Markers are sometimes embedded in

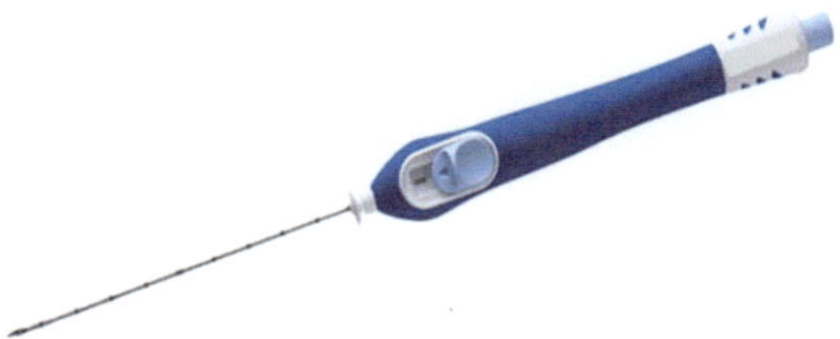

Fig. 12.11 Marker insertion systems Deployment system containing marker

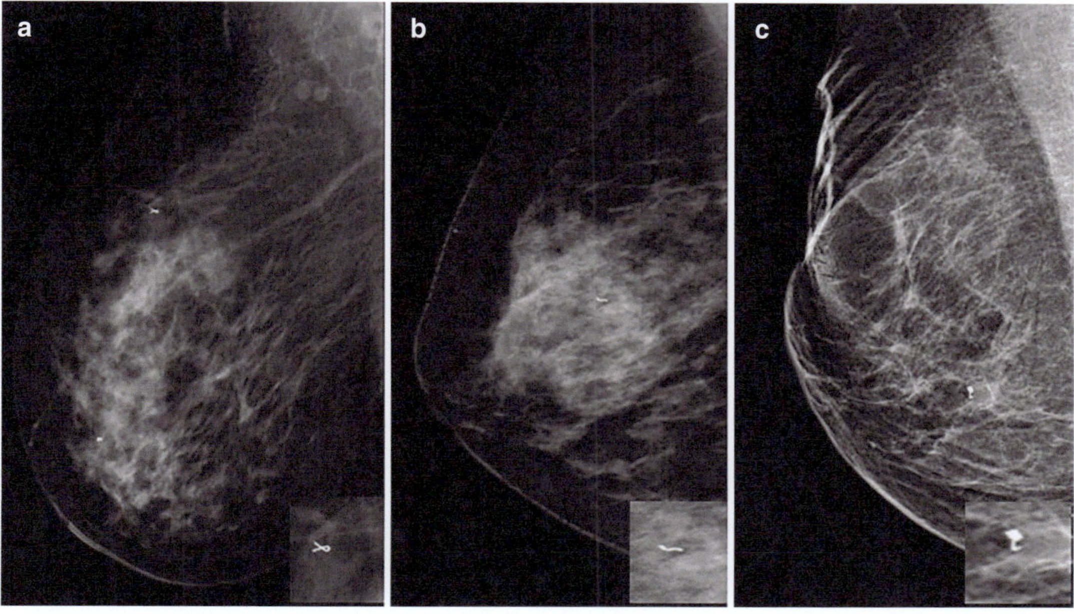

Fig. 12.12 Various shapes of clips (magnified in inset images) (**a**) Ribbon clip, (**b**) Comma clip, (**c**) Coil clip

a collagen or polyvicryl material, which is sonographically visible for several weeks, thus allowing subsequent MR imaging and US-guided preoperative localization in the event of a malignant diagnosis. Some clip markers have a small amount of nickel—these are not advised for use in patients with nickel allergy. Also, there have been some reports of inflammatory reactions due to collagen-embedded markers and some centers prefer to use nonembedded markers, which are also MR-compatible [10].

Clips come preloaded within needles with a push mechanism used for deployment. It is advisable to completely evacuate blood and fluid from the biopsy cavity using suction after vacuum-assisted excision or biopsy, in order to prevent clip migration.

The clip is deployed by pushing the plunger and the empty needle is withdrawn.

12.3.4 Localization

Indications

- Small, impalpable, screen detected or incidentally found breast cancers
- DCIS presenting as microcalcification
- Cancers that have shown good response to neoadjuvant chemotherapy and are no longer palpable
- Cancer in a breast where multiple lesions are present (in order to target the correct lesion for excision)
- (Rarely) lesions not proven to be cancer but requiring diagnostic (incisional) biopsy

12.3.4.1 Wire Localization

Wires have been the mainstay for localization of breast cancers for very many years for the indications mentioned above. A schematic illustration of technique of wire localization is shown in Fig. 12.13. Needle-wire systems with a variety of needle lengths (3–15 cm) and introducers (16–20 gauge) are available in single-use sterilized packages. The distal end of the wire can have different configurations, including hook, barb, or pigtail configurations (Fig. 12.14), to anchor the wire in or near the target [9].

The advantages of wires are that most are cheap, easily available, have few contra-indications and localization in experienced hands is a safe and effective technique. Ideally, wire insertion needs planning with the surgeon and keeping in mind the surgical incision or local reconstructive/cosmetic procedure being attempted. The main disadvantage of wires is the need for insertion on the day of surgery. This adds a delay to the operative pathway. There is also increased patient discomfort and stress on the day

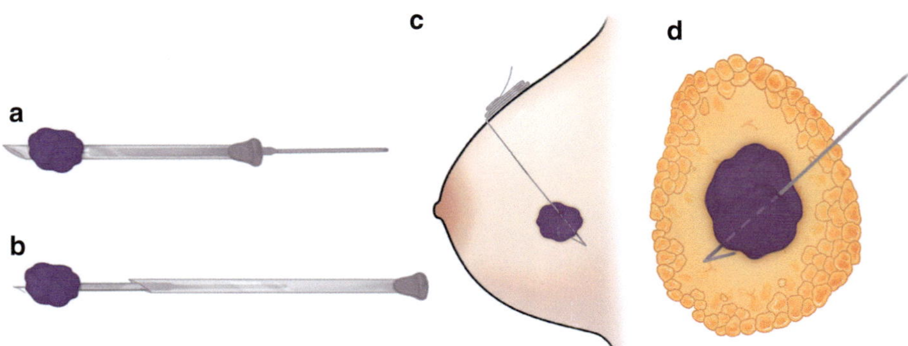

Fig. 12.13 Schematic representation showing technique of wire localisation. (**a**) The needle is localized at the distal aspect of the lesion to be localized. (**b**) Wire is advanced through the needle and hooked to the lesion and the needle is withdrawn. (**c**) Postprocedural appearance—wire hooked to the lesion. (**d**) Postoperative specimen where wire is excised in toto with the lesion

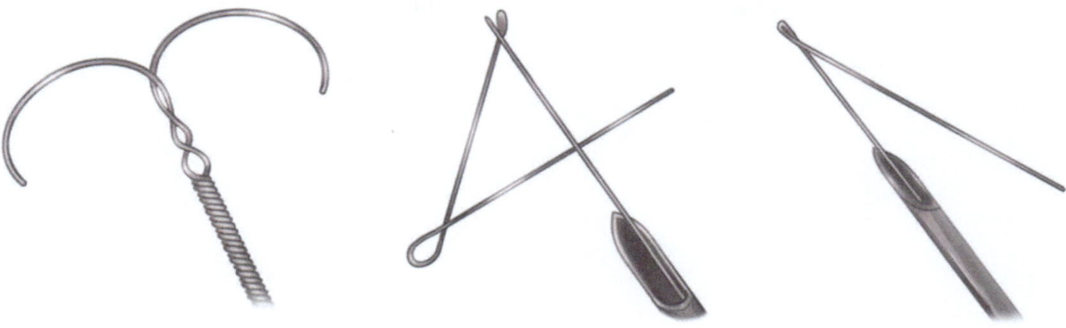

Fig. 12.14 Different types of wire tips

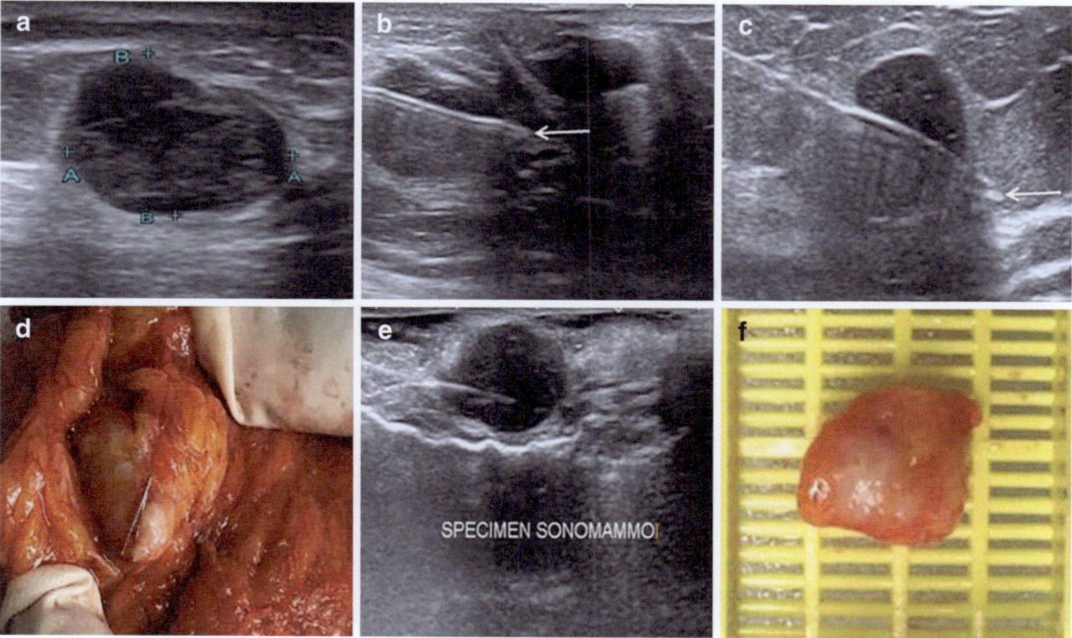

Fig. 12.15 (**a**) USG reveals a hypoechoic mass in the left breast subareolar region. (**b**) Wire localization needle is advanced through the mass till the distal margin (arrow). (**c**) wire hook noted just outside the distal margin of mass. (**d**) Intraoperative image showing wire inside the lesion. (**e**) Ultrasound of the excised specimen shows lesion removed in toto. (**f**) Gross specimen. HPE—Benign intraductal papilloma

of the operation. In addition, wires risk displacement and may need further localization and once deployed, most wires cannot be re-positioned.

More recently, a number of vendors have marketed wires that allow for retraction and redeployment thus obviating the need for a second wire placement due to incorrect wire placement. These are understandably slightly more expensive than conventional wires. Few examples of clinical applications of wire localisation are shown in Figs. 12.15, 12.16, 12.17, 12.18, and 12.19.

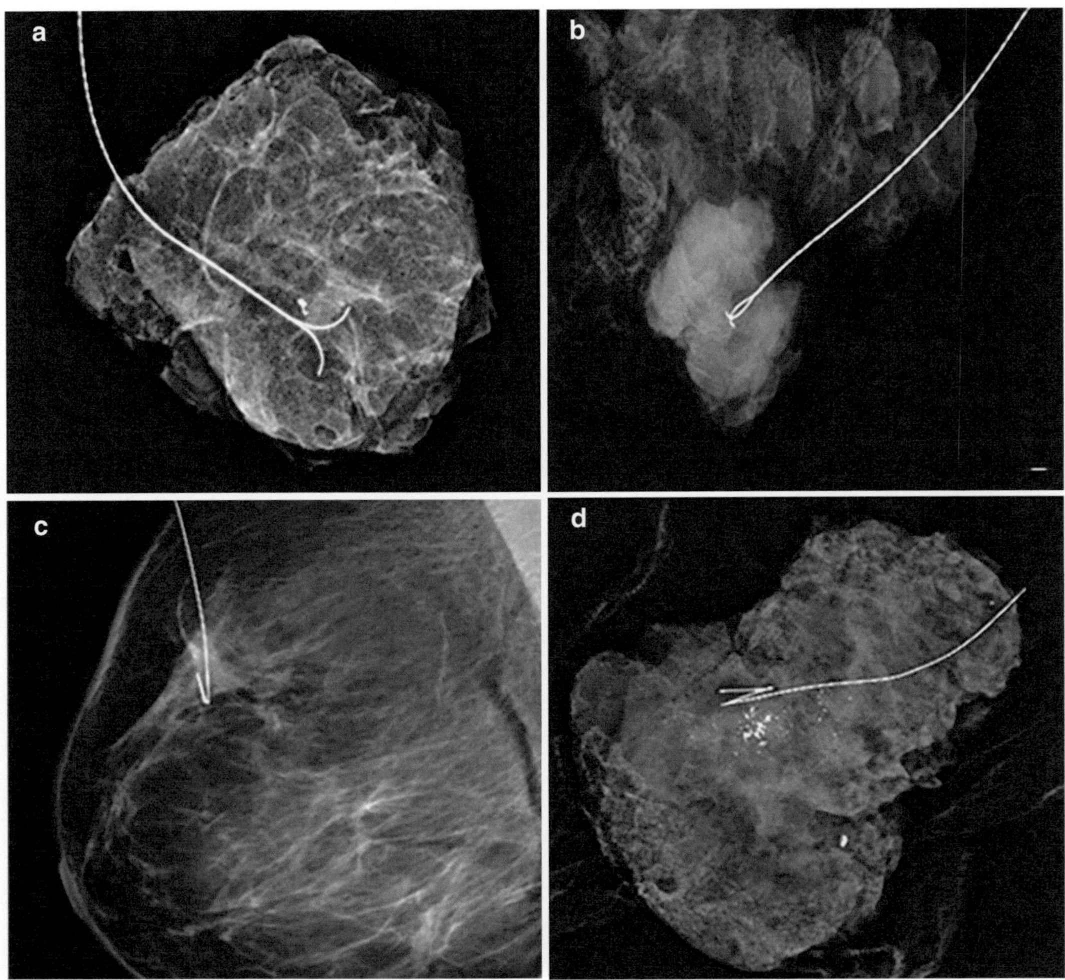

Fig. 12.16 Wire tips with different configurations. (**a**) Specimen X-ray with wire tip adjacent to mass (clip marker seen within mass), (**b**) specimen X-ray with wire tip within the mass, (**c**) wire within mass seen on check film of right breast, (**d**) specimen X-ray with wire tip in area of microcalcification

12.3.4.2 Non-wire Localization (ROLL)

ROLL Technique

Radio-guided occult lesion localization (ROLL) has been in in use since the 1990s and was started soon after radioisotope injection for sentinel node biopsy. The approach involves the intratumoral injection of a small amount of nuclear radiotracer under guidance by ultrasonography or stereotactic mammography. Radioactivity allows for the radiolabeling of the lesion and subsequent surgical excision guided by a handheld gamma ray detection probe. ROLL has gained popularity on account of several advantages associated with a reduced excision volume, more accurate centricity of a lesion within the surgical specimen, better cosmetic results, and a higher percentage of tumor-free margins. The disadvantages of ROLL include a short window for surgery necessitating injection on the day of surgery, need for access to radioactive material requiring a license and relatively complicated methods of obtaining and disposal of tracer.

A recognition of the drawbacks of localization using wires and ROLL has resulted more recently in newer nonwire localizations.

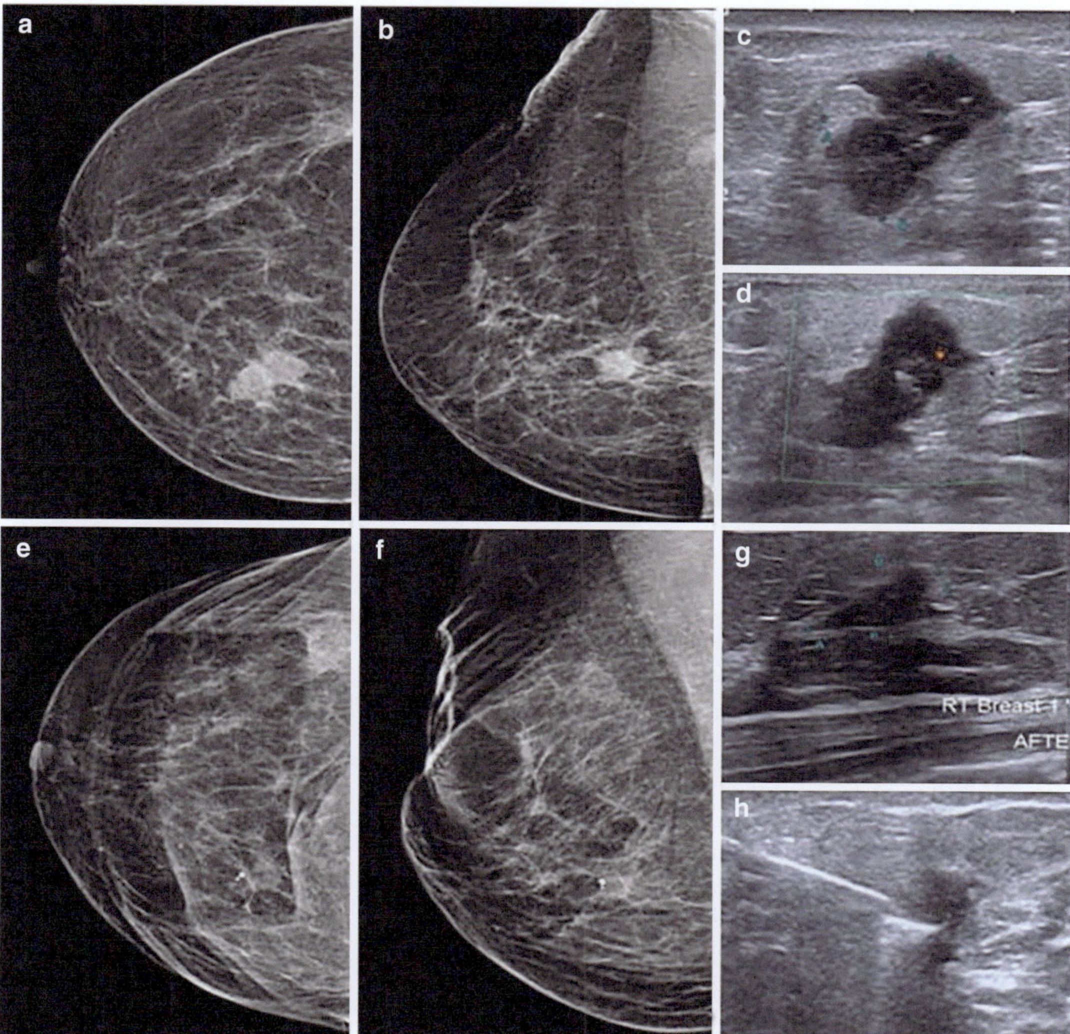

Fig. 12.17 (**a**, **b**) Irregular high density mass in the lower inner quadrant of right breast. (**c**, **d**) USG showing irregular hypoechoic mass with mild internal vascularity. HPE—Invasive mammary carcinoma. (Marker clip was placed in view of small size of the lesion) (**e**, **f**) Post neoadjuvant chemotherapy follow up mammogram images showed near complete regression of the mass (clip aids in identifying the location of the tumor). (**g**) Residual mass on ultrasound. (**h**) USG Wire localization of the mass. (**i**, **j**) Right mammogram confirming the location of wire in close proximity to the clip. (**k**, **l**) Specimen X-ray (**k**) and specimen sonogram (**l**) showing excision of the mass in toto along with the wire and clip. (**m**) Gross specimen showing clip in situ. (**n**) Clip removed from the mass

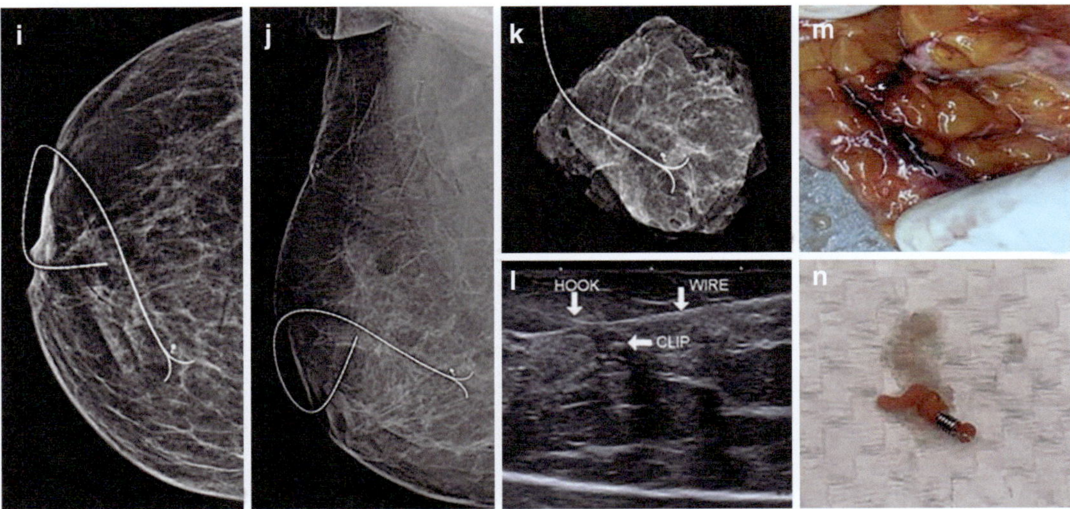

Fig. 12.17 (continued)

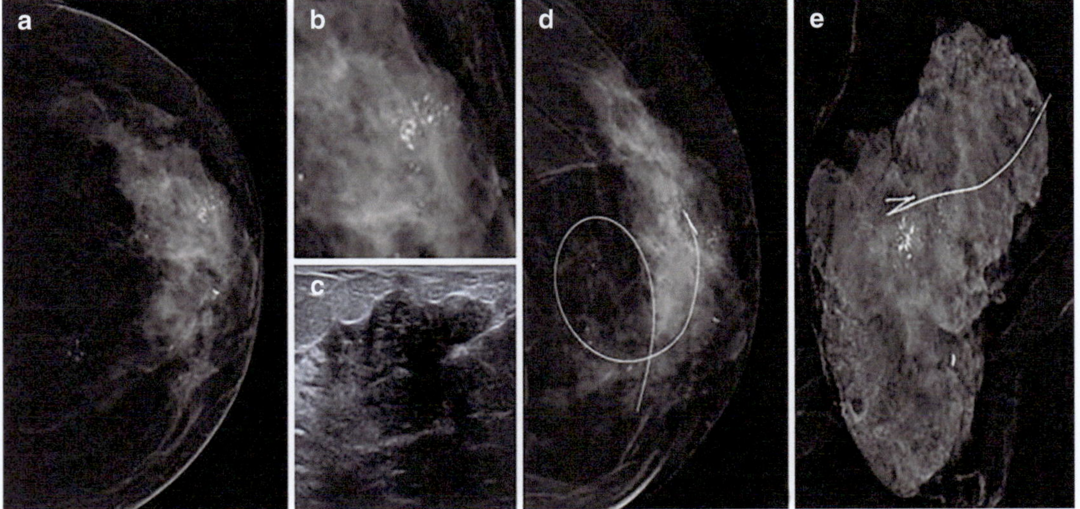

Fig. 12.18 (**a**) Xray mammogram reveals clustered micro calcifications in the outer left breast. (**b**) Magnified image revealing suspicious calcifications. (**c**) Ultrasound reveals irregular hypoechoic mass. (**d**) Check mammogram shows wire in the vicinity of calcifications. (**e**) Specimen X-ray showing complete excision of the calcification with wire in situ. HPE—DCIS

12.3.4.3 Newer Nonwire Localizations

A number of alternatives to wire localization have become available in recent years. Deployment may be under mammographic, ultrasound, or CT guidance [11].

Some of these include [11, 12]

- Iodine 125 (125I) radioactive seeds (Advantage I-125; IsoAid, Port Richey, Fla)
- Radar reflectors (Savi SCOUT; Cianna Medical, Aliso Viejo, Calif),
- Magnetic seed markers (Magseed; Endomagnetics, Cambridge, England)
- RFID tags (LOCalizer; Hologic, Marlborough, Mass)

Each of these systems has 3 components: a single-use sterilized 5–12-mm-long device pre-

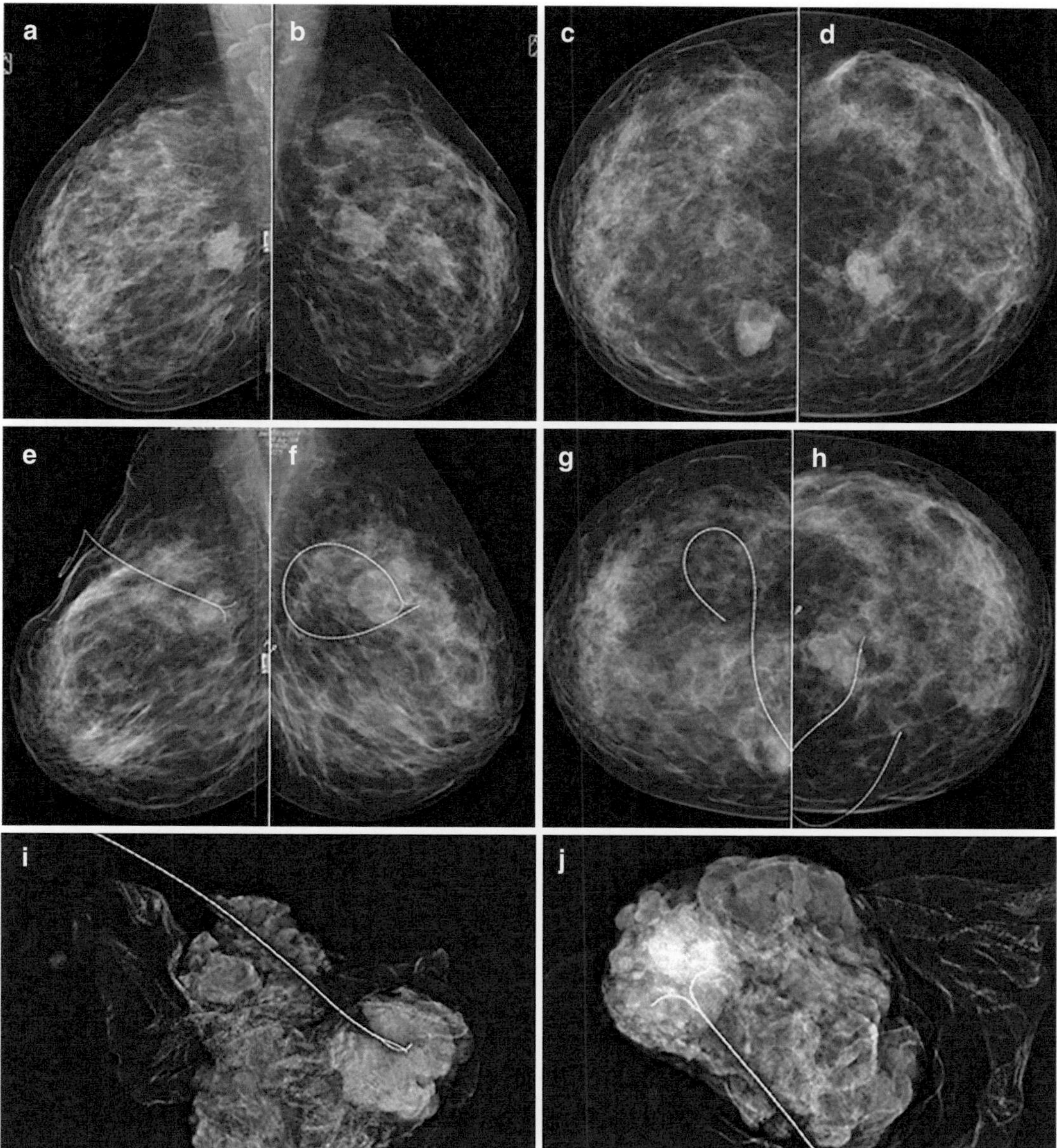

Fig. 12.19 (**a**, **c**) CC and MLO view of X-ray mammogram reveal suspicious mass in the upper inner quadrant right breast. (**b**, **d**) CC and MLO view of X-ray mammogram reveal suspicious mass in the upper inner quadrant left breast. (**e**–**h**) Lesions are wire localized and check X-ray mammogram reveals wire in situ. (**i**, **j**) Specimen mammogram reveals complete excision of the mass with wires in situ

loaded in a 12–18-g needle introducer, a reusable small console, and a dedicated handheld intraoperative probe [12].

Nonwire localization systems use send-receive technology at a specific wavelength in the electromagnetic spectrum. The probe is used in the operating room to detect the localization device in the breast. The console emits real-time audio and visual feedback that aids the surgeon as he or she continues the dissection and advance closer to the target.

Although comparative cost is one of the downsides (most systems cost between 4 and 20 times more than conventional wires), the major advantage of these localization techniques is the absence of a wire. As these localizers remain effective for long (most are effective >30 days, I 125 needs insertion no more than 5 days prior to surgery), need for insertion on the day of surgery is obviated.

Iodine 125, radar reflectors, and magnetic seed systems (Fig. 12.20) utilize reusable probes and can also be used for sentinel node procedures. Of these I 125 can be used with existing probes for sentinel node biopsy. (RFID is as yet unlicensed for axillary node surgery.)

The disadvantages include cost as previously mentioned and in case of RFID, disposable probe needs to be used during surgery. Localizers such as I 125 and RFID require support from the nuclear medicine department for transport and disposal of radioactive material used. This also increases the time taken to set up such a service. Radar reflectors may cause nickel allergy as they are made of Nitinol. Also, although all of these are MRI-compatible, the magnetic seed causes a large susceptibility artifact (sometimes as large as 5 cm), making images nondiagnostic. The magnetic seed is contraindicated in patients with implanted cardiac devices. In addition, nonmagnetic surgical tool-kit is needed when operating on these patients to avoid signal interference.

12.3.5 Therapeutic Procedures

Indications

1. Cyst
2. Abscess
3. Postoperative collection

Breast intervention includes therapeutic aspiration for benign lesions such as cysts—aspiration is performed for symptomatic relief (Fig. 12.21).

Aspiration of infected material (Fig. 12.22) from a breast abscess yields material for microbiology and many a times avoids operative intervention altogether.

Similarly, aspiration of postoperative collections (seromas, hematomas, infected collections) gives symptomatic relief and the sample obtained can be subjected to microbiological evaluation to guide antibiotic treatment as appropriate.

Although nonradiological aspiration can be performed, when performed under ultrasound guidance, it allows for better targeting especially in cases where the fluid may be in pockets. Also in cases of implant reconstruction ultrasound guidance is always considered safe.

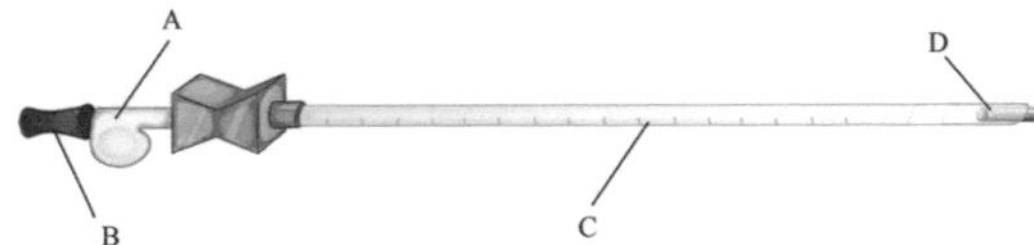

Fig. 12.20 Magseed—A—Safety bung made of rubber—prevents accidental deployment of seed, B—Plunger, C—Hollow needle containing plunger and Magseed, D—Needle tip for release of seed

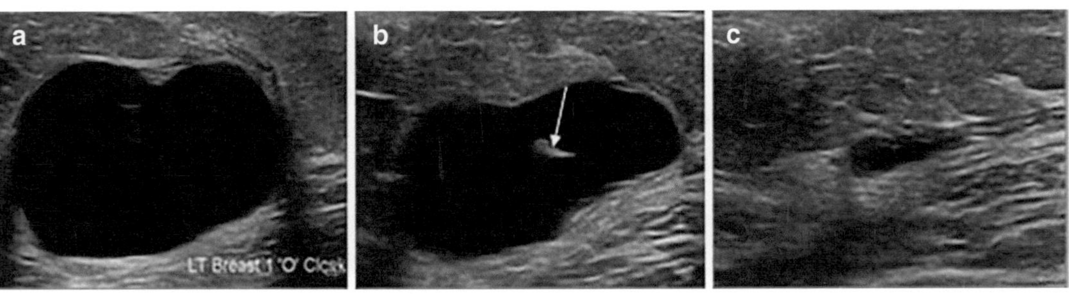

Fig. 12.21 (**a**) USG reveals a thin-walled cyst in left breast. (**b**) Needle tip is noted within the cyst (arrow). (**c**) Post aspiration image shows near-complete resorption of cyst

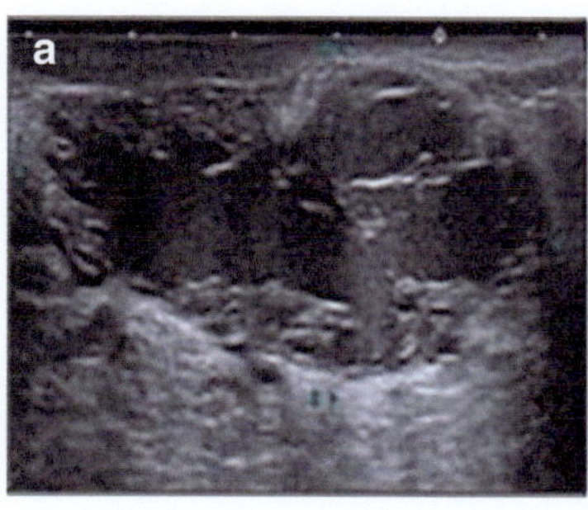

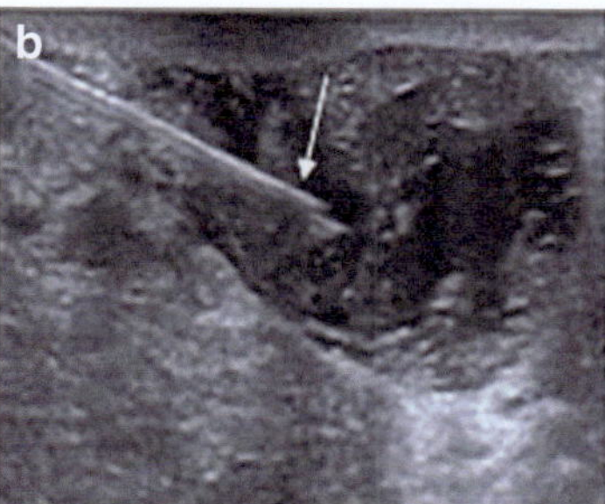

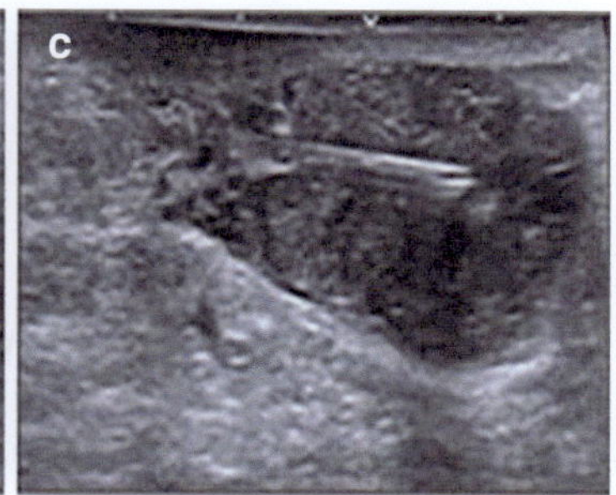

Fig. 12.22 (**a**) USG reveals a thick-walled abscess in right breast. (**b**) shows needle tip (arrow) within the liquid component of the abscess. (**c**) Postaspiration image shows near-complete aspiration of the liquid component. Note that more solid material may liquefy over time and patient may benefit from further aspiration at a later date

In addition, inflammatory corticosteroid (triamcinolone) may be injected into the seroma cavity in order to eliminate the cavity and prevent recurrent seroma collection [13].

References

1. ACR Practice Parameter for the Performance of Stereotactic-Guided Breast Interventional Procedure. 11. https://www.acr.org/-/media/ACR/Files/Practice-Parameters/stereo-breast.pdf.
2. Bassett L, Winchester DP, Caplan RB, Dershaw DD, Dowlatshahi K, Evans WP, et al. Stereotactic core-needle biopsy of the breast: a report of the Joint Task Force of the American College of Radiology, American College of Surgeons, and College of American Pathologists. Breast J. 1997;3(6):317–30.
3. Melotti MK, Berg WA. Core needle breast biopsy in patients undergoing anticoagulation therapy. Am J Roentgenol. 2000;174(1):245–9. https://doi.org/10.2214/ajr.174.1.1740245.
4. Somerville P, Seifert PJ, Destounis SV, Murphy PF, Young W. Anticoagulation and bleeding risk after core needle biopsy. Am J Roentgenol. 2008;191(4):1194–7.
5. Helbich TH, Rudas M, Haitel A, Kohlberger PD, Thurnher M, Gnant M, Wunderbaldinger P, Wolf G, Mostbeck GH. Evaluation of needle size for breast biopsy: comparison of 14-, 16-, and 18-gauge biopsy needles. Am J Roentgenol. 1998;171(1):59–63.
6. Nath ME, Robinson TM, Tobon H, Chough DM, Sumkin JH. Automated large-core needle biopsy of surgically removed breast lesions: comparison of samples obtained with 14-, 16-, and 18-gauge needles. Radiology. 1995;197(3):739–42.
7. Fishman JE, Milikowski C, Ramsinghani R, Velasquez MV, Aviram G. US-guided core-needle biopsy of the breast: how many specimens are necessary? Radiology. 2003;226(3):779–82. https://doi.org/10.1148/radiol.2263011622.
8. de Lucena CE, Dos Santos Júnior JL, de Lima Resende CA, do Amaral VF, de Almeida Barra A, Reis JH. Ultrasound-guided core needle biopsy of breast masses: how many cores are necessary to diagnose cancer? J Clin Ultrasound. 2007;35(7):363–6. https://doi.org/10.1002/jcu.20380.
9. Parker SH, Klaus AJ. Performing a breast biopsy with a directional, vacuum-assisted biopsy instrument. Radiographics. 1997;17(5):1233–52.
10. Mahoney MC, Newell MS. Breast intervention: how I do it. Radiology. 2013;268(1):12–24.
11. Kapoor MM, Patel MM, Scoggins ME. The wire and beyond: recent advances in breast imaging preoperative needle localization. Radiographics. 2019;39(7):1886–906.
12. Hayes MK. Update on preoperative breast localization. Radiol Clin. 2017;55(3):591–603.
13. Rieka T, et al. Triamcinolone reduces seroma re-accumulation in the extended latissimus dorsi donor site. J Plast Reconstr Aesthet Surg. 2008;61(6):636–42.

Part IV

Pathological Considerations in Breast Masses

13 Handling of Breast Core Biopsies and Processing

Archana B, Leena Dennis Joseph, and Sandhya Sundaram

Abstract

With advances in imaging, surgery, and molecular testing, breast conservation surgeries, excisions, and wire localized specimens have gained popularity. A definitive pathologic diagnosis is the cornerstone to guiding appropriate treatment. This requires a proper handling of tissue specimens received in the pathology laboratory. Breast grossing techniques are important for providing accurate information on critical parameters required for tumor staging such as tumor size, margin, and lymph node status. Here, we provide a practical simplified approach to grossing breast specimens.

Keywords

Specimens · Breast excision · Mastectomy · Margins · Orientation

A. B (✉) · L. D. Joseph · S. Sundaram
Department of Pathology, Sri Ramachandra Medical College, Chennai, India
e-mail: archanab@sriramachandra.edu.in; leenadennisj@sriramachandra.edu.in

13.1 Introduction

Grossing of breast specimens has been evolving since a few decades with the advent of newer techniques of sampling like image-guided biopsies [1]. Proper grossing and handling of breast specimens with appropriate submission of tissue sections are essential for an accurate histopathologic diagnosis. This requires a multidisciplinary team approach involving pathologists, radiologists, and surgeons. Breast specimens could be received for evaluation as core needle (tru-cut, ultrasound guided or stereotactic), excisional biopsies (with or without wire localization), or as mastectomy specimens.

13.2 Fixation of Specimens

Fixation of specimens should be done in 10% neutral buffered formalin immediately after collection. With biomarker testing gaining importance in the prognosis and treatment of breast cancer, recent guidelines have recommended a rapid transport and fixation of specimens with a cold ischemia time less than 1 hour, fixation not less than 6 hours or not more than 72 hours [2]. The volume of the fluid should be ten times the volume of the tissue for an adequate fixation. The fixation time depends on the size of the specimen with the fixation rate being 1 mm of tissue penetration per hour. Mastectomies and excision specimens need to be

B. Dev, L. D. Joseph (eds.), *Holistic Approach to Breast Disease*,
https://doi.org/10.1007/978-981-99-0035-0_13

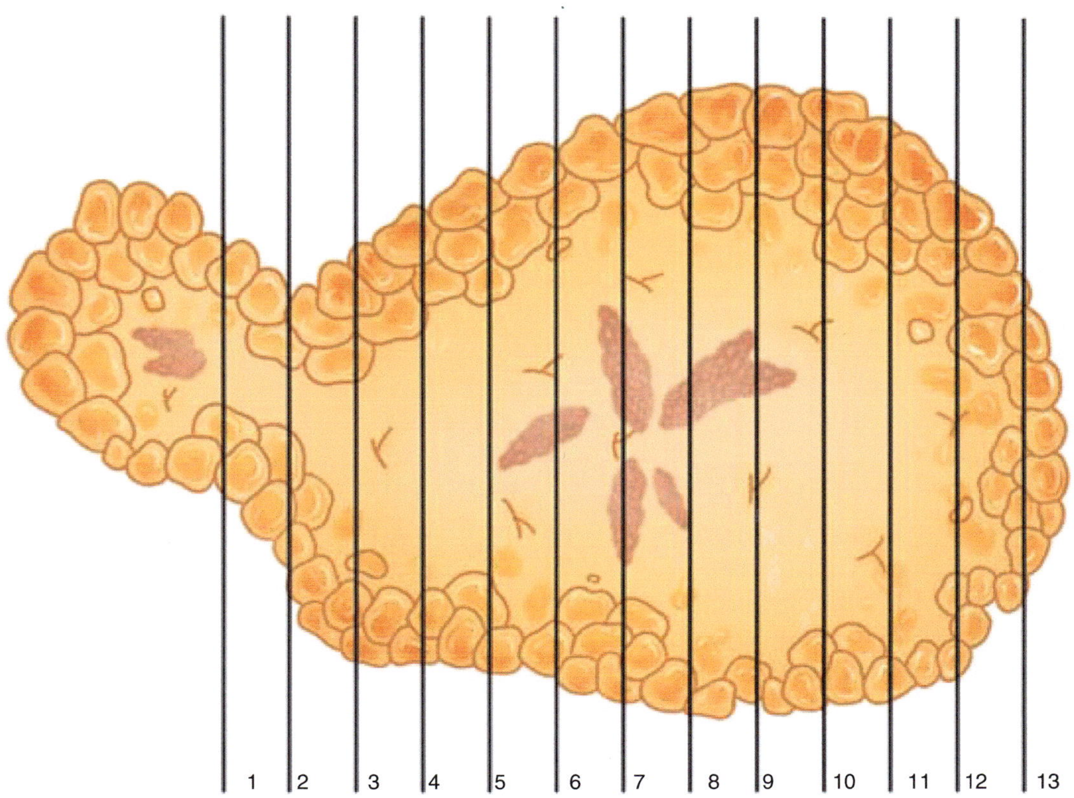

Fig. 13.1 Diagrammatic representation of slicing of the breast specimen every 0.5 cm intervals during fixation of the specimen

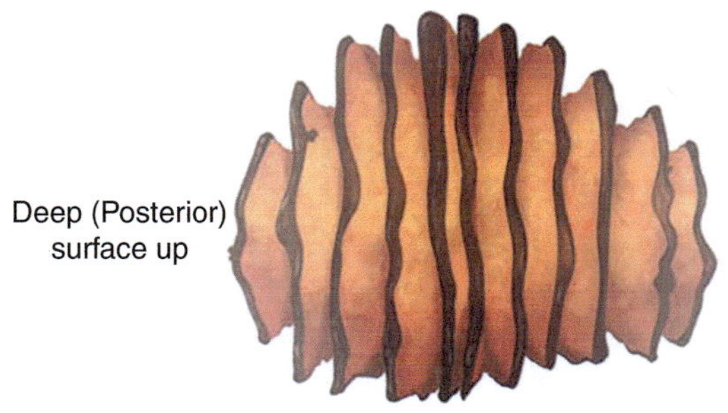

Fig. 13.2 Diagrammatic representation of the sliced breast tissue

sliced at 0.5 cm intervals, not cutting through the skin [3]. The posterior/deep resected margin can be inked prior to slicing. A gauze/tissue paper may be placed in between each slice to ensure diffusion of the fixative (Figs. 13.1 and 13.2).

Overnight fixation is ideal for proper processing of tissues. Carnoy's fixative is used for enhancing the detection of lymph nodes in cancer specimens. It is composed of 60% ethanol, 30% chloroform, and 10% glacial acetic acid, which dissolves lipids from the tissue, allowing lymph nodes to be easily identified [4].

13.3 Special Considerations in the Grossing of Specimens

In case of needle biopsies, it is important to describe the number of cores, color, size, and place the cores parallel to each other wrapped in a filter paper. Eosin can be used to identify cores, which are too small to be visualized with the naked eye.

For excision biopsy, it is important to orient the specimen, ink entirely to assess the margins, weigh, measure the specimen, and describe the external surface. It is also important to describe the lesion with respect to its consistency, growth pattern, necrotic/hemorrhagic areas, and assess distance from margins by making parallel cuts along the long axis of the specimen (1 cut/cm).

13.4 Sampling of Specimens

Specimens such as incisional or excisional biopsies may be received in the Pathology laboratory. The lesion must be sampled adequately (one section per cm of the lesion) along with normal fibrous tissue, skin, and nipple areola complex if included. For multiple lesions, it is advisable to submit sections of tissue in between the lesions to check for multifocality.

13.5 Excision Specimens

Specimens need to be oriented and must be inked appropriately to assess the margins. Discussion with the surgeon and understanding the orientation in relation to the sutures will help in handling the specimens accurately. Surgeons may prefer to mark the superior margin with a short suture and lateral margin with a long suture for uniformity. Each margin may be inked with a different color, or a standard method of inking may be adopted for all specimens to identify distance of tumor from margins (Fig. 13.3). Margins may be submitted as shave or perpendicular based on the distance of tumor from the margins (shave/en face if lesion is away and perpendicular if lesion is close).

Tissue samples in excision specimens are submitted from the medial to lateral aspect after making serial sections. In addition to a detailed description, a photograph or drawing may be included in the grossing report to indicate where the sections were taken from. Samples need to be included from the lesion, all the margins - perpendicular (if lesion is close), parallel/en face (if lesion is away) and from the adjacent normal tissue. Large slices may need to be sectioned further before placing them in the tissue cassette (Fig. 13.4).

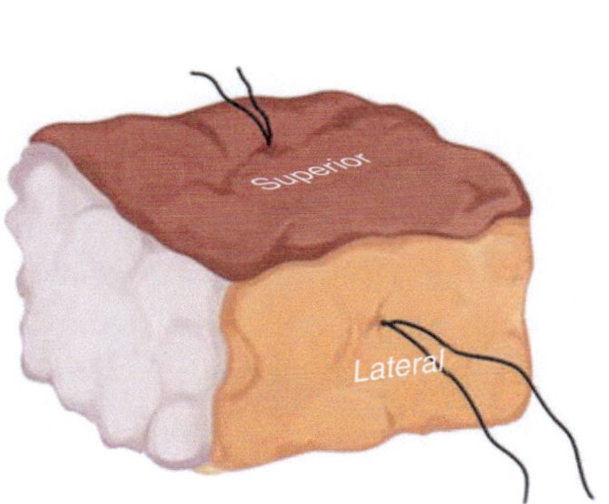

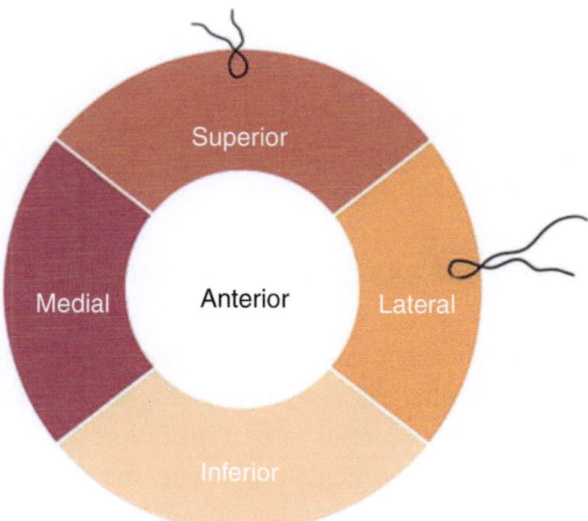

Fig. 13.3 Diagrammatic representation of orientation of specimens based on the position of sutures and inking of margins with different colors

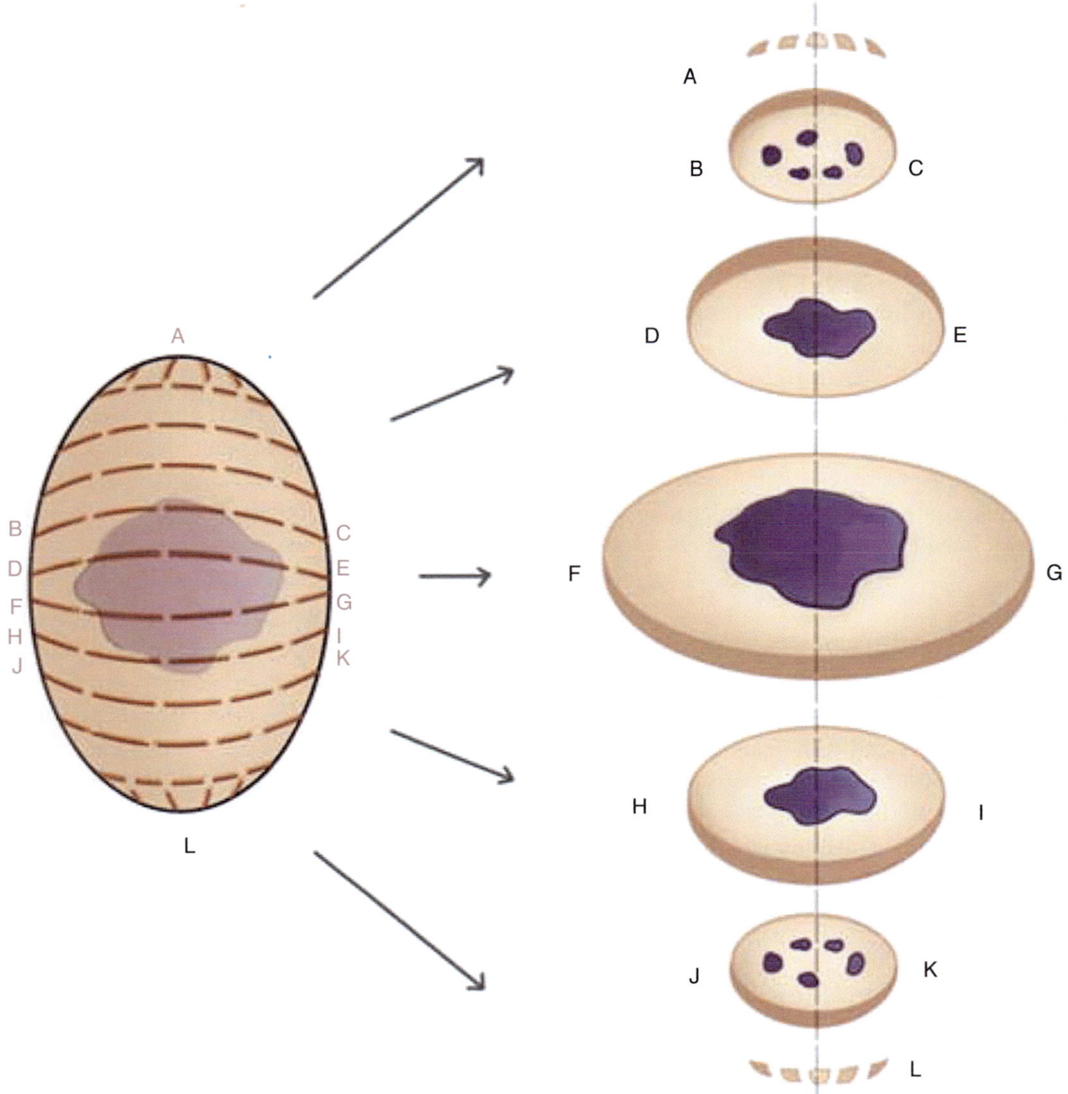

Fig. 13.4 Diagrammatic representation of sections to be submitted in excision specimens

13.6 Wire Localized Specimens

In case of excisions of mammographic nonpalpable lesions that are wire localized at the mammographically abnormal site, a pathologist should discuss the specimen details with the clinicians and receive a copy of the specimen radiograph along with the interpretation. Specimens should be oriented, inked, and margins need to be assessed (Fig. 13.5). Specimens should be bisected along the plane of the wire. Then, one must describe the specimen as done with other excision specimens, sample adequately, and appropriately from the area localized by the wire. Extensive sampling is especially needed in proven Ductal Carcinoma in Situ (DCIS) and Atypical Ductal Hyperplasia (ADH) cases. In large specimens, it may be sufficient to examine initial sections before submitting more tissue. Microscopic sections that need to be submitted are like excision specimens.

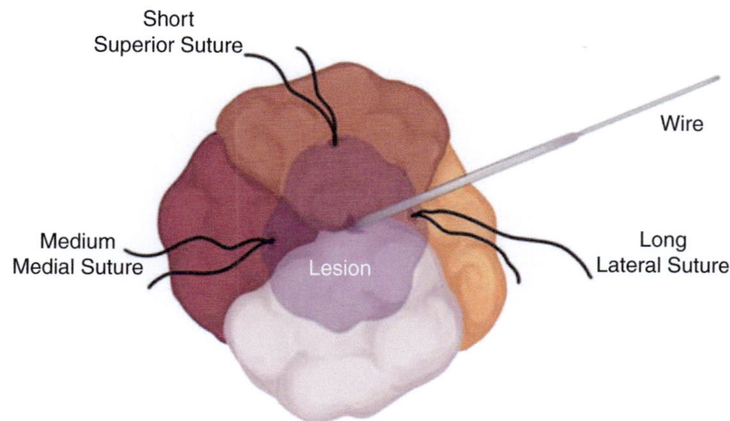

Fig. 13.5 Excisional biopsy of a wire localized specimen

13.7 DCIS

Measuring the extent of DCIS is challenging but extremely important as it directly impacts patient management. No standardized method is available. However, few methods that can be followed include serial sequential sampling method, which is the most accurate method and involves mapping the location of each block on the sliced specimen radiograph and calculating the extent through 3D reconstruction [5]. Other methods include calculating size based on areas of calcification, recording the number of blocks involved by DCIS and multiplying that number by 0.3 cm, and measuring the largest extent of DCIS on a single slide (Fig. 13.6). Microscopic sections are to be submitted from the mass, margins, and normal tissue. In tissues containing mammographic calcifications, entire tissue must be submitted. In the absence of a palpable mass, random bits may be initially submitted, or the specimen may be entirely submitted.

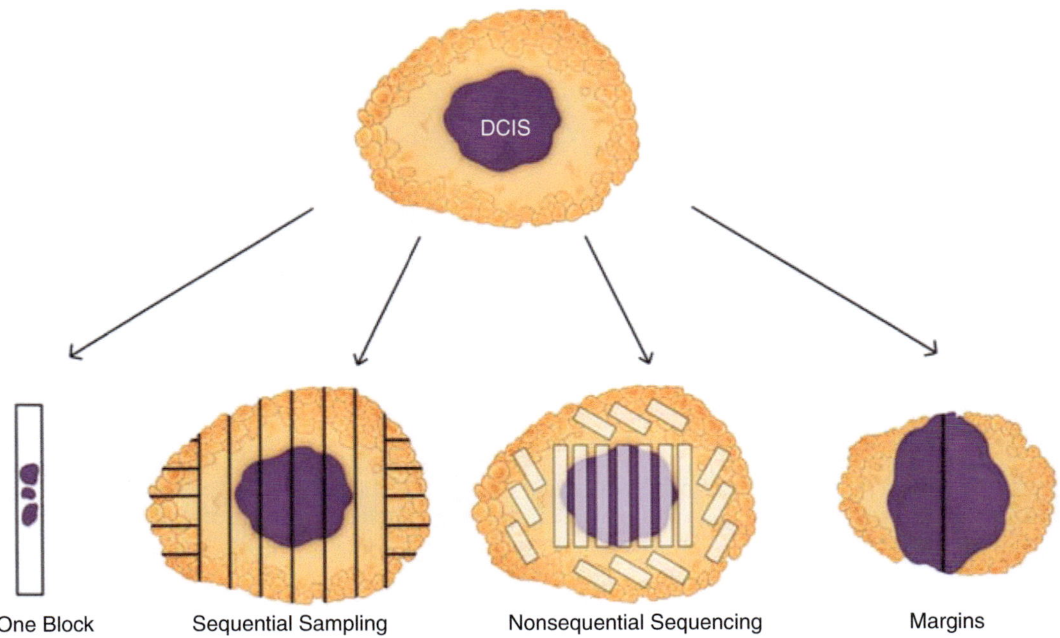

Fig. 13.6 Methods of estimating the size of DCIS

13.8 Mastectomy Specimens

Types of mastectomies include subcutaneous, simple, skin sparing, nipple sparing, modified radical (with axillary dissection), radical (with pectoralis muscle), and prophylactic mastectomy [3]. Care must be taken to orient the specimen, weigh and measure the specimen, describe the skin and nipple areola complex, ink the deep resected margin, and separate the axillary tail if included. The axillary tail must be placed in alcohol to look for nodes. Serial sectioning at 0.5 cm interval is of prime importance. One must look for key features like the size, color, location, and distance from margins (skin and deep margin). In multiple lesions, one must describe the distance between the lesions and submit sections from the intervening tissue after mapping. Nipple sectioning usually includes one perpendicular section; alternatively, it can be amputated in case of abnormal nipple or a history of Paget's disease. Cases in which a prior excision or core biopsy has been performed may be challenging. Hence, radiological correlation and identification of the tumor bed is crucial during sampling.

Cassettes need to be given as follows: one each from nipple areola, deep margin (perpendicular section), skin/scar, lesion bits (1 bit/cm of tumor), one section from each of the 4 quadrants, nipple, and lymph nodes (Fig. 13.7). Checklist formats can be made use of for better reproducibility.

Nipple-sparing mastectomies are processed like other mastectomies. Specimens are oriented, weighed, and measured, following which the entire anterior margin is inked, serially sectioned, and submitted entirely to ensure a negative margin. Other margins are processed as usual. Evaluation of crucial margins is challenging during frozen sections due to histologic freezing artifact; institutional policies may be adopted for evaluating these procedures.

Prophylactic mastectomies may be performed in genetically susceptible women who have mutations in BRCA1 or BRCA2 genes. Correlation with radiological findings and appropriate examination of the specimen is essential. Submission of sections may be based on gross findings in the absence of which representative sections from each quadrant may be submitted [6].

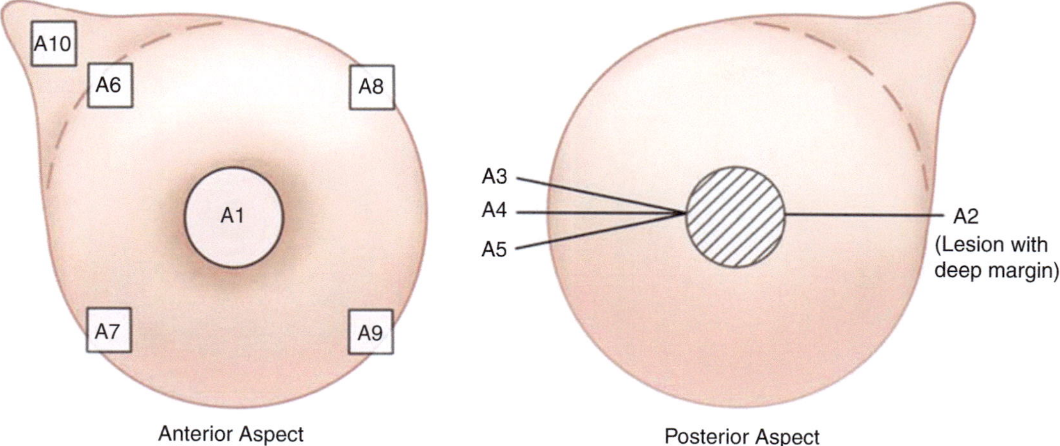

Fig. 13.7 Diagrammatic representation of a sample mastectomy specimen with presence of a 3 cm tumor in the subareolar region (note: scored area is represented as tumor). Examples of bits given from the lesion are as follows: A1—Nipple areola, A2—tumor with deep resected margin, A3 to A5—Tumor bits, A6 to A9—bits from other quadrants, A10—bit from axilla including lymph nodes (more to be given based on the number of nodes identified)

Reduction mammoplasties are mostly bilateral and received as multiple fragments of tissue. It is considered therapeutic if the specimen weighs above 300 g and cosmetic if lesser [3]. Incidence of carcinomas is rare in these specimens. Two sections from each side must be submitted, and any suspicious areas may be additionally sampled. Care must be taken to identify the correct laterality.

13.9 Lymph Node Sampling

Evaluation of lymph nodes in the entire specimen is critical and is an important prognostic indicator. An adequate amount of time needs to be dedicated for retrieving nodes from specimens. The axillary tail containing maximum number of nodes can be placed in alcohol or Bouin's fixative to dissolve the fat and help identify nodes. This process may yield maximum number of nodes required for staging. Ten to twenty nodes are ideal in axillary dissections; if lesser nodes are retrieved, then it is mandatory to have a second look at the specimen. Size of the largest node needs to be recorded, and large nodes must be bisected and completely submitted. Recording the total number of nodes during submission and recording the exact number of nodes placed in each cassette avoids confusion in counting the total number.

References

1. Huo L. A practical approach to grossing breast specimens. Ann Diagn Pathol. 2011;15(4):291–301.
2. Hammond EH, Hayes DF, Dowsett M, Allred DC, Hagerty KL, Badve S, et al. American Society of Clinical oncology/college of American Pathologists guideline recommendations for immunohistochemical testing of estrogen and progesterone receptors in breast cancer. Arch Pathol Lab Med. 2010;134:907–22.
3. Lester SC. Manual of surgical pathology. 3rd ed. Edinburgh: Elsevier; 2006.
4. Selvi R. Breast pathology: approach to handling of surgical resection specimens and reporting. In: Breast diseases. New Delhi: Springer; 2015. p. 223–228
5. Grin A, Horne G, Ennis M, O'Malley FP. Measuring extent of ductal carcinoma in situ in breast excision specimens: a comparison of 4 methods. Arch Pathol Lab Med. 2009;133(1):31–7.
6. Coopey SB, Smith BL. The nipple is just another margin. Ann Surg Oncol. 2015;22(12):3764–6.

14 Pathology Reporting Template

Archana B, V. Pavithra, and Leena Dennis Joseph

Abstract

Pathology reporting of breast cancer specimens need to have all the key essential elements required to plan optimal patient management. These reports serve as an important basis of communication between different departments and hence need to be absolute in all aspects. It is therefore essential to have a comprehensive checklist to avoid missing data, thereby ensuring completeness of the final report. The College of American Pathologists (CAP) have brought out useful checklists ensuring the accomplishment of a perfect report containing all useful information for planning patient care. Here is a summary of key features that can be incorporated in the checklist, which also includes scoring for biomarker reporting and the recently adopted Residual cancer burden (RCB) index for assessing prognosis in patients who have received neoadjuvant chemotherapy.

A. B (✉) · V. Pavithra · L. D. Joseph
Department of Pathology, Sri Ramachandra Medical College, Chennai, India
e-mail: archanab@sriramachandra.edu.in; pavithrav@sriramachandra.edu.in; leenadennisj@sriramachandra.edu.in

Keywords

Breast cancer · Pathology · Report · Biomarker · Scoring · Treatment effect

14.1 Introduction

Pathology reports contain crucial information in deciding the diagnosis, therapy, and prognosis of patients with breast cancers. They serve as an important medium of communication between the Clinician and Pathologist in planning patient care and a vital source of information for researchers and epidemiologists [1]. The use of Template Based Synoptic Reports (TBSRs) of breast resection specimens has brought out a list of essential data required by clinicians, thereby ensuring completeness of data, and reducing missing elements in pathology reports [2]. Professional institutions like the College of American Pathologists (CAP) have brought out valuable reporting templates that assist Pathologists in providing accurate relevant information while reporting surgical cancer specimens of the breast. CAP checklists of reporting are readily available at the CAP website with regular revision and updating of these checklists based on proposed guidelines [3]. Reporting via these checklists is, however, variable based on clinical preference, individual style of reporting, and institutional and regional policies [4].

B. Dev, L. D. Joseph (eds.), *Holistic Approach to Breast Disease*,
https://doi.org/10.1007/978-981-99-0035-0_14

14.2 Pathology Reporting Template for Resected Breast Specimens with Invasive Carcinoma

Below is a reference template which is adopted from the College of American Pathologists (CAP) Protocol for the Examination of Resection Specimens from Patients with Invasive Carcinoma of the Breast [5]:

Surgical pathology cancer case summary-checklist

1. **Procedure**
2. **Specimen Laterality**
3. **Tumor Site**

   Specify the quadrant and the specific clock positions.
4. **Tumor Size**

   Greatest dimension of largest invasive focus >1 mm (specify exact measurement in mm), Additional dimensions: ___ × ___ mm

   (For microinvasion <1 mm)
5. **Histologic Type**

   Special types should contain at least 90% pure pattern
6. **Histologic Grade (Nottingham Histologic Score)** (Fig. 14.1)

   Only microinvasion present (not graded)

   Glandular (Acinar)/Tubular Differentiation

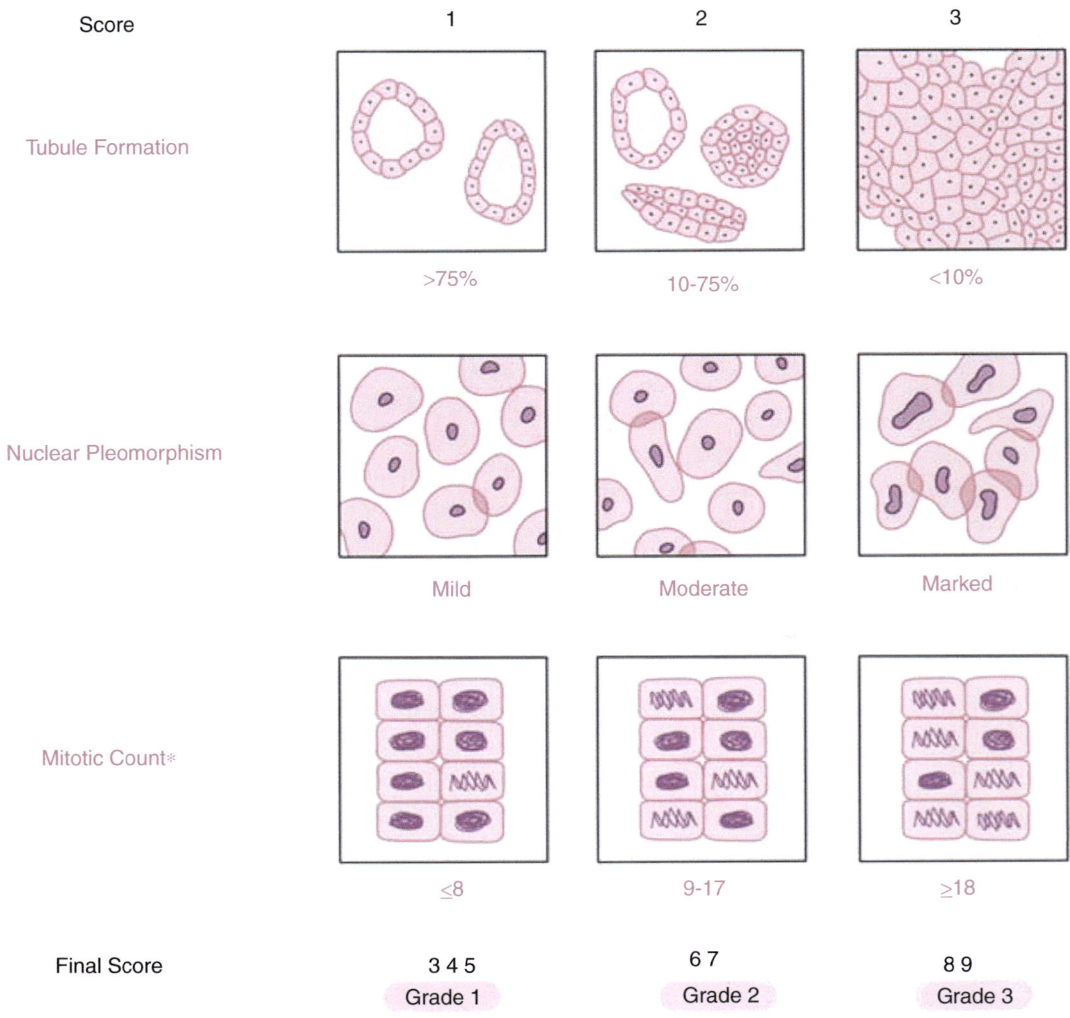

Fig. 14.1 Nottingham histologic score for grading invasive mammary carcinoma

- Score 1 (>75% of tumor area forming glandular/tubular structures)
- Score 2 (10–75% of tumor area forming glandular/tubular structures)
- Score 3 (<10% of tumor area forming glandular/tubular structures)

Nuclear Pleomorphism

- Score 1 (nuclei small with little increase in size in comparison with normal breast epithelial cells, regular outlines, uniform nuclear chromatin, little variation in size)
- Score 2 (cells larger than normal with open vesicular nuclei, visible nucleoli, and moderate variability in both size and shape)
- Score 3 (vesicular nuclei, often with prominent nucleoli, exhibiting marked variation in size and shape, occasionally with very large and bizarre forms)

Mitotic Rate

- Score 1 (<12 mitosis/10 high power fields)
- Score 2 (12–24 mitosis/10 high power fields)
- Score 3 (>25 mitosis/10 high power fields)

Overall Grade

- Grade 1 (scores of 3, 4, or 5)
- Grade 2 (scores of 6 or 7)
- Grade 3 (scores of 8 or 9)

7. **Tumor Focality** (Fig. 14.2)

   In cases with multiple invasive carcinomas, size, grade, histologic type, and the results of studies for estrogen receptor (ER), progesterone receptor (PR), and HER2 should pertain to the largest invasive carcinoma.
8. **Ductal Carcinoma In Situ**

   Specimen Laterality
   Tumor Site
   Size (Extent) of DCIS
   Histologic Type
   - Ductal carcinoma in situ, Paget's disease (DCIS involving nipple)

   Architectural Patterns

   - Comedo
   - Pagets disease (DCIS involving nipple skin)
   - Cribriform
   - Micropapillary
   - Papillary
   - Solid

   Nuclear Grade

   - Grade I (low)
   - Grade II (intermediate)
   - Grade III (high)

   Necrosis

   - Not identified
   - Present, focal (small foci or single cell necrosis)
   - Present, central (expansive "comedo" necrosis)

9. **Lobular Carcinoma In Situ (LCIS)**
10. **Tumor Extension**

    Skin

    - Invasive carcinoma directly invades into the dermis or epidermis without skin ulceration (this does not change the T classification.).
    - Invasive carcinoma directly invades into the dermis or epidermis with skin ulceration (classified as T4b).
    - Satellite skin foci of invasive carcinoma are present (i.e., not contiguous with the invasive carcinoma in the breast) (classified as T4b).

    Nipple
    Skeletal Muscle
    Note: Invasion into pectoralis muscle is not considered chest wall invasion, and cancers are not classified as T4a unless there is invasion deeper than this muscle

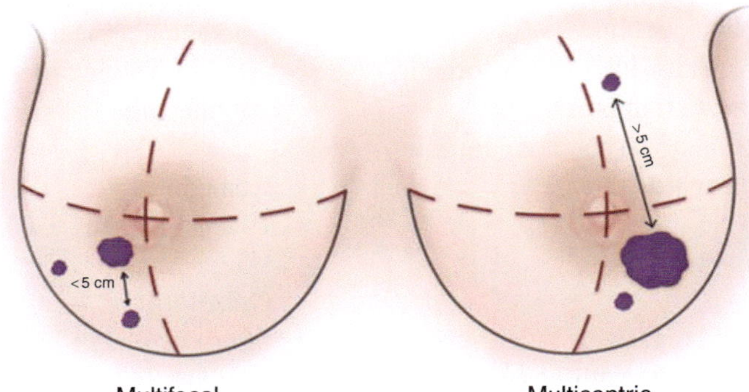

Fig. 14.2 Differentiating between multifocal and multicentric breast carcinoma. In multifocal carcinoma the final grade, histologic subtype, size and molecular profile should pertain to the largest invasive foci. Multiple carcinomas should be prefixed with "m" in the TNM staging. However, bilateral carcinomas should be staged separately

11. **Margins**

    Applicable to DCIS also. Distance from closest margin and specify the closest margin. Distance from other margins (anterior, posterior, superior, inferior, medial, lateral) in millimeters (mm).
12. **Lymphovascular invasion (LVI) and dermal lymphovascular invasion**

    Please note: Use Rosen criteria for LVI based on (1) endothelial lining, (2) LVI should be outside the border of invasive carcinoma, (3) tumor emboli will not conform to the contours of the vessel space, (4) invasion in lymphatic vessel adjacent to blood vessel. This could be confirmed with IHC for CD31 or CD34 [6].
13. **Microcalcifications**; in DCIS/invasive carcinoma or nonneoplastic tissue.
14. **Regional Lymph Nodes involvement** (Fig. 14.3)

    - Number of Lymph Nodes with Macrometastases (>2 mm)
    - Number of Lymph Nodes with Micrometastases (>0.2–2 mm and/or >200 cells)
    - Number of nodes with Isolated Tumor Cells (ITCs) (0.2 mm or less OR 200 cells or less). ITCs are excluded from positive node count for N classification
    - Size of the largest nodal metastatic deposit
    - Extranodal Extension
    - Number of sentinel nodes examined (if applicable)
15. **Distant Metastasis:** Mention the site involved
16. **Treatment Effect in the Breast**

    - No definite response to presurgical therapy in the invasive carcinoma.
    - Probable or definite response to presurgical therapy in the invasive carcinoma.
    - No residual invasive carcinoma is present in the breast after presurgical therapy.

    Treatment Effect in the Lymph Nodes (required if nodes are submitted and it is known that the patient had presurgical therapy)

    - No definite response to presurgical therapy in metastatic carcinoma
    - Probable or definite response to presurgical therapy in metastatic carcinoma
    - No lymph node metastases. Fibrous scarring or histiocytic aggregates, possibly related to prior lymph node metastases with pathologic complete response
    - No lymph node metastases and no fibrous scarring or histiocytic aggregates in the nodes

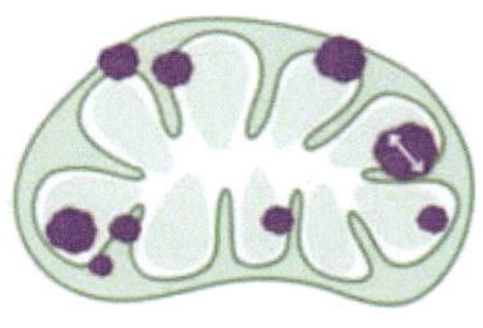

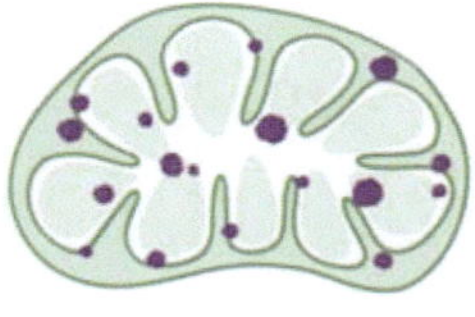

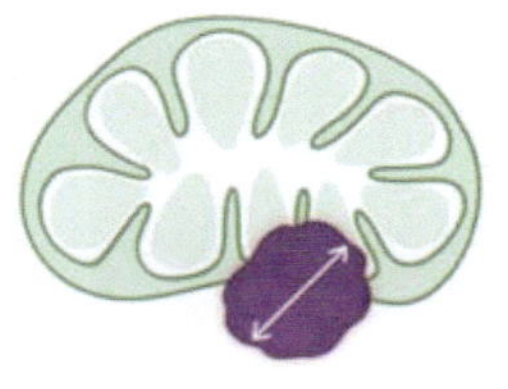

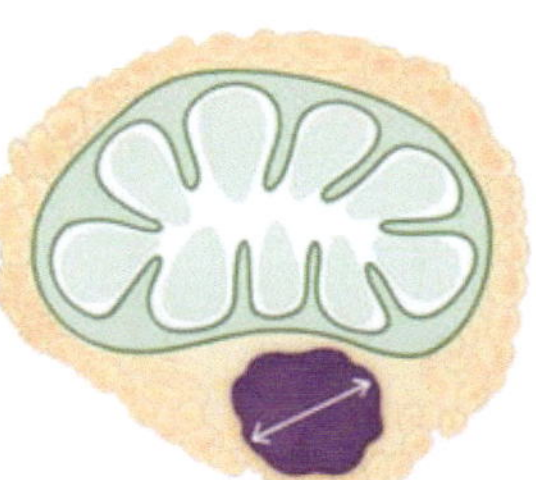

Fig. 14.3 Types of lymph node metastases

Residual cancer burden [7]

Residual cancer burden post neoadjuvant chemotherapy predicts long-term outcome in breast cancer. It is calculated by an online calculator freely available to all Pathologists (www.mdanderson.org/breastcancer_RCB), which categorizes patients into four groups (RCB 0–III) based on tumor bed and lymph nodes. RCB score of 0 corresponds to pathological complete response. RCB I corresponds to minimal burden, RCB II moderate burden, and RCB III extensive burden [8]. Though it has not been incorporated in the CAP protocol, this index scores high in its clinical usefulness for assessing prognosis and in decision making.

17. **Pathologic Stage Classification (pTNM, AJCC 8th Edition)** (Fig. 14.4)

TNM Descriptors (required only if applicable)

m (multiple foci of invasive carcinoma)
r (recurrent)
y (posttreatment)

Primary Tumor (pT)

pTX: Primary tumor cannot be assessed
pT0: No evidence of primary tumor
pTis (DCIS): Ductal carcinoma in situ
pTis (Paget): Paget disease of the nipple not associated with invasive carcinoma and/or DCIS in the underlying breast parenchyma
pT1: Tumor ≤20 mm in greatest dimension
pT1mi: Tumor ≤1 mm in greatest dimension
pT1a: Tumor >1 mm but ≤5 mm in greatest dimension (round any measurement >1.0–1.9–2 mm)
pT1b: Tumor >5 mm but ≤10 mm in greatest dimension
pT1c: Tumor >10 mm but ≤20 mm in greatest dimension
pT2: Tumor >20 mm but ≤50 mm in greatest dimension
pT3: Tumor >50 mm in greatest dimension
pT4: Tumor of any size with direct extension to the chest wall and/or to the skin (ulceration or skin nodules)
pT4a: Extension to the chest wall; invasion or adherence to pectoralis muscle in the absence of invasion of chest wall structures does not qualify as T4
pT4b: Ulceration and/or ipsilateral macroscopic satellite nodules and/or edema (including peau d'orange) of the skin that does not meet the criteria for inflammatory carcinoma
pT4c: Both T4a and T4b are present
pT4d: Inflammatory carcinoma

Regional Lymph Nodes Modifier (required only if applicable)

(sn): Sentinel node(s) evaluated. If six or more nodes (sentinel or non-sentinel) are removed, this modifier should not be used.
(f): Nodal metastasis confirmed by fine needle aspiration or core needle biopsy.

Regional Lymph Nodes (pN)

pNX: Regional lymph nodes cannot be assessed (e.g., not removed for pathological study or previously removed)

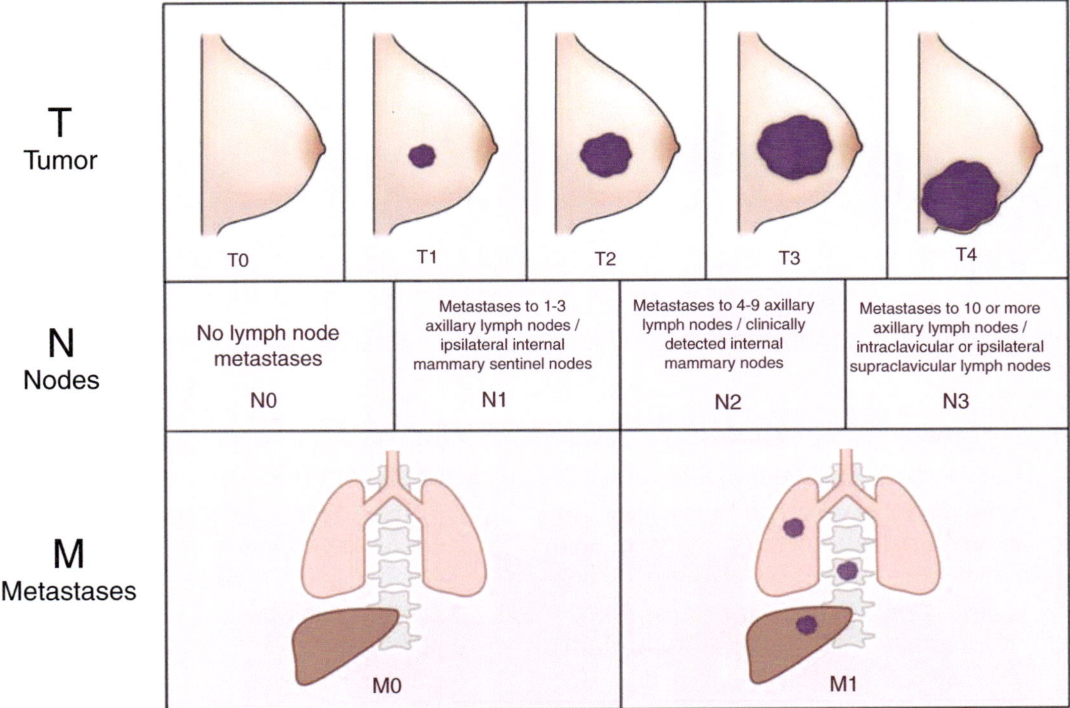

Fig. 14.4 Diagrammatic representation of the TNM staging of breast carcinoma

pN0: No regional lymph node metastasis identified or ITCs (isolated tumor cells) only

pN0 (i+): ITCs only (malignant cell clusters no larger than 0.2 mm) in regional lymph node(s)

N0 (mol+): Positive molecular findings by reverse transcriptase polymerase chain reaction (RT-PCR); no ITCs detected

pN1mi: Micrometastases (approximately 200 cells, larger than 0.2 mm, but none larger than 2.0 mm)

pN1a: Metastases in 1–3 axillary lymph nodes, at least 1 metastasis larger than 2.0 mm

pN1b: Metastases in ipsilateral internal mammary sentinel nodes, excluding ITCs

pN1c: pN1a and pN1b combined

pN2a:Metastases in 4–9 axillary lymph nodes (at least 1 tumor deposit larger than 2.0 mm)

pN2b: Metastases in clinically detected internal mammary lymph nodes with or without microscopic confirmation; with pathologically negative axillary nodes

pN3a: Metastases in 10 or more axillary lymph nodes (at least 1 tumor deposit larger than 2.0 mm) or metastases to the infraclavicular (Level III axillary lymph) nodes

pN3b: pN1a or pN2a in the presence of cN2b (positive internal mammary nodes by imaging); or pN2a in the presence of pN1b

pN3c: Metastases in ipsilateral supraclavicular lymph nodes

Table 14.1 ALLRED scoring for ER and PR. The Intensity and Proportion scores are added together. Scores of 0 and 2 are Negative. Scores 3–8 are Positive

Positive cells %	Proportion score	Intensity	Intensity score
0	0	None	0
<1	1	Weak	1
1–10	2	Intermediate	2
11–33	3	Strong	3
34–66	4		
>67	5		

Distant Metastasis (pM) (required only if confirmed pathologically in this case)

pM1: Histologically proven metastases larger than 0.2 mm

18. **Breast Biomarker reporting**

Estrogen Receptor (ER)/Progesterone Receptor (PR)

- Positive if >1% of cells demonstrate nuclear positivity, mention the percent positivity
- Average intensity of staining: Weak, Moderate, Strong

ASCO and CAP have recommended using scoring systems like the Allred scoring (Table 14.1) for reporting immunohistochemical results of ER and PR [9]. Other scoring systems like the H score provide an overall score ranging from 0 to 300 based on the percentiles of staining (weak, moderate, or strong).

HER2 by Immunohistochemistry

Negative (Score 1+)
Equivocal (Score 2+)
Positive (Score 3+)

HER2 by in situ Hybridization

Negative (not amplified)
Positive (amplified)
Equivocal
(Additional information can be added like number of observers, number of invasive tumor cells counted, average number of HER2 signals per cell, average number of CEP17 signals per cell, HER2:CEP17 ratio)

Ki-67%

Percentage of cells with nuclear positivity

Androgen Receptor (AR)

Positive or negative (nuclear positivity)

EGFR/CK5

Positive or negative (cytoplasmic/membranous)

Note: Additional ancillary studies for E cadherin, p63, p53, etc., may be performed based on specific tumor types

14.3 Reporting Template for Trucut Biopsy

Trucut biopsies are frequently received in the Pathology department. It should contain adequate information so that the Clinician can plan the appropriate management. Reporting of trucut biopsies should include the following:

- Tumor laterality based on clinical examination
- Histological type
- Histological grade (Nottingham histologic grade)
- DCIS/LCIS
- Lymph vascular invasion
- Ancillary biomarker test results (Panel of ER, PR, Her 2 neu, Ki67%, AR, EGFR/CK5)

References

1. Kadivar M, Rahimabad PK. Missing elements in surgical pathology reports: breast, colon and stomach cancers. Asian Pac J Cancer Prev. 2016;17(3):1469–72.
2. Aumann K, Niermann K, Asberger J, Wellner U, Bronsert P, Erbes T, Hauschke D, Stickeler E, Gitsch G, Kayser G, Werner M. Structured reporting ensures complete content and quick detection of essential data in pathology reports of oncological breast resection specimens. Breast Cancer Res Treat. 2016;156(3):495–500.
3. Goldsmith JD, Siegal GP, Suster S, Wheeler TM, Brown RW. Reporting guidelines for clinical laboratory reports in surgical pathology. Arch Pathol Lab Med. 2008;132(10):1608–16.
4. Lester SC, Bose S, Chen YY, Connolly JL, de Baca ME, Fitzgibbons PL, Hayes DF, Kleer C, O'Malley FP, Page DL, Smith BL. Protocol for the examination of specimens from patients with ductal carcinoma in situ of the breast. Arch Pathol Lab Med. 2009;133(1):15–25.
5. College of American Pathologist. Protocol for the examination of resection specimens from patients with invasive carcinoma of the breast version: breast invasive resection 4.5.0.1. Northfield: CAP; 2021.
6. Rosen PP. Tumor emboli in intramammary lymphatics in breast carcinoma: pathologic criteria for diagnosis and clinical significance. Pathol Ann. 1983;18:215–32.
7. Yau C, Osdoit M, van der Noordaa M, Shad S, Wei J, de Croze D, Hamy AS, Laé M, Reyal F, Sonke GS, Steenbruggen TG. Residual cancer burden after neoadjuvant chemotherapy and long-term survival outcomes in breast cancer: a multicentre pooled analysis of 5161 patients. Lancet Oncol. 2022;23(1):149–60.
8. Symmans WF, Wei C, Gould R, Yu X, Zhang Y, Liu M, Walls A, Bousamra A, Ramineni M, Sinn B, Hunt K. Long-term prognostic risk after neoadjuvant chemotherapy associated with residual cancer burden and breast cancer subtype. J Clin Oncol. 2017;35(10):1049.
9. Fitzgibbons PL, Dillon DA, Alsabeh R, Berman MA, Hayes DF, Hicks DG, Hughes KS, Nofech-Mozes S. Template for reporting results of biomarker testing of specimens from patients with carcinoma of the breast. Arch Pathol Lab Med. 2014;138(5):595–601.

Overview of Immunohistochemistry in Breast Lesions

15

V. Pavithra, Sandhya Sundaram, and Archana B

Abstract

Many advances and extensive analysis had been focused around the diagnostic protocol development in breast carcinoma over a decade. Testing for various markers on the initial biopsies, prior to definitive surgery, assists in planning management and is critical for the increasing number of cases in which neoadjuvant chemotherapy is being considered. This chapter will discuss on the current immunohistochemistry recommendations on prognostic marker testing of breast carcinoma.

Keywords

Immunohistochemistry · Prognostic marker · Breast cancer

15.1 Hormone Receptor Testing [1]

15.1.1 Estrogen Receptor (ER) and Progesterone Receptor (PgR) Testing

Normal breast epithelial cells have these receptors for estrogen and progesterone, which promotes the proliferation under their influence. Most of the breast carcinomas also express these receptors and may be stimulated to grow by these hormones. Removal of endogenous hormones by oophorectomy or blocking hormonal action pharmaceutically (e.g., with tamoxifen or aromatase inhibitors) can slow or prevent tumor growth and prolong survival.

Hormone receptor status is determined primarily to identify patients who may benefit from hormonal therapy. About 75–80% of invasive breast cancers are positive for ER and PgR (Table 15.1), including almost all well-differentiated cancers and most moderately differentiated cancers and studies have shown a substantial survival benefit from endocrine therapy among patients with ER-positive tumors. True ER-negative, PgR-positive carcinomas are extremely rare, but patients with such tumors are also considered eligible for hormonal therapy. Receptor status is only a weak prognostic factor.

V. Pavithra (✉) · S. Sundaram · A. B
Department of Pathology, Sri Ramachandra Medical College, Chennai, India
e-mail: pavithrav@sriramachandra.edu.in; archanab@sriramachandra.edu.in

B. Dev, L. D. Joseph (eds.), *Holistic Approach to Breast Disease*,
https://doi.org/10.1007/978-981-99-0035-0_15

Table 15.1 Reporting results of Estrogen Receptor (ER) and Progesterone Receptor (PgR) testing (American Society of Clinical Oncology [ASCO] and College of American Pathologists [CAP] guidelines) [2]

Result	Criteria	Comments
Positive	Immunoreactive tumor cells present (≥1%)	Invasive carcinomas with 1–10% of cells staining for ER (not PR) should be reported as "Low Positive" and the comment to be added in the report is as follows: "The cancer in this sample has a low level (1–10%) of ER expression by immunohistochemistry (IHC). There is limited data on the overall benefit of endocrine therapies for patients with low level (1–10%) ER expression, but they currently suggest possible benefit, so patients are considered eligible for endocrine treatment. There are data that suggest invasive cancers with these results are heterogeneous in both behavior and biology and often have gene expression profiles more similar to ER-negative cancers" The Low Positive applies only to invasive carcinoma, and it is not to be used for Progesterone receptor or DCIS
Negative	<1% immunoreactive tumor cells present	

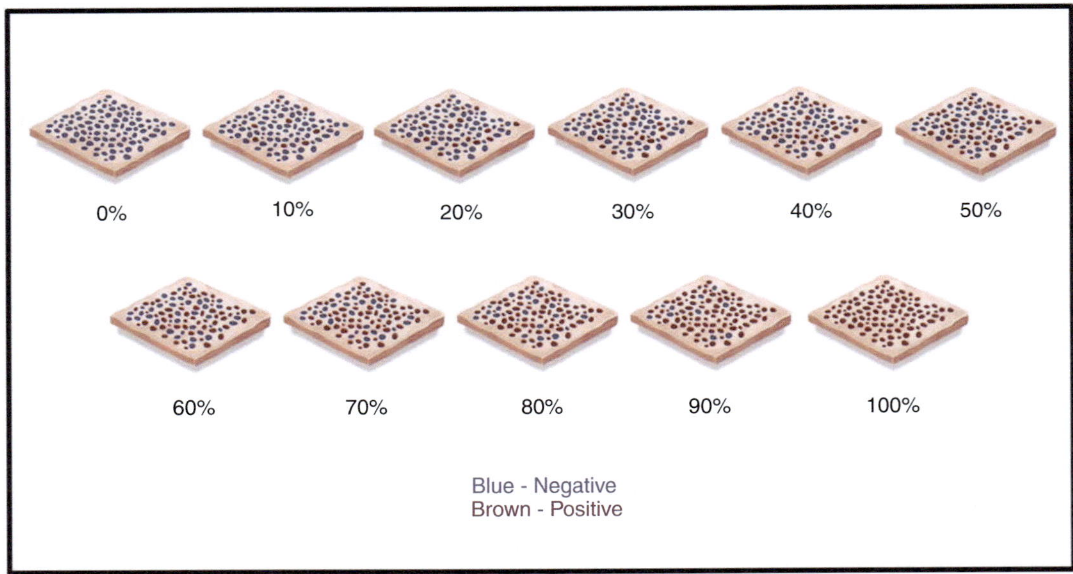

Fig. 15.1 Quantification of immunohistochemical findings. The percentage of positive cells can be visually estimated

15.1.2 Quantification of ER and PgR

- Number of positive cells: The number of positive cells can be reported as a percentage or within discrete categories (Fig. 15.1).
- Intensity: Refers to degree of nuclear positivity (i.e., pale to dark) (Fig. 15.2).

Two methods of quantifying ER by using both intensity and percentage of positive cells are the Allred score (Table 15.2) and the H score (Table 15.3). The two systems classify carcinomas into similar, but not identical, groups [2].

15.1.3 HER2 (*ERBB2*) Testing

A subset of breast carcinomas (approximately 15–20%) overexpress human epidermal growth factor receptor 2 (HER2; HUGO nomenclature

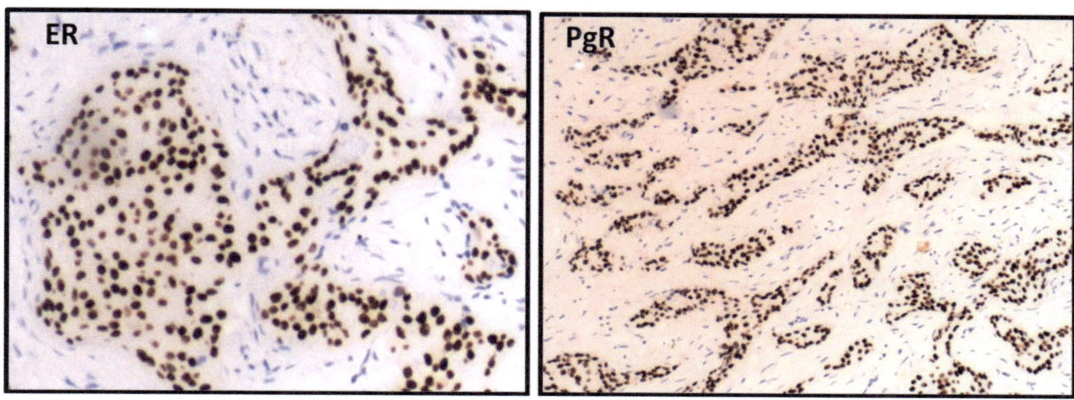

Fig. 15.2 Immunohistochemistry ER (Estrogen Receptor) and PgR (Progesterone Receptor): nuclear positivity

Table 15.2 Allred Score[a] for estrogen and progesterone receptor evaluation

Proportion score	Positive cells %	Intensity	Intensity score
0	0	None	0
1	<1	Weak	1
2	1–10	Intermediate	2
3	11–33	Strong	3
4	34–66		
5	≥67		

[a] The Allred score combines the percentage of positive cells and the intensity of the reaction product in most of the carcinoma cases. The two scores have to be added together for a final score. Scores of 0 and 2 are considered negative. Scores of 3–8 are considered positive

Table 15.3 H score[a] for estrogen and progesterone receptor evaluation

	Calculation of H score	
Cell signal	Percentage of cells	Value multiplied
Cells with no signal		% × 0 = 0
Cells with weak signal		% × 1 =
Cells with moderate signal		% × 2 =
Cells with strong signal		% × 3 =
Total score =		

[a] The H score is determined by multiplying the percentage of cells demonstrating ER and PgR each intensity (scored from 0–3) and adding the results. There are 300 possible values. In this system, <1% positive cells is considered to be a negative result

ERBB2). Protein overexpression is usually due to gene amplification. Assays for gene copy number, mRNA quantity, and protein generally give similar results; gene amplification correlates with protein overexpression in about 95% of cases. In a small subset of carcinomas (probably <5%), protein overexpression may occur by different mechanisms. Overexpression is both a prognostic and predictive factor.

HER2 status is primarily evaluated to determine patient eligibility for anti-HER2 therapy. It may identify patients who have a greater benefit from anthracycline-based adjuvant therapy.

Methods: HER2 status can be determined in formalin-fixed, paraffin-embedded tissue by assessing protein expression on the membrane of tumor cells using IHC (Table 15.4) (Fig. 15.3) or by assessing the number of HER2 gene copies using in situ hybridization (ISH) (Tables 15.5 and 15.6). When both IHC and ISH are performed on the same tumor, the results should be correlated.

Table 15.4 Reporting results of HER2 Testing by Immunohistochemistry (IHC) (ASCO and CAP guidelines) [2]

Result	Criteria
Negative (Score 0)	No staining observed *or* Membrane staining that is incomplete and is faint/barely perceptible and within ≤10% of tumor cells
Negative (Score 1+)	Incomplete membrane staining that is faint/barely perceptible and within >10% of tumor cells[a]
Equivocal (Score 2+)[b]	Weak to moderate complete membrane staining in >10% of tumor cells *or* Complete membrane staining that is intense but within ≤10% of tumor cells[a]
Positive (Score 3+)	Complete membrane staining that is intense and > 10% of tumor cells[a]

[a] Readily appreciated using a low-power objective and observed within a homogeneous and contiguous population of invasive tumor cells

[b] Correlation with histologic and other biomarker results. If the HER2 test is negative by IHC, but the tumor has characteristics associated with HER2 positivity (see above), repeating the test by ISH should be considered.

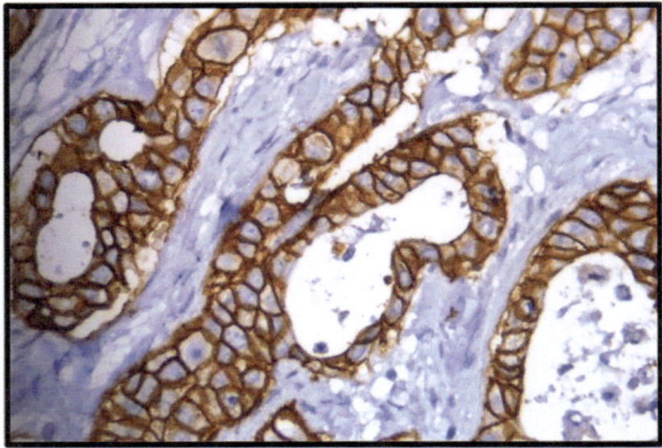

Fig. 15.3 Immunohistochemistry HER2 (ERBB2) receptor: membrane positivity

Table 15.5 Reporting results of *HER2* testing by in situ hybridization (single-probe assay)

Result	Criteria (single-probe assay)
Negative	• Average HER2 copy number <4.0 signals/cell • Average HER2 copy number ≥4.0 and <6.0 signals/cell and concurrent IHC 0, 1+ or 2+ • Average HER2 copy number ≥4.0 and <6.0 signals/cell and concurrent dual probe ISH Group 5
Positive	• Average HER2 copy number ≥6.0 signals/cell • Average HER2 copy number ≥4.0 and <6.0 signals/cell and concurrent IHC 3+ • Average HER2 copy number ≥4.0 and <6.0 signals/cell and concurrent dual probe ISH Group 1

Table 15.6 Reporting results of *HER2* testing by in situ hybridization (dual-probe assay) (Fig. 15.4)

Result	Criteria (dual-probe assay)
Negative	• Group 5
Negative[a] (see comment)	• Group 2 and concurrent IHC 0–1+ or 2+ • Group 3 and concurrent IHC 0–1+ • Group 4 and concurrent IHC 0–1+ or 2+
Positive[a]	• Group 2 and concurrent IHC 3+ • Group 3 and concurrent IHC 2+ or 3+ • Group 4 and concurrent IHC 3+
Positive	• Group 1

[a] For Groups 2–4 final ISH results are based on concurrent review of IHC, with recounting of the ISH test by a second reviewer if IHC is 2+ (per 2018 CAP/ASCO Update recommendations)

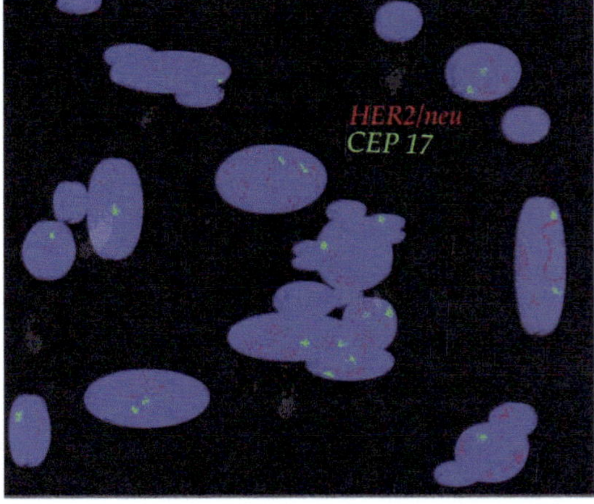

Fig. 15.4 HER2 Testing by in situ hybridization (dual-probe assay)

15.1.4 HER2 (ERBB2) Testing by Immunohistochemistry

Must order reflex test (same specimen using ISH) or order a new test (new specimen if available, using IHC or ISH).

15.1.5 HER2 Testing by In Situ Hybridization [2]

Fluorescence in situ hybridization (FISH), chromogenic in situ hybridization (CISH), and silver-enhanced in situ hybridization (SISH) studies for *HER2* determine the presence or absence of gene amplification. Some assays use a single probe to determine the number of HER2 gene copies present, but most assays include a chromosome enumeration probe (CEP17) to determine the ratio of HER2 signals to copies of chromosome 17. Although 10–50% of breast carcinomas have more than 2 CEP17 copies, only 1–2% of carcinomas show true polysomy (i.e., duplication of the entire chromosome).

Reporting guidelines: ASCO and CAP have issued recommendations for reporting the results of HER2 testing by ISH.

Dual Probe ISH Group Definitions

- Group 1 = HER2/CEP17 ratio ≥ 2.0; ≥4.0 HER2 signals/cell
- Group 2 = HER2/CEP17 ratio ≥ 2.0; <4.0 HER2 signals/cell
- Group 3 = HER2/CEP17 ratio < 2.0; ≥6.0 HER2 signals/cell
- Group 4 = HER2/CEP17 ratio < 2.0; ≥4.0 and <6.0 HER2 signals/cell
- Group 5 = HER2/CEP17 ratio < 2.0; <4.0 HER2 signals/cell

15.2 Other Markers [3]

15.2.1 Epidermal Growth Factor Receptor

Epidermal growth factor receptor (EGFR, also HER1) (Fig. 15.5) is a type 1 tyrosine kinase receptor that is expressed in normal breast. The frequency of detection by immunohistochemistry, which has membranous staining in breast cancers, varies between different studies and can range from 15% to >60%.The presence of EGFR in breast cancers is associated with a lack of ER and poor prognostic features. Tyrosine kinase inhibitors of EGFR, such as gefitinib, are now available for targeted therapy.

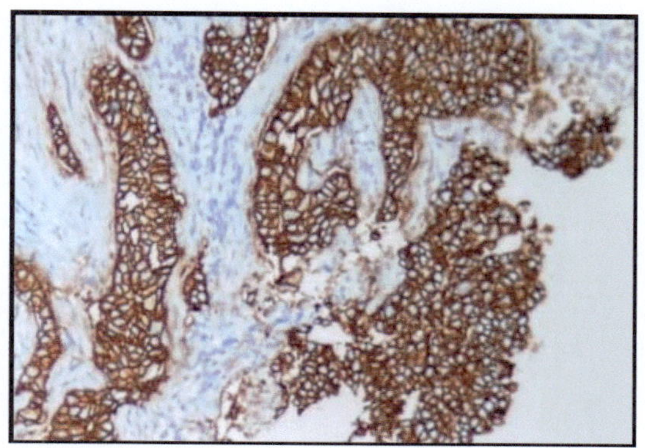

Fig. 15.5 Immunohistochemistry epidermal growth factor receptor (EGFR): membrane positivity

15.2.2 Basal Markers

Immunohistochemistry markers often used for identifying basal-like tumors include basal cytokeratins (CK5/6, CK5, CK14, and CK17). In particular, positivity of CK5/6 can be helpful in diagnosing ER$^-$/PR$^-$/HER2$^-$ poorly differentiated or undifferentiated invasive carcinomas of the breast as basal-like triple-negative breast cancers, especially in the core biopsy setting in which in situ lesions may be absent. In addition, a small proportion of high-grade DCIS cases demonstrate a triple-negative phenotype (ER$^-$/PR$^-$/HER2$^-$), and those lesions more commonly show expression of CK5/6 and/or EGFR. CK5/6 and EGFR positivity also helps in a diagnosis of basal-like DCIS, which may represent a precursor lesion to an invasive, basal-like TNBC.

High-level expression of CK5/6 and EGFR may have a role in the development of nodal or distant metastases in basal-like TNBCs and may be predictive of metastatic disease.

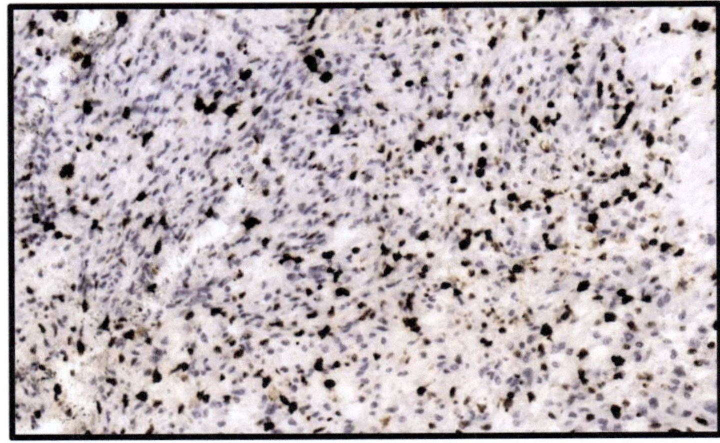

Fig. 15.6 Immunohistochemistry Ki 67 proliferative marker: nuclear positivity

15.2.3 Proliferation Marker

The **Ki-67** antigen is expressed in the nucleus of cells (Fig. 15.6) in all phases of the cell cycle and is a useful marker of cell proliferation and is used for prognostication.

Changes in Ki-67 expression following preoperative endocrine treatment can predict long-term outcome.

Other proliferation markers that have been evaluated immunohistochemically in breast cancer include **cyclin E**, **cyclin D1**, **p21**, and **p27**, but there is no strong evidence for their use as predictive markers outside of clinical research.

15.2.4 Androgen Receptor

Androgen receptor (AR) expression has been shown to have prognostic implications in breast cancers, and higher AR expression levels have been associated with higher expression of ER or PR, lower nuclear grade, and smaller tumors, with lower risk of recurrence and death. Significant differences in AR protein nuclear expression (Fig. 15.7) have been detected in the various molecular subtypes of breast cancers. Triple-negative breast cancers, which are by nature ER^-, characteristically have much lower frequency of AR expression compared with ER^+ breast cancers.

15.2.5 Apoptotic Proteins and p53

As with proliferation markers, there have been many immunohistochemical studies evaluating expression of apoptotic proteins including **bcl-2**, **bax**, **bcl-x**, and **survivin**, but for various reasons including availability of suitable antibodies, methods of evaluation, and lack of strong evidence, these are not suitable as routine predictive markers.

p53 has been considered as a potential predictor of response of breast cancers to chemotherapy, but much of the data comes from mutation analysis. Immunohistochemistry detects stabilized p53 protein, which may reflect a mutation but will not detect protein truncation mutations; there are also problems in evaluation and defining what is positive.

15.2.5.1 GATA 3

GATA3, a zinc-binding transcription factor that regulates the differentiation of many human tissue types, including the mammary gland, is a novel, sensitive, and specific marker for primary breast carcinomas with up to 94% sensitivity, especially for those that are ER positive. GATA3 has been widely used as a breast marker in routine clinical practice and is particularly useful in the workup of metastatic TNBCs, because ER, PR, or HER2 by IHC cannot serve as markers for detection.

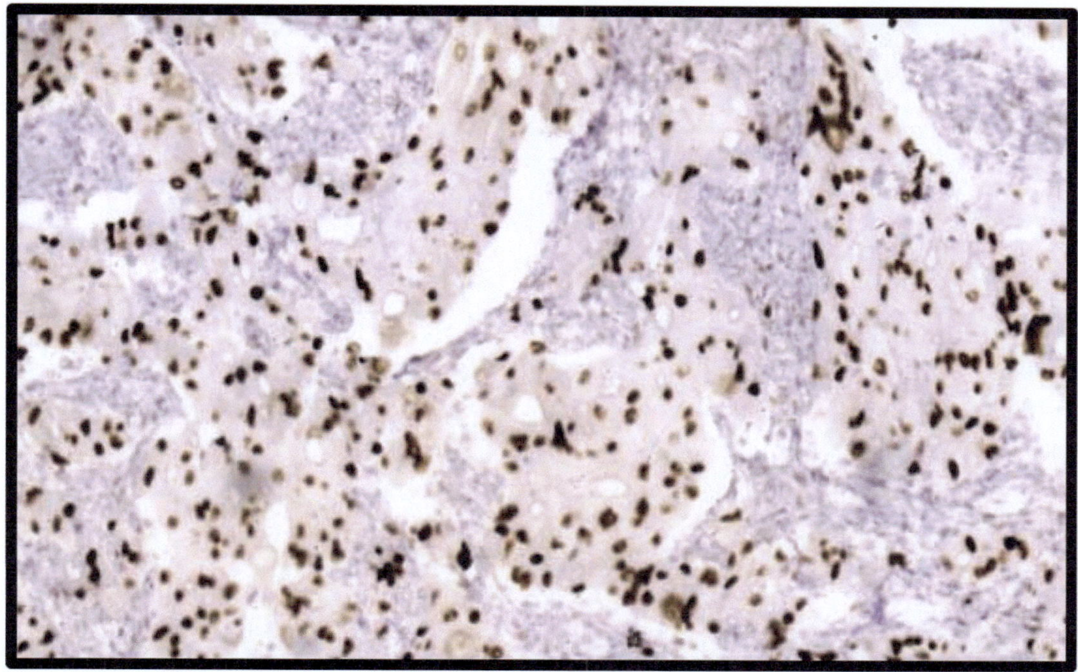

Fig. 15.7 Immunohistochemistry androgen receptor (AR): nuclear positivity

15.2.5.2 PELP1

PELP1 is a novel coregulator of nuclear hormone receptors that has a role in driving breast cancer and enhancing metastatic potential. In addition, the diffuse, strong nuclear immunoreactivity of PELP1 in triple-negative breast cancer (TNBC) suggests that PELP1 may be a potential molecular target for treatment of TNBC.

15.2.5.3 Cyclin E

Cancer proliferation is fundamentally related to an altered regulation of the cell cycle, and cyclin E is an important regulator of the cell cycle and its overexpression was associated with a poor prognosis in breast cancer. Cyclin E protein expression was higher in TNBCs than in non-TNBCs, and it was positively correlated with Ki-67 expression in both TNBCs and non-TNBCs. These findings suggest that cyclin E expression may be associated with tumor aggressiveness in TNBCs.

15.2.5.4 p16 [4]

p16 normally acts as a cyclin-dependent kinase (CDK) inhibitor by inactivating CDK4/6 and preventing the phosphorylation of retinoblastoma (Rb). p16 is a tumor suppressor protein, which plays an important role in cell cycle regulation. p16 by IHC is widely used as a surrogate marker for high-risk HPV infection in diagnosing high-grade dysplasia and squamous cell carcinoma of the cervix and the oropharynx. Recent studies demonstrated that a strong and diffuse p16 expression was seen in the majority of triple-negative breast cancers.

15.2.6 Myoepithelial Markers [5]

The myopeithelial markers that most effectively combine sensitivity, specificity, and ease of interpretation include smooth muscle myosin heavy chains, calponin, p75, p63 (Fig. 15.8), P-cadherin, basal cytokeratins, maspin, Smooth Muscle Myosin Heavy Chains (SMMHC), and CD10. The most common use of myoepithelial markers is to establish the presence or absence of an invasive carcinoma.

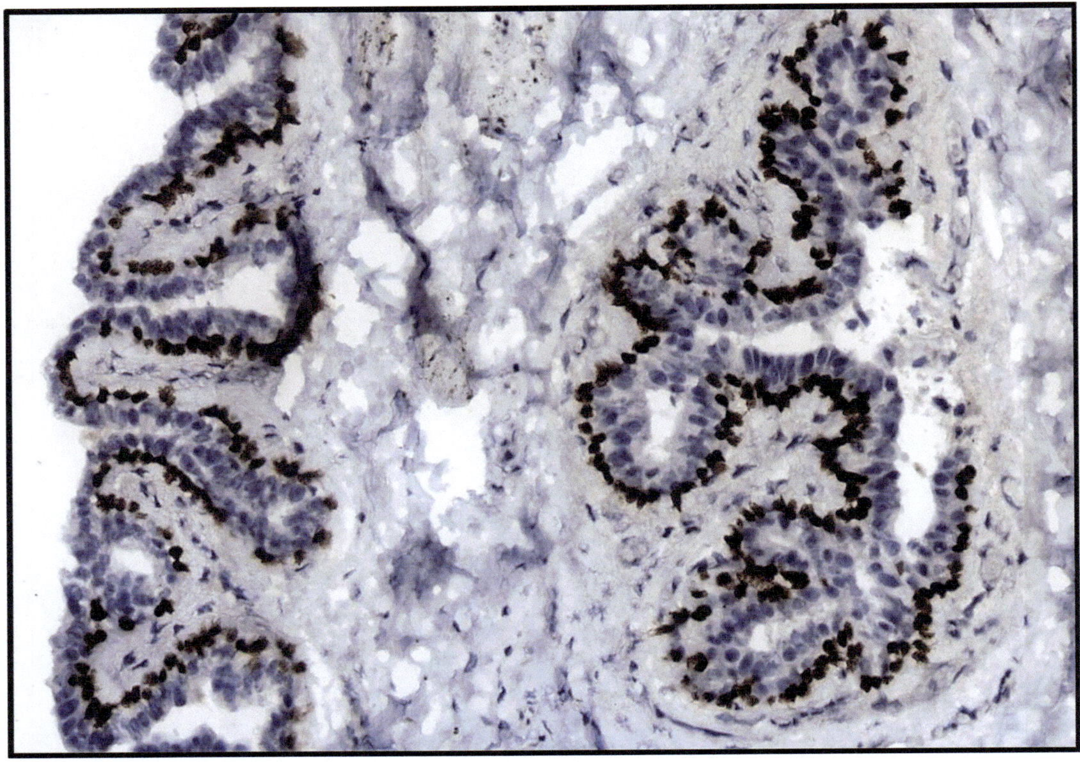

Fig. 15.8 Immunohistochemistry p63 (Myoepithelial Marker): nuclear positivity

References

1. Walker RA. Immunohistochemical markers as predictive tools for breast cancer. J Clin Pathol. 2008;61(6):689–96.
2. Breast Biomarker Reporting—CAP Protocol 2021.
3. Hagemann IS. Molecular testing in breast cancer: a guide to current practices. Arch Pathol Lab Med. 2016;140(8):815–24.
4. Bohn OL, Fuertes-Camilo M, Navarro L, Saldivar J, Sanchez-Sosa S. p16INK4a expression in basal-like breast carcinoma. Int J Clin Exp Pathol. 2010;3(6):600–7.
5. Liu H. Application of immunohistochemistry in breast pathology: a review and update. Arch Pathol Lab Med. 2014;138(12):1629–42.

16 Molecular Classification of Breast Cancer and Liquid Biopsy

V. Pavithra, Sandhya Sundaram, and Mala Gera

Abstract

There are underlying genetic alterations and the biological events involved in cancer development and progression that are quite complex. A detailed biological characterization of genomic alterations may aid prognostication with risk stratification and thus tailoring better treatment plans for patients. In this chapter, molecular testing with liquid biopsy is provided for novel targeted treatment directed at the underlying molecular aberrations, driving individual tumor growth. Many molecular research studies have provided evidence to support the existence of multiple pathways of development in breast cancers; different subgroups are associated with specific patterns of genetic alterations.

Keywords

Genomic alterations · Liquid biopsy · Molecular · Breast cancer

V. Pavithra (✉) · S. Sundaram
Department of Pathology, Sri Ramachandra Medical College, Chennai, India
e-mail: pavithrav@sriramachandra.edu.in

M. Gera
Clinipath Labs, Osborne Park, WA, Australia

16.1 Molecular Pathways of Carcinogenesis

The breast cancers recently are therapeutically approached and treated on the basis of the classification of breast carcinoma by molecular analysis (Table 16.1).

ER-positive cancers frequently exhibit deletions of 16q and gains of 1q, which are uncommon in ER-negative cancers and the latter group also tends to be unstable with a high incidence of p53 mutations, HER2 amplifications, and BRCA1 dysfunction. New evidence has also emerged to suggest that ER-positive tumors can progress from low to high grade with up to 50% of Grade 3 tumors harboring identical 16q and 1q alterations as grade 1 ER-positive cancers, indicative of a common pathway of carcinogenesis.

Current evidence also indicates that lobular cancers are genetically very similar to ductal cancers; they also exhibit 16q and 1q alterations but additionally reveal loss of E-cadherin expression in the lobular phenotype. Flat epithelial atypia, atypical ductal hyperplasia, and lobular in situ neoplasias also show similar molecular profiles and frequently coexist in the same tumor, pointing to a common pathway of progression in low-grade lesions.

B. Dev, L. D. Joseph (eds.), *Holistic Approach to Breast Disease*,
https://doi.org/10.1007/978-981-99-0035-0_16

Table 16.1 Classification of breast carcinoma based on immunohistochemistry/molecular analysis [1]

Intrinsic subtype	Gene profile	Molecular findings	IHC phenotype	Histologic subtypes
Luminal A	High expression of luminal epithelial genes and ER-related genes	Mutations in PI3CKA, MAPK3K1 and GATA 3; CCDN1 amplification	ER+, PgR ≥20%, Her2-, Ki67 low	Tubular carcinoma, low-grade IDC-NST, classic ILC
Luminal B	Low expression of luminal epithelial genes and ER-related genes but high level of proliferation and Her2-related genes than luminal A	Similar to Luminal A with high TP53 and RB pathways inactivation as well as Myc-related and FOXM1-related transcription	ER+, PgR ≤20%, Her2+ or Ki67 high	IDC-NST Micropapillary carcinoma Pleomorphic ILC
Her2 neu enriched	High expression of Her2 neu-related genes and low expression of ER-related genes	Her2 amplicon and EGFR/Her2 signal protein signature	ER–, PgR, Her2+	High-grade IDC-NST, pleomorphic ILC
Basal like	High expression of basal epithelial and proliferation genes, low expression of Her2-related and ER-related genes	Mutation in TP53, losses in RB1 and BRCA 1, amplification of MYC, high PI3K/AKT pathway activation	ER–, PgR–,Her2–	High-grade IDC-NST, metaplastic carcinoma, medullary carcinoma, adenoid cystic carcinoma

IDC NST invasive ductal carcinoma nonspecific type, *ILC* invasive lobular carcinoma

16.2 Prognostic and Predictive Molecular Tests in Breast Carcinoma

On the basis of the commercially available kits, further prognostic and predictive factors are assessed in breast carcinoma for the clinical utility (Table 16.2).

Several multigene assays have been developed in an attempt to identify the low-risk and high-risk subset of patients. Oncotype DX (Genomic Health, Redwood City, CA) and MammaPrint are the most common tests in routine use.

A 70 gene prognostic signature forms the basis for the MammaPrint™ assay (Agendia BV, Amsterdam, The Netherlands); this assay uses microarray-based gene expression profiling. The Microarray In Node-negative Disease may Avoid ChemoTherapy (MINDACT) uses standard clinico-pathologic prognostic factors and 70-gene MammaPrint assay to assess patients for adjuvant therapy.

A 21-gene multiplex high-throughput, real-time, reverse-transcriptase–polymerase-chain-reaction (RT-PCR) method on fixed, paraffin-embedded archival tumor blocks form the basis for the ONCOTYPE DX test. The test is used to determine the 10-year risk of disease recurrence in ER-positive, lymph-node-negative tumors by using a continuous variable algorithm and assigning a tripartite Recurrence Score (RS). The test comprises a panel of 16 cancer-related genes and 5 reference genes. Proliferation-related and ER pathways were found to maximally influence the RS calculation followed by the HER2 pathway. The assay has now been studied in lymph-node-positive patients with promising results. DNA microarrays require the use of fresh or snap-frozen tissue, restricting their clinical usefulness.

Current National Comprehensive Cancer Network (NCCN) guidelines advise chemotherapy for patients with a high recurrence score. An intermediate RS proves a problem, as it represents a therapeutic gray zone.

The cost of these assays is high compared with traditional pathology testing; their benefit over conventional clinicopathologic predictive factors is limited to cancers with intermediate features. The RS calculation used in Oncotype DX testing primarily relies on proliferation-related markers followed by ER, PR, and HER2.

There is now evidence suggesting that algorithms based on conventional factors, such as levels of ER, PR, and HER2, as assessed by IHC, histologic grade, and proliferation index markers, such as Ki67, may be used to predict RS.

Table 16.2 Commercially available prognostic/predictive multigene tests for invasive breast carcinoma

	Mamma print	PAM50 (breast bioclassifiers)	MapQuant Dx/simplified	Oncotype Dx	Breast cancer index	Endo predict
Analysis	Microarray	qRT-PCR	Microarray/qRT-PCR	qRT-PCR	qRT-PCR	qRT-PCR
Tissue type	Fresh /frozen	FFPE	Fresh /frozen/FFPE	FFPE	FFPE	FFPE
Assay	70-gene signature	50-gene signature	97-gene signature or 8 gene PCR	21 gene RS	2 gene	8 cancer 3 control
Clinical indications	0–3 nodes positive <5 cm All ages ER+/–	Stage I–III All ages ER+/–	ER+ Histologic grade 2	ER+ 0 to 3 nodes positive Treated with Tamoxifen	ER+ Node negative All ages	Early stage ER+ Her2 breast cancer treated with Tamoxifen
Prognostic/ predictive value	Prognostic for early distant recurrence within first 5 years after diagnosis Predictive for chemoresponse in poor prognostic group	Prognostic based on molecular subtypes Predictive for tamoxifen benefit luminal cancers	Prognostic in ER + tumor Predictive for chemoreponse in high genomic grade index (GGI) tumor	Prognostic for distant recurrence in 10 years Predictive for chemoresponse in high recurrence group patients	Prognostic in ER + tumors Predictive for tamoxif-en response in low risk group	Prognostic in Her2 + tumors Predictive for early and late relapse

FFPE formalin fixed paraffin embedded

16.3 Liquid Biopsy: Breast Carcinoma

The diagnosis of breast cancer is often not simple, as the disease presents late and an accurate diagnosis can be made only with a tissue biopsy from the tumor itself. Accessing the tumor can be done only with procedures such as an ultrasound or CT-guided biopsy and excision biopsy. These procedures are invasive and are associated with their fair share of complications. Over the last decade, a new diagnostic tool—liquid biopsy—has been introduced as an alternative to tissue biopsies. The diverse molecular architecture of breast cancer can be thoroughly screened using newly developed liquid biopsy methods. This highly sensitive technology developed for the analysis of liquid biopsy makes serial biopsies in cancer patients possible through noninvasive approach [2].

In the course of formation of the tumor, various components are released into the blood, which include circulating tumor cells (CTCs), circulating tumor DNA (ctDNA), cell-free RNA (cfRNA), tumor educated platelets, and exosomes following apoptosis and necrosis [3] (Table 16.3), which can be easily accessible from samples such as blood, urine, CSF, sputum, and saliva.

Liquid biopsy exclusively forms a complementary to or an alternative to high-risk invasive tumor sampling as it is quick with minimal pain/risk, less invasive and comprehensive tissue profile can be obtained.

Table 16.3 Liquid biopsy components [2]

	Characteristics	Isolation/analytical techniques	Applications	Limitations
Circulating tumor cells (CTC)	Released from tumor	Size selection via multiorifice flow fractionation/surface marker enrichment via CellSearch platform	– Helps in early cancer detection – Prognosis – Monitor treatment – Prediction of recurrence	– Low plasma concentration – Difficulty in differentiating primary tumor/metastatic tumor
Circulating tumor DNA (ct DNA)	– ctDNA is a subcategory of cfDNA – Copies the genetic profile of tumor	Qualitative analysis (via next-generation Sequencing, molecular barcodes)	– Helps in early cancer detection – Minimal residual disease detection – Longitudinal screening – Detection of heterogeneity	– Low ctDNA:cfDNA ratio at early-stage cancer – Lack of detection for low allele frequencies – Difficult to analyze RNA and proteins
Cell free DNA (cf DNA)	– Concentration increases with cancer – Much high in concentration than CTC	Quantitative analysis (droplet digital PCR, molecular barcodes)	– Helps in early cancer detection – Disease stage and prognosis	– Low sensitivity and specificity
Cell free RNA (cf RNA)	– mRNA and miRNA from tumor – Much high in concentration than ctDNA	Quantitative analysis (RT-qPCR) and qualitative analysis (Microarrays and Next-Generation Sequencing)	– Genetic profile expression – Epigenetic alterations	– Less analysis of intergenic DNA – Inability to isolate due to size limitations – No reliable methods

Table 16.3 (continued)

	Characteristics	Isolation/analytical techniques	Applications	Limitations
Tumor educated platelets (TEP)	– No nucleus – Presence of mRNA/miRNA – Helps in intravasation of metastatic tumor cells – Factors for angiogenesis secreted	– TEP—RNA sequencing	Helps in early cancer detection	– Less source of research in the field – Difficult in identification between TEPs and platelets if it is noncancerous – No reliable methods
Exosome	– Carriers for intercellular communication (plays a role in metastasis) – Sheds by exocytosis of multivesicular bodies in both tumor cells/healthy cells	– qRT-PCR – Microarrays	Metastasis and tumor growth	– Difficult in identification between tumor-derived and healthy exosomes – No reliable methods

16.4 Utilization [4]

It is a game changer and in breast clinics, it can be utilized for

- Early diagnosis in high-risk and general population of patients
- Longitudinal monitoring to know the status of metastasis, development of resistance, or for response to treatment
- Targeted treatment based on genetic profile
- Predicting recurrence

16.5 Methodology

Sequences of ctDNA extracted from blood samples can be analyzed through targeted and nontargeted sequencing techniques. Targeted sequencing is used for the analysis of known breast cancer-related loci, while nontargeted whole-genome sequencing (WGS) is adopted as a method to identify novel variations with no pre-existing knowledge. Analysis of ctDNA consists of quantitative and qualitative studies. Quantitative analysis of ctDNA using droplet digital polymerase chain reaction (ddPCR) assay is performed on the basis of the correlation between disease stage and ctDNA: cfDNA concentration ratio [5]. On the other hand, qualitative studies use Next-Generation Sequencing (NGS) to examine ctDNA for variations in cancer hotspots or the entire genome to examine early-stage disease, response to treatment, and prognosis. Detection of single-nucleotide variations is generally performed through sensitive methods such as BEAMing and ddPCR assays, while WGS is used to detect copy number variations (CNVs) and chromosomal instabilities [6]. Analysis of single-locus hotspots is achieved through ddPCR assays, but this approach is limited when searching for a large number of variants or when looking for novel variants. For these applications, next-generation sequencing (NGS) could potentially help, but the challenge is that the allele frequency of ctDNA mutations in the pool of cfDNA is the same as the range of the NGS technology error rate. This shortcoming can be resolved with molecular barcoding technology; in this method, unique molecular barcodes or tags are added into every DNA fragment in order to keep track of possible PCR and sequencing artifacts (Fig. 16.1) This method

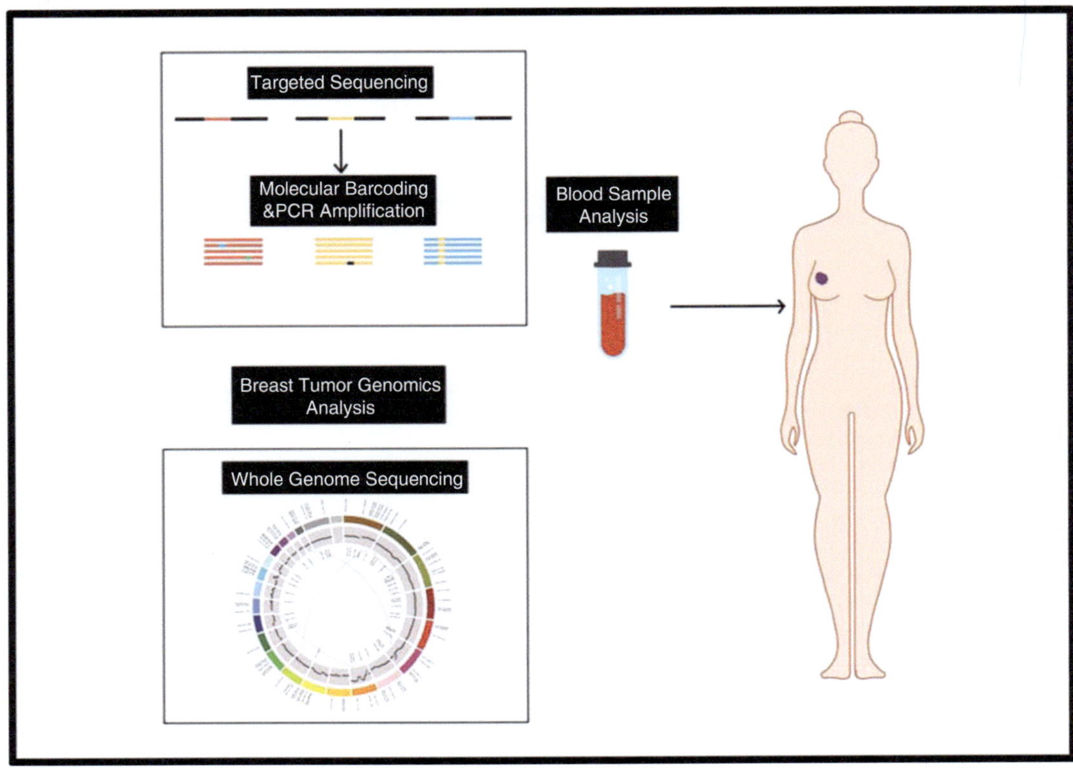

Fig 16.1 Schematic process for analysis of liquid biopsy samples

increases the accuracy of variation identification for very low allele frequencies [7].

In conclusion, breast cancer possesses high levels of heterogeneity and is usually prone to clonal evolution underpinning drug treatment. The heterogeneity in breast cancer can cause major problems in drug selection, increasing the need for more personalized therapy, which can be achieved through liquid biopsy, which can also create new horizons for the screening and management of breast cancer. Future perspective studies are required to overcome few disadvantages of this method and also to establish standardized protocols for its utilization in clinical settings.

References

1. Tsang JYS, Tse GM. Molecular classification of breast cancer. Adv Anat Pathol. 2020;27:27–35.
2. Alimirzaie S, Bagherzadeh M, Akbar MR. Liquid biopsy in breast cancer: a comprehensive review. Clin Genet. 2019;95:643–60.
3. Jahr S, Hentze H, Englisch S, et al. DNA fragments in the blood plasma of cancer patients: quantitations and evidence for their origin from apoptotic and necrotic cells. Cancer Res. 2001;61(4):1659–65.
4. Pérez-Callejo D, Romero A, Provencio M, Torrente M. Liquid biopsy based biomarkers in non-small cell lung cancer for diagnosis and treatment monitoring. Transl Lung Cancer Res. 2016;5(5):455–65.
5. Van Ginkel JH, Huibers MMH, van Es RJJ, de Bree R, Willems SM. Droplet digital PCR for detection and quantification of circulating tumor DNA in plasma of head and neck cancer patients. BMC Cancer. 2017;17:428.
6. Zare F, Dow M, Monteleone N, Hosny A, Nabavi S. An evaluation of copy number variation detection tools for cancer using whole exome sequencing data. BMC Bioinform. 2017;18:286.
7. Peng Q, Vijaya Satya R, Lewis M, Randad P, Wang Y. Reducing amplification artifacts in high multiplex amplicon sequencing by using molecular barcodes. BMC Genomics. 2015;16(1):589.

Part V

Benign Breast Disorders

17 Inflammatory Lesions

Harini Gnanavel, Leena Dennis Joseph, Mohana Priya, Anupama Chandrasekharan, and Bhawna Dev

Abstract

Inflammatory and reactive conditions of the breast are relatively uncommon among benign breast lesions and may present with clinical and radiologic abnormalities akin to malignant processes. Hence, core biopsy should be performed to exclude the possibility of malignancy. In most cases, the diagnosis based on microscopy is clear, but in fragmented core biopsy samples, some conditions may mimic malignancy. Conversely, some malignancies can also simulate benign inflammatory or reactive conditions.

Keywords

Inflammatory · Mastitis · Ectasia · Abscess · Granulomatous

H. Gnanavel (✉) · A. Chandrasekharan · B. Dev
Department of Radiology, Sri Ramachandra Institute of Higher Education and Research, Chennai, India
e-mail: harini@sriramachandra.edu.in; bhawnadev@sriramachandra.edu.in

L. D. Joseph
Department of Pathology, Sri Ramachandra Institute of Higher Education and Research, Chennai, India
e-mail: leenadennisj@sriramachandra.edu.in

M. Priya
Department of Surgery, Sri Ramachandra Institute of Higher Education and Research, Chennai, India
e-mail: mohanapriyadr@sriramachandra.edu.in

17.1 Imaging

The most useful imaging modality in inflammatory conditions is ultrasound, since x-ray mammogram may be painful while compression is given during imaging, thereby degrading image quality. An acceptable compromise must be found between the need for sufficient image quality and the pain caused to the patient by breast compression. But X ray mammogram can provide crucial information for diagnosing and managing the patients' condition like architectural distortion and calcification. Bilateral mammography is always recommended in order to compare the healthy and affected breasts. Breast MRI is performed in few cases where inflammatory carcinoma is suspected or the findings are indeterminate on other modalities or instances to find the extent of the tumor [1].

17.2 Fat Necrosis

It is a benign nonsuppurative inflammatory process of the adipose tissue [2].

Clinical presentation—Fat necrosis can clinically mimic malignancy. It is frequently a result of trauma, but also sometimes seen as a consequence of surgery or radiation therapy. Traumatic necrosis occurs more often in overweight women and women with pendulous/larger breasts. Patients usually present with a painless mass with

B. Dev, L. D. Joseph (eds.), *Holistic Approach to Breast Disease*,
https://doi.org/10.1007/978-981-99-0035-0_17

retraction or dimpling of the overlying skin, as a result of fibrotic bands between necrotic tissue and skin [3].

17.2.1 Radiology

Mammogram: Lipid cysts are pathognomonic of fat necrosis. A lipid cyst is a round or oval, smooth-bordered, lucent mass with a thin calcific rim (Figs. 17.1 and 17.2). Other mammographic presentations of fat necrosis include microcalcifications (branching, rod-like calcifications, pleomorphic calcifications), coarse calcifications (Fig. 17.1), irregular, dense spiculated mass, focal asymmetry, and focal nonlucent mass. These findings may mimic malignancy and require precise history taking and further evaluation with histopathological correlation wherever necessary [4].

Ultrasound: The common presentation seen is a well-defined hypoechoic lesion with peripheral echogenic calcific rim representing an oil cyst (Figs. 17.1 and 17.2) [5].

17.2.1.1 BI-RADS Category

BI-RADS 2—Oil cyst, cyst with egg shell calcification

BI-RADS 3—microcalcifications, focal asymmetry, and focal nonlucent mass—illustrated by relevant surgical history

BI-RADS 4—if no history is elicited

17.2.2 Pathology

17.2.2.1 Gross Examination

Early lesions present as hemorrhage in the indurated fat. After several weeks, the lesion becomes demarcated and forms a distinct yellow gray and focally reddish tumor. Secondary changes of cystic degeneration and calcification can also occur.

17.2.2.2 Histopathology

Microscopically, fat necrosis is seen as disruption of fat cells, accompanied by hemorrhage and influx of histiocytes. Later there are multinucleated histiocytes, hemosiderin deposition, and calcification with admixture of inflammatory cells (Fig. 17.3). Further the lesion develops fibrosis at the periphery and center may be cystic, squamous metaplasia may be noted in the ducts and lobules.

Localised hemorrhagic necrosis of skin and breast can be seen secondary to anticoagulant therapy [3].

17.2.3 Treatment/Management

Major concern in breast fat necrosis is to rule out malignancy. It is more of a diagnosis of exclusion. All patients should be subjected to imaging—ultrasound or mammogram followed by core needle biopsy. Palpable areas of fat necrosis may enlarge, remain unchanged, regress, or resolve. It usually does not necessitate any surgical treatment, and clinical follow-up is sufficient in the patient population in whom pain is not present and cosmesis is not the primary concern. However, if fat necrosis is confirmed, and it does not resolve and/or it causes pain or distortion in the breast shape, surgical removal is an option. In the case of a solid mass and/or breast distortion, treatment options depend on the size of the anticipated defect after excision. A small defect may be addressed with either excision alone or excision with fat grafting and/or local tissue rearrangement. For a large defect such as those due to partial flap loss after reconstruction, a more significant tissue debridement and reconstruction may be necessary [6].

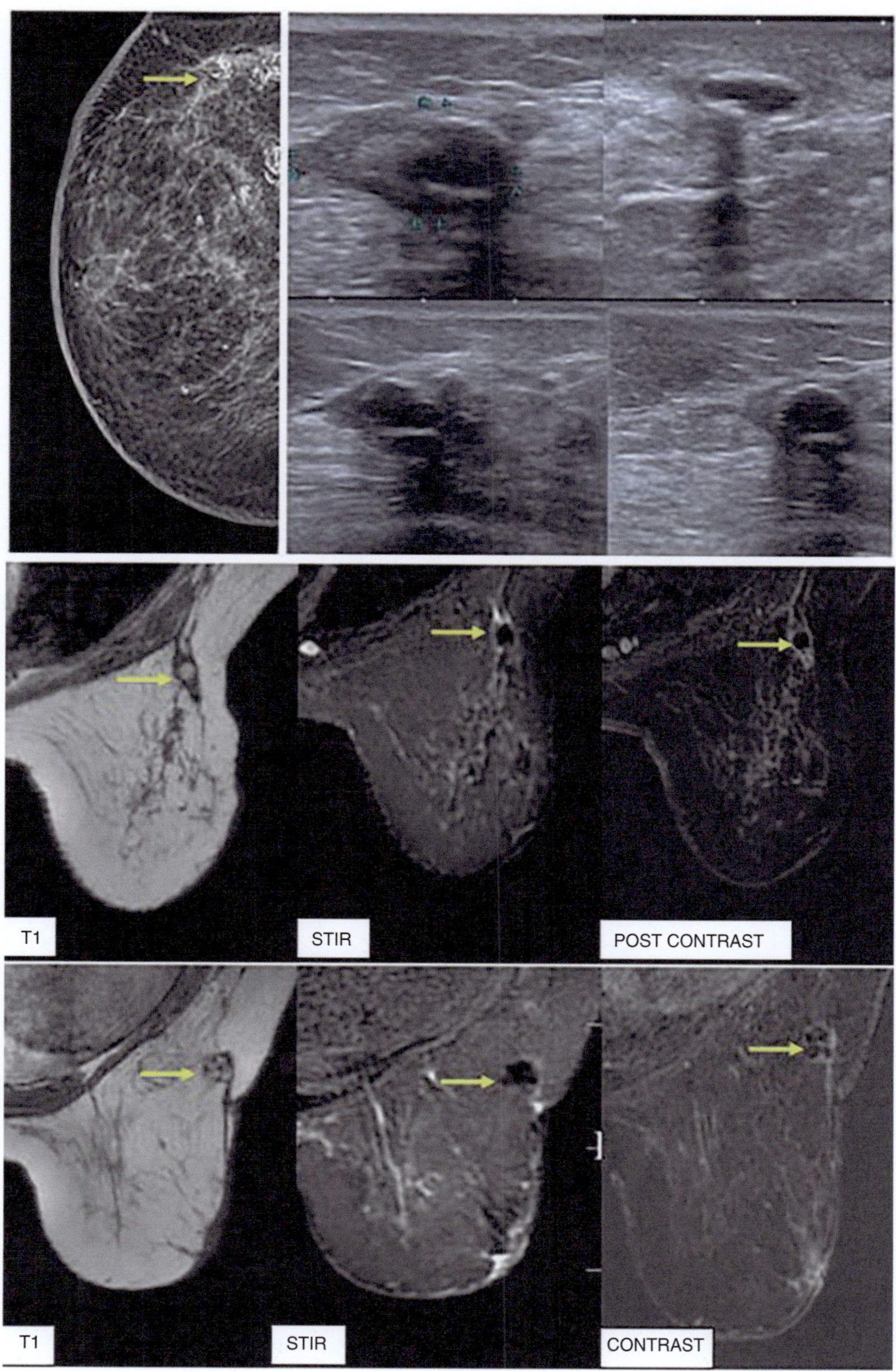

Fig. 17.1 Imaging of a patient with history of post breast conservation surgery (BCS). X ray mammogram showing oil cyst (yellow arrow). Ultrasound showing central hypoechogenicity with rim calcification. MRI showing suppression of fat on STIR images centrally with peripheral hypointensity indicating an oil cyst

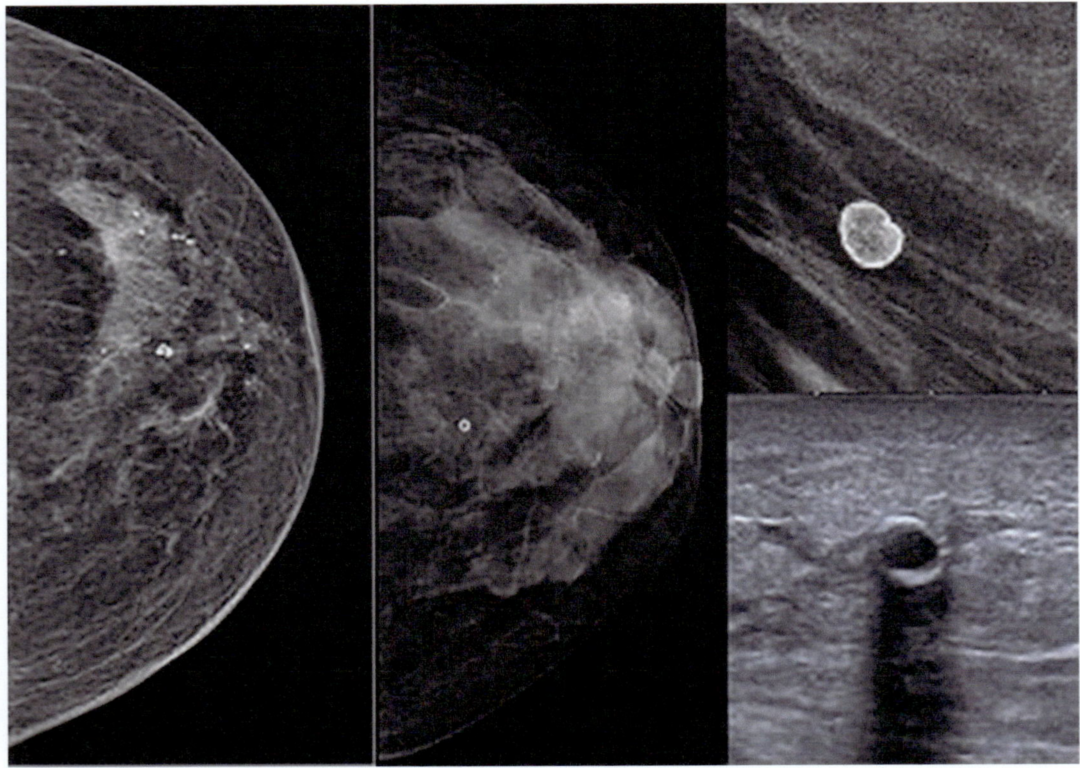

Fig. 17.2 X-ray mammogram and USG showing oil cyst with peripheral rim calcification

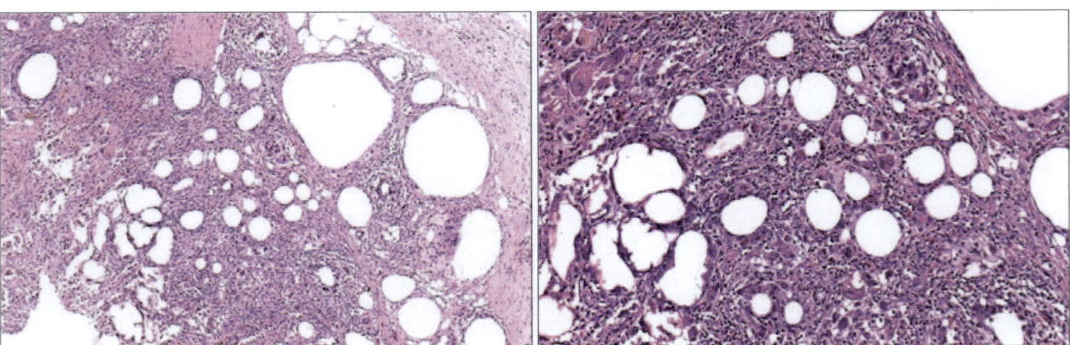

Fig. 17.3 Photomicrograph showing foci of foamy macrophages and multinucleated giant cells

17.3 Breast Infarct

Clinical presentation—Mammary infarction may present as a firm mass, which may or may not be painful. Breast infarct commonly develops as a discrete mass, during pregnancy or postpartum. This firm mass can also clinically mimic malignancy [7].

Etiology of breast infarction has not been established, but possible causes are localized thrombosis due to insufficient local vascularity. The increased frequency during pregnancy or lactation is probably due to compression of a local artery by enlarged ducts; however, none of these have been completely accepted. Infarcts can be seen with fibroadenoma, sclerosing adenosis, and papillomas.

17.3.1 Radiology

Imaging features of breast infarction are nonspecific.

Ultrasound: It can be seen as a mass with lobulated margins or a mass with heterogenous echotexture showing acoustic shadowing. (Comparison with previous reports is necessary whenever available to look for sudden increase in changes). However, isolated infarcts are rare [8].

17.3.2 Histopathology

Microscopically, infarcts present as areas of coagulative necrosis (Fig. 17.4), at times as liquefactive necrosis. There may be a variable inflammatory response with hemosiderin and fibrosis [7].

17.3.3 Treatment

If core needle biopsy is suggestive of infarct and patient is symptomatic, an excision biopsy of the lump can be done. If it is suspicious, then an on-table frozen section is recommended. Once malignancy is ruled out, excision of the lump will suffice [7].

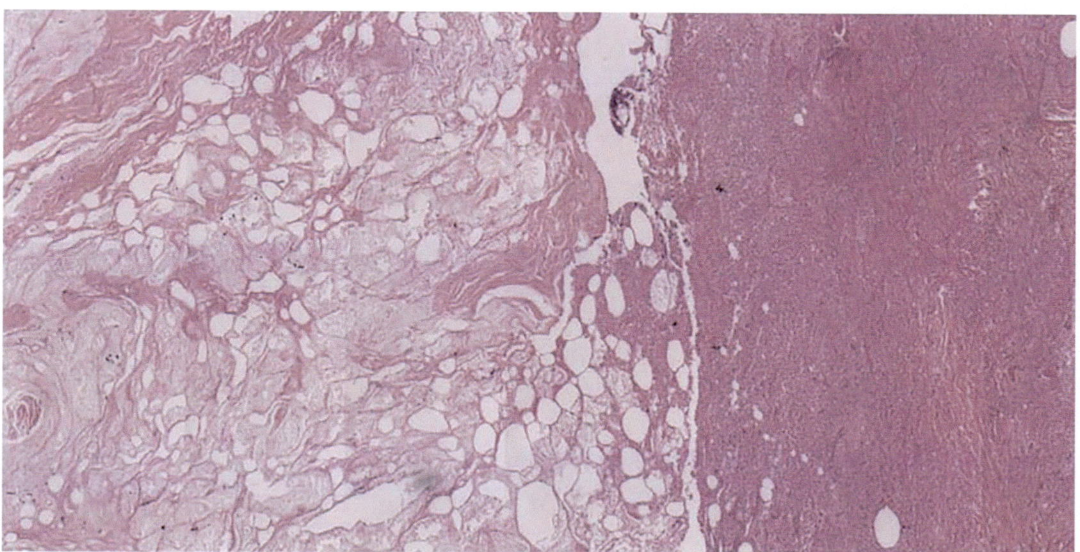

Fig. 17.4 Photomicrograph showing breast tissue with foci of coagulative necrosis

17.4 Galactocele

A galactocele is a benign lesion defined as an encysted collection of milk products usually associated with pregnancy and lactation [9].

Clinical presentation: Galactocoele presents as solitary or multiple circumscribed masses, which may be unilateral or bilateral. Clinically, the firm lesion may suggest carcinoma [10]. Patient may present with tender breast lump during lactation or painless firm lump several days after stopping lactation.

17.4.1 Radiology

Mammogram: Depending on the percentage of fat and protein in breast milk, mammographic findings may vary, which can be seen as follows.

1. Pseudolipoma: With higher fat content, it can be seen as a completely radiolucent mass (Fig. 17.5).
2. Cystic mass with fat-fluid level (Fig. 17.6): Low concentration of fat content rises up and the liquid sinks to the bottom. It is a diagnostic finding that is usually seen in the mediolateral oblique view of mammography.
3. Pseudo-hamartoma: In later stages when the milk has become old, lipid does not separate from liquid and shows radiologic features similar to hamartoma [9]. It will be seen as an oval or round shaped mass, with inhomogeneous radio-opaque and radiotransparent areas reflecting the presence of tissues of different density [11].

Ultrasound: It varies depending on the time of presentation. In the acute phase, it may appear as an anechoic unilocular simple cyst or a multilocular cyst with thin septation. The intensity of hypoechogenicity increases gradually due to the interface between the fat and water components. The common diagnostic key features are that of a well-defined lesion with low level internal echoes, and shows posterior acoustic enhancement (Fig. 17.6). Galactoceles being rich in nutrients, sometimes, can get infected and the surrounding parenchyma may appear heterogeneous and show increased vascularity [9].

Intervention: On fine needle aspiration, milk-like thick fluid is found and sometimes, purulent material is noticed if lesion is infected [9]. Surgical excision is done rarely.

17.4.1.1 BI-RADS Category

BI-RADS 2—Galactocele, pseudo lipoma, pseudo hamartoma

BI-RADS 3—Infected galactocele, sometimes pseudo hamartoma

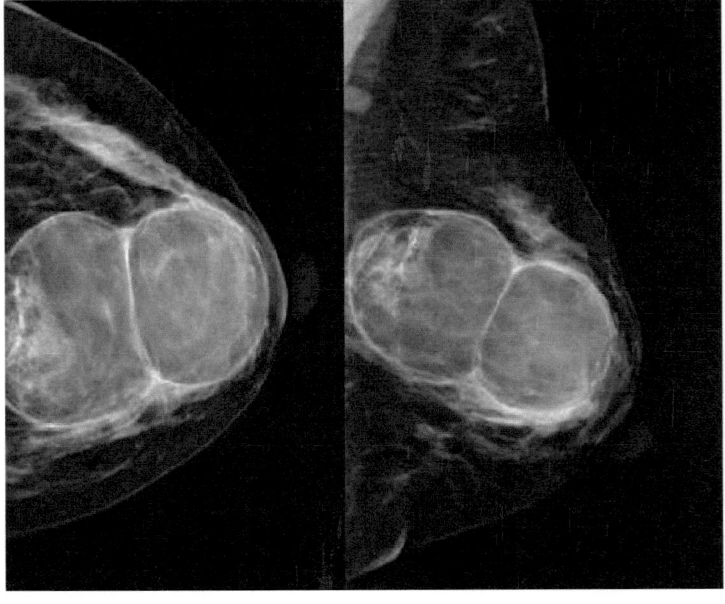

Fig. 17.5 X-ray mammogram showing a galactocele—radiolucent mass with well-defined margins

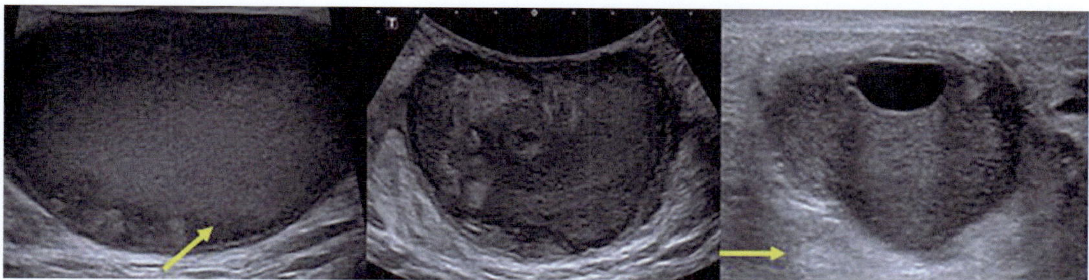

Fig. 17.6 Ultrasound showing galactocele with low level internal echoes. Note the fat fluid level (arrow in first image) and posterior acoustic enhancement (arrow in third image)

17.4.2 Pathology

17.4.2.1 Gross Examination

The lesion is composed of cysts that contain fluid contents resembling milk.

17.4.2.2 Histopathology

Microscopic examination shows dilated cysts, lined by cuboidal or flat epithelial cells with cytoplasmic vacuolization. Apocrine metaplasia may be seen. Inspissated secretions are seen within the cysts. Leakage of the fluid can elicit inflammation, even a granulomatous reaction at times [10]

17.4.3 Treatment

In patients presenting with cystic masses, ultrasound-guided aspiration of the fluid content is done and sent for cytology. For patients with recurrence/cysts with internal echoes, surgical excision is done.

17.5 Plasma Cell Mastitis

Plasma cell mastitis is a benign breast condition that occurs due to calcification of inspissated secretions. Though the cause is unclear, a suggested etiology is aseptic inflammation of the breast that occurs due to extravasation of intraductal secretions into periductal connective tissue. It commonly affects middle-aged nonpregnant and nonlactating females [12].

Clinical presentation—The patient presents with acute onset of redness, pain, and a thick nipple discharge in the acute phase. This will be followed by an edema of the overlying skin with persistent nipple discharge. At times, there may be a retracted nipple, with an ipsilateral axillary node enlargement, which, clinically and radiologically, mimics malignancy. Cases have been reported in the male breast also, where it clinically resembled gynecomastia [13]. In chronic phase it may be an incidental imaging finding presenting without any clinical symptoms.

17.5.1 Radiology

Mammogram: In acute stage, the findings are nonspecific. In chronic stage, it has a classical appearance of large rod-like branching calcifications (Fig. 17.7) radiating from the nipple due to inspissated calcified intra-ductal content. It is usually bilateral. When it heals completely, it produces scar and skin retraction, mimicking a malignancy. The close differential is DCIS, which shows fine linear branching calcification in linear or segmental distribution and is usually unilateral.

Ultrasound: May present as dilated ducts with echogenic material within and surrounding increased vascularity or it may not show any changes on ultrasound [14].

17.5.1.1 BI-RADS Category

BI-RADS 2- Bilateral Rod Like Calcification

17.5.2 Pathology

17.5.2.1 Histopathology

This lesion is characterized by a marked, diffuse plasma cell infiltrate surrounding ducts as well as

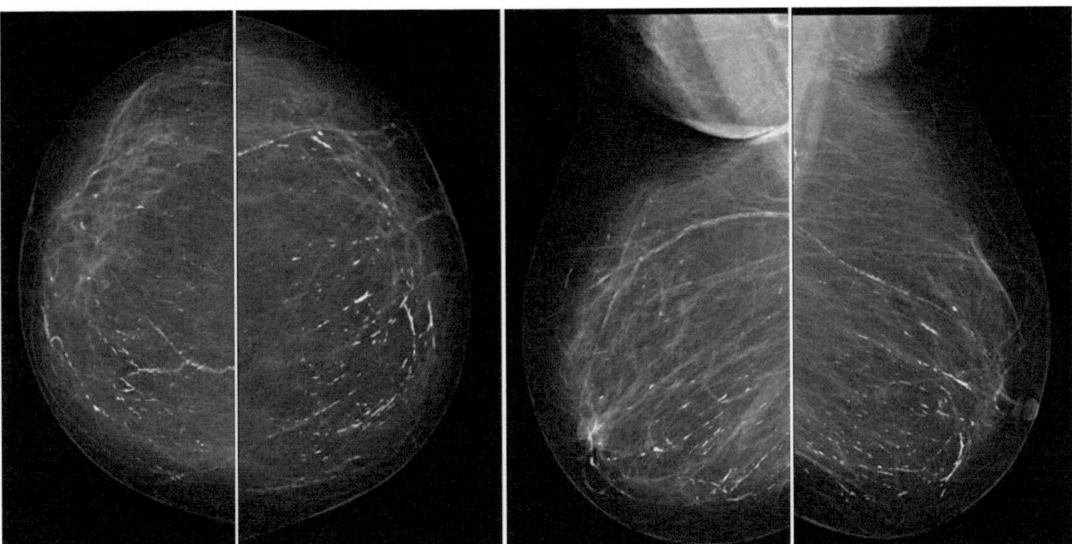

Fig. 17.7 X-ray mammogram showing diffuse rod-like calcification in both breasts

lobules. Interleukin-6 (IL-6) is a proinflammatory cytokine produced mostly by the lymphocytes, fibroblasts, and myeloid cells and has been characterized as a potent activator of Signal Transducer and Activator of Transcription 3 (STAT3). IL-6/STAT3 signaling pathway is vital not only for the differentiation of plasma cells but also for plasma cell survival [15]. There is a variable hyperplastic ductal epithelium, with foci of histiocytic infiltrate and granulomatous reaction to the desquamated epithelium and lipid material. Lymphocytes and neutrophils are also present [16].

17.5.3 Treatment

The primary concern is to rule out malignancy. For those presenting with discharge and nipple retraction, focused excision of the lesion and correction of the nipple retraction is done.

17.6 Mammary Duct Ectasia

Clinical presentation—This condition may present with spontaneous, intermittent nipple discharge, causing anxiety to the patients, who are mostly postmenopausal women. The secretions are usually clear, yellow, green, or brown. Stasis of secretion and leakage can elicit periductal inflammation. This can lead to duct sclerosis, obliteration, and ectasia. Cigarette smoking has been associated with periductal mastitis. Long-standing lesions may be palpable as doughy, worm-like masses beneath the nipple. Nipple retraction can be another sign, which can point toward malignancy [17].

17.6.1 Radiology

First-line Imaging modalities used to evaluate the duct include ductography (not used much in present days and is surpassed by US), ultrasound of the breasts. X-ray Mammogram and MRI are second-line modalities for evaluating the duct.

Mammogram: On mammography, duct ectasia may appear as radio-dense serpentine tubular structures converging on the nipple-areolar complex and its visibility depends on the overall density of the breast parenchyma as well as the extent of the dilatation. Ductal calcifications can be picked up accurately than any other modality [18].

Ultrasonography: The ultrasound appearance of ducts varies between individuals, within areas of the same breast, and according to the lactational state of the patient. On US, ducts are usually not visualized and if visible they are seen as tubular anechoic or hypoechoic wider at the level

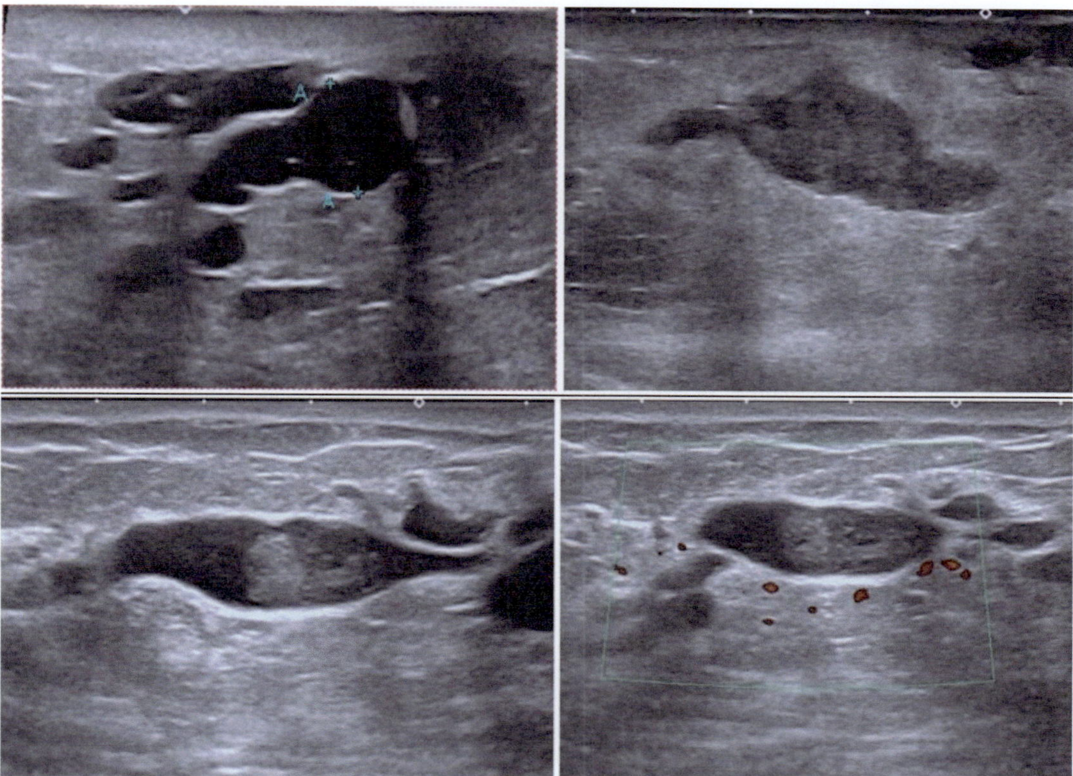

Fig. 17.8 Ultrasound showing dilated duct with no internal component (first image). Ultrasound showing dilated duct with internal echoes and no internal vascularity on color Doppler in other images

of the nipple, then taper more distally as they arborize peripherally. Normal ducts are collapsed or up to 1–2 mm in diameter.

Duct ectasia is defined as a duct measuring greater than 2 mm in diameter or the ampullary portion measures greater than 3 mm in diameter. The common location where ductal ectasia is noted is the retro-areolar region. On ultrasound it is seen as anechoic smooth-walled branching structures that taper peripherally. It can be filled with fluid, thick secretions or cellular debris (Fig. 17.8).

Ultrasound features that favour a malignant process include a peripheral location of the duct ectasia, irregularity of the duct margin, focal thickening of the duct wall, and the presence of adjacent hypoechoic tissue, whereas a central location favours a benign process [18].

MRI: On MR normal ducts blend in with the background breast parenchyma and are not visible. In ductal ectasia, it will be visible on nonenhanced T1-weighted images as high-signal-intensity branching tubular structures (due to proteinaceous or sometimes haemorrhagic material within). There is no associated enhancement seen. On subtraction images, subtle areas of ductal wall enhancement can indicate active inflammatory process, a mass lesion, or possibly malignancy [18].

Other ductal abnormalities include blocked ducts, inflammatory infiltrates, periductal mastitis, apocrine metaplasia, papilloma (discussed later).

17.6.1.1 BI-RADS Category

BI-RADS 2—Simple duct ectasia or with internal debris

BI-RADS 4—With echogenic solid internal component or focal wall thickening

17.6.2 Pathology

17.6.2.1 Histopathology

The dilated ducts are filled with intraluminal contents, ranging from eosinophilic (granular or amor-

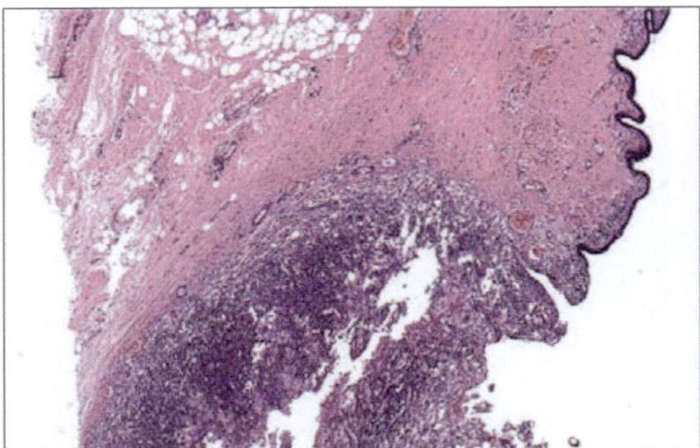
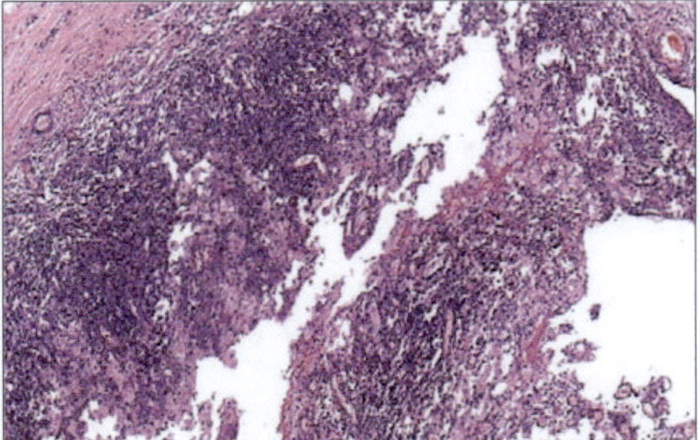

Fig. 17.9 Photomicrograph showing dilated duct with inflammation in the wall. Photomicrograph showing foamy macrophages admixed with inflammatory cells

phous) proteinaceous material to an admixture of lipid-containing histiocytic cells and desquamated duct epithelial cells (Fig. 17.9) Cholesterol crystals and calcifications may be found amid such debris. There may be neutrophils and lymphocytes, in the event of intense inflammation [17].

Disruption of ectatic ducts is accompanied by discharge of stagnant material (including cholesterol crystals) in periductal tissue, causing periductal inflammation. Cholesterol granuloma is an uncommon complication of periductal mastitis [16].

17.6.3 Treatment

Nipple discharge is checked for cytology and imaging is done. For patients with persistent single duct discharge, microdochectomy is done either through circumareolar or radial incision. Total duct/cone excision is done for older women with multiduct involvement with or without nipple inversion.

17.7 Granulomatous Lobular Mastitis

Granulomatous lobular mastitis, also known as nonpuerperal mastitis or Idiopathic Granulomatous Mastitis (IGM), is a benign rare chronic inflammatory breast disease characterized by sterile noncaseating lobulo-centric granulomatous inflammation. It affects parous premenopausal women [19].

Clinical presentation—This is another inflammatory disease of the breast, with no specific etiologic agent identified. Patient may present with a lump that is firm to hard with skin changes like peaud'orange, skin ulceration, or features of abscess. This lesion also clinically mimics malignancy [20].

17.7.1 Radiology

Mammogram: The mammographic findings are nonspecific and varied or may appear normal. The most common appearance is focal asymmetry or irregular mass. Additional ancillary findings include axillary adenopathy and focal skin thickening or edema, in contrast to inflammatory breast cancer, which characteristically involves more than one-third of the breast skin. Calcifications may be present.

Ultrasound: Most frequent presentation is a large irregular hypoechoic parallel mass with tubular extensions. Other presentations may include a circumscribed hypoechoic parallel mass, heterogeneous breast parenchyma and parenchymal distortion with acoustic shadowing but without a discrete mass. The tubular extensions demonstrate how granulomatous mastitis insinuates around the breast lobules rather than destroying it. Posterior acoustic features may vary in different cases. The lesions and the surrounding tissue may show variable vascularity on color flow imaging (Fig. 17.10). Ancillary US findings include skin thickening and edema, subcutaneous fat obliteration, and axillary ade-

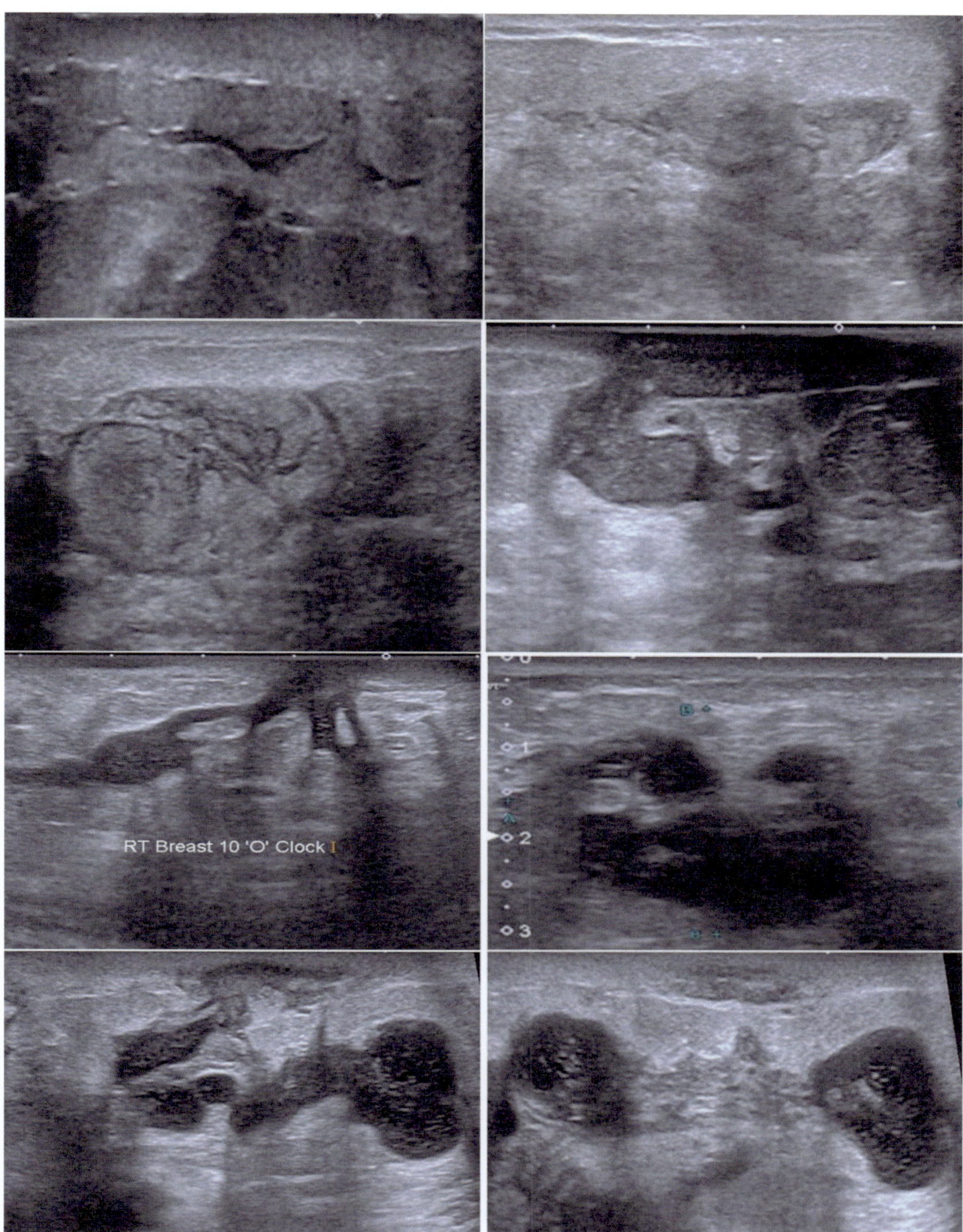

Fig. 17.10 US showing various stages of granulomatous mastitis

nopathy (smooth reactive cortical thickening with preserved fatty hilum or with calcification) (Fig. 17.11). In some cases, ultrasound may be normal even in the presence of positive mammogram findings.

MRI: The sensitivity of this modality is high; however, it is less commonly used. On contrast MRI, it is visualized as a heterogeneously enhancing mass or rim-enhancing lesions. It can also be seen as a segmental nonmass enhance-

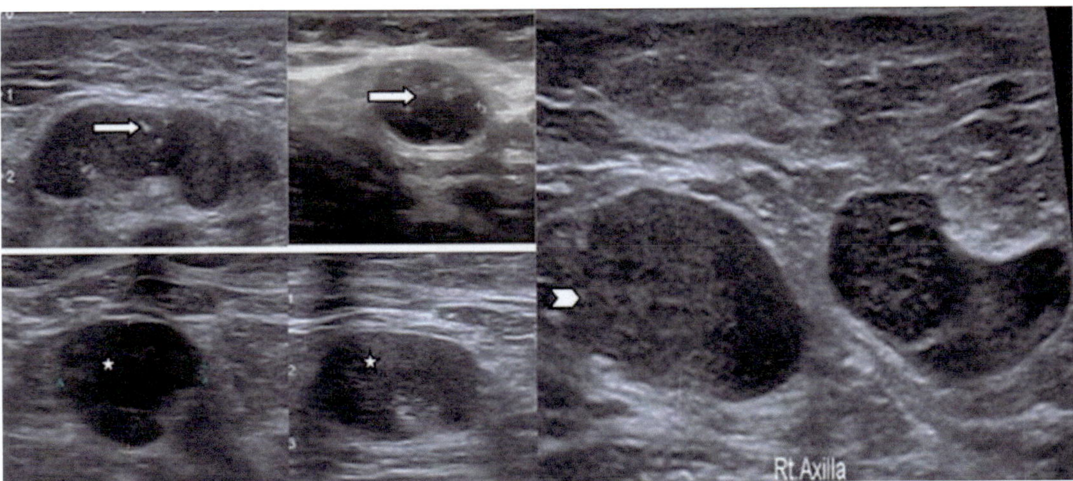

Fig. 17.11 US showing lymphnode with calcification (arrow), with thickened cortex (star) and lost fatty hilum (arrow head)—different presentations in various patients of granulomatous mastitis

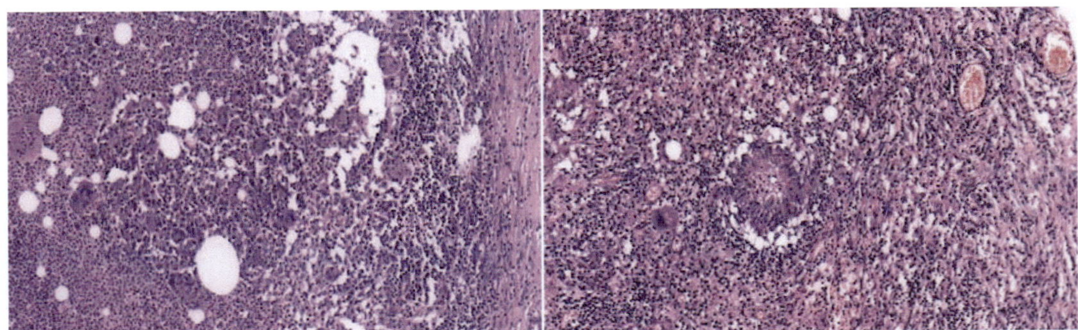

Fig. 17.12 Photomicrograph showing epithelioid granulomas surrounded by lymphocytes and many multinucleated giant cells

ment rather than regional enhancement. Some small lesions demonstrate confluency, T2 hyperintensity, and rim enhancement presumed to represent microabscesses [19].

17.7.1.1 Bi-RADS Category

BI-RADS 3—Focal asymmetry on mammogram, circumscribed hypoechoic parallel mass on ultrasound

BI-RADS 4—Irregularly shaped mass on mammogram and ultrasound

17.7.2 Pathology

17.7.2.1 Histopathology

Light microscopy shows epithelioid granulomas, centered on lobules. The epithelioid histiocytes are admixed with langerhan giant cells, plasma cells, and, occasionally, eosinophils (Fig. 17.12) [1]. Fat necrosis, abscess formation, and fibrosis may lead to effacement of the lobular distribution of confluent lesions. These granulomas have to be differentiated from other inflammatory conditions, like tuberculosis, sarcoidosis, cat scratch disease, etc. [20].

17.7.3 Treatment

To date, there is no agreed gold standard treatment for Idiopathic Granulomatous Mastitis. The clinical management often starts with tests to eliminate microbial infection and, when microbial infection can be ruled out, long-term oral steroid treatment or surgery is administered [21]. Although many patients prefer breast-preserving treatment to surgery, systemic steroid treatments can have severe side effects and may not be suitable for patients with diabetes, glaucoma, heart disease, hypertension, or obesity. More importantly, as the recurrence rate of patients who undergo surgical resection is much lower than that of patients who undergo nonsurgical treatment, it has been suggested that surgery is more effective in preventing recurrence [22].

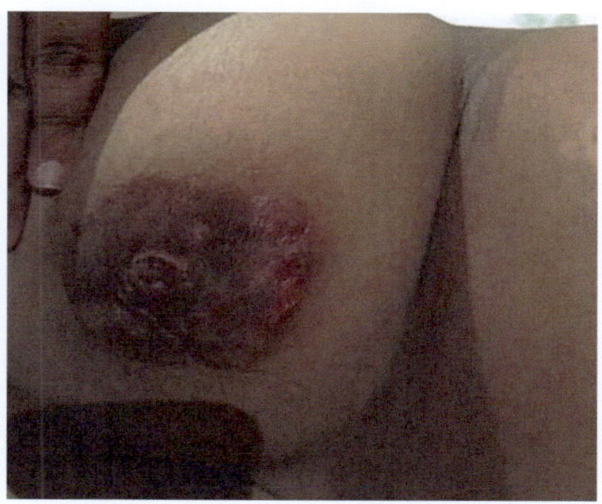

Fig. 17.13 Clinical picture showing ulceration (sinus), and skin redness

17.8 Tuberculous Granulomatous Mastitis

Breast tuberculosis is a very rare disease and constitutes only 0.025–1.04% of all breast diseases. Its prevalence has been estimated to be 0.1% of breast lesions examined histologically, and it constitutes about 3–4.5% of surgically-treated breast diseases in developing countries [23]. The breast may become infected in a variety of ways: (1) haematogenous, (2) lymphatic, (3) spread from contiguous structures, (4) direct inoculation, and (5) ductal infection. Despite the high prevalence of tuberculosis, mammary cells offer great resistance to the survival and multiplication of *Mycobacterium tuberculosis*. Breast tuberculosis was first classified into five different types by Mckeown and Wilkinson: (1) Nodular tubercular mastitis, (2) Disseminated or confluent tubercular mastitis, (3) Sclerosing tubercular mastitis, (4) Tuberculous mastitis obliterans, and (5) Acute miliary tubercular mastitis. Later on, breast tuberculosis was reclassified as nodular, disseminated, and abscess varieties. The sclerosing type, mastitis obliterans, and miliary variety are of historical importance only [24].

Clinical presentation—Varied presentation like breast lump, mastitis, mastalgia, sinus (Fig. 17.13) in the breast, axillary lump and breast abscess is seen. High degree of suspicion is required for diagnosis of breast tuberculosis.

FNAC or core needle biopsy or biopsy of sinus opening confirms the diagnosis of breast tuberculosis in suspected lesions. Culture methods like BACTEC, mycobacterial growth indicator tube (MGIT) helps in rapid detection of early mycobacterial growth (5–14 days as compared to 2–8 weeks with conventional methods).

17.8.1 Radiology

The imaging presentations are varied and similar to granulomatous lobular mastitis as mentioned in earlier section (Fig. 17.14).

17.8.2 Histopathology

Tuberculosis can be diagnosed on histopathology by presence of epithelioid cell granulomas and caseous necrosis.

17.8.3 Treatment

Once the diagnosis of tuberculosis is confirmed, patient is started on Antituberculous drugs based on newer RNTCP guidelines. For patients presenting with breast abscess, nondependent drainage of abscess is done [25]. Rarely, excision is done if there is no response to Antituberculous drugs or if malignancy cannot be ruled out.

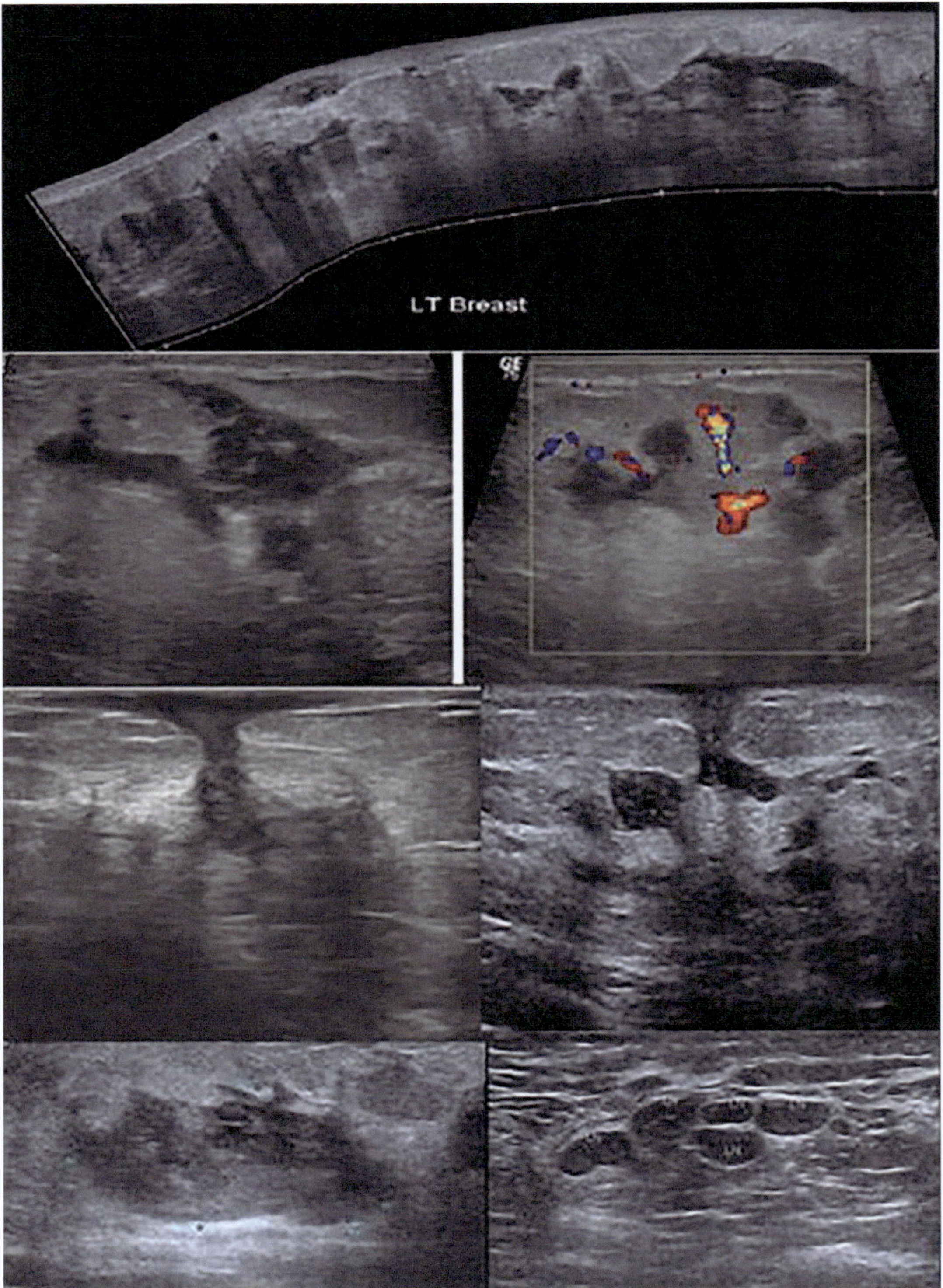

Fig. 17.14 Ultrasound images showing various presentations of tuberculos mastitis as inflammatory changes, sinus tracts and lesion with internal echoes

17.9 Sarcoidosis

Sarcoidosis is an immunologic disease that may affect the lungs, lymph nodes, skin, spleen, and liver. Primary breast involvement is very rare and is secondary to a well-known systemic involvement. Age of onset is third and fourth decades of life [26].

Clinical presentation—Systemic sarcoidosis may affect the breast, which is usually seen in young women, in their early third decade. The firm to hard masses may be mistaken clinically for malignancy [27].

17.9.1 Radiology

Mammogram: Breast sarcoidosis shows an irregular or ill-defined, often spiculated mass mimicking a malignancy. Although small, well-defined round masses have also been described. The latter finding may represent intramammary lymph node involvement. Calcifications are generally absent.

Ultrasound: Irregular hypoechoic mass (mimicking a malignancy) is the most common presentation [26].

17.9.2 Pathology

17.9.2.1 Histopathology

Microscopically, there are confluent naked granulomas, forming nodules in the mammary parenchyma with asteroid and schaumann bodies. Differential diagnoses include idiopathic granulomatous mastitis, tuberculosis, fungal infection, cat-scratch disease, and sarcoid-like reactions to cancer [27].

17.9.3 Treatment

Sarcoidosis of breast can be diagnosed only after excluding other diseases causing granulomatous inflammation like fungal, tuberculosis, and foreign body. If needed, image-guided biopsy is done to confirm the diagnosis. Treatment is similar to pulmonary sarcoidosis.

17.10 Inflammatory Pseudotumors

Clinical presentation—Yet another firm mass in the breast parenchyma, which can cause confusion with malignancy. Most patients with IgG4 mastitis are also included in this category, which is seen in premenopausal women who present with unilateral, palpable, painless mass.

17.10.1 Radiology

Imaging findings are nonspecific for this condition and histopathology remains the gold standard.

17.10.2 Pathology

17.10.2.1 Histopathology

Localized nodular lesions of the breast, composed of interlacing bundles of bland myo-fibroblastic cells with a prominent inflammatory cell infiltrate composed mainly of lymphocytes, plasma cells, and histiocytes. IgG4-related disease is characterized by mass-forming IgG4-dominant plasma cells associated with fibrosclerosis and obliterative phlebitis [28].

17.10.3 Treatment

Wide local excision is the treatment. Steroids have been used in few cases but its use is not routinely warranted.

17.11 Vasculitis

Clinical presentation—The presentation of vasculitis often resembles carcinoma clinically. These lesions, which can present as mass, may vary from giant cell arteritis, wegener's granulomatosis, polyarteritis, sarcoidosis to dermatomyositis. Inflammation of the veins, as seen in superficial thrombophlebitis or Mondor's disease, presents as a subcutaneous painless or painful and tender cord-like swelling [29].

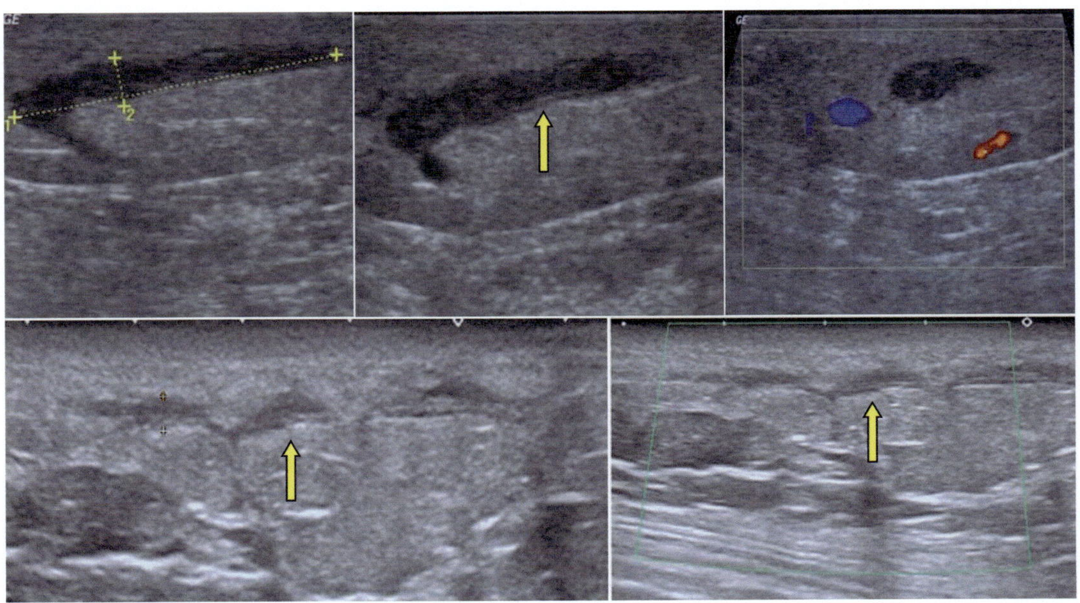

Fig. 17.15 A long linear tubular hypoechoic structure in the superficial plane with irregular margins and no flow on color Doppler (arrows)

17.11.1 Radiology

There are no pathognomonic features on imaging to pick up vasculitis in breast.

One specific entity seen is the Mondor's disease and is a benign condition characterized by superficial thrombophlebitis of the mammary region and anterior chest wall. Anatomically, the affected veins include the lateral thoracic, thoraco-epigastric, and superior epigastric.

Mammogram: Finding is a dilated tubular high density close to skin that may potentially be mistaken for a dilated duct.

Ultrasound: The thrombosed vessel is seen in the superficial plane as a long, tubular, anechoic structure with beaded appearance and shows no flow on color Doppler (Fig. 17.15).

Bilaterality is rare and is located mostly in the upper outer quadrant of the breast. A thrombosed vein is longer than a duct, shows beaded appearance, and does not terminate at the areola [30].

The other conditions as mentioned above are uncommon in breast.

17.11.2 Pathology

17.11.2.1 Histopathology

Histologic examination of biopsies in patients with vasculitis has revealed inflammatory cells infiltrating small- and medium-sized vessels. Patterns of vascular inflammation may be granulomatous or nongranulomatous, with or without necrosis of vessel wall. Granulomatous vasculitis is more associated with generalized diseases like giant cell arteritis or wegener's granulomatosis. Usually, nongranulomatous conditions may be seen as isolated single organ disease [29].

17.11.3 Treatment

Most of isolated breast vasculitis regress spontaneously. Persistent lesion or if malignancy cannot be ruled out excision is done. If it is associated with systemic vasculitis, then treatment is steroid or immunosuppressive therapy.

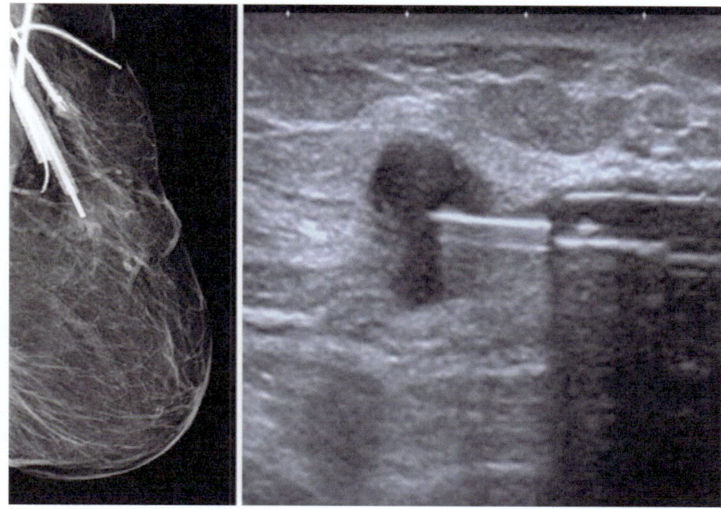

Fig. 17.16 X-ray mammogram showing pacemaker leads extending into breast parenchyma. US showing the leads with granuloma formation in the tip

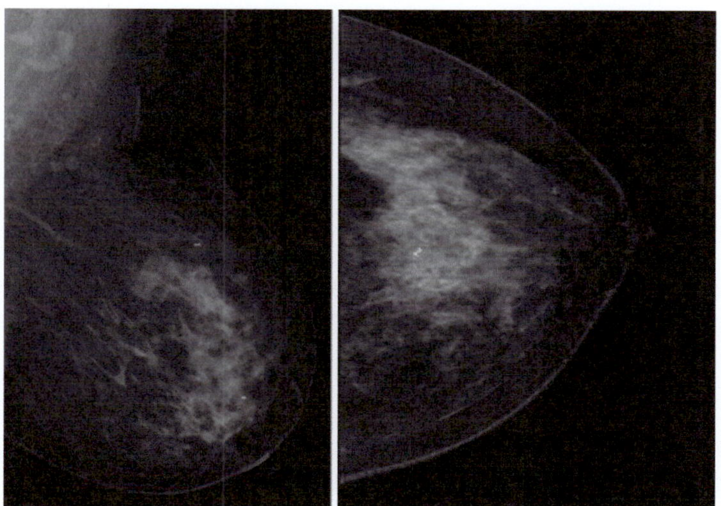

Fig. 17.17 X-ray mammogram showing clip/marker

17.12 Foreign Bodies

Clinical presentation—Extraneous material like paraffin injection or silicone implant can also elicit an inflammatory response in the breast. These substances will present as a hard, nodular mass, which closely mimics malignancy, but a proper history helps in identifying this entity [31].

17.12.1 Radiology

Foreign bodies that we encounter in breast include the following:

Breast implants (Fig. 17.16), implant rupture, medical devices like guide wire, breast clips (Fig. 17.17), ventriculoperitoneal shunt, pacemaker (Fig. 17.18) and miscellaneous objects like acupuncture needles, lead contained in go-yak (Chinese herbal treatment), nipple piercing, etc. [32].

Mammogram: A wide range of nonspecific features depending on the material type and its size.

Ultrasound: Foreign bodies show echogenic appearance with posterior acoustic shadowing. There may be a hypoechoic halo that may represent edema, hematoma, or granulation tissue (Fig. 17.18) with minimal surrounding vascularity [33].

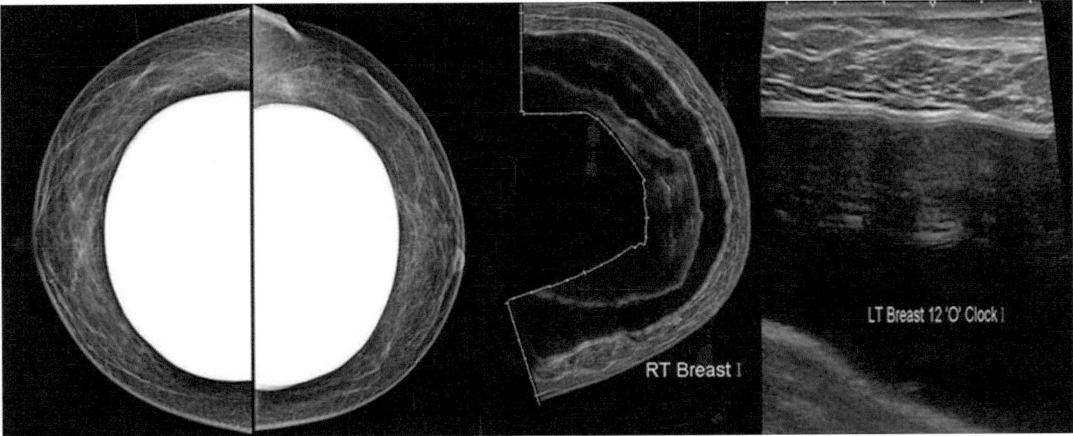

Fig. 17.18 X ray mammogram ultrasound showing bilateral breast implant

17.12.2 Pathology

17.12.2.1 Histopathology

Light microscopy shows a dense foreign body reaction, at times, with granulomas and adjacent areas of fat necrosis. There may also be areas of fibrous scar tissue; histiocyte response; foreign body giant cell reaction to extruded or exposed material including synovial-like metaplasia; and calcification [31].

17.12.3 Treatment

Removal of the foreign body is done if warranted.

17.13 Diabetic Mastopathy

Clinical presentation—Usually, insulin-dependent diabetic patients present with fibrous tumor in the breast parenchyma, forming stromal proliferation called diabetic mastopathy. These patients present with palpable, firm to hard tumor, detected in one or both breasts. These masses are ill defined and nontender and mimic malignancy [34].

17.13.1 Radiology

Radiological appearance in diabetic mastopathy is frequently mistaken for carcinoma. Multifocal or bilateral breast involvement is not uncommon.

Mammogram: It is seen as ill-defined masses (Fig. 17.19) or as multiple asymmetric areas.

Ultrasound: Diabetic mastopathy manifests as an ill-defined hypoechoic lesion with significant posterior acoustic shadowing (Fig. 17.19).

Diagnosis is usually made on histology and imaging findings are not confirmatory [14].

17.13.1.1 BI-RADS Category

BI-RADS 4—irregular hypoechoic mass

17.13.2 Pathology

17.13.2.1 Histopathology

Microscopy shows a collagenous stroma with keloid like features and prominent myofibroblasts. Perivascular lymphocytic infiltrates (Fig. 17.20), predominantly B cell type, are characteristic of diabetic mastopathy [35].

17.13.3 Treatment

No specific treatment is needed except for glycemic control for this condition. Malignancy is ruled out by imaging and histopathology. Patient is advised to do a breast self-examination and come for yearly clinical follow-up.

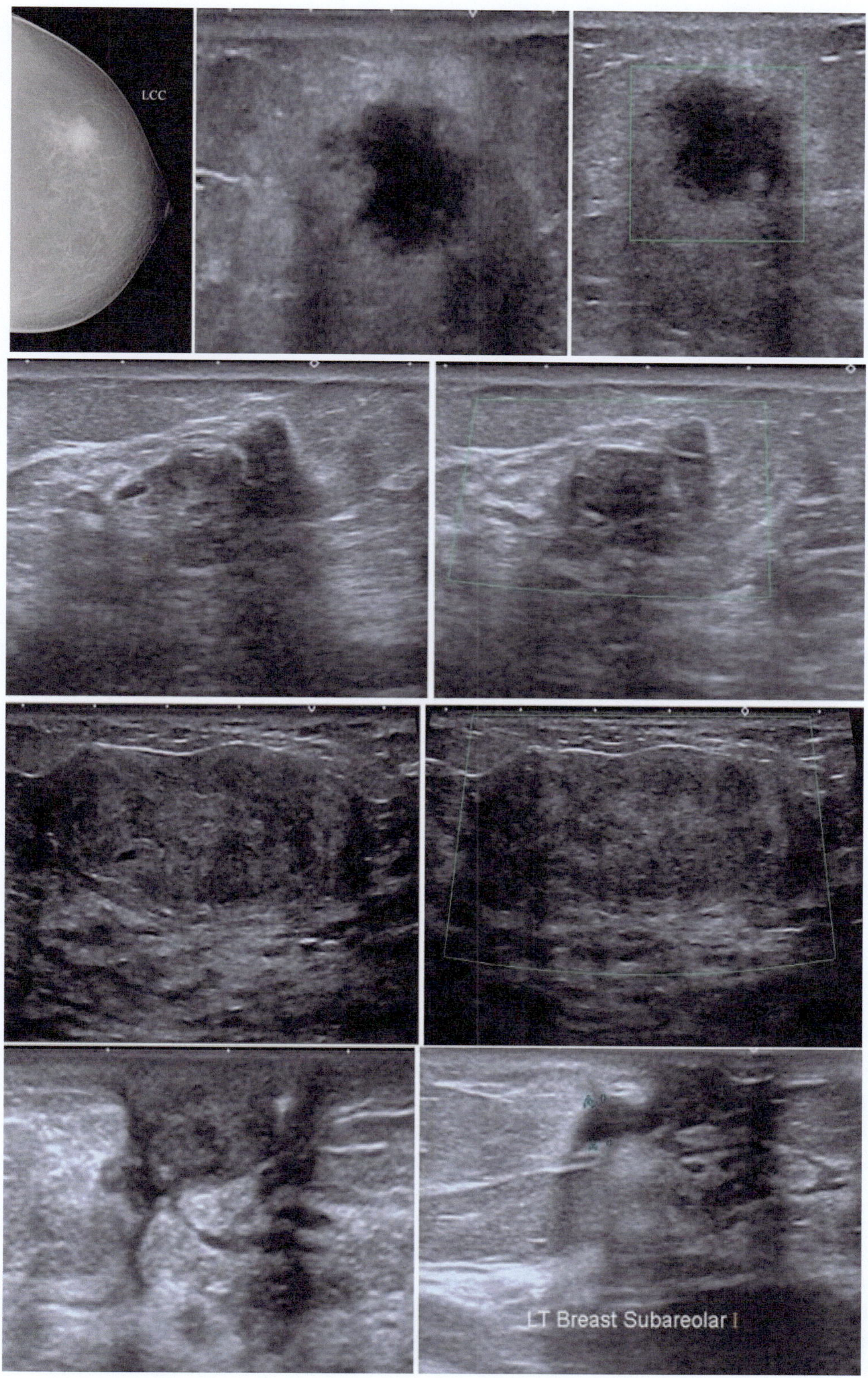

Fig. 17.19 X-ray mammogram and ultrasound showing various presentations of diabetic mastopathy

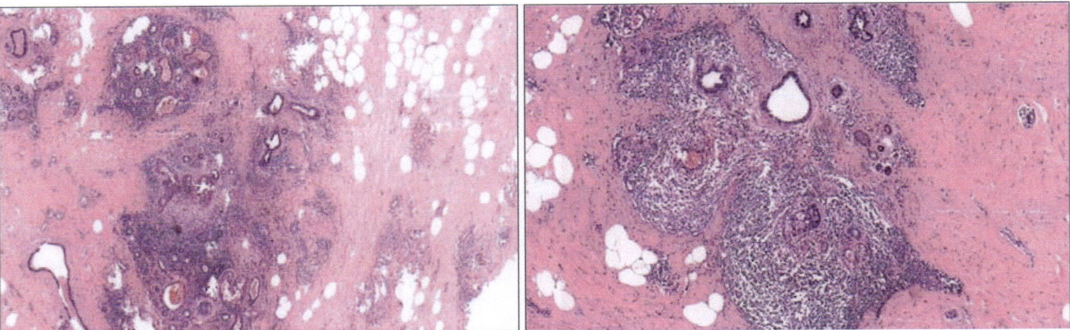

Fig. 17.20 Photomicrograph showing dense lymphoplasmacytic infiltrate around lobules

17.14 Breast Abscess

Clinical presentation—Breast abscess is typically caused by either an inflammatory reaction to an infectious process (bacteria, fungus or parasite) or, less commonly as a reaction to a foreign substance within the body. This can be lactational or nonlactational. Breast abscess typically presents as a painful mass (Fig. 17.21) and overlying skin is warm and tender [36].

17.14.1 Radiology

Breast abscess can either be central (peri-areolar) or peripheral.

Mammogram: It may show skin thickening, an asymmetry, a mass, or distortion and none of these are specific. On the other hand, the presence of suspicious microcalcifications should lead to a biopsy to rule out carcinoma [37].

Ultrasound: Nonpuerperal abscess in acute evolving stage appears as an ill-defined area of altered echotexture with increased echogenicity, inflammation of surrounding fat, hypoechoic areas in the glandular parenchyma, and associated mild skin thickening (Fig. 17.22). Inflammatory axillary lymph nodes may also be seen and show mild-to-moderate circumferential cortical thickening and increased vascularity on color flow imaging. In later stages, it can appear as a thick-walled hypoechoic collection of variable shapes and sizes and is usually multiloculated, with echogenic debris (Fig. 17.19) and increased peripheral vascular flow. Ideally, no vascularity should be seen within the collection. Acoustic enhancement is present due to fluid content [37].

17.14.1.1 BI-RADS Category

BI-RADS 3—Thick-walled hypoechoic collection with echogenic debris

BI-RADS 4A—Ill-defined area of altered echotexture, inflammation of surrounding fat

17.14.2 Pathology

17.14.2.1 Histopathology

The most common bacterial organism is *Staphylococcus aureus*, although various other organisms can also lead to abscess formation. Microscopically, infections and inflammations can present as abscess formation, which may be a cavity with abundant neutrophils and necrotic debris. There is a notable destruction of tissue along with presence of fibrin. The cavity may be rimmed by granulation tissue formation.

During the cytopathological analysis, the aspirates will usually contain yellow purulent material. In thick cellular smears, acute inflammation could be observed with and without fat necrosis, macrophages, multinucleated giant cells (Fig. 17.23), and debris [38].

Mycotic infections in the breast can present as suppurative granulomas or as an abscess formation, where the fungal organisms can be demonstrated by histochemical stains or fungal cultures, for species identification, which could be histoplasmosis, blastomycosis, cryptococcosis, aspergillus, etc.

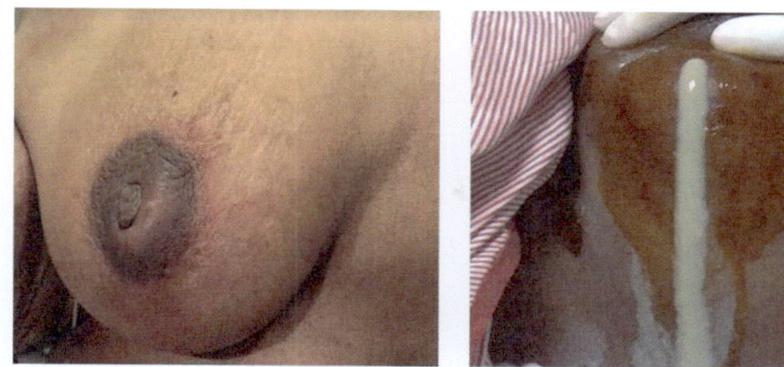

Fig. 17.21 Clinical picture in a patient with breast abscess showing redness and swelling and a clinical picture showing pus being drained from breast abscess

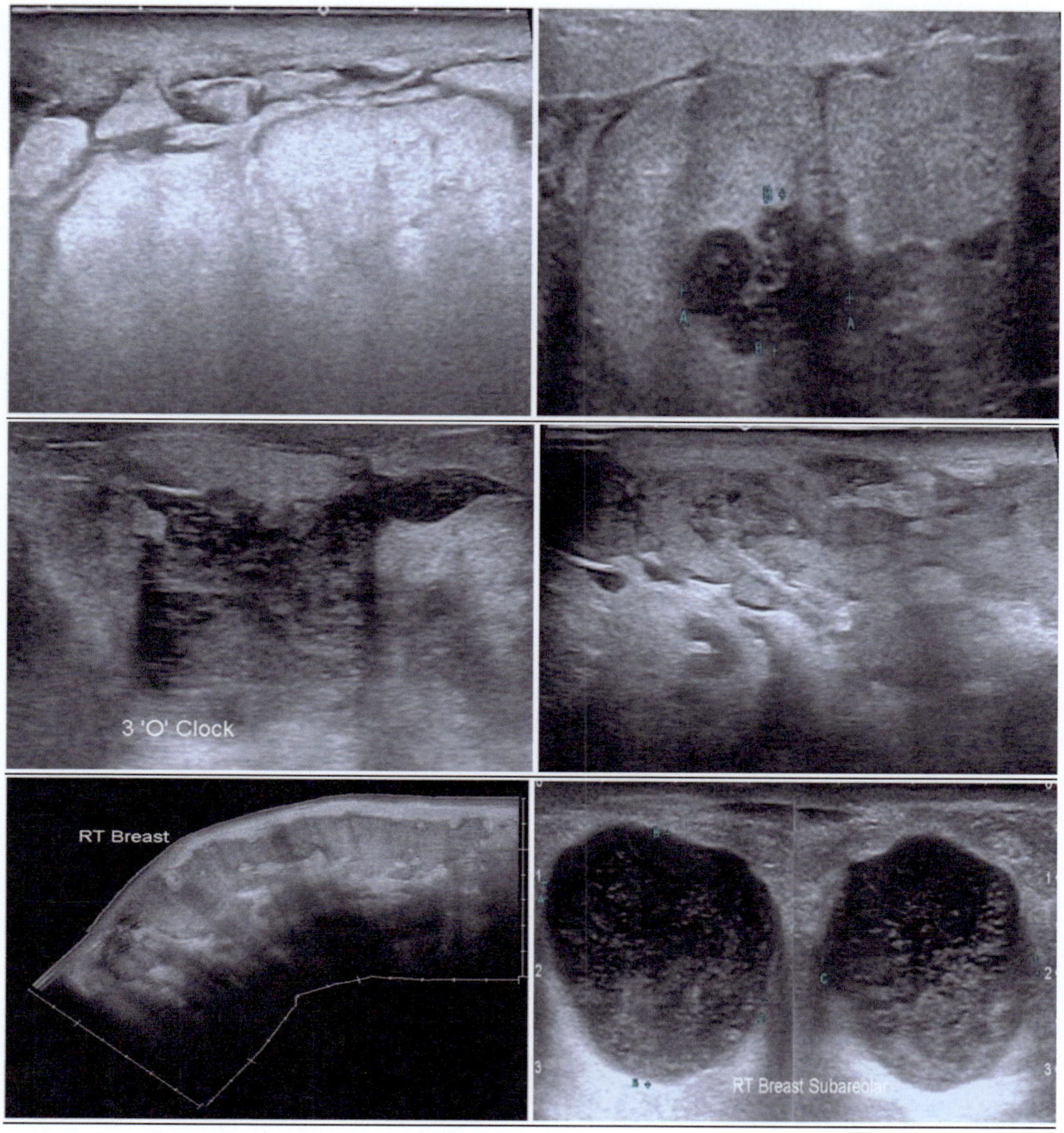

Fig. 17.22 Ultrasound showing various stages of breast abscess

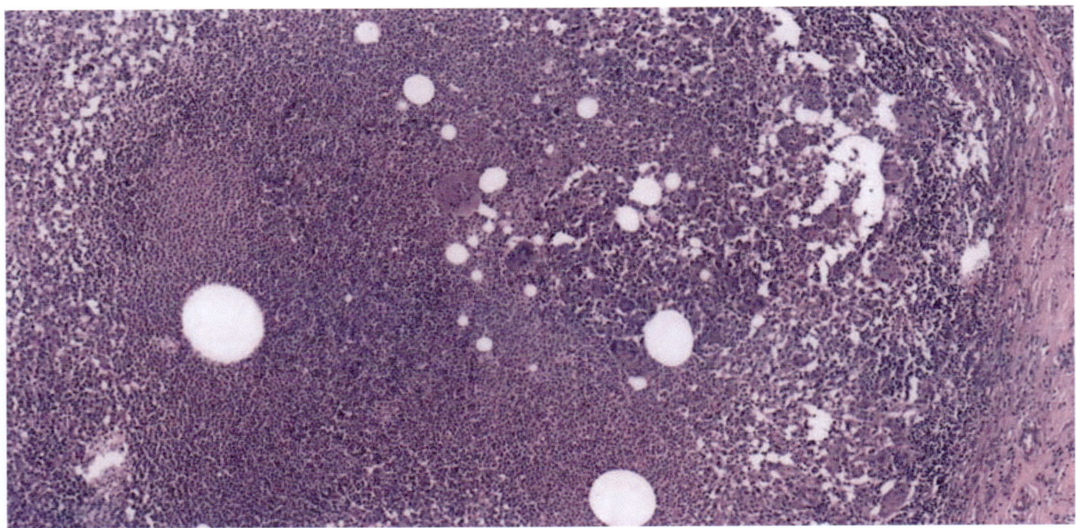

Fig. 17.23 Photomicrograph showing sheets of neutrophils admixed with few giant cells

Breast parenchyma could also host parasitic infections and mycobacterial organisms, like *Mycobacterium tuberculosis*. Other organisms, like actinomycosis, nocardia, and cat scratch disease, have also been reported. Any of these organisms can present as a breast abscess or subareolar abscess, mimicking malignancy.

Tuberculous mastitis is a rare clinical entity and usually affects women from the Indian subcontinent and Africa. It often mimics breast carcinoma and pyogenic breast abscess clinically and radiologically, may both coexist [39].

17.14.3 Treatment

Historically, incision and drainage was considered the standard of care for abscesses. Although this method yields a lower recurrence rate, it is more invasive than needle aspiration and frequently results in scarring with structural damage and poor cosmetic outcomes. Fine-needle aspiration should be considered as first-line therapy for abscesses smaller than 5 cm owing to its lower risks, followed by incision and drainage if recurrence occurs. Although success has been reported with oral antistaphylococcal antibiotics and serial aspiration, surgical excision may be required for infected or obstructed lactiferous ducts and provides a lower rate of recurrence for nonpuerperal abscess and mastitis [40].

For persistent lesions, treatment options may include ultrasound-guided needle aspiration, percutaneous drainage catheter, and/or surgical drainage. Loculations are associated with failure of resolution with aspiration, regardless of abscess volume. Vacuum-assisted biopsy is a viable option for the management of lactational breast abscesses and has been associated with a shorter healing time than simple needle aspiration. Furthermore, percutaneous catheter drainage may be considered for larger abscesses [41, 42].

References

1. Lepori D. Inflammatory breast disease: the radiologist's role. Diagn Interv Imaging. 2015;96(10): 1045–64.
2. Atasoy MM, Ören NC, Ilica AT, Güvenç İ, Günal A, Mossa-Basha M. Sonography of fat necrosis of the breast: correlation with mammography and MR imaging. J Clin Ultrasound. 2013;41(7):415–23.
3. Kerridge W, Kryvenko O, Thompson A, Shah B. Fat necrosis of the breast: a pictorial review of the mammographic, ultrasound, CT, and MRI findings with histopathologic correlation. Radiol Res Pract. 2015;2015:1–8.
4. Hogge JP, Robinson RE, Magnant CM, Zuurbier RA. The mammographic spectrum of fat necrosis of the breast. Radiographics. 1995;15(6):1347–56.
5. Upadhyaya VS, Uppoor R, Shetty L. Mammographic and sonographic features of fat necrosis of the breast. Indian J Radiol Imaging. 2013;23(4):366.

6. Genova R, Waheed A, Garza RF, editors. Breast fat necrosis. Treasure Island, FL: StatPearls Publishing; 2022. https://www.ncbi.nlm.nih.gov/books/NBK542191/
7. Han B, Zhang H, Jiang P, Zheng C, Bi L, Lu LU, Fan Z. Breast infarction during pregnancy and lactation: a case report. Exp Ther Med. 2015;10(5):1888–92. https://doi.org/10.3892/etm.2015.2756. Epub 2015 Sep 21. PMID: 26640567; PMCID: PMC4665851
8. Sabate JM, Clotet M, Torrubia S, Gomez A, Guerrero R, de Las Heras P, Lerma E. Radiologic evaluation of breast disorders related to pregnancy and lactation. Radiographics. 2007;27(Suppl_1):S101–24.
9. Yu JH, Kim MJ, Cho H, Liu HJ, Han SJ, Ahn TG. Breast diseases during pregnancy and lactation. Obstet Gynecol Sci. 2013;56(3):143–59.
10. Kemp JD, Holcomb KZ, Sperling LC. Xanthogranulomatous reaction to a ruptured galactocele. J Cutan Pathol. 2010;37(9):973–6.
11. Presazzi A, Di Giulio G, Calliada F. Breast hamartoma: ultrasound, elastosonographic, and mammographic features. Mini pictorial essay. J Ultrasound. 2015;18(4):373–7.
12. Katic V, Stosic D, Rankovic A, Simonovic M, Todorovic J. Plasma cell mastitis resembling a breast cancer: a case report and review of the literature. J Infect Dis Ther. 2017;5(346):2332–0877.
13. Palmieri A, d'Orazi V, Martino G, Frusone F, Crocetti D, Amabile MI, Monti M. Plasma cell mastitis in men: a Single-center experience and review of the literature. In vivo. 2016;30:727–32.
14. Leong PW, Chotai NC, Kulkarni S. Imaging features of inflammatory breast disorders: a pictorial essay. Korean J Radiol. 2018;19(1):5–14.
15. Liu Y, Zhang J, Zhou YH, Jiang YN, Zhang W, Tang XJ, Ren Y, Han SP, Liu PJ, Xu J, He JJ. IL-6/STAT3 signaling pathway is activated in plasma cell mastitis. Int J Clin Exp Pathol. 2015;8(10):12541–8. PMID: 26722442; PMCID: PMC4680387
16. Brogi E, Hoda SA, Koerner FC, Rosen PP, editors. Rosens diagnosis of breast pathology by needle core biopsy. 4th ed. Philadelphia, PA: Wolters Kluwer Health; 2017. p. 84.
17. D'Alfonso TM, Ginter PS, Shin SJ. A review of inflammatory processes of the breast with a focus on diagnosis in core biopsy samples. J Pathol Transl Med. 2015;49(4):279–87. https://doi.org/10.4132/jptm.2015.06.11. Epub 2015 Jul 15. PMID: 26095437; PMCID: PMC4508565
18. Ferris-James DM, Iuanow E, Mehta TS, Shaheen RM, Slanetz PJ. Imaging approaches to diagnosis and management of common ductal abnormalities. Radiographics. 2012;32(4):1009–30.
19. Pluguez-Turull CW, Nanyes JE, Quintero CJ, Alizai H, Mais DD, Kist KA, Dornbluth NC. Idiopathic granulomatous mastitis: manifestations at multimodality imaging and pitfalls. Radiographics. 2018;38(2):330–56.
20. Jiang L, Li X, Sun B, Ma T, Kong X, Yang Q. Clinicopathological features of granulomatous lobular mastitis and mammary duct ectasia. Oncol Lett. 2020;19(1):840–8. https://doi.org/10.3892/ol.2019.11156. Epub 2019 Nov 28. PMID: 31885718; PMCID: PMC6924204
21. Gautier N, Lalonde L, Tran-Thanh D, El Khoury M, David J, Labelle M, et al. Chronic granulomatous mastitis: imaging, pathology and management. Eur J Radiol. 2013;82:e165–75.
22. Kayahan M, Kadioglu H, Muslumanoglu M. Management of patients with granulomatous mastitis: analysis of 31 cases. Breast Care. 2012;7:226–30.
23. Puneet SK, Tiwary RR, Sanjay SS. Breast tuberculosis: still common in India. Internet J Trop Med. 2005;2(2):1540–2681.
24. Akcan A, Akyildiz H, Deneme MA, Akgun H, Aritas Y. Granulomatous lobular mastitis: a complex diagnostic and therapeutic problem. World J Surg. 2006;30:1403–9.
25. Thyagarajan M, Nallasivam M, Singh B. Bacilli in the breast. Int Surg J. 2017;4:3344–6.
26. Sabaté JM, Clotet M, Gómez A, De Las Heras P, Torrubia S, Salinas T. Radiologic evaluation of uncommon inflammatory and reactive breast disorders. Radiographics. 2005;25(2):411–24.
27. Panzacchi R, Gallo C, Fois F, Dalpiaz G, Cucchi MC, DegliEsposti R, Foschini MP. Primary sarcoidosis of the breast: case description and review of the literature. Pathologica. 2010;102(3):104–7.
28. Cheuk W, Chan AC, Lam WL, et al. IgG4-related sclerosing mastitis: description of a new member of the IgG4-related sclerosing diseases. Am J Surg Pathol. 2009;33:1058–64.
29. Lee JY, Joo M. Isolated breast vasculitis manifested as breast oedema with suggestive sonographic findings: a case report with imaging findings. J Med Ultrason. 2017;44:191–5. https://doi.org/10.1007/s10396-016-0753-6.
30. Shetty MK, Watson AB. Mondor's disease of the breast: sonographic and mammographic findings. Am J Roentgenol. 2001;177(4):893–6.
31. Yeoh G, Russell P, Jenkins E. Spectrum of histological changes reactive to prosthetic breast implants: a clinopathological study of 84 patients. Pathology. 1996;28(3):232–5.
32. Moon SJ, Park YM, Kim SJ, Jung HK, Lee SJ, Choo HJ. Various foreign bodies seen on mammography Eur Congress Radiol. 2014.
33. Shah AT, Jankharia BB. Imaging of common breast implants and implant-related complications: a pictorial essay. Ind J Radiol Imaging. 2016;26(2):216.
34. Neetu G, Pathmanathan R, Weng NK. Diabetic Mastopathy: a case report and literature review. Case Rep Oncol. 2010;3(2):245–51. https://doi.org/10.1159/000318641. PMID: 20740205; PMCID: PMC2920008
35. Ely KA, Tse G, Simpson JF, Clarfeld R, Page DL. Diabetic mastopathy. A clinicopathologic review. Am J Clin Pathol. 2000;113(4):541–5.
36. Fahrni M, Schwarz EI, Stadlmann S, Singer G, Hauser N, Kubik-Huch RA. Breast abscesses: diagnosis, treatment and outcome. Breast Care. 2012;7(1):32–8.

https://doi.org/10.1159/000336547. Epub 2012 Feb 21. PMID: 22553470; PMCID: PMC3335354
37. Trop I, Dugas A, David J, El Khoury M, Boileau JF, Larouche N, Lalonde L. Breast abscesses: evidence-based algorithms for diagnosis, management, and follow-up. Radiographics. 2011;31(6):1683–99.
38. D'Alfonso TM, Ginter PS, Shin SJ. A review of inflammatory processes of the breast with a focus on diagnosis in Core biopsy samples. J Pathol Transl Med. 2015;49(4):279–87. PMCID: PMC4508565 PMID: 26095437
39. Tauro LF, Martis JS, George C, Kamath A, Lobo G, Hegde BR. Tuberculous mastitis presenting as breast abscess. Oman Med J. 2011;26(1):53–5. https://doi.org/10.5001/omj.2011.14. PMID: 22043382; PMCID: PMC3191622
40. Falco G, Foroni M, Castagnetti F, Marano L, Bordoni D, Rocco N, Marchesi V, Iotti V, Vacondio R, Ferrari G. Ultrasound-guided percutaneous catheter drainage of large breast abscesses in lactating women: how to preserve breastfeeding safely. Breastfeed Med. 2016;11:555–6. (ISSN: 1556-8342)
41. Kang YD, Kim YM. Comparison of needle aspiration and vacuum-assisted biopsy in the ultrasound-guided drainage of lactational breast abscesses. Ultrasonography. 2016;35(2):148–52. (ISSN: 2288-5919)
42. Lam E, Chan T, Wiseman SM. Breast abscess: evidence based management recommendations. Expert Rev Anti-Infect Ther. 2014;12(7):753–62.

18 Fibroepithelial Lesions of the Breast

Priya K. Palanisamy, Archana B, Bhawna Dev, and Ramya Ramakrishnan

Abstract

Fibroepithelial lesions of the breast are a spectrum of pathologies ranging from common, benign entity like fibroadenomas to uncommon and malignant pathologies like malignant phyllodes. These biphasic neoplasms of the breast are usually seen in women during the third and fourth decades. In this chapter, we brief the demographics, clinical, imaging, and pathological features of these fibroepithelial lesions to aid in the diagnosis and management.

Keywords

Fibroadenoma · Phyllodes tumor · Borderline · PASH · Lactating adenoma

P. K. Palanisamy (✉) · B. Dev
Department of Radiology, Maidstone and Tunbridge Wells NHS Trust, Kent, UK
e-mail: bhawnadev@sriramachandra.edu.in

A. B
Department of Pathology, Sri Ramachandra Institute of Higher Education and Research, Chennai, India
e-mail: archanab@sriramachandra.edu.in

R. Ramakrishnan
Department of Surgery, Sri Ramachandra Institute of Higher Education and Research, Chennai, India
e-mail: ramya.r@sriramachandra.edu.in

18.1 Introduction

Fibrous lesions of the breast are the most commonly encountered lesions in clinical practice. These are predominantly composed of prominent stromal elements with varying amounts of glandular epithelium. These include

1. Fibroadenoma
2. Phyllodes Tumor
3. Benign mesenchymal breast lesions—like Fibromatosis, Pseudo-angiomatous stromal hyperplasia, Focal fibrosis
4. Diabetic fibrous mastopathy
5. Mammary Hamartoma

Some fibrous lesions like Phyllodes tumor have malignant potential. Pathologically, they are classified into low -grade (Benign) lesion, borderline and high grade (Malignant) Lesions. There is no specific imaging feature in mammography or ultrasound (USG), which aids in differentiating the Malignant fibrous lesions from benign Fibroadenomas. A radio pathological correlation is required to better enable the differentiation between the benign fibrous lesions of the breast from the ones, which require surgical resection [1].

B. Dev, L. D. Joseph (eds.), *Holistic Approach to Breast Disease*,
https://doi.org/10.1007/978-981-99-0035-0_18

18.2 Fibroadenoma

These are the commonest benign Fibroepithelial tumors of the breast. It develops from the **Terminal Duct Lobular Unit (TDLU)**, which are the basic units of histological assessment (Fig. 18.1).

Clinical presentation: Commonly palpable lesion found in adolescent girls and young women. About 15% of cases have multiple fibroadenomas at presentation [2].

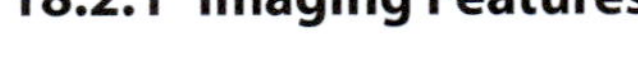

18.2.1 Imaging Features

Mammogram—Well defined round, oval, or lobulated equal density masses with smooth or obscured margins (Fig. 18.2a, b). A hypoechoic halo can be seen peripherally due to optical illusion called the Mach effect. Calcifications are seen in **involuting fibroadenoma**, occurring typically in postmenopausal women. Initially, the calcification starts in the periphery as dots, which later coalesce in the center to form the pathognomonic **Popcorn Calcification** (Fig. 18.2c, d).

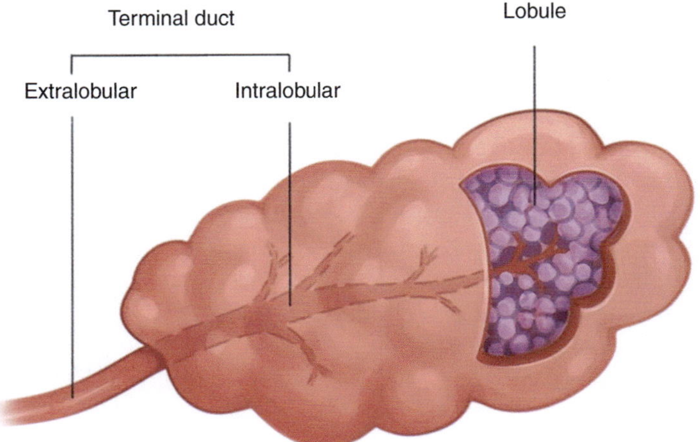

Fig. 18.1 Pictorial representation of terminal duct lobule of the breast

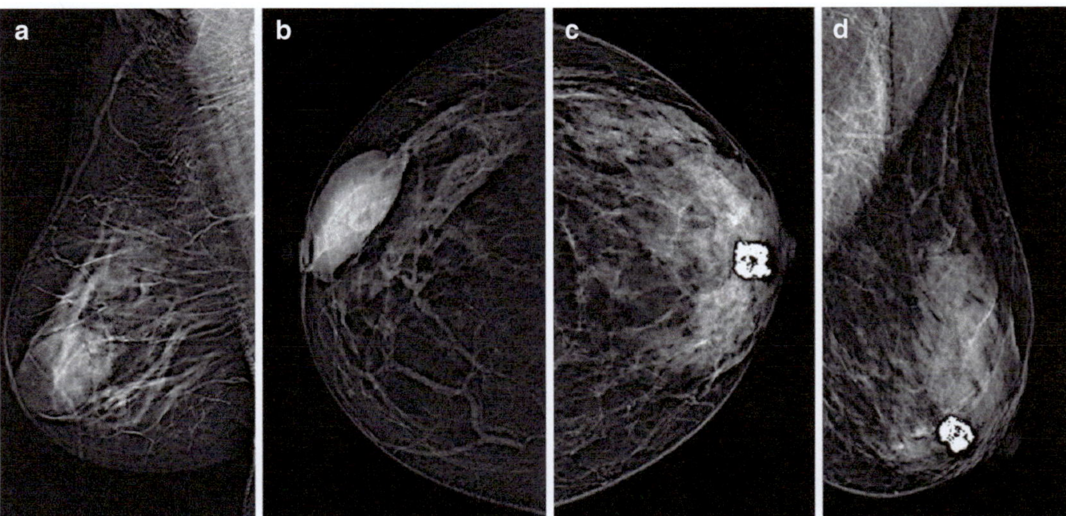

Fig 18.2 (**a**, **b**) MLO and CC view of the right breast shows an oval circumscribed equal density mass in the subareolar region. A hypodense halo (arrow) seen around the periphery of the mass suggestive of the benign nature of mass (**c**, **d**) CC and MLO of the left breast shows benign coarse calcification—**popcorn calcification**

These calcifications can vary from benign dystrophic to coarse pleomorphic calcifications. However, all circumscribed masses with calcifications should not be dismissed as benign fibroadenoma, rather any suspicious calcification even in a circumscribed mass should warrant further evaluation with ultrasound and if needed biopsy. Most often a fibroadenoma in a mammogram can have nonspecific features and may require further evaluation.

Contrast-Enhanced Spectral Mammography (CESM): May or may not show enhancement and if enhancement is present can be variable. Ultimately, the decision to biopsy secondary to enhancing mass in CESM depends on combination of morphological features in mammogram and USG.

Ultrasound—oval/elliptical in shape, parallel, circumscribed with smooth margins, and uniform echotexture (hypoechoic or isoechoic) (Fig. 18.3a). Has few thin fibrous internal septations and variable posterior features, which can vary from posterior shadowing in case of hyalinized fibroadenoma and posterior enhancement in a epithelialized fibroadenoma (Fig. 18.3b, c). Internal vascularity within a fibroadenoma is variable. Most of them have thin echogenic pseudocapsule, which is nothing but the compressed surrounding breast stroma. On elastography, the stiffness of fibroadenoma is variable.

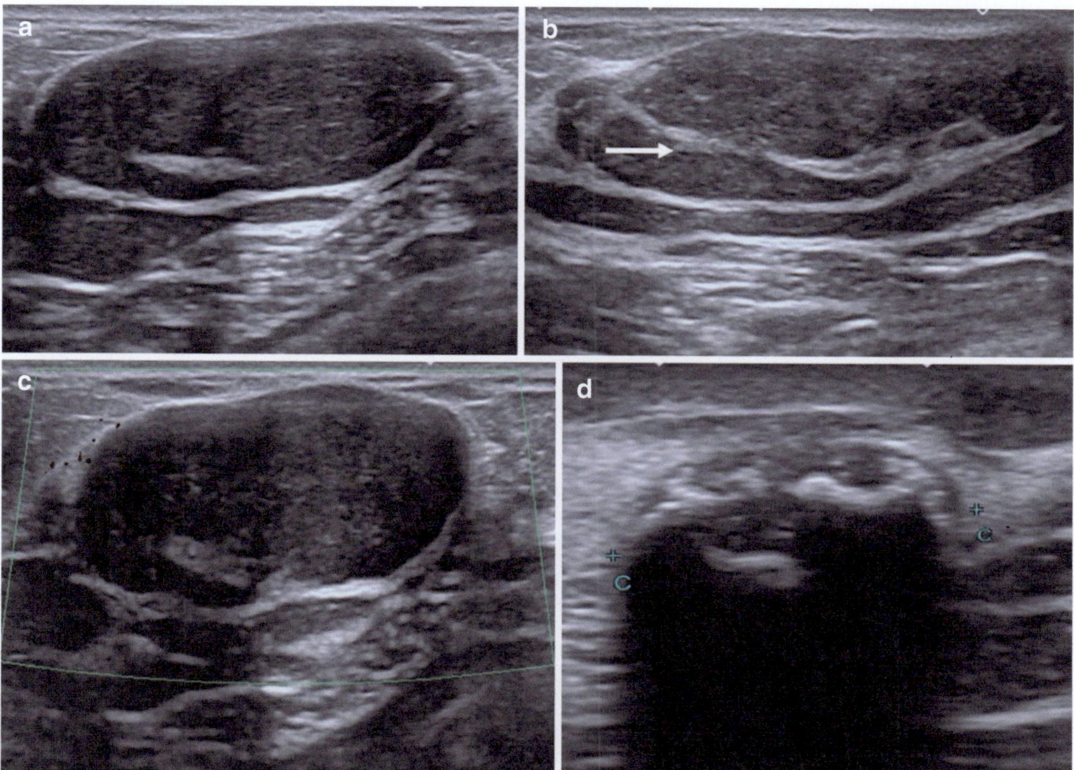

Fig. 18.3 Ultrasound image demonstrates a well-defined paraellely oriented oval hypoechoic fibroadenoma with thin echogenic capsule in the periphery (**a**). Common feature of fibroadenoma on USG is echogenic thin internal septations as shown with arrow in (**b**). Posterior enhancement (arrow) with mild marginal vascularity on doppler (**c**). Typical feature of an involuting fibroadenoma with coarse popcorn calcification showing dense posterior shadowing in USG (**d**)

NOTE: Calcified involuting fibroadenomas are benign masses and do not require further workup with USG/biopsy (Fig 18.3d). Noncalcified isodense circumscribed masses in mammogram require USG correlation.

MRI: Variable signal intensities depend on the hyalinization of the mass. Sclerotic or hyalinized fibroadenoma is T2 hypointense and cellular or myxoid fibroadenoma is T2 hyperintense. Fibroadenomas have a variable enhancement pattern, myxoid fibroadenoma has a homogenous enhancement pattern, and sclerotic variant shows no or minimal enhancement. Typical fibroadenoma shows the Type I kinetic curve (rapid initial enhancement, persisting in delayed phase). Classical fibroadenoma has nonenhancing T2 dark internal septations within [3] (Figs. 18.4 and 18.5).

18.2.2 Atypical features of fibroadenoma

Most often a benign fibroadenoma may present with atypical imaging features making these suspicious (BI-RADS-4 and above), which requires further evaluation with biopsy and histopathological confirmation. These atypical imaging features range from irregular shape (Fig. 18.6a), indistinct/lobulated margins (Fig. 18.6b), posterior acoustic shadowing in the absence of calcification and cystic internal spaces (Fig. 18.6c).

BI-RADS category and management: Involuting fibroadenoma with popcorn calcifications, are considered as **BI-RADS 2 (Benign)** masses and do not require interval imaging follow-up or CNB/Fine-needle Aspiration. Noncalcified parallel masses with smooth margins, are categorized as **BI-RADS 3 (probably benign)** and requires interval follow-

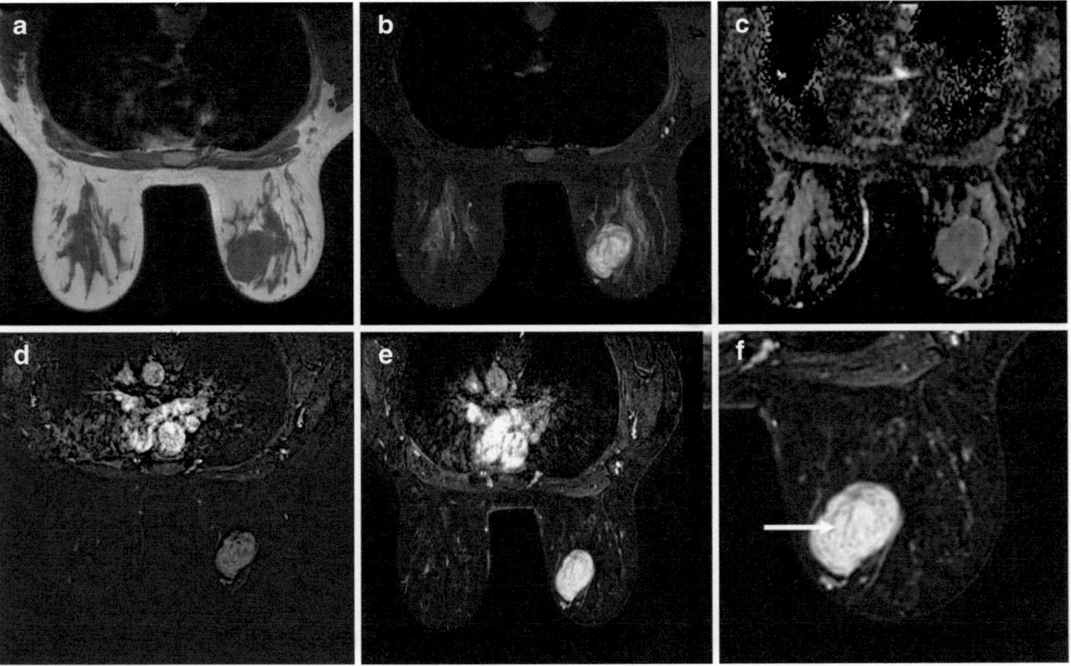

Fig. 18.4 MRI appearance of a typical fibroadenoma in a 35-year female: Mass on T1 sequence appears homogenously hypointense (**a**), hyperintense on T2 sequence with T2 dark internal septations (**b**), and no diffusion restriction on ADC sequence (**c**). On dynamic T1 postcontrast subtracted images, the fibroadenoma shows early enhancement in early phase (**d**) and progressive enhancement in the late phase (**e**). The classic appearance of the nonenhancing internal septations of the fibroadenoma demonstrated with an arrow in the magnified late phase postcontrast subtracted images (**f**)

Fig. 18.5 Dynamic contrast MRI breast of the same 35-year-old female, (**a**) Mass shows areas of neovascularity, the color code mapping demonstrates Type 1 Kinetic Curve with progressive benign type of enhancement on Time Intensity Curve (TIC) with ROI within the neovascular region (**b**, **c**) corresponding to the histopathological diagnosis of fibroadenoma

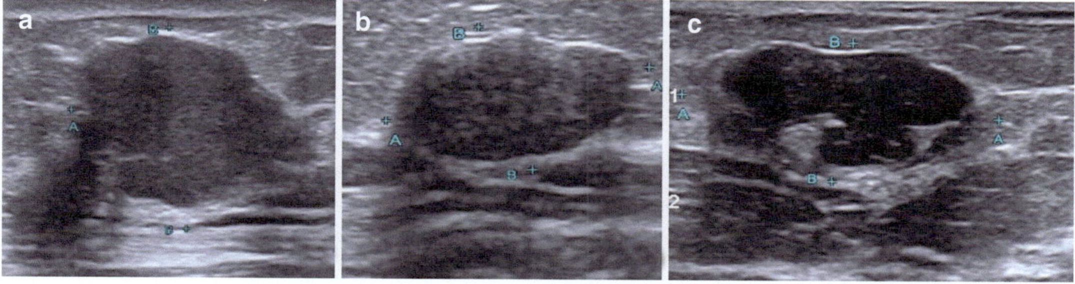

Fig. 18.6 Atypical feature of fibroadenoma—Irregular margins (**a**), smooth macrolobulated margins with posterior shadowing seen in epithelized fibroadenoma (**b**). A complex fibroadenoma with internal cystic spaces (**c**)

up according to ACR guidelines of BI-RADS 3 masses at 6 months interval for 2 years without core biopsy. If there is 20% or more growth in the size of the lesion at any point during the follow-up imaging, a biopsy is recommended (even if previously biopsied and proven to be fibroadenoma). As mentioned earlier, the presence of any atypical/suspicious imaging features (**BI-RADS 4 and above**) in the masses warrants biopsy and pathological correlation.

Asymptomatic patient with biopsy suggestive of benign fibroadenoma needs no further follow-up or excision. In symptomatic patients, the option of surgical or minimally invasive procedures like Vacuum-Assisted Excision (VAE) and ablation can be offered. However, if the size of the fibroadenoma is >3 cm only surgical excision is recommended.

18.2.3 Histopathology

Gross findings—Fibroadenomas are bosselated with a smooth surface externally. Cut surface is firm, grey white with slit-like spaces (Fig. 18.7a). Some can have a gelatinous appearance, tiny cysts may also be noted.

Microscopy (Fig. 18.7b, c)—They are well circumscribed. Proliferation of glandular and stromal components is noted. Ducts are lined by inner epithelial and outer myoepithelial cells. Two patterns of growth are noted: intracanalicular and peri canalicular. Intracanalicular pattern is seen when the abundant stroma compresses ducts into slit like lumens. When ducts are not compressed by stroma, they comprise the pericanalicular pattern. Stroma can undergo myxoid change. Epithelial components may show squamous metaplasia, apocrine metaplasia, and cyst formation similar to fibrocystic disease.

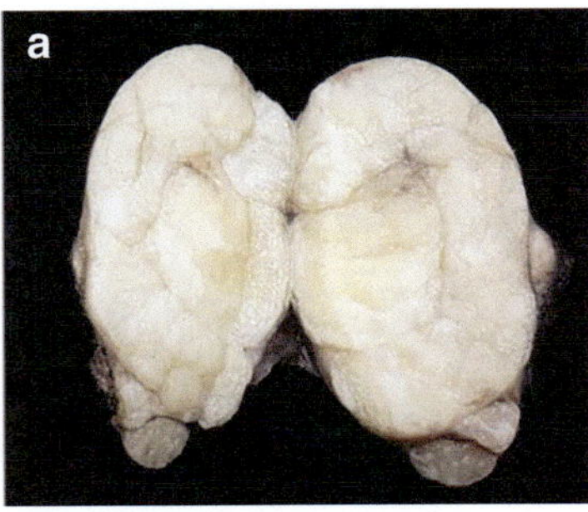

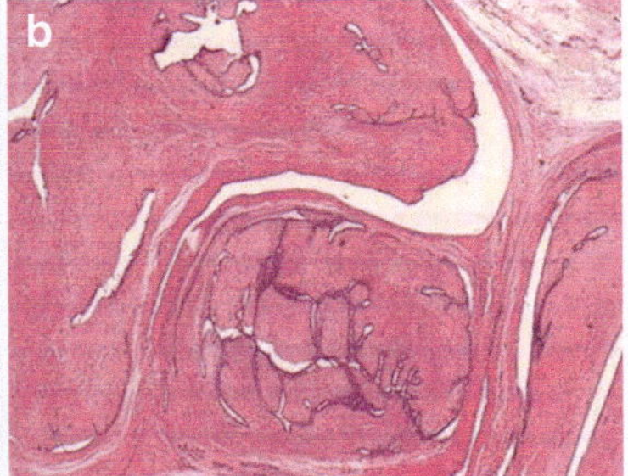

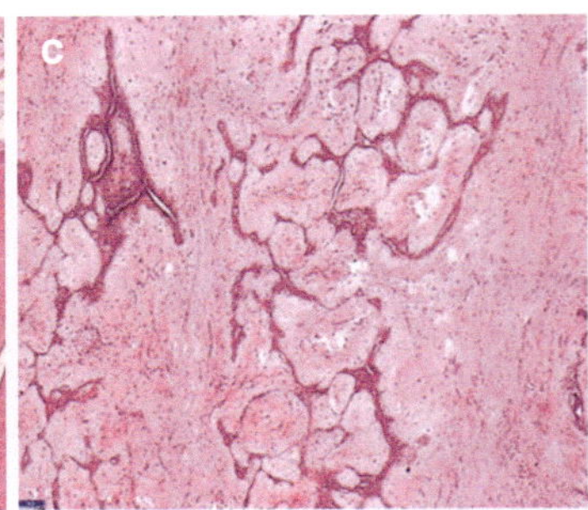

Fig. 18.7 Gross image of fibroadenoma showing a circumscribed gray white lesion with slit like spaces (**a**), Pictomicrograph of a H&E-stained section demonstrating a circumscribed lesion with compressed ducts surrounded by prominent stroma (5×) (**b**), Pictomicrograph of a fibroadenoma with myxoid changes (20×) (**c**)

18.2.4 Variants of fibroadenoma [3]

Juvenile fibroadenoma: is seen primarily in adolescent girls. Imaging features are similar to fibroadenoma, except that these are generally **larger in size during the presentation and show rapid growth rate**. Grossly, they are indistinguishable from the adult variety and their sizes may vary from 2 to 22 cms. Microscopically, they are differentiated by increased stromal hypercellularity and epithelial hyperplasia with or without mild atypia. Epithelial hyperplasia can have a lactiform, papillary, solid, lobular-terminal ductal or, cribriform pattern [4] In contrast to the typical fibroadenoma, these usually require surgical excision due to the rapid growth rate and larger size (Fig. 18.8).

Tubular adenoma: Rare and is seen in younger women as noncalcified well-circumscribed mass and menopausal women as an irregular suspicious mass with microcalcification, which requires biopsy. It is a histological variant of peri canalicular fibroadenoma with florid adenosis like epithelial proliferation. Microscopically, they are composed of closely packed round to oval glands lined by epithelial and myoepithelial cells, which may contain secretions in their lumen [5].

Lactating Adenoma [6]: is a benign stromal tumor and is typically seen during the third trimester of pregnancy through the period of lactation. Primarily, these are considered as a variant of fibroadenoma or tubular adenoma, which has undergone hormonal influence during lactation. Clinically, these are firm, nontender, mobile masses. About 5% of the lactating adenoma can undergo infarction. Imaging appearance is similar to a classic fibroadenoma. This may have inspissated milk within, which appears as hyperechoic foci showing posterior enhancement (Fig. 18.9) in USG and radiolucent areas in Mammography secondary to the fat content in the milk. Microscopically, they are fibroadenomas with secretory hyperplasia characterized by cuboidal cells having foamy to finely vacuolated cytoplasm [7] (Fig 18.9c). These are treated conservatively as most of the lactating adenomas usually regress spontaneously after the period of lactation.

Complex fibroadenoma: It has a relative risk of about 3.10 times higher for developing invasive breast cancer than 2.17 times risk in patients with classical fibroadenoma [8]. In USG, it shows internal heterogeneity with cysts and punctate echogenic foci (Fig. 18.6c). Microscopically, fibroadenomas with sclerosing adenosis, cysts, epitheliosis, papillary apocrine hyperplasia, and calcifications are termed "complex fibroadenoma" as they have a relatively higher chance of developing breast cancer [7]. These warrant interval imaging follow up/biopsy.

> **NOTE**: Fibroadenoma is very rare in males, as they have very few Terminal Duct Lobular Units (TDLU).

Fig. 18.8 A 15-year-old girl presented with rapidly increasing size of both breasts, causing severe discomfort. Clinical picture shows grossly enlarged breasts with severe skin congestion and tortuous superficial vessels (**a**). T1 sequence showing multiple iso- to hypointense masses completely replacing the breast parenchyma on both side (**b**), hyperintense with dark internal septations on T2 sequence (**c**). On postcontrast coronal sequence (**d**) these masses show enhancement with non-enhancing septae. Coronal MIP sequence (**e**) shows multiple superficial arteries supplying these masses. Biopsy and surgical pathology confirmed multiple juvenile fibro adenomatosis

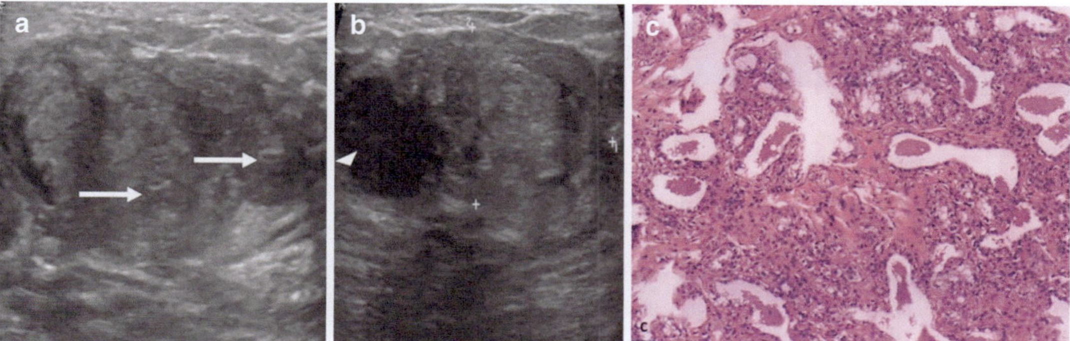

Fig. 18.9 A 32-year-old lactating woman with tender lump in the left breast, shows an ill-defined mass with indistinct margins showing multiple echogenic foci (arrow in **a**) and area of cystic spaces within (arrowhead in **b**). On aspiration no pus could be aspirated and biopsy performed was suggestive of lactating adenoma showing closely packed glands with vacuolated cytoplasm and secretions (40×) (**c**)

18.3 Phyllodes Tumor

These were originally described as **Cystosarcoma Phyllodes**, due to their leaf-like pattern of growth. These are rare yet clinically significant fibroepithelial lesions of the breast, accounting for about 1% of all breast neoplasms [9]. They may be benign, borderline, and malignant in nature. About 75% of the incidence is benign, 25% borderline, and only 10% are malignant.

Clinical presentation: It occurs between the age group from 12 to 80 years, with a peak at 30 to 40 years. This lesion presents as a large mass with rapid growth when compared to fibroadenomas. Skin ulcerations may be seen in larger masses. Since borderline and malignant subtypes have a propensity for **local recurrence and hematogenous metastasis**, it is treated like other high-grade sarcomas with surgical resection, chemotherapy, and adjuvant radiotherapy. The overall 5-year survival rate of phyllodes tumors is 90%. However, high-grade phyllodes have only 65% five year survival rate [1].

18.3.1 Imaging Features

Mammogram: Round, lobulated, well-circumscribed high-density masses, which can mimic fibroadenoma (Fig. 18.10). Calcifications if present are dystrophic and coarse. Can be larger in size (more than >3 cm) and larger size could help in differentiating potential malignant phyllodes from benign.

Ultrasound: Though very similar to fibroadenoma in appearance, the presence of intralesional clefts and cystic spaces favor phyllodes tumor more in USG (Fig. 18.10c, d). It is possible to differentiate borderline and malignant subtypes by USG, as they can be seen as larger irreg-

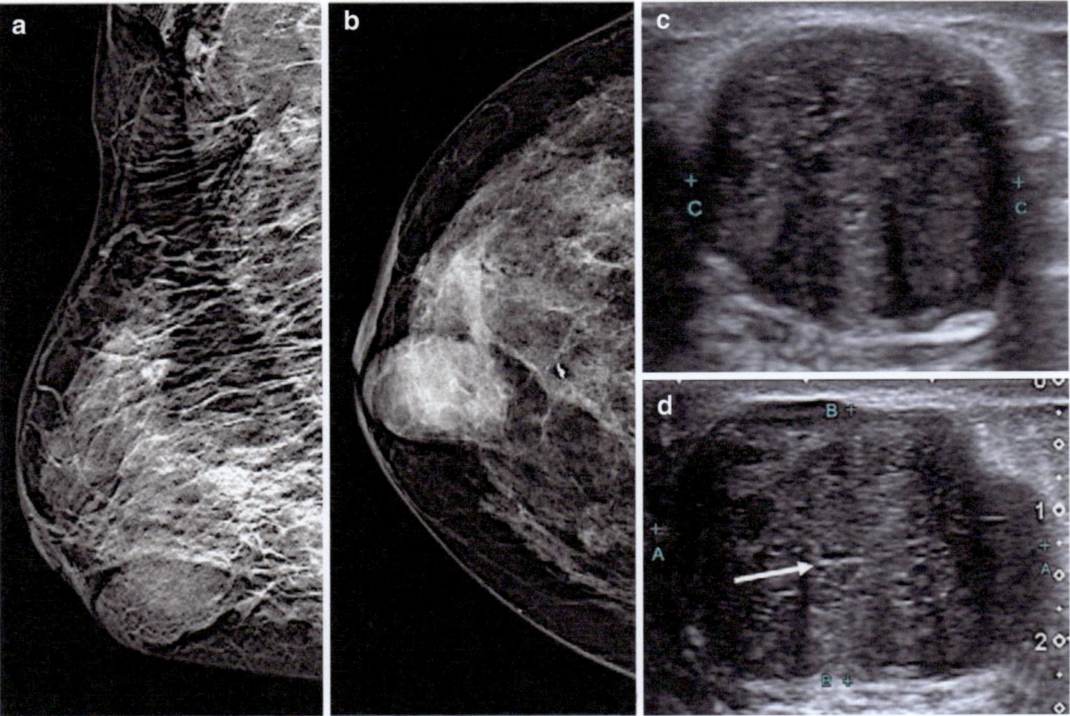

Fig. 18.10 A 45-year-old with palpable lump in the left breast which was proven to be benign phyllodes on biopsy. MLO (**a**) and CC view (**b**) mammograms of the right breast shows a round to oval equal dendity mass with smooth lobulated margins in the lower central region 6'o clock position of right breast. The mammographic features are similar to a fibroadenoma). On ultrasound (**c**), hypoechoic mass with lobulated margins and **(d)** subtle cleft like cystic spaces within the center of the mass (arrow) are seen

ular masses with uncircumscribed margins and may have larger cystic spaces within secondary to the necrosis, nature of these masses. Shows variable vascularity on doppler and variable stiffness on elastography.

MRI: Oval, lobulated masses with circumscribed margins showing homogenous T2 high to intermediate signal intensity with T2 hyperintense cystic necrotic spaces/hemorrhage within secondary to the rapid growth. May show rapid tumor enhancement with washout in a malignant phyllodes and slow progressive enhancement in benign phyllodes, but these features can overlap. MRI is mostly used to acquire information about the tumor extent, chest wall invasion, and possible satellite lesions before surgical excision.(Fig. 18.11).

NOTE: In a study by Libermann et al. [10], it was found phyllodes tumor larger than 3 cm and increased age had a higher likelihood of malignancy. They were also able to evaluate the **doubling time of phyllodes tumours and found malignant variant was 36 days and that of benign variants is 211 days**.

BI-RADS category and management: Imaging is not reliable in differentiating cellular fibroadenoma from benign phyllodes tumor as both show similar imaging features. Core needle biopsy is preferred over fine needle aspiration in evaluating such masses. Follow-up imaging becomes man-

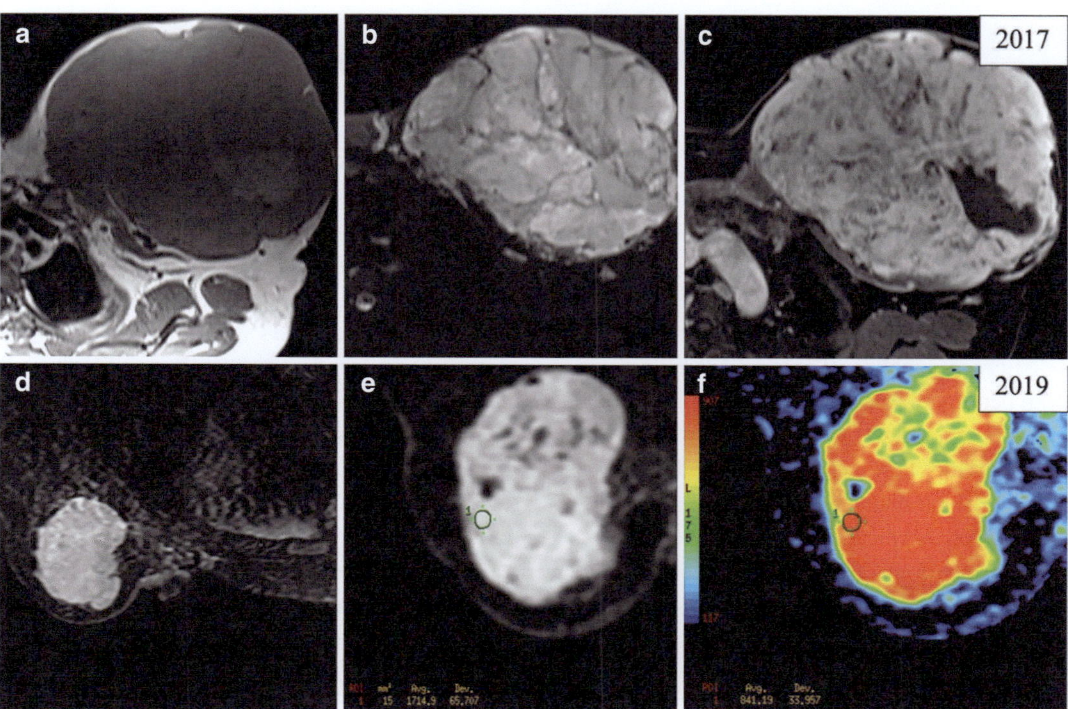

Fig. 18.11 A 45-year-old woman presented with rapidly enlarging left breast in 2017 underwent mastectomy for the biopsy proven malignant phyllodes tumor. MRI breast T1 sequence shows a large lobulated hypointense mass with focal hyperintensity suggestive of hemorrhage (**a**), heterogeneously T2 hyperintense with multiple dark clefts (**b**). On contrast administration shows rapid enhancement (**c**). The patient presented to the clinic with recurrence in the left mastectomy site after two years (**d**). Rapidly enhancing mass after contrast administration (**e**) and dynamic contrast sequence with color mapping shows malignant type of enhancement (**f**). No distant metastasis was found

datory as the malignant variant tends to grow rapidly with a median doubling time of about 36 days and has hematogenous metastasis, unlike other breast malignancies.

Benign subtype: which are generally less than 3 cm in size with smooth well circumscribed margins in mammogram and USG, are considered as BI-RADS 3 lesions and requires interval follow up after core biopsy.

Borderline and malignant subtype: presents as more than 3 cm in size irregular masses with uncircumscribed margins, are considered as BI-RADS-4 and requires core needle biopsy (CNB). These lesions require surgical excision with 1 cm clear margins to prevent recurrence. The patient needs to be on imaging follow-up for 5 years post-surgery. Large lesions might require mastectomy, as borderline and malignant phyllodes need to be treated as soft tissue sarcomas. Distant metastasis needs to be ruled out and they are unlikely to have nodal metastasis.

18.3.2 Histopathology

Gross features—They are well-circumscribed but unencapsulated. The cut surface is firm, bulging, grey tan, may have a cut cabbage appearance. Areas of necrosis, cysts, myxoid changes may be noted (Fig. 18.12).

Microscopically (Fig. 18.12)—This arise from periductal stroma with few lobular elements. Expansion and cellular stromal components are characteristic. Periductal stromal condensation is noted. Mitotic activity may also be increased in these areas. Atypical ductal hyperplasia may be noted in phyllodes tumors. Elongated cleft lined by epithelium is a feature. Phyllodes tumor may be benign, borderline, or malignant based on some features like stromal overgrowth, borders, cellularity, and mitosis (Table 18.1).

18.3.3 Immunohistochemistry

Stroma is positive for vimentin, actin, CD34, desmin, VEGF (Vascular Endothelial Growth Factor), they are reported to be more positive in the stroma of malignant phyllodes. Ki67 labeling index indicates the proliferative activity of stromal cells and is increased with higher-grade histologic type of phyllodes and also helps in differentiating it with fibroadenoma in which the Ki67% is relatively lower [12].

Differentiating fibroadenoma from phyllodes tumor (Table 18.2): Though both fibroadenoma and phyllodes tumor are fibroepithelial tumors, Phyllodes tumors has rapid growth with malignant potential warranting surgical resection. In contrast, fibroadenoma does not usually require removal, making the preoperative diagnosis imperative.

18.3.4 Miscellaneous Fibroepithelial Lesions of Breast

Fibromatosis: Also known as extra-abdominal desmoid tumor. Develops in pectoralis fascia and causes retraction of the skin and nipple. **On mammogram** seen as a round or irregular mass with spiculated margins. **Histologically**, these have bland spindle cells with interspersed fibroblasts and collagen. Requires complete surgical excision.

Pseudo Angiomatous Stromal Hyperplasia (PASH) [13]: Commonly seen in women of reproductive age and Premenopausal women on hormonal therapy, especially progesterone as it causes proliferation of myofibroblasts.

Imaging features of PASH may appear similar to a fibroadenoma (Fig. 18.13). Hence core needle/excision biopsy is needed for histological diagnosis.

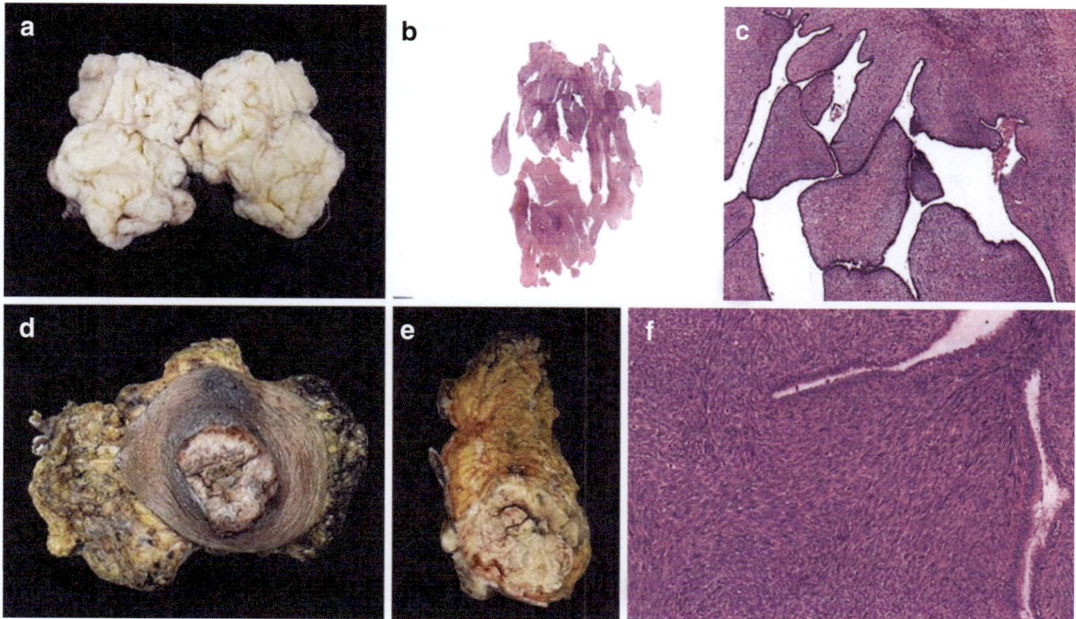

Fig. 18.12 Gross image of the cut surface of a benign phyllodes tumor, which appears circumscribed, grey white with cleft like spaces resembling a leaf-like pattern (**a**), H&E stained pictomicrograph showing a benign phyllodes tumor arranged in a leaf-like architectural pattern (1.5×) (**b**), Borderline phyllodes showing a moderately cellular stroma surrounding the ducts,(10×) (**c**), Gross image of a malignant phyllodes tumor, which is fungating (**d**), cut surface of a malignant phyllodes tumor shows a fairly circumscribed bosselated lesion with areas of hemorrhage and necrosis (**e**), H&E stained pictomicrograph of a malignant. Phyllodes tumor showing stromal cellularity, stromal overgrowth (**f**)

Table 18.1 Pathological difference between benign, borderline, and malignant phyllodes tumor of breast [11]

	Benign	Borderline	Malignant
Mitoses/10 HPF	0–4	5–10	>10
Tumor borders	Pushing	Pushing or focally infiltrative	Diffusely infiltrative, permeative
Stromal atypia	None to mild	Mild to moderate	Marked
Stromal overgrowth	None	Focal/moderate	Marked/diffuse
Stromal cellularity	Mild	Moderate	Marked/high
Malignant heterologous stromal elements	None	None	Present

Histologically: these are mesenchymal lesions that may be mistaken for angiosarcoma. They have the proliferation of fibroblasts and myofibroblasts forming slit-like spaces admixed with benign breast ducts. The bland spindle cells that line these spaces are strongly positive for vimen-

Table 18.2 Summary of difference between fibroadenoma and phyllodes tumor

	Fibroadenoma	Phyllodes tumor
Age	Younger females Peak incidence at 20–30 years of age	Older patients Peak incidence at 40–50 years
Clinical presentation	A palpable lesion with stable or minimal growth	Rapid growth. Tends to recur. The borderline and malignant phyllodes has rapid doubling time and hematogenous distant metastasis unlike other breast malignancies
Histology	Epithelial and stromal components	Double layered epithelial component arrayed into clefts with surrounding **stromal hypercellularity** protruding into the epithelial lining as a classic "**leaf-like**" pattern
Mammogram	Oval or round equal density masses with circumscribed margins Pop-corn type of calcification seen in involuting Fibroadenoma	Borderline and malignant subtypes are commonly seen as irregular masses with obscured or uncircumscribed margins
Ultrasound	Cystic spaces not seen commonly **BI-RADS 3**	Intralesional cystic and cleft like spaces are specific to Phyllodes **Benign subtype: BI-RADS 3** **Borderline and malignant subtype: BI-RADS 4**
Histopathology	• Duct-like spaces surrounded by fibrous stroma • No mitosis • Stromal overgrowth and stromal infiltration absent	• Leaf-like architecture with **increased stromal cellularity** (one high power field shows an absence of epithelial component) • Increased mitosis • Stromal overgrowth and stromal infiltration present
Management	Doesn't require core needle biopsy (CNB) and surgical resection	Requires core needle biopsy (CNB), aggressive subtypes (borderline and malignant types) requires surgical excision with 1 cm or greater margin clearance without axillary dissection and consideration for chemotherapy and adjuvant radiotherapy

tin and CD34 and negative for cytokeratin and factor VIII [14].

Management: The treatment of tumoral PASH is wide local excision. Follow-up imaging is crucial in PASH, as they are known to recur and have synchronous malignancies in the same or contralateral breast.

Focal fibrosis: Similar to pseudo angiomatous lesions occurring in premenopausal women, as firm masses containing collagenous stroma with a less glandular component.

Diabetic fibrous mastopathy: occur typically in young women about 20 years after the onset of insulin-dependent diabetes mellitus. **Clinically** presents as firm nontender mass.

Imaging features: **On mammogram**, it is often seen as dense asymmetry or irregular mass. Typically **US** images show dense and multiple acoustic shadowing within (Fig. 18.14a–c). There is no associated risk of developing fibromatosis or breast cancer.

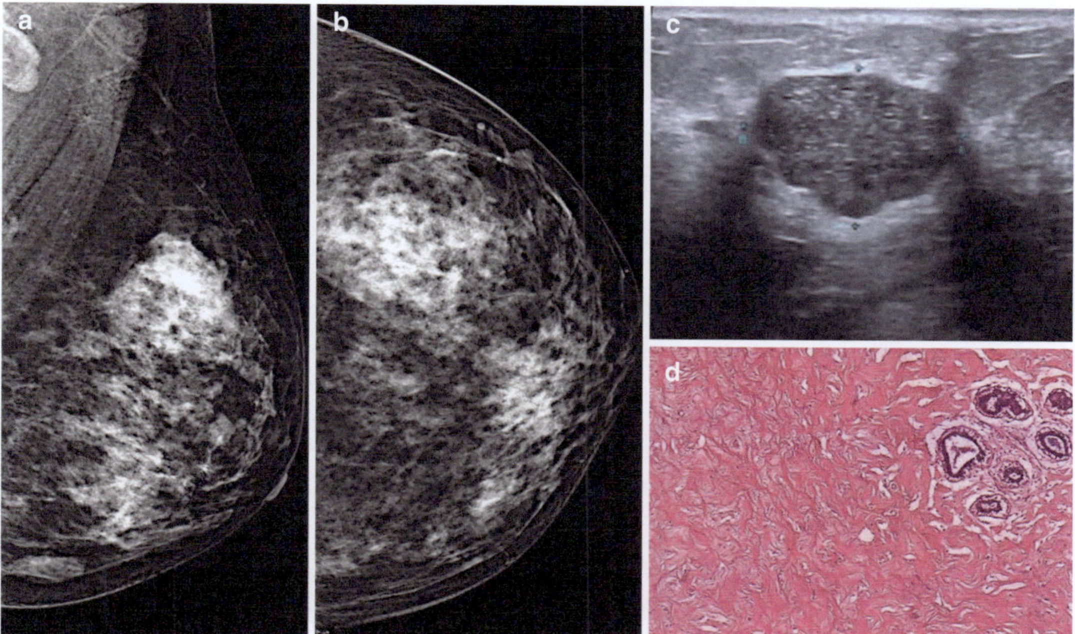

Fig. 18.13 A 42-year-old woman with biopsy proven PASH, mammogram (MLO and CC views) of left breast shows ill-defined isodense mass with indistinct margins in the upper outer quadrant (**a**, **b**). On ultrasound shows lobulated margins with posterior enhancement (**c**). H&E (20×) shows anastomosing spaces lined by myofibroblasts in a dense collagenous keloid like stroma (**d**)

Histopathology (Fig. 18.14d): Grossly no evidence of tumor noted, masses may be firm to hard. On cut-surface, the lesion is gray white homogeneous almost indistinguishable from surrounding breast parenchyma. Microscopically, the lesion is composed of lymphocytes (mostly B cells) and few plasma cells, clustered around ducts, lobules, and blood vessels. Stroma is collagenous with prominent myofibroblasts that appear epithelioid [15].

Mammary hamartoma: It is a relatively uncommon benign mass of the breast with a reported incidence of 0.1–0.7%. The hamartoma is a proliferation of fibrous and adenomatous nodular elements in fat surrounded by a capsule of connective tissue.

Clinical presentation: These are found in premenopausal women mostly in their 40s. They present as painless, usually mobile, soft to firm masses commonly found in the outer breast quadrants. About 60% of breast hamartomas are nonpalpable and are diagnosed radiologically.

Imaging features: **Mammogram**—They always appear as a benign mass with sharp margins and a thin capsule, which is evident if there is fat surrounding the lesion. Lobulated densities dispersed within encapsulated fat give the hamartomas their characteristic "**Slice Of Salami/ Breast within breast**" appearance [16] (Fig. 18.15). If they have little fat, they may mimic fibroadenomas. Calcifications are rare

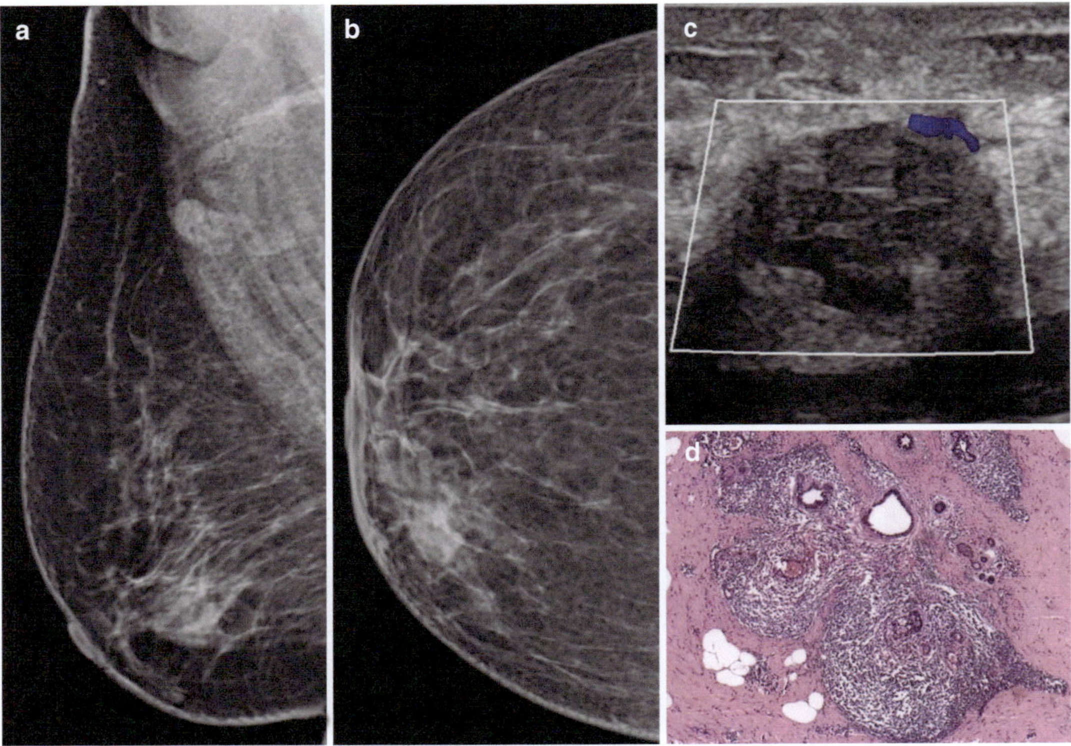

Fig. 18.14 A 45-year-old women with Type 1 diabetes with biopsy confirmed diabetic mastopathy in right breast. Right breast MLO and CC view (**a**, **b**) of right breast shows a dense mass with indistinct margins in the sub-areolar region. On high-resolution USG, it has irregular margin with posterior shadowing and minimal peripheral vascularity with surrounding echogenic inflammatory changes (**c**). (**d**) H&E stained pictomicrograph showing periductal and perilobular lymphocytic infiltration in a diabetic mastopathy (20×)

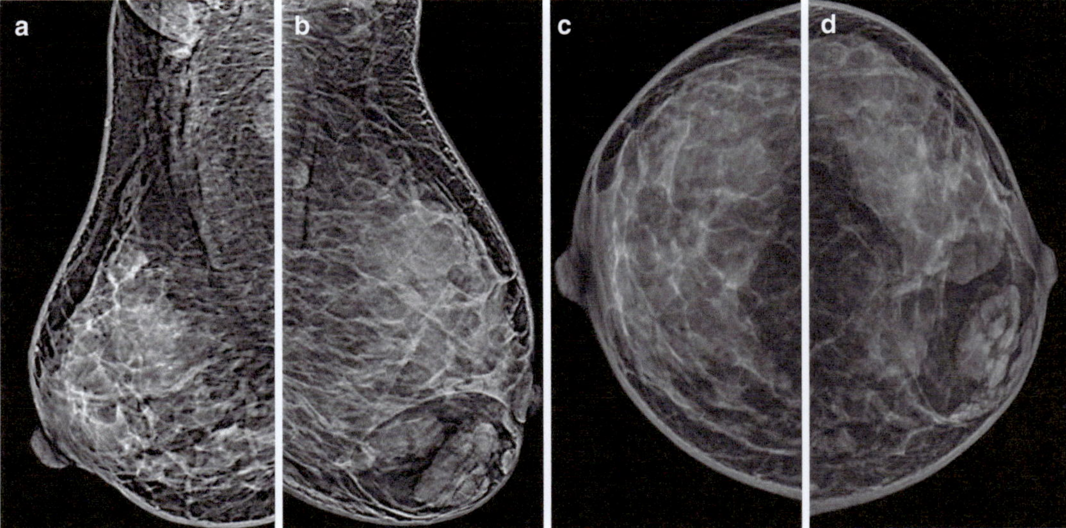

Fig. 18.15 A 40-year-old asymptomatic woman who had her first screening mammogram of both breasts. MLO (**a**, **b**) and CC views of both breasts (**c**, **d**) show a well-defined ovoid mixed density mass in the left breast lower inner quadrant containing soft tissue and fat density within—classic of hamartoma "**Breast within Breast appearance**"

mammographic findings, if present are smooth amorphous or round calcifications.

Ultrasound: They are sharply defined with sonolucent zones as well as echo producing fibrous structures within.

MRI: It is usually not recommended for these lesions. They appear as well-circumscribed mass, which displaces the surrounding breast tissue and contains fibrous as well as glandular tissue on T2 imaging. The fibro glandular component shows enhancement following intravenous gadolinium administration.

Histopathology: Hamartomas have two variants—**adenolipoma** and **chondrolipoma**. On gross examination, adenolipomas are soft, circumscribed and surrounded by a thin fibrous capsule. Cut surface has a variegated pattern of fat and fibrous tissue. Microscopically, it consists of mature adipose tissue and breast parenchyma (normal lobules and ducts) in different proportions surrounded by a pseudocapsule comprising of compressed breast tissue. Chondrolipomas comprise of hyaline cartilage and mature adipose tissue. Grossly, it is soft, rubbery circumscribed lobulated that is gray white to glistening white in color. Microscopically, islands of hyaline cartilage, focal calcification, mature adipose tissue, and breast parenchyma are noted. Similar to adenolipoma, it has a pseudocapsule [17].

Management: Breast hamartomas are usually left alone untill otherwise patient feels lump or pain, in such case excision is considered curative.

References

1. Goel NB, Knight TE, Pandey S, Riddick-Young M, de Paredes ES, Trivedi A. Fibrous lesions of the breast: imaging-pathologic correlation. Radiographics. 2005;25(6):1547–59.
2. Foster ME, Garrahan N, Williams S. Fibroadenoma of the breast: a clinical and pathological study. J R Coll Surg Edinb. 1988;33(1):16–9.
3. Klinger K. Fibroadenoma: from imaging evaluation to treatment. J Am Osteopath Coll Radiol. 2019;8(2):14.
4. Mies C, Rosen PP. Juvenile Fibroadenoma with atypical epithelial hyperplasia. Am J Surg Pathol. 1987;11(3):184–90.
5. Moross T, Lang AP, Mahoney L. Tubular adenoma of breast. Arch Pathol Lab Med. 1983;107(2):84–6.
6. Ravikanth R, Kamalasekar K. Imaging of lactating adenoma: differential diagnosis of solid mass lesion in a lactating woman. J Med Ultrasound. 2019;27(4):208–10.
7. O'Hara MF, Page DL. Adenomas of the breast and ectopic breast under Lactational influences. Hum Pathol. 1985;16(7):707–12.
8. Dupont WD, Page DL, Parl FF, Vnencak-Jones CL, Plummer WD, Rados MS, Schuyler PA. Long-term risk of breast cancer in women with Fibroadenoma. N Engl J Med. 1994;331(1):10–5.
9. Tse GMK, Niu Y, Shi H-J. Phyllodes tumor of the breast: an update. Breast Cancer. 2009;17(1):29.
10. Liberman L, Bonaccio E, Hamele-Bena D, Abramson AF, Cohen MA, Dershaw DD. Benign and malignant Phyllodes tumors: mammographic and sonographic findings. Radiology. 1996;198(1):121.
11. Joshi M, Reddy SJ, Nanavidekar M, Russo JP, Russo AV, Pathak R. Core biopsies of the breast: diagnostic pitfalls. Indian J Pathol Microbiol. 2011;54(4):671–82.
12. Shin SJ, Rosen PP. Ki-67 index is diagnostically useful in distinguishing benign fibroepithelial lesions in young females. lab invest. 2006;86:42A.
13. Rafeek N, Dev B, Thambidurai L, Satchidanandam A. Tumoral Pseudoangiomatous stromal hyperplasia: radiological and pathological correlation with review of literature. Egypt J Radiol Nuclear Med. 2017;48(1):147–52.
14. Guray M, Sahin AA. Benign breast diseases: classification, diagnosis, and management. Oncologist. 2006;11(5):435–49.
15. Dorokhova O, Fineberg S, Koenigsberg T, Wang Y. Diabetic Mastopathy, a Clinicopathological correlation of 34 cases. Pathol Int. 2012;62(10):660–4.
16. Farrokh D, Hashemi J, Ansaripour E. Breast hamartoma: mammographic findings. Iran J Radiol. 2011;8(4):258–60.
17. Rosen PP. Rosen's breast pathology. Philadelphia, PA: Lippincott; 2009.

19 Fibrocystic Disorders

Leena Dennis Joseph, Bhawna Dev, Mehak Garg, and Ramya Ramakrishnan

Abstract

Fibrocystic disorders of the breast are the most common benign breast diseases found predominantly in women aged 30–50 years with a spectrum of diseases ranging from simple cyst to solid lesions like usual ductal hyperplasia. These disorders are usually asymptomatic and are detected incidentally or if the patient presents with breast lump or pain. The clinical, radiological, and pathological evaluation is done then for an effective management.

L. D. Joseph (✉)
Department of Pathology, Sri Ramachandra Institute of Higher Education and Research, Chennai, India
e-mail: leenadennisj@sriramachandra.edu.in

B. Dev
Department of Radiology, Sri Ramachandra Institute of Higher Education and Research, Chennai, India
e-mail: bhawnadev@sriramachandra.edu.in

M. Garg
Fellow in Breast Imaging, Department of Radiology, Sri Ramachandra Institute of Higher Education and Research, Chennai, India

R. Ramakrishnan
Professor Department of Surgery, Sri Ramachandra Institute of Higher Education and Research, Chennai, India
e-mail: ramya.r@sriramachandra.edu.in

Keywords

Fibrocystic disorders · Simple cyst · Breast lump

19.1 Introduction

FibroCystic Change (FCC) of the breast is a benign alteration in the terminal ductal lobular unit of the breast and is a most common benign breast condition frequently observed in women aged 20–50 years, with a peak in the perimenopausal age group.

Fibrocystic changes in breast is not a distinct entity, this term encompasses a spectrum of lesions ranging from various forms of cysts, fibrosis, apocrine metaplasia, adenosis, and hyperplasia [1, 2] (Fig. 19.1).

The pathophysiology of these changes is determined by the response of the breast tissue to the monthly hormonal imbalances, particularly by estrogen predominance and progesterone deficiency, which results in hyperproliferation of the connective tissue (fibrosis), which may or may not be preceded by epithelial proliferation.

Multiple analogous terms are used for fibrocystic changes like Aberrations of Normal Development and Involution (ANDI): Bloodgood's disease, chronic cystic mastitis, cystic hyperplasia, cystic mastopathy, fibroadenosis, fibrocystic changes, hyperplastic cystic

B. Dev, L. D. Joseph (eds.), *Holistic Approach to Breast Disease*,
https://doi.org/10.1007/978-981-99-0035-0_19

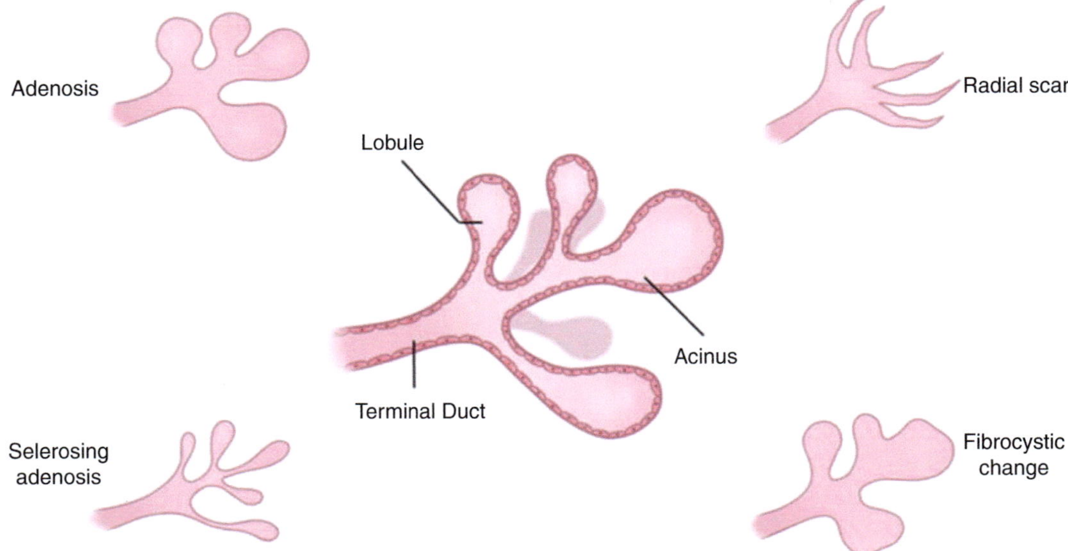

Fig. 19.1 Schematic representation of findings seen in fibrocystic changes—the normal terminal ductal lobular unit, adenosis—enlargement and multiplication of TDLUs, sclerosing adenosis, and radial scar appearing as distorted TDLU [3]

disease, Konig's disease, mammary dysplasia, mammary dystrophy, Reclus'disease, Schimmelbusch's disease, and sclerocystic disease [1, 4].

Clinical presentation: They are very common and can occur in women of any age, with a peak incidence in the 30–50 years age group. The usual presentation is vague pain, heaviness, lump (commonly related to the menstrual cycle), redness, or unusual nipple discharges, which may be dull yellow, greenish to blackish in color.

On physical examination: Most breast cysts are nonpalpable, asymptomatic and are incidental findings on routine imaging [5] Cysts that are apparent clinically, classically, present as lumps that are smooth, soft to firm, mobile, and sometimes tender. Cysts under tension can be firm to hard on examination and may be associated with significant tenderness. A cluster of cysts can present as a tender area of nodularity. Benign cysts are typically mobile within the glandular breast tissue, chest wall, and skin and rubbery in texture. Except for cysts with inflammatory changes, discomfort and tenderness are rarely experienced in fibrocystic changes [6].

Spectrum of Fibrocystic Changes

1. Cysts
   (a) Simple cysts
   (b) Clustered microcysts
   (c) Complicated cysts
   (d) Complex cysts
2. Solid appearing lesions
   (a) Radial scar
   (b) Complex sclerosing lesion
   (c) Sclerosing adenosis
   (d) Usual ductal hyperplasia (UDH)
   (e) Epithelial hyperplasia

Note: Term fibrocystic change is not used in imaging; instead, findings should be described as simple cyst, multiple simple cysts, clustered cysts, complicated cysts, complex cysts, mass, architectural distortion as seen on X-ray mammogram or ultrasound.

19.1.1 Imaging

19.1.1.1 X-ray Mammogram

Dense Breast: Fibrocystic changes are most commonly seen in patients with dense fibroglandular pattern (type C or type D) due to the presence of fibrosis (proliferation of connective tissue). Dense fibroglandular parenchyma generally obscures fine details and underlying mass lesions.

Cysts: These are usually seen as round or oval shaped, equal to high density lesions with circumscribed margins or some with obscured margins due to overlapping with surrounding dense fibroglandular tissue. Usually, they are multiple, of varying sizes, and are bilateral. Few cysts may show a lucent halo (**halo sign**) around, signifying them to be more likely benign. Microscopically, these dilated cysts are lined by ductal and myoepithelial cells. The dilated cysts may be filled with eosinophilic secretions and the lining cells may show apocrine change. Different types of cysts are simple, complicated, complex, or clustered (Fig. 19.2).

Calcifications: The other common presentation of benign fibrocystic changes on mammogram is—**diffuse round calcifications**, which occur due to calcium oxalate deposition in cysts. These are benign sedimented calcifications in macro-/microcysts. Lobular pattern of rounded calcifications is most commonly encountered in pathology arising from the lobular unit of terminal duct lobular unit (TDLU) [7].

On CC (cranio-caudal view)—they appear as round punctate grouped calcifications and in **true lateral projection** (medio-lateral view), they give the appearance of tea-cup-like configuration (Figs. 19.3 and 19.4).

Some cyst walls may show **rim-like calcifications**, which is again a benign feature and does not warrant any further investigation.

Sometimes amorphous type of calcifications may also be noted and, in such cases, follow-up is of utmost importance.

Microscopically, calcification may be visualized as amorphous basophilic material, which may be in the foci of secretions or in the cyst lining or in the stroma.

> **Note**: X-ray mammogram cannot differentiate solid from cystic lesion, additional imaging with ultrasound is required to differentiate both, and hence, ultrasound is of immense help in differentiating and categorizing the lesions in suspected fibrocystic changes of breast.

19.1.1.2 Ultrasound

The simple cysts are the most common imaging finding in FCC on ultrasound [8]. They are usually multiple and bilateral, either single or clustered together.

Simple Cyst has four features—anechoic, circumscribed, thin walled round or oval with posterior acoustic enhancement (Fig. 19.5).

BI-RADS Category and Management: BI-RADS 2

Treatment: The usual protocol is routine follow-up. Cyst aspiration is performed in cases either

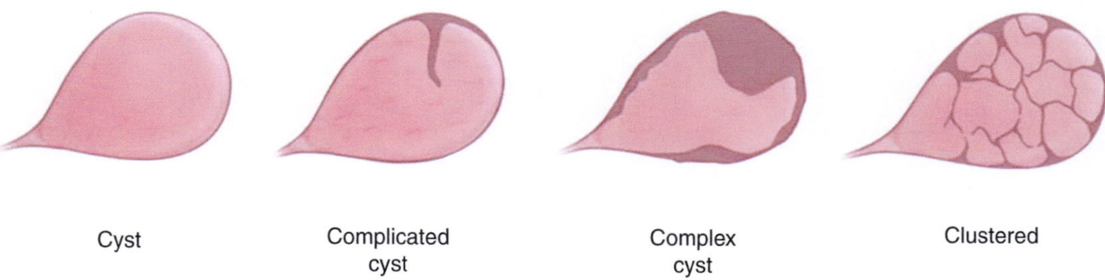

Fig. 19.2 Different types of cysts: simple, complicated, complex, and clustered

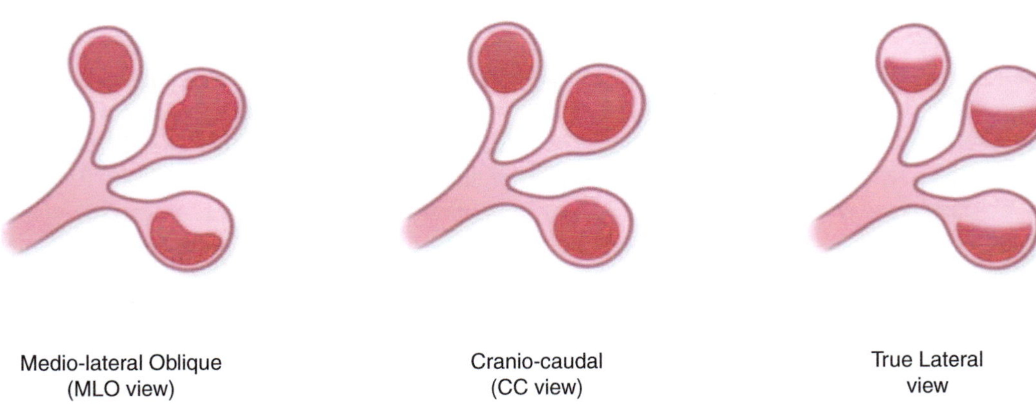

Fig. 19.3 Round calcifications in different views on mammogram

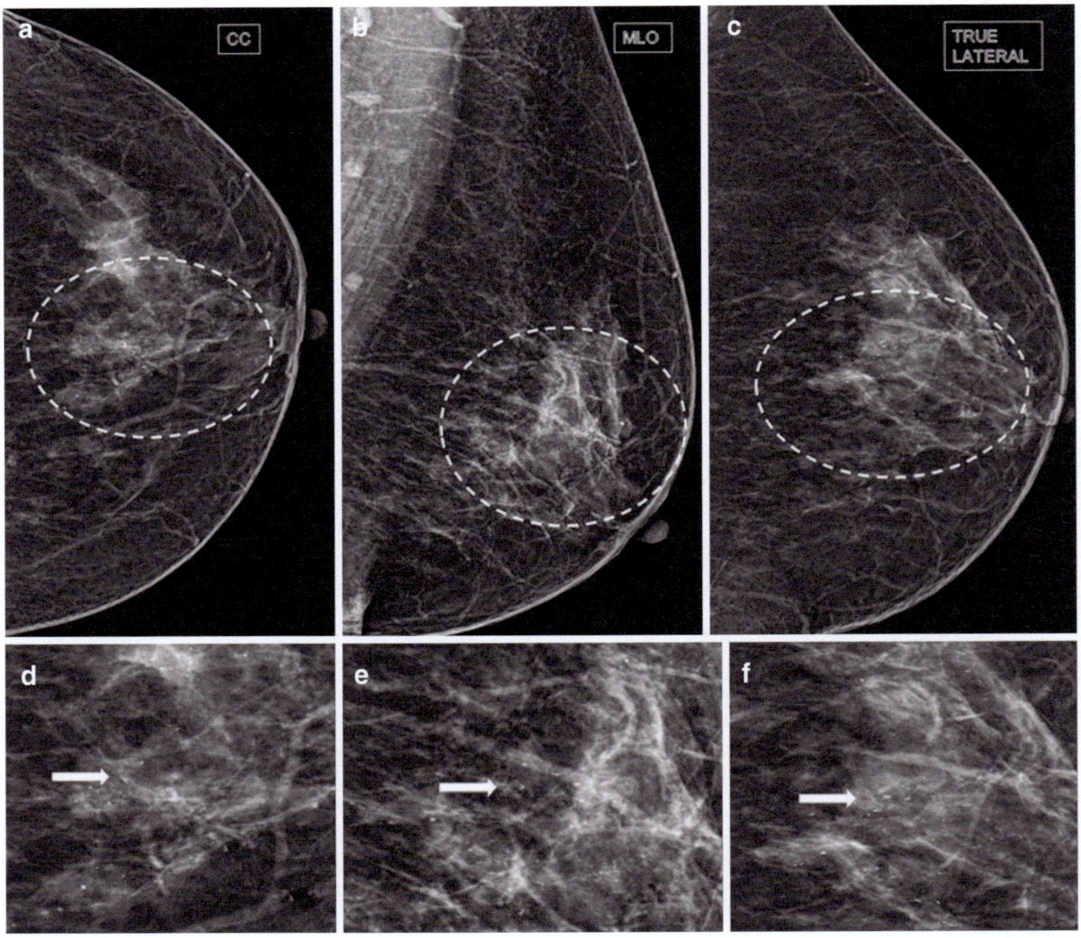

Fig. 19.4 (**a**, **b**) CC and MLO view showing segmental distribution of punctate calcifications (**d**, **e**) zoomed view of the same in a patient with fibrocystic disease (**c**) true lateral projection showing tea cup appearance of calcifications (**f**) zoomed view of the same

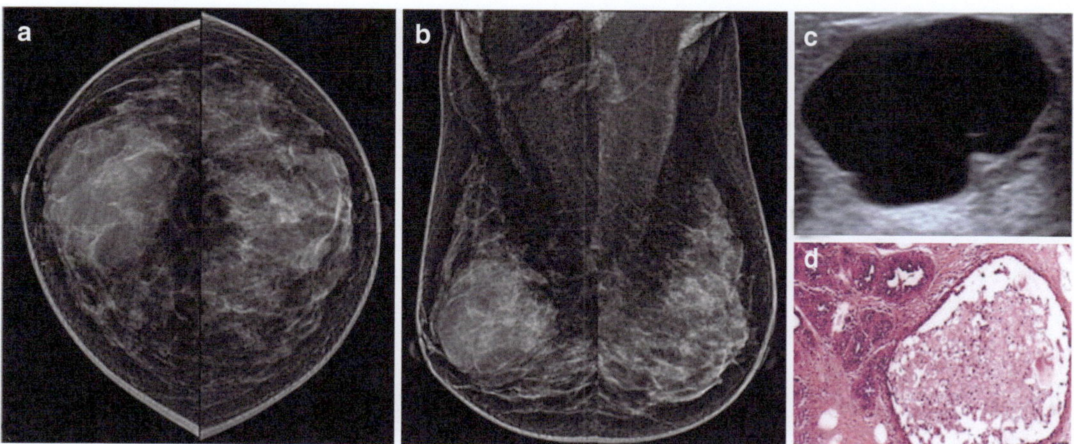

Fig. 19.5 Imaging findings in a simple cyst (**a**, **b**) X-Ray mammogram (right CC, MLO) shows oval equal density lesion with circumscribed margins in comparison to normal left side. (**c**) USG in the same patient: oval anechoic cystic lesion with posterior acoustic enhancement. (**d**) HPE image: dilated cyst with foamy macrophages in the lumen

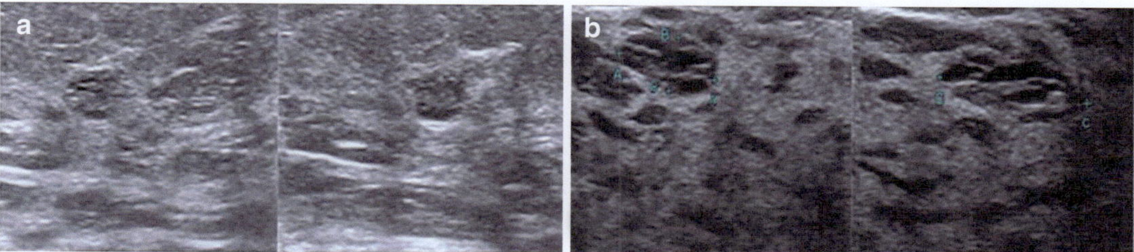

Fig. 19.6 USG findings of cluster of microcysts (**a**, **b**) Cluster of anechoic cysts (each cyst less than 2–3 mm) noted in two different patients

for symptomatic relief or to allay a patient's anxiety.

Clustered microcysts: A cluster of anechoic cysts, each anechoic cyst within the cluster measures <2–3 mm with thin (<0.5 mm) intervening septations and no discrete solid components (Fig. 19.6).

Complicated cysts: Round or oval circumscribed cystic lesion with thick septations or thick walls. Cyst may contain throughout homogeneous low level internal echoes or fluid-fluid or fluid-debris level, which changes its position with shift in patient's position. Sometimes, surrounding edema may be noted if the cyst is inflamed or fluid from the cysts has leaked. Minimal vascularity in the cyst wall may be seen in a few cases (Figs. 19.7 and 19.8).

BI-RADS category and management: If clustered cysts/complicated cyst are multiple in breasts, that is, two in one breast and at least one in contralateral breast, they can be labeled as BI-RADS 2. If these are single, then they are categorized as BI-RADS 3 and short-term 6-month follow-up ultrasound is recommended.

Complex Cysts: Cysts with features like thick irregular wall, thick septations (>0.5 cm) and solid/mural component are defined as complex cysts (Figs. 19.9 and 19.10). Berg et al. have categorized complex cystic masses into four classes on the basis of their US features: Type 1 masses have a thick outer wall, thick internal septa, or both; type 2 masses contain one or more intracystic masses; type 3 masses contain mixed cystic and solid components and are at least 50% cystic;

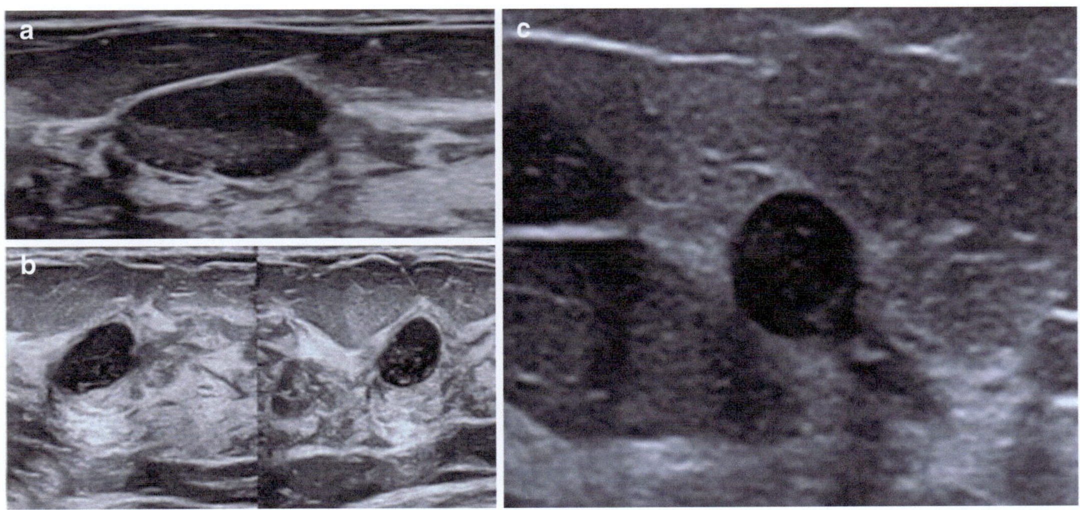

Fig. 19.7 USG findings in complicated cysts (**a**–**c**) Thin walled cysts in three different patients showing internal debris with fluid debris level in (**a**)

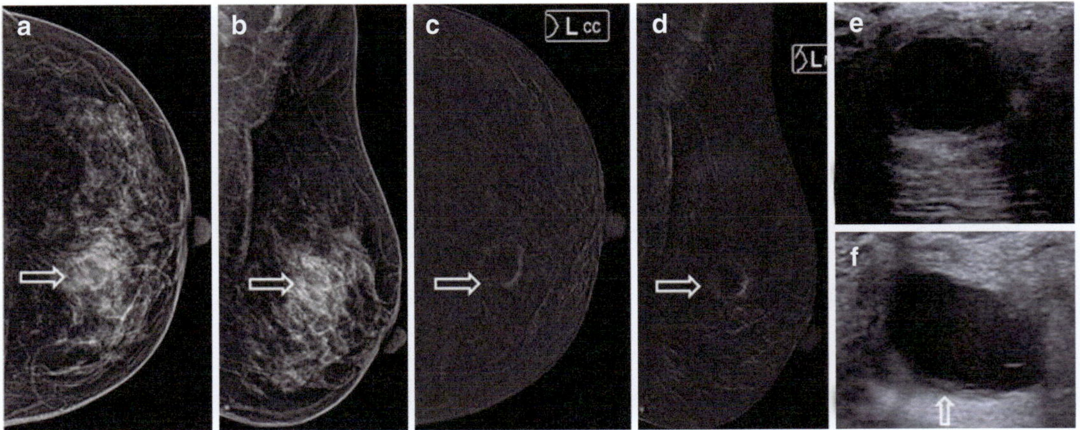

Fig 19.8 (**a**, **b**) CC and MLO view of left breast of a 50-year-old patient with complaint of painful lump in left breast showing an oval equal density partly circumscribed lesion in inner central quadrant (**c**, **d**) contrast-enhanced mammogram (recombined images) in same patient where the lesion shows smooth peripheral rim enhancement (**e**, **f**) USG shows a thick wall cyst with low lying internal echoes-complicated cyst

and type 4 masses are predominantly (at least 50%) solid with eccentric cystic foci [9].

BI-RADS category & Management BI-RADS 4A/4B/4C. It is essential to have a radiological & pathological concordance in BI-RADS 4 lesions. Ultrasound is the modality of choice to do either 14 gauge core biopsy or vacuum-assisted biopsy for particular lesion. The evaluation of mobility and flow of the internal contents within the cystic mass is a good approach to differentiate a complex cyst and a complicated cyst [10].

> **Note**: In few cases in BI-RADS 4A category where its almost certain along with other features that it might not be malignant, patients may be kept on a close short-term follow-up in consensus with a referring physician.

Differential Diagnosis: Common benign causes of complex cystic masses include fibro-

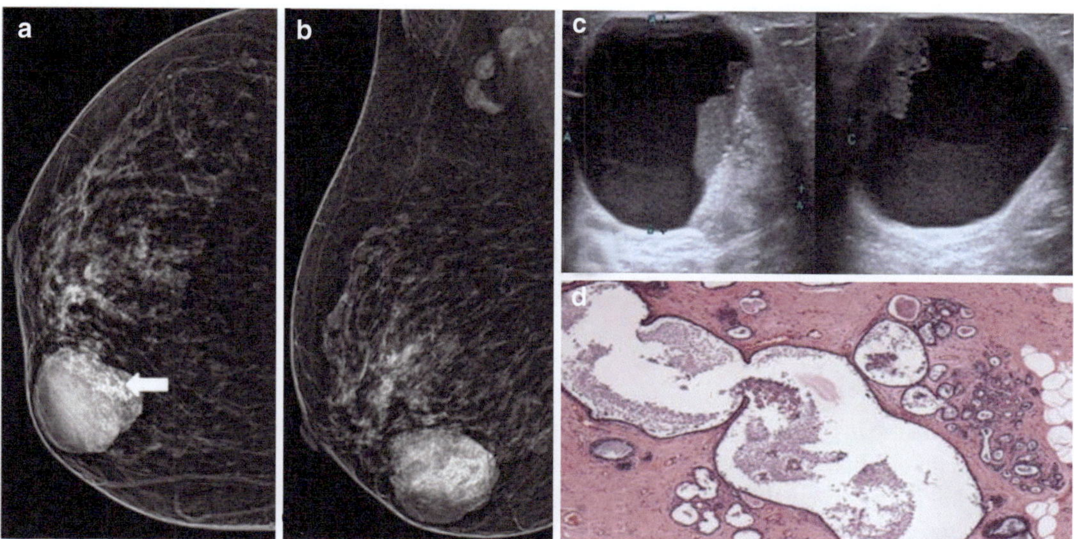

Fig. 19.9 Imaging findings in a complex cyst: (**a**, **b**) Mammogram (CC, MLO view) showing an irregular high density mass with circumscribed margins in lower inner quadrant with suspicious amorphous and coarse heterogeneous calcifications within (marked with white arrow). (**c**) USG findings in same patient shows a solid cystic mass (type 3 mass-50% is cystic component). (**d**) Histopathology showing multiple dilated cysts of varying sizes, most of them containing secretions

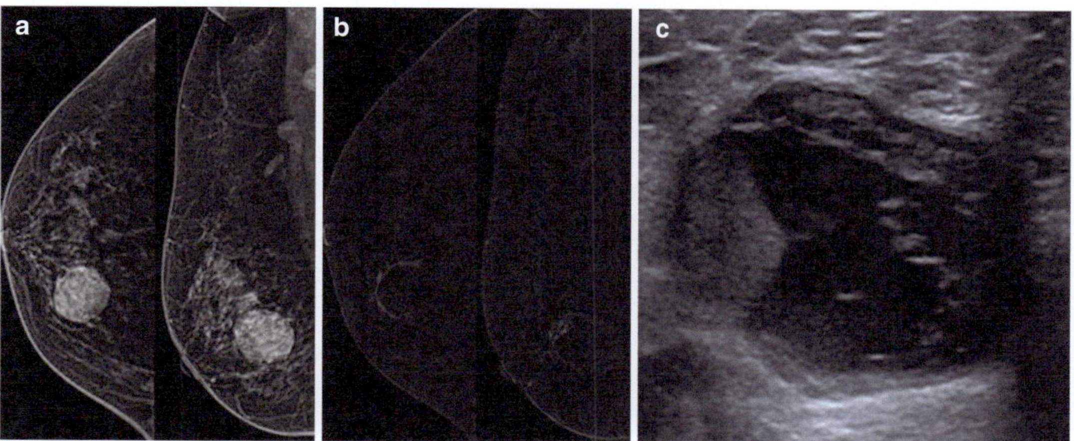

Fig. 19.10 (**a**) CC and MLO view of right breast of a 65-year-old patient with complaint of palpable lump in right breast showing a round equal density circumscribed lesion in lower inner quadrant (**b**) contrast-enhanced mammogram (recombined images) in same patient where the lesion shows peripheral enhancement with enhancing mural solid nodule within. (**c**) USG showed a complex cyst with internal solid papillary mass

cystic changes, intraductal or intracystic papilloma without atypia and fibroadenoma. Atypical findings include atypical ductal hyperplasia, lobular neoplasia, and atypical papilloma. Complex cysts may also be seen in malignant conditions including DCIS, infiltrating ductal carcinoma, and infiltrating lobular carcinoma [10].

19.1.2 The Role of Cytology and Surgery

Fluid from atypical cysts should be sent for cytological assessment unless the cyst drains fully with aspiration, leaving no sonographic abnormality postaspiration or the cyst fluid is not macroscopically blood stained.

Surgery is rarely indicated for breast cysts. It is reserved for

- Palpable cysts that recur despite repeated aspiration
- Cysts that appear to have an intracystic solid lesion on imaging
- Lesions that do not resolve completely with aspiration and show atypical or suspicious cytology

Educating and reassuring the patient is very important in the management of breast cysts, as most cysts are asymptomatic incidental findings on ultrasound that are unlikely to cause the patient any problems [5].

19.1.3 Histopathology

Breast cysts are fluid-filled widening of the terminal duct lobular units (TDLUs), lined with a single layer of epithelium [11] Microscopically these dilated cysts are lined by ductal and myoepithelial cells. The dilated cysts may be filled with eosinophilic secretions and the lining cells may show apocrine change. **Apocrine metaplasia** is characterized by abundant granular eosinophilic cytoplasm with apical snouts. On histopathology, fibrocysticbreastchangescanbecategorisedasfollows-

Nonproliferating
- Simple cysts
- Papillary apocrine metaplasia

Proliferating without atypia
- Usual ductal hyperplasia (UDH)
- Columnar cell hyperplasia (blunt duct adenosis)
- Sclerosing adenosis
- Radial scar

Proliferating with atypia
- Flat epithelial atypia (FEA)
- Atypical ductal hyperplasia (ADH)
- Atypical lobular hyperplasia (ALH)

19.1.4 Proliferating with/Without Atypia

Columnar cell lesions (CCLs) are clonal alterations of the terminal duct lobular units, which are characterized by enlarged and dilated acini lined by columnar epithelial cells. The lesions that come under flat epithelial atypia is characterized by low-grade cytological atypia. These lesions are usually detected incidentally as grouped, amorphous calcifications on mammography. CCL may represent the earliest change in low grade breast neoplasia pathway, which may progress to ADH or DCIS. On microscopic examination, the acini are lined by columnar epithelial cells which may have apical snouts. If they present as one to two cell layer thick, it is called columnar cell change and if more layers are present, it is called columnar cell hyperplasia. Cytological atypia is usually not seen, if present it is called flat epithelial atypia.

Flat Epithelial Atypia (FEA) presents on histopathology, with one to several layers of mildly atypical cuboidal to columnar cells, with apical snouts.

CCLs and FEA may be seen in association with other changes, like cysts and other epithelial proliferative lesions.

19.2 Solid Appearing Changes

Fibrocystic changes can also present as solid changes/masses. Most of the solid changes can be either sclerosing or non sclerosing adenosis. These generally present as architectural distortion/solid masses with few mimicking malignancy [12, 13].

Radial scar/Complex sclerosing lesion—Radial scar is a lesion represented by stellate configuration of a fibroelastic core with entrapped ducts and lobules [14]. If the same lesion is larger than 10 mm, it is referred to as complex sclerosing lesion.

19.2.1 Imaging

X-ray mammogram: Usually these lesions are picked up incidentally on screening mammogram as most of the patients are asymptomatic.

These often appear as mass, asymmetry, architectural distortion (Fig. 19.11), spiculated lesion with central lucent hub (black star as described by Dr. Tabar) as compared to the malignant lesions where the center of the lesion is opaque/white representing solid tumor mass (white star as described by Dr. Tabar). Complex sclerosing lesions also have long spicules as compared to spicules of malignant mass. These lesions may appear different on different views unlike malignant lesions which will have the same appearance in different views [7].

The lesions may sometimes also present with amorphous, punctate, pleomorphic, fine linear branching calcifications; distribution of these calcifications may give insight to their malignant potential. Some lesions may present as mass along with calcifications.

Ultrasound: They may appear as a solid oval or round mass with hyperechoic center representing sclerosis [7] or may appear as irregular non circumscribed microlobulated or angular mass with or without posterior acoustic shadowing (Fig. 19.12). Focal posterior acoustic shadowing without mass configuration is considered to be suspicious for malignancy [15].

MRI: has a 97.6–100.0% negative predictive value for differentiating between benign and malignant radial scar lesions [16]. Contrast-

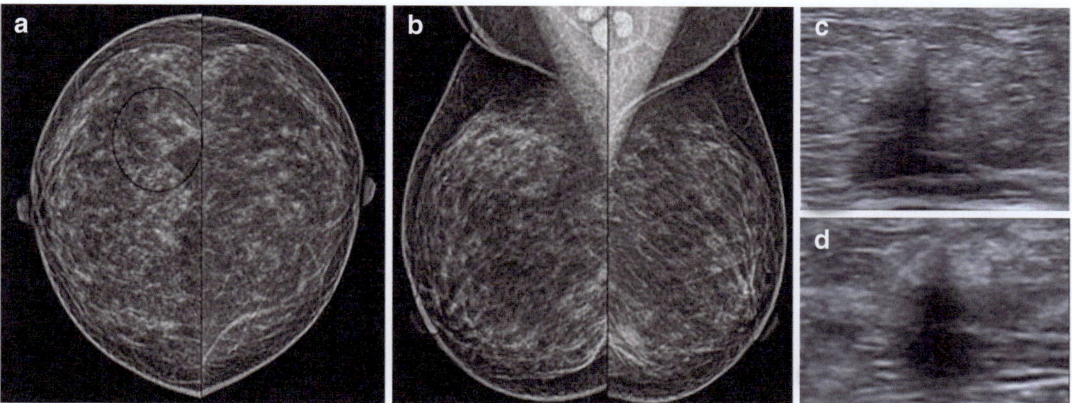

Fig. 19.11 Imaging findings in radial scar: (**a**, **b**) Mammogram (CC, MLO view) shows architectural distortion in right breast in retro mammary region (seen only on CC view). (**c**) USG breast in same patient shows an irregular hypoechoic taller than wider lesion with posterior acoustic shadowing. (**d**) zoomed USG image of the same mass

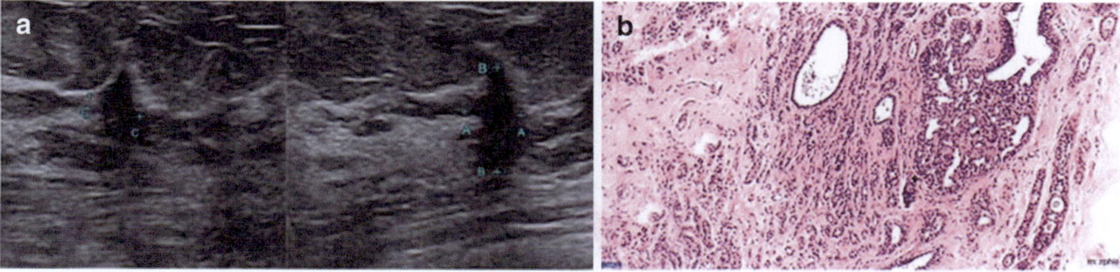

Fig. 19.12 Imaging findings in sclerosing adenosis: (**a**) USG shows an irregular taller than wider hypoechoic lesion with indistinct margins with no internal vascularity. (**b**) HPE of same patient came as sclerosing adenosis with small tubular ducts, compressed by stroma

enhanced MR mammogram (CE-MRM) is recommended in all cases where X-ray mammogram is suspicious for radial scar. The enhancing lesion at CE-MRI most probably indicates the lesion is malignant or there is an associated malignancy with the lesion. Nonenhancement may indicate the presence of a single radial scar, which should be kept under close monitoring in order to exclude associated foci of carcinoma [17].

BI-RADS category and management: BI-RADS 4A/4B image-guided core biopsy or vacuum-assisted biopsy is performed for tissue diagnosis.

Differential Diagnosis: Invasive carcinoma has overlapping radiological features, making the diagnosis of radial scars challenging for radiologists.

Histopathology: Adenosis and benign sclerosing lesions are characterized by a lobulo centric proliferation of tubules and acini, with both epithelial and myoepithelial cell layer. Benign sclerosing lesions also have a central sclerotic focus, from which the glandular structures appear to spread out. **Sclerosing adenosis** is a kind of hyperplastic proliferation of glandular component of breast, which can occur as a focal or generalized proliferation of ducts and it may be accompanied by various forms of hyperplasia and even carcinoma.

Microscopically, the lesion has an oval to round configuration with central accentuation of cellularity. High power examination shows elongated and compressed glands formed by atrophied epithelial cells with preservation of myoepithelial layer and surrounded by sclerosed stroma. The ductules are small, round to somewhat angular, and generally uniform in size. Microcalcifications may be seen at times. The stromal collagen may compress the ductules, which may create an impression of invasion. At times, there may be a solid or cord-like growth pattern. The lesion may be seen extending into the adjacent adipose tissue; however, lobulocentric architecture is preserved.

Note: Radial scars are benign changes on histopathology, even though on imaging, these may show features suggestive of malignancy; however, histologically, they show a stellate fibroelastic core with entrapped ducts and radial epithelial structures.

Usual ductal hyperplasia (UDH): Hyperplasia is overgrowth of cells that line the lobules or ducts inside the breast. It as such is not malignant, but some types of hyperplasia are associated with higher risk of developing breast carcinoma.

Hyperplasia can be of two types: usual ductal hyperplasia (UDH) or atypical ductal hyperplasia (ADH).

UDH: In UDH, there is overgrowth of cells lining the ducts in breast, but cells look very close to the normal cells. Risk of breast carcinoma is half to double the risk in a woman with no breast abnormalities.

ADH: The cells look more distorted and abnormal and can be either atypical ductal hyperplasia or atypical lobular hyperplasia. The risk of breast carcinoma is 4–5 times higher than normal woman.

Out of the 2 types of hyperplasia, UDH falls under the category of fibro-cystic changes of breast and is a pathological diagnosis. There is no evidence of any clinically palpable lump or pain. Mammogram may have changes in form of either a lesion or architectural distortion. UDH is mainly investigated further to distinguish it from ADH. UDH is not a premalignant condition itself but requires follow-up/excision biopsy.

UDH is characterized by a cohesive proliferation of benign cells that display a haphazard orientation with respect to one another. It shows the presence of secondary lumina or fenestrations. These lumina are peripherally located and are usually slit-like. The cells are irregularly arranged with indistinct borders, nuclear grooves, and intranuclear cytoplasmic pseudoinclusions. Blunt duct adenosis is characterized by an increase in the size and number of epithelial cells. Sclerosing adenosis can also be noted in areas of UDH, where there is an increased number and size of the acini within the TDLU accompanied by stromal hyperplasia [18, 19].

Epithelial hyperplasia—Breast ducts are lined by two layers of epithelial cells, luminal and basal cells. Any increase in cell number within ductal space is regarded as epithelial hyperplasia. Based on cytomorphology and presence of nuclear atypia, the lesions are subclassified as typical or atypical hyperplasia. The diagnosis of **atypical epithelial hyperplasia** (AEH) increases with breast cancer screening. AEH is divided into three groups: atypical ductal hyperplasia, columnar cell lesions with atypia, lobular neoplasia.

Atypical duct hyperplasia is an intraductal epithelial proliferative lesion with cytological and architectural features resembling a low-grade DCIS. There is a partial involvement of ductal spaces with or without microcalcifications. There is a presence of evenly spaced monotonous cells containing rounded nuclei with dense chromatin. The architectural patterns are also quite distinct from DCIS, with presence of rigid bridges, bars, and arcades of uniform thickness.

Diagnostic difficulty arises when duct spaces are uniformly involved by an intraductal proliferation, with the cytological features of a DCIS. In such situations, it is very difficult to distinguish ADH from DCIS. When the lesion is less than or equal to 2 mm in contiguous extent, it is classified as ADH. The cells in ADH are strongly and diffusely positive for ER and lack staining for high-molecular-weight cytokeratin as CK5/6. However, UDH shows uniform staining for ER and high-molecular-weight cytokeratins.

19.2.2 Imaging

There are no specific features of usual ductal hyperplasia, atypical epithelial hyperplasia on imaging as it is a histopathological diagnosis.

X-ray mammogram may show a circumscribed or noncircumscribed mass or mass with calcifications or architectural distortion (Fig. 19.13) or asymmetric density [20]. It can also manifest as a group of microcalcifications [21].

Ultrasound: may appear as microlobulated mass with mild hypoechogenicity and no posterior features [20].

MRI: can show a focus of enhancement.

Molecular Breast Imaging Or Breast Specific Gamma Imaging: can show radiotracer uptake.

BI-RADS categorization & Management: **BI-RADS 4A/4B** image-guided core biopsy or vacuum-assisted biopsy is performed for tissue diagnosis.

Usually, FCCs are benign breast diseases and are usually associated with no increased risk for cancer if only cysts, apocrine metaplasia, sclerosing adenosis, fibrosis, and mild hyperplasia (more than 2 but less than 4 cells

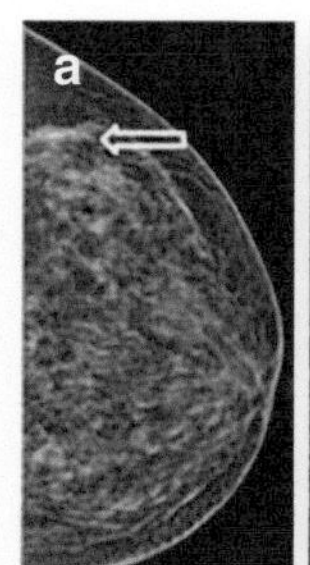

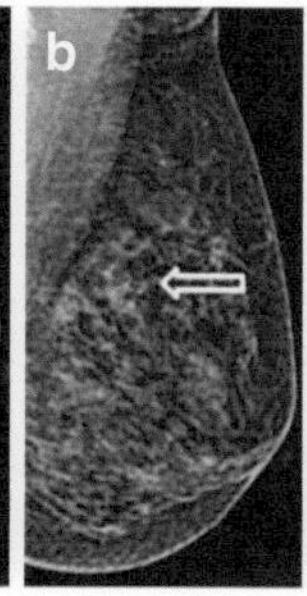

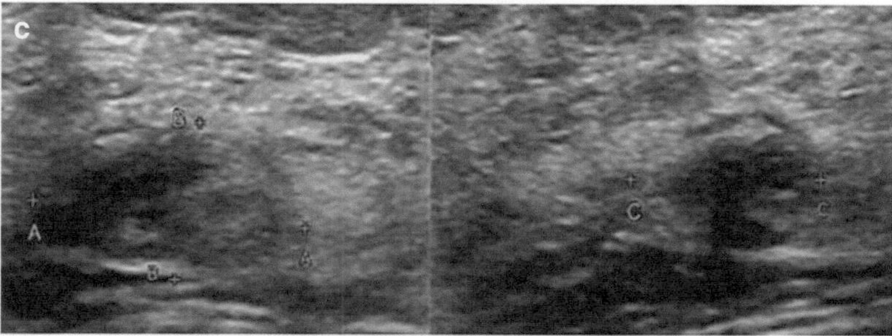

Fig. 19.13 Imaging findings in patient with usual ductal hyperplasia (**a**, **b**) Mammogram (CC, MLO view) left breast shows an area of architectural distortion in the upper outer quadrant (marked with arrow). (**c**) USG breast in the same patient shows an irregular solid cystic mass with indistinct margins, which on biopsy came as usual ductal hyperplasia

thick) exist, so these can be labeled as BI-RADS 2 and kept on regular follow-up (after 1 year). There is slightly increased risk of breast carcinoma (1.5–2 times) if moderate or florid hyperplasia (Usual ductal hyperplasia) is found, which is labeled as BI-RADS 4A/B and after biopsy can be kept on follow-up. There is moderately increased risk of breast carcinoma (five times) if atypical hyperplasia (AH), regardless of ductal or lobular, is found in the FCC, which needs surgical excision [22].

19.3 Conclusion

Fibrocystic changes encompass a broad spectrum of lesions ranging from completely benign simple cysts to premalignant conditions like atypical ductal hyperplasia. Thus, a detailed clinical evaluation with mammogram and ultrasound breast followed by cytology and histopathology correlation of suspicious lesions (BI-RADS 3/4) is of utmost importance in diagnosing a patient with fibrocystic disease and appropriate follow-up accordingly.

References

1. Pina L. Fibrocystic disease, breast. In: Baert AL, editor. Encyclopedia of diagnostic imaging. Heidelberg: Springer; 2008. p. 708–9. https://doi.org/10.1007/978-3-540-35280-8_943.
2. Guinebretière JM, Menet E, Tardivon A, Cherel P, Vanel D. Normal and pathological breast, the histological basis. Eur J Radiol. 2005;54(1):6–14.
3. Selvi R. Breast diseases: imaging and clinical management. New Delhi: Springer; 2015.
4. Hughes LE. Problems of concept and nomenclature of benign disorders of the breast. In: Hughes LE, Mansel RE, Webster DJT, editors. Benign disorders and diseases of the breast. Concepts and clinical management. London: Saunders; 2000. p. 1–5.
5. Brennan M, Houssami N, French J. Management of benign breast conditions. Austr Fam Physician. 2005;34(4):253–5.
6. K Malherbe, S Fatima Fibrocystic breast disease. In: StatPearls [Internet]. Treasure Island (FL): StatPearls Publishing; 2019. ncbi.nlm.nih.gov.
7. Henrot P, Leroux A, Barlier C, Genin P. Breast microcalcifications: the lesions in anatomical pathology. Diagn Interv Imaging. 2014;95:141–52.
8. Guray M, et al. Benign breast diseases: classification, diagnosis, and management. Oncologist. 2006;11:435–49.
9. Berg WA, Campassi CI, Ioffe OB. Cystic lesions of the breast: sonographic-pathologic correlation. Radiology. 2003;227(1):183–91.
10. Doshi DJ, March DE, Crisi GM, Coughlin BF. Complex cystic breast masses: diagnostic approach and imaging-pathologic correlation. Radiographics. 2007;27:S53–64.
11. Athanasiou A, Aubert E, Vincent Salomon A, Tardivon A. Complex cystic breast masses in ultrasound examination. Diagn Interv Imaging. 2014;95:169–79.
12. Taskin F, et al. Sclerosing adenosis of the breast: radiologic appearance and efficiency of core needle biopsy. Diagn Interv Radiol. 2011;17:311–6.
13. Lee K, Chan JKC, Gwi E. Tubular adenosis of the breast: a distinctive benign lesion mimicking invasive carcinoma. Am J Surg PatholAm J Surg Pathol. 1996;20:46–54.
14. Eusebi V, Millis RR. Epitheliosis, infiltrating epitheliosis, and radial scar. Semin Diagn Pathol. 2010;27(1):5–12.
15. Stavros AT. Breast ultrasound. Philadelphia: Lippincott; 2004. p. 589–93.
16. Linda A, Zuiani C, Furlan A, Lorenzon M, Londero V, Girometti R, Bazzocchi M. Nonsurgical management of high-risk lesions diagnosed at core needle biopsy: can malignancy be ruled out safely with breast MRI? AJR Am J Roentgenol. 2012;198(2):272–80. https://doi.org/10.2214/AJR.11.7040.
17. Federica Pediconi MD, Rossella Occhiato MD, Venditti F, et al. Radial scars of the breast: contrast-enhanced magnetic resonance mammography appearance. Breast J. 2005;11(1):23–8.
18. Jeon-Hor Chen, , Orhan Nalcioglu, Min-Ying Su, Fibrocystic change of the breast presenting as a focal lesion mimicking breast cancer in MR imaging. J Magn Reson Imaging. 2008; 28(6): 1499–1503.
19. Stachs A, Stubert J, Reimer T, Hartmann S. Benign breast disease in women. Dtsch Arztebl Int. 2019;116:565–74. https://doi.org/10.3238/arztebl.2019.0565.
20. Mesurolle B, Perez JCH, Azzumea F. Atypical ductal hyperplasia diagnosed at Sonographically guided Core needle biopsy: frequency, final surgical outcome, and factors associated with underestimation. Am J Roentgenol. 2014;202:1389–94. https://doi.org/10.2214/AJR.13.10864.
21. Helvie MA, Hessler C, Frank TS, Ikeda DM. Atypical hyperplasia of the breast: mammographic appearance and histologic correlation. Radiology. 1991;179:759–64.
22. Dupont WD, Page DL. Risk factors for breast cancer in women with proliferative breast disease. N Engl J Med. 1985;312(3):146–51.

Part VI

Approach to Papillary Neoplasms

Papillary Masses of the Breast

20

M. C. Sheela, V. Pavithra, Ramya Ramakrishnan,
Bhawna Dev, and Sandhya Sundaram

Abstract

Papillary masses of the breast comprises overlapping spectrum of benign and malignant masses. The clinical and imaging findings cannot reliably differentiate between these masses, necessitating histopathological correlation for appropriate clinical management and follow-up.

Keywords

Papilloma · Atypical papilloma · Papillary DCIS · Papillary carcinoma · Solid cystic mass of breast

20.1 Introduction

Papillary masses of the breast consist of a varied group of masses, which include benign intraductal papilloma (IDP), papilloma with atypia (atypical papilloma), intraductal papilloma (IDP) with DCIS, papillary DCIS, and variants of papillary carcinoma. The differentiation of benign papilloma from the malignant papillary masses on imaging is difficult at times, due to varied spectrum and overlapping imaging appearances. The papillary masses of the breast can be broadly classified as in Fig. 20.1.

M. C. Sheela (✉) · B. Dev
Department of Radiology, Sri Ramachandra Institute of Higher Education and Research, Chennai, India
e-mail: sheelamc@sriramachandra.edu.in; bhawnadev@sriramachandra.edu.in

V. Pavithra · S. Sundaram
Department of pathology, Sri Ramachandra Institute of Higher Education and Research, Chennai, India
e-mail: pavithrav@sriramachandra.edu.in

R. Ramakrishnan
Department of Surgery, Sri Ramachandra Institute of Higher Education and Research, Chennai, India
e-mail: ramya.r@sriramachandra.edu.in

B. Dev, L. D. Joseph (eds.), *Holistic Approach to Breast Disease*,
https://doi.org/10.1007/978-981-99-0035-0_20

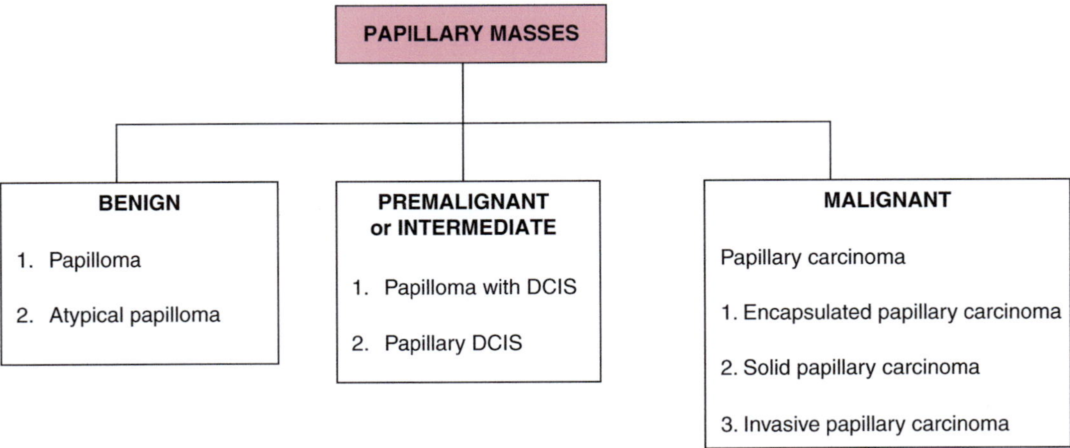

Fig. 20.1 Broad classification of papillary masses of breast

20.2 Benign Masses

This includes benign papilloma and atypical papilloma.

20.2.1 Benign Papilloma

20.2.1.1 Introduction

The most common age group is between the fifth and sixth decades with the usual presentation as a serous, serosanguineous or watery type of nipple discharge. The most common cause of bloody nipple discharge is an intraductal papilloma [1].

These lesions rarely undergo malignant transformation [2]. However, the risk of developing breast carcinoma in a woman who has an intraductal papilloma is a matter of debate.

20.2.1.2 Clinical Presentation

The intraductal papilloma can be solitary or multiple.

Solitary intraductal papilloma is mostly centrally located/in the retro-areolar region and manifests as nipple discharge. The discharge is usually spontaneous from a single duct and is unilateral.

Multiple intraductal papillomas are located peripherally in the breast. They are less common than solitary papilloma and usually present as a palpable mass. They are more often associated with hyperplasia, atypia, DCIS, invasive cancer, sclerosing adenosis, and radial scars [3].

20.2.1.3 Imaging Features

Galactography

In a normal galactogram, contrast material diffuses and fills branching ductal systems extending toward the chest wall. Normal ducts have a branching, smooth-tapering appearance (Fig 20.2a, b). Papilloma appears as a focal filling defect and may completely obstruct further filling with contrast material beyond the level of obstruction (Fig. 20.2c). As galactography is an invasive procedure, it 'i rarely performed nowadays.

Mammogram

Small solitary papillomas are difficult to identify due to relative denser breast tissue in the retro-areolar region. Larger masses appear as well-circumscribed equal density masses (Fig. 20.3) with no ominous features like microcalcifications or surrounding architectural distortions.

Ultrasound

These masses appear as a round or oval well-circumscribed solid mass with an adjacent dilated duct (Fig. 20.4) or a dilated duct with an internal echogenic component or a solid cystic mass (Fig. 20.5). On Doppler study, the solid component shows a vascular feeding pedicle, which helps in differentiating from an inspissated secretion.

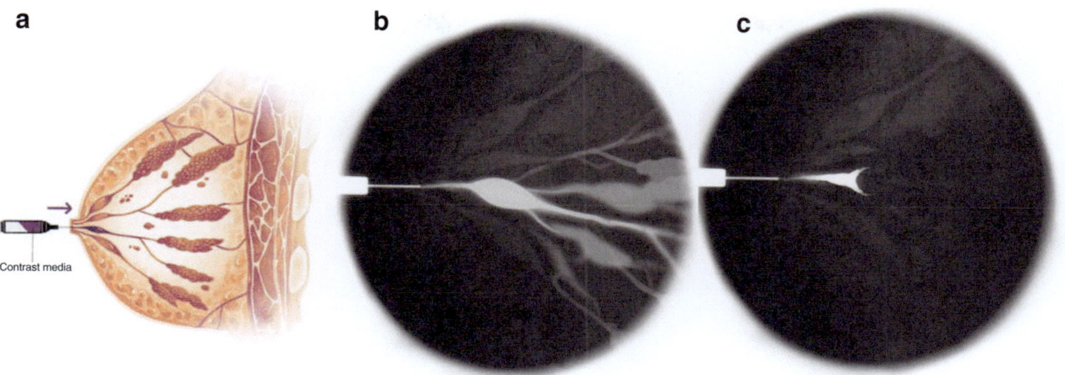

Fig. 20.2 Diagrammatic representation of galactogram. (**a**) Contrast media is injected into the duct. (**b**) Galactogram reveals uniform opacification of the duct with smooth tapering of the duct. (**c**) Galactogram reveals focal smooth filling defect (claw sign/meniscus sign) with no contrast opacification distal to the obstruction

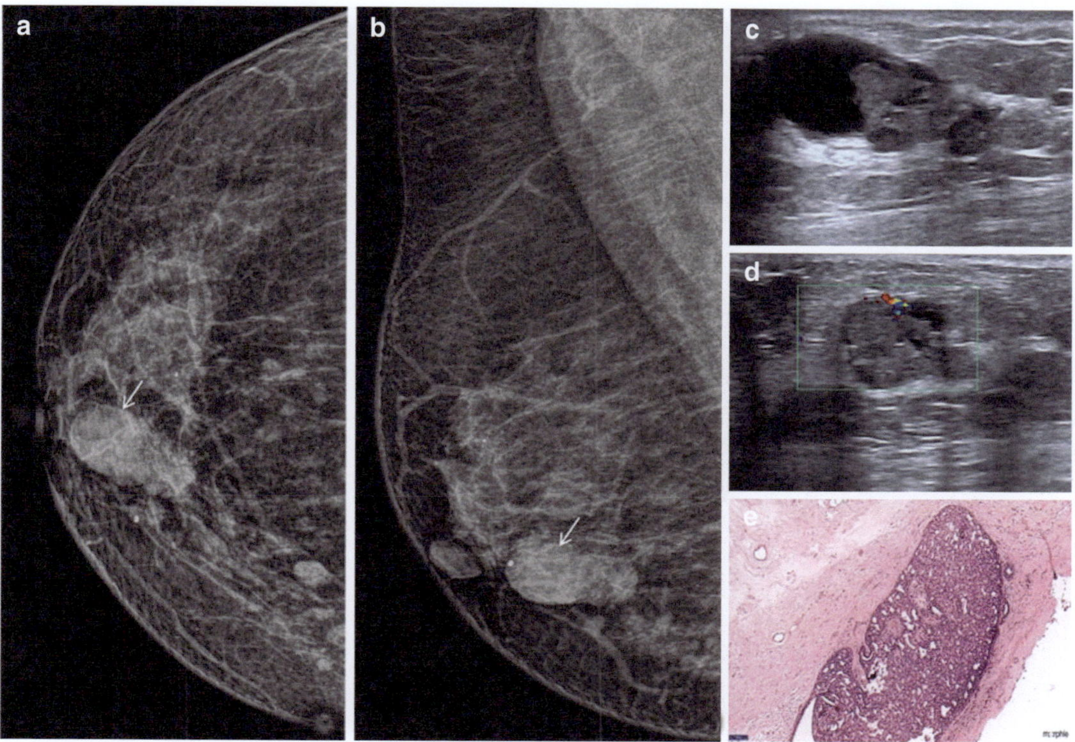

Fig. 20.3 Benign intraductal papilloma. (**a**, **b**) CC and MLO view of the right breast shows a circumscribed oval equal density mass in the retro-areolar region (Arrow). (**c**) USG reveals a dilated duct with intraductal solid component, which shows internal vascularity within (**d**). (**e**) H & E: Well-circumscribed lesion with intraductal papillary proliferation of ductal and myoepithelial cells ×100

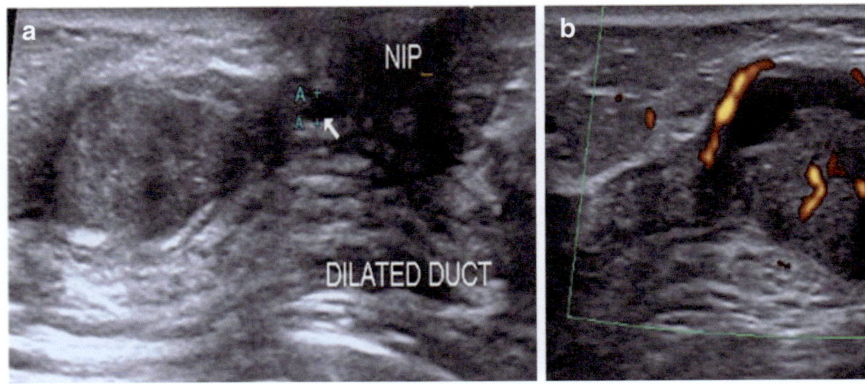

Fig. 20.4 Benign intraductal papilloma. (**a**) USG reveals a circumscribed oval isoechoic solid mass, almost completely filling the duct with a proximal dilated duct in subareolar region (**b**). (**b**) Doppler shows increased vascularity within the solid component.

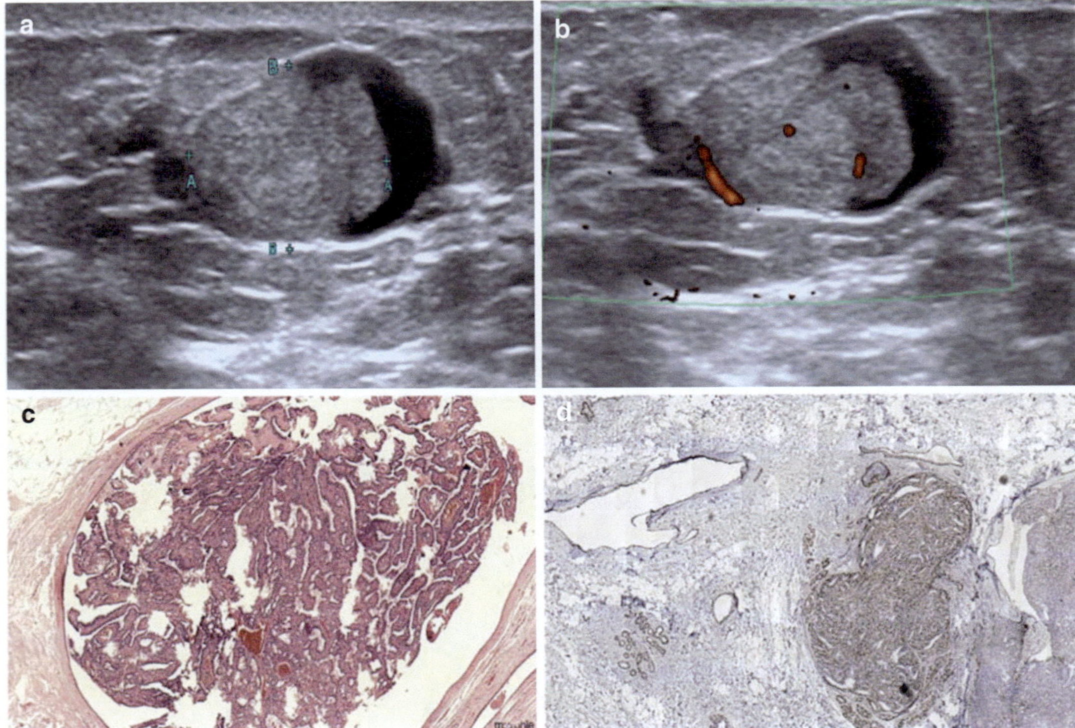

Fig. 20.5 Benign intraductal papilloma. (**a**) USG reveals a solid cystic mass with increased vascularity in the solid component in (**b**). (**c**) H & E: Papillary architecture and fibrovascular cores covered by benign inner myoepithelial and outer epithelial layers ×100—(**d**) Immunohistochemistry-p63: Shows positivity within the papillae and at the periphery ×40

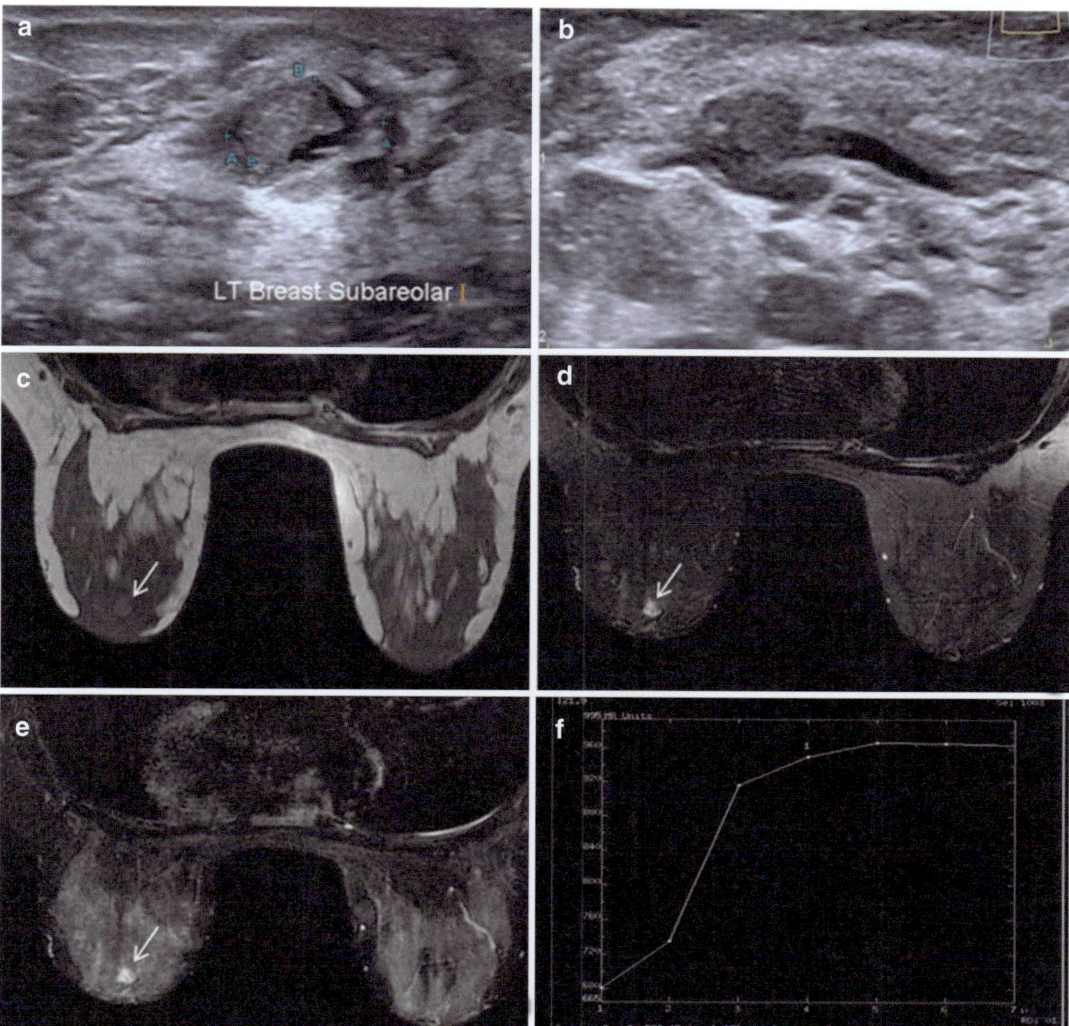

Fig. 20.6 Benign intraductal papilloma. (**a**, **b**) USG reveals a dilated duct with echogenic component within. (**c**) T1W Image shows an iso to hyperintense mass (arrow), (**d**) appearing hyperintense (arrow) on T2W Fat-saturated images. (**e**) postcontrast study showing intense enhancement (arrow) (**f**) type II time kinetic curve for the same mass

20.2.1.4 Magnetic Resonance Imaging (MRI)

MRI is usually performed in patients with inconclusive findings in mammography and ultrasound. It may appear as a well-circumscribed oval or round mass or an irregular mass, or a solid and cystic mass; they may also be occult at imaging [4].

On T1W sequence: Circumscribed hyperintense or isointense mass within a dilated duct (Fig. 20.6).

On T2W sequence: Iso- or hyperintense mass and may show adjacent dilated ducts.

On postcontrast scans, they appear as well-defined enhancing nodules. Sometimes, the masses are better appreciated in subtracted images only.

Kinetic evaluation can reveal progressive, plateau, or washout-type enhancement, which makes it difficult to differentiate from malignant massses.

20.2.1.5 BI-RADS Category

The usual BI RADS category assigned is **BI RADS 4 A**.

20.2.1.6 Pathology [5]

Gross Presentation: Central papilloma may form well-circumscribed round tumor of papillary fronds attached by one or more pedicles to the wall of the dilated duct. The size of central papilloma varies from few millimeters to >5 cm. Focal necrosis or hemorrhage may be present. In contrast, peripheral papillomas are usually grossly occult unless they are associated with other findings.

Microscopy: Histologically, the benign intraductal papillomas (IDP) are well circumscribed with intraductal proliferation comprising of broad and blunt fronds with papillary architecture and fibrovascular cores, covered by benign inner myoepithelial and outer epithelial layers. The epithelium is of columnar morphology and/or displays Usual Ductal Hyperplasia (UDH) and/or apocrine metaplasia.

Immunohistochemistry: The myoepithelial markers (p63, p40, Calponin, SMA, CK5/6, CK14, or SMMHC) may be variably prominent but is uniformly present, both at the periphery and within the papillae.

Differential Diagnosis: Depending on the histopathological context, the differential diagnosis for papilloma may include the spectrum of papillary lesions—intraductal papilloma with Atypical Ductal Hyperplasia (ADH)/Ductal Carcinoma In Situ (DCIS), papillary DCIS/intraductal papillary carcinoma (in particular the dimorphic subtype, because globoid cells may mimic myoepithelium), encapsulated papillary carcinoma, solid papillary carcinoma and tall cell carcinoma with reversed polarity as well as adeno-myoepithelioma or fibroepithelial tumors with polypoid stromal architecture, nipple adenoma, and sweat gland hidradenoma papilliferum.

> Rarely, papillomas have been described in axillary lymph nodes as a form of benign epithelial inclusions.

20.2.2 Papilloma with Atypia (Atypical Papilloma)

This entity is purely a pathological diagnosis. The clinical presentation and imaging features are indistinguishable from a benign intraductal papilloma (Fig. 20.7).

20.2.3 Pathology [6]

Microscopy: Intraductal papilloma with atypical ductal hyperplasia is the same as atypical papilloma. One should use the same criteria to diagnose atypical ductal hyperplasia (ADH) in a papilloma that we used to diagnose ADH elsewhere in the breast. Typically, the IDP with atypia exhibits focal solid or cribriform epithelial expansion of small (0.3 cm) size and composed of small, monotonous epithelial cells.

Immunohistochemistry: On immunohistochemistry, the foci of atypia are negative for high-molecular-weight cytokeratin (CK) 5/6 and diffusely positive for estrogen receptor (ER).CK 5 is a better stain to distinguish usual ductal hyperplasia, which will be positive versus ADH in a papilloma where CK5 is negative.

20.2.4 Clinical Management of Benign Papillary Lesions

The preferred management following the diagnosis of papillary masses of the breast based on core needle biopsy (CNB) has been contentious. Surgical excision of papillary masses is widely recommended especially for those with atypia due to their high association with malignancy. However, the case is not the same as the treatment of papillary masses without atypia. Discrepancy as to the upgradation rate from a papillary mass without atypia to a cancer diagnosis has been noted, ranging from 2% to 33% [7]. The reason for this discrepancy has been intensively investigated. Factors, such as mass size, nipple discharge, and palpable disease, have been reported to be associated with upgrading; however, results are not consistent.

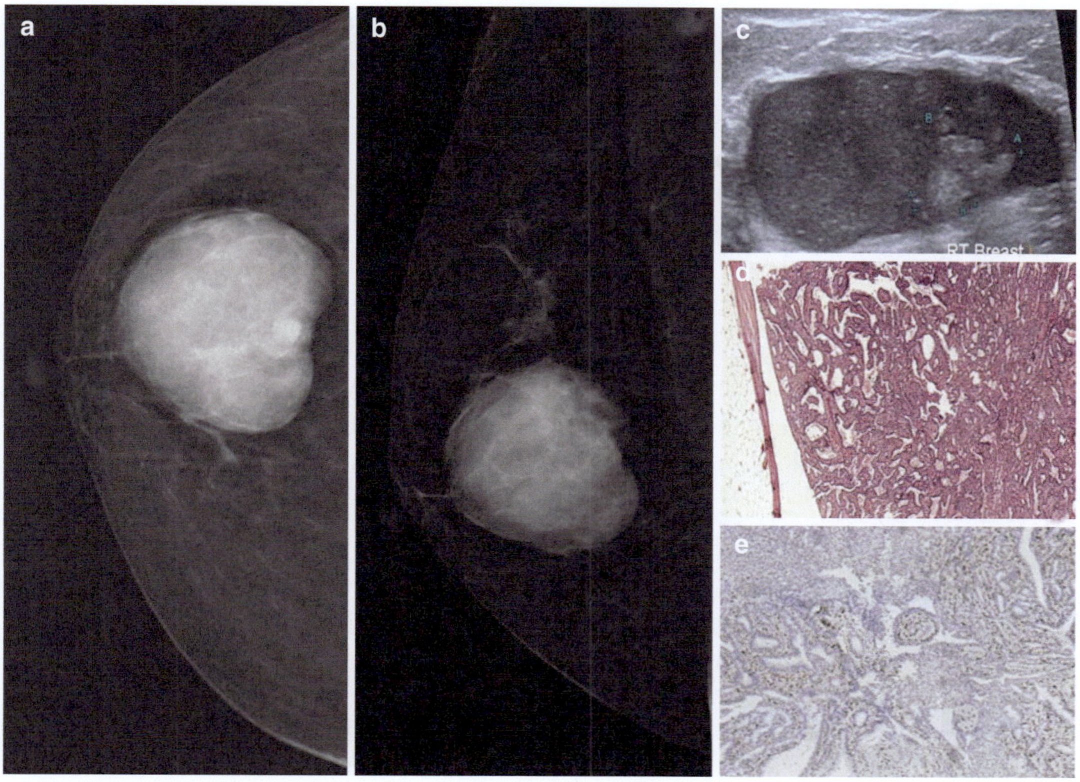

Fig. 20.7 Atypical papilloma. (**a**, **b**) CC and MLO view of the right breast shows a circumscribed high density mass in the retro-areolar region. (**c**) USG reveals a complex cyst with echogenic solid component within. (**d**) H & E: Intraductal papilloma with atypical ductal hyperplasia composed of small, monotonous epithelial cells. ×100 (**e**) Immunohistochemistry: A foci of atypia is negative for p63 staining ×100

Vacuum-assisted biopsy (VAB) is considered more accurate in terms of both sensitivity and specificity than CNB. Some have proposed conservative management of papillary masses of the breast by VAB instead of open biopsy. Chang et al. performed US-guided VAB to remove lesions, none of which were reclassified as high risk [8]. Wyss et al. also demonstrated that VAB of papillomas did not underestimate the pathology when compared to excision biopsy [9]. Given that VAB is less invasive, less expensive, and quicker to perform, it may be preferred over open biopsy, which is the current gold standard in treating papillary lesions.

Patients with low-risk benign papillomas diagnosed by CNB and without significantly bothersome symptoms (e.g., copious nipple discharge or an anxiety provoking mass) can be safely followed. High-risk papillomas, particularly those with atypia, should generally be excised to rule out coexisting cancer, and these patients should continue to have close surveillance along with consideration of possible chemoprevention [10].

20.3 Premalignant/Intermediate Lesions

This include papilloma with DCIS and papillary DCIS.

20.3.1 Papilloma with DCIS

20.3.1.1 Clinical Presentation

The usual clinical presentation is bleeding per nipple with or without a palpable mass.

20.3.1.2 Imaging Features

Mammogram

Papillomas associated with DCIS and papillary DICS may appear identical to benign papillomas on all imaging modalities. Although indeterminate calcifications within a papilloma could suggest the presence of DCIS [11], similar microcalcifications may also be observed with infarction, hemorrhage, or fibrosis.

Ultrasound

It may appear as well-circumscribed round or oval solid mass or as a solid cystic mass with mild vascularity on doppler study.

MRI

The role of MRI in evaluating these papillomas is uncertain [12]. However, in papillomas with DCIS, MRI may be useful in defining the extent of DCIS involvement in the surrounding tissues.

20.3.1.3 Bi-RADS Category

It usually is categorized under BI RADS 4A.

20.3.1.4 Pathology [13]

Microscopy: Intraductal papillomas, which exhibit foci of architectural and cytological atypia, which would be diagnosed as DCIS elsewhere in the breast, are designated as Intraductal papilloma with DCIS. These are usually larger than 0.3 cm and have a solid or cribriform growth pattern with monotony and readily identifiable cell borders.

Immunohistochemistry: The involved foci of atypia will show CK5/6 positivity and ER being diffusely positive.

20.3.2 Papillary DCIS

It is also known as intraductal papillary carcinoma. This noninvasive diffuse form of papillary carcinoma tends to be multifocal, involving the terminal ductal lobular unit and growing within dilated ducts.

20.3.2.1 Clinical Presentation

Papillary DCIS most commonly affects women in their fifth and sixth decades of life, usually not palpable.

20.3.2.2 Imaging Features [14, 15]

Mammogram

Most sensitive modality for this entity. On mammogram, this tumor most commonly presents as single group or as multiple grouped amorphous or pleomorphic microcalcifications (Fig. 20.8), and less frequently as a circumscribed mass. It may also present as an area of asymmetric density, with or without calcification.

Ultrasound

Usually, the ductal distension is noted, which is secondary to the presence of tumor within or it may present as a hypoechoic mass (Fig. 20.8) with or without microcalcifications. In young patients, when ultrasound is performed as a first step examination, it can detect the associated microcalcifications, especially when the underlying breast tissue is diffusely hypoechoic. In these situations, irrespective of patient's age, mammogram should be indicated in order to analyze the morphology of calcifications.

MRI: It may show nonmass-like enhancement.

20.3.2.3 Pathology [16]

Gross Presentation

The gross appearance of papillary DCIS in a subareolar location is difficult to distinguish from that of encapsulated papillary carcinoma as the two lesions may coexist.

Microscopy

Papillary DCIS consists of an intraductal neoplastic epithelial proliferation lining arborizing fibrovascular cores, devoid of myoepithelium. Unlike encapsulated and solid papillary carcinomas, papillary DCIS shows an intact myoepithe-

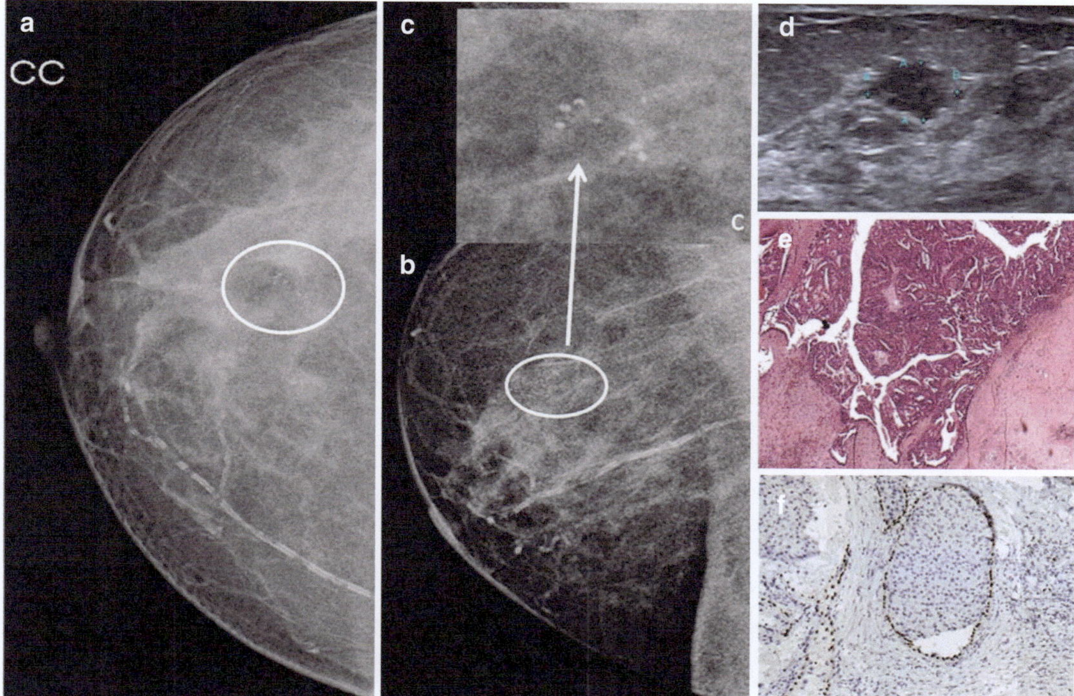

Fig. 20.8 Papillary DCIS. (**a**, **b**) X-ray mammogram reveals grouped pleomorphic microcalcifications. (**c**) Magnified view of the suspicious microcalcifications. (**d**) USG reveals an irregular spiculated subcentimeter mass. (**e**) H & E: Intraductal neoplastic epithelial proliferation lining arborizing fibrovascular cores with intact myoepithelial layer in the periphery ×200. (**f**) Immunohistochemistry p63: Shows only peripheral positive staining ×100

lial layer at the epithelial-stromal interface of the periphery of the involved ducts. The epithelial proliferation may partially or completely fill the spaces between the papillae. Compared with other types of DCIS, papillary DCIS is less commonly associated with comedo necrosis.

Immunohistochemistry: The papillary DCIS too exhibits diffuse positivity of CK5/6 in the myoepithelium, which is present at the periphery of the duct and will be sparse to absent within the papillae and ER will be positive.

Differential Diagnosis

- Apocrine metaplasia
- Encapsulated papillary carcinoma: In this lesion, there is absence of myoepithelial cells within the papillae and at the periphery of the duct spaces.
- Intraductal papilloma: It has fibrovascular core with both epithelial and myoepithelial cells.

20.3.3 Management of Premalignant/Intermediate Lesions

There is universal agreement that surgical excision is required when an atypical papillary mass, papillary ductal carcinoma in situ, or papillary intraductal carcinoma is present in a core needle biopsy specimen [17].

20.4 Papillary Carcinoma

Papillary carcinoma is an uncommon variant of breast cancer representing just 1–2% of breast carcinomas.

20.4.1 Clinical Presentation

It is most commonly detected in postmenopausal women and arises in the retro-areolar region in almost 50% of patients.

Research has been carried out to identify the possible risk factors for malignant papillomas, including patient age on diagnosis, lesion location, and the presence of nipple discharge, tumor size and radiologic findings. The impact of age was controversial, some showed a higher underestimation rate in patients age under 50 years, whereas others concluded differently [18, 19]. Peripherally located [20] and larger papillomas [8, 18, 19] are also more likely to be underestimated to be benign than centrally located and smaller papillomas.

The variants of papillary carcinoma are:

- Encapsulated papillary carcinoma
- Solid papillary carcinoma
- Invasive papillary carcinoma

20.5 Encapsulated Papillary Carcinoma

It was previously referred to as intracystic or encysted papillary carcinoma.

20.5.1 Clinical Presentation

Encapsulated papillary carcinoma presents in postmenopausal women, mainly with an average age between 55 and 67 years old [21]. Many cases were also described in the male population in the literature, and it is the second most common type of breast cancer in men [22]. Clinically, it frequently presents as a benign mass. The tumor can also manifest with a bloody nipple discharge, and in some cases, it can be asymptomatic and is revealed on screening mammogram. Axillary node involvement is infrequent [23]. This mass may be uni- or multifocal and can be found as a pure form or may be associated with ductal carcinoma in situ or invasive carcinoma.

20.5.2 Imaging Features [24]

20.5.2.1 Mammogram

Mammographic findings are often nonspecific. It is usually a round, oval, or lobulated circumscribed mass, mostly seen in the retro-areolar region (Fig. 20.9). There may be associated spiculations and nipple retraction, which can be due to invasion or secondary to sclerosis or inflammation of the surrounding tissue.

Multiple masses may be present, often within one quadrant. Occasionally, satellite nodules, pleomorphic microcalcifications are noted.

20.5.2.2 Ultrasound

It is seen as either single or multiple predominantly cystic/solid cystic masses. The cyst may be with or without internal septa; the solid papillary masses have an irregular branching pattern with peripheral fronds. The tumor demonstrates posterior acoustic enhancement due to its predominantly cystic component. The presence of fluid-debris levels in the cyst is secondary to spontaneous bleeding. Encapsulated papillary carcinoma may be diagnosed with ultrasound only if they do not occupy the entire cyst lumen, else it is not possible to differentiate from other solid masses.

Color Doppler shows vascularity within the solid component.

The size of the intracystic solid component, the heterogeneous echotexture, and an irregular border of the solid papillary mass are suspicious for malignancy.

20.5.2.3 MRI

The tumor usually appears as a round or oval mass with well-defined margins. The solid component is seen as nodular mass or multiple

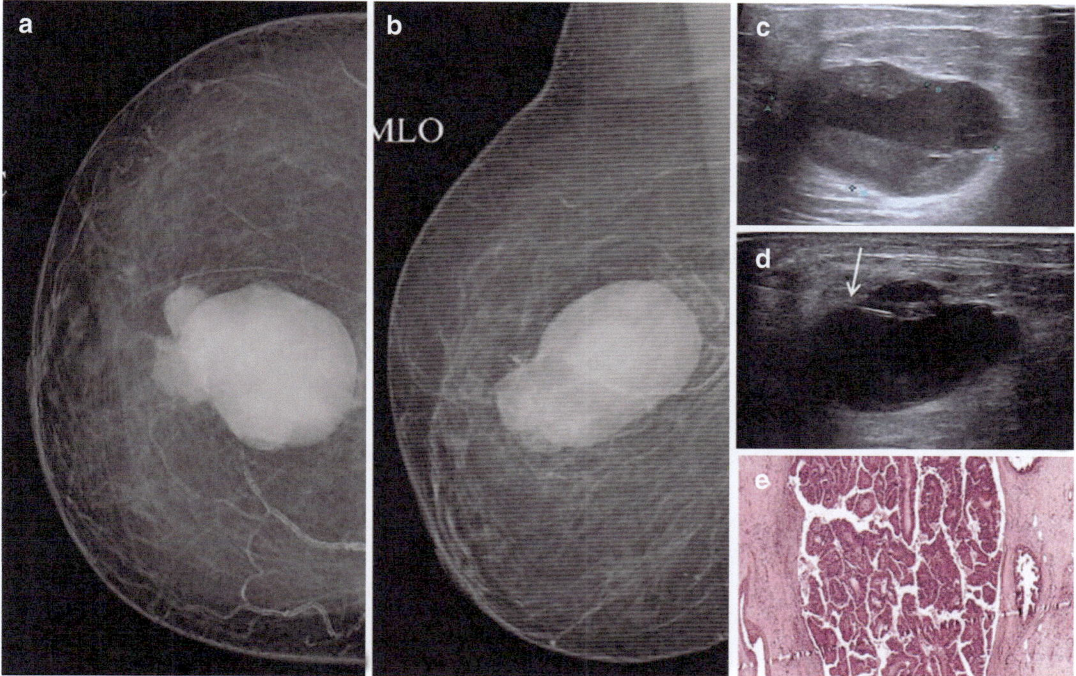

Fig. 20.9 Encapsulated papillary carcinoma. (**a**, **b**) X-ray mammogram reveals a circumscribed high-density mass in the right breast. (**c**) USG reveals a circumscribed solid cystic mass. (**d**) USG guided tru cut biopsy from the solid component (arrow). (**e**) H & E: Papillary mass within a cystic space with multiple delicate fibrovascular stalks consisting of monomorphic population of neoplastic epithelial cells and no myoepithelial cells ×100

nodules of intermediate signal intensity projecting from the periphery into the lumen. The cystic component shows varied signal intensities i.e., if the contents of the cyst are serous, it will have low signal intensity on T1 and high signal on T2-weighted images and if the cyst has hemorrhagic contents, it will be hyperintense on both T1- and T2-weighted images and fluid-fluid levels may be seen on T2-weighted images.

Contrast-enhanced MR imaging show intense enhancement of the cyst walls, septa, and mural nodules.

Dynamic MR imaging shows a significant increase in signal intensity at a peak of 3 min, a finding that indicates malignancy, in contrast to benign papillomas, which show early and rapid uptake of gadolinium contrast material.

Hence, the round or oval shape with smooth margins and the mixture of solid and cystic components are the main features that allow differentiation of encapsulated papillary carcinoma from other types of cancer.

20.5.3 BI-RADS Category

It is characterized under category **BI-RADS 4 A/B/C**.

20.5.3.1 Pathology

Gross Presentation: Encapsulated papillary carcinoma is often observed as a friable mass within a cystic space mostly seen in the central and subareolar region.

Microscopy: Encapsulated papillary carcinoma usually consists of a papillary mass within a cystic space; less often, it is composed of an aggregate of close nodules. The tumor has a rounded, pushing border and is typically surrounded by a fibrous capsule of varying thickness. The lesion consists of multiple delicate fibrovascular stalks covered by a monomorphic population of neoplastic epithelial cells with low- or intermediate-grade nuclei and no myoepithelial cells. Frank invasion in this setting is defined as the presence of neoplastic elements that permeate beyond the fibrous capsule with an irregular infiltrative appearance, most often taking the form of Invasive breast carcinoma-No special type.

Immunohistochemistry: The neoplastic epithelial component does not express high-molecular-weight cytokeratins. Staining for multiple myoepithelial markers demonstrates the absence of myoepithelial cells. Encapsulated papillary carcinomas express ER and (usually) PR, lack ERBB2 (HER2) gene amplification, and demonstrate a low to occasionally moderate Ki-67 proliferation index.

Differential Diagnosis: The differential diagnosis includes solid papillary carcinoma, papillary ductal carcinoma in situ, invasive papillary carcinoma, and papilloma with superimposed ductal carcinoma in situ, as well as the rare cases of benign hyperplastic papillary apocrine lesions that present as papillary cystic lesions lined by benign apocrine cells, devoid of nuclear atypia or necrosis, in which a myoepithelial cell layer may be absent.

20.5.4 Clinical Management

Core needle biopsy of the intracystic mass under ultrasound guidance has been used by many authors for distinguishing benign from malignant papillary lesions, but it has a low accuracy for distinguishing between in situ or invasive papillary carcinoma, because the site of biopsy is generally central, while the invasion is usually found in the periphery of the tumor [23]. Therefore, surgical excision is preferred for adequate histologic diagnosis and treatment [25].

Surgical excision is recommended after core-needle biopsy if there is atypia, high-risk lesion, positivity for malignancy, or imaging-histological discordance. Biopsy excision is often performed directly when papillary carcinoma is suggested on ultrasound or mammography.

There are no evidence-based guidelines for treatment of IPC. There is no randomized controlled trial comparing breast-conserving surgery to mastectomy. However, many case reports and retrospective studies showed excellent prognosis with conservative surgery without axillary dissection in IPC not associated to DCIS or microinvasion lesions [26].

Sentinel node biopsy may be an excellent alternative to full axillary dissection in patients with IPC and associated invasive carcinoma [27]. There is also lack of evidence about the role of adjuvant therapy.

20.6 Solid Papillary Carcinoma

Solid papillary carcinoma (also known as neuroendocrine breast carcinoma in situ; spindle cell ductal carcinoma in situ; neuroendocrine ductal carcinoma in situ; endocrine ductal carcinoma in situ) is a variant of papillary carcinoma, which occurs primarily in postmenopausal women, mainly during the seventh decade of life or later.

20.6.1 Imaging Features

20.6.1.1 Mammogram

Papillary carcinomas are round, oval, or lobulated in shape. The margins are usually well defined but may be poorly defined in areas of invasion. As there is minimal perilesional fibrotic reaction, spiculations are rarely seen. It may be associated with pleomorphic microcalcifications (Fig. 20.10) but may occasionally have a coarse or stippled appearance.

20.6.1.2 Ultrasound

It is seen as a hypoechoic solid mass or a complex cystic mass with septations or a cyst with a mural nodule. Doppler imaging often shows internal vascularity in the solid component.

20.6.1.3 MRI

No adequate literature is available due to the rarity of the lesions. It may appear as irregular enhancing nodules or enhancing complex solid cystic mass. However, there is a significant overlap in the morphology and kinetic curves with those of benign papillomas. MRI may help in the surgical planning of multiple papillary lesions [28].

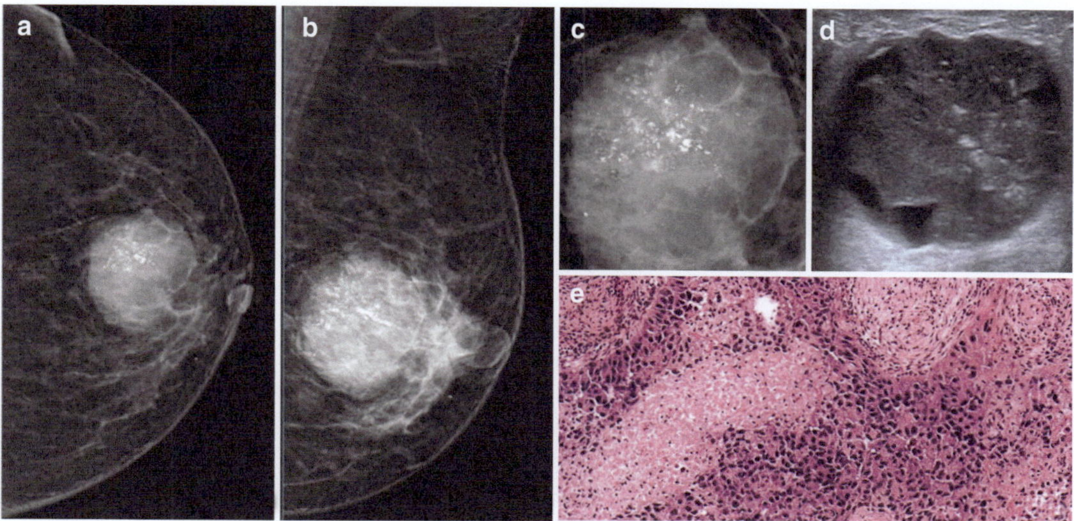

Fig. 20.10 Solid papillary carcinoma. (**a**, **b**) X-ray mammogram revealing a circumscribed solid lesion in the retro-areolar region with pleomorphic microcalcifications within. (**c**) Magnified X-ray view of the mass and suspicious calcifications. (**d**) USG showing a heteroechoeic solid lesion with few cystic spaces and microcalcifications within. (**e**) H & E: Proliferation of monotonous population of round- to spindle-shaped epithelial cells with moderate nuclear atypia around tumor necrosis with no myoepithelial cells ×100

20.6.2 BI-RADS Category

The BI RADS category assigned **BI RADS 4C/5**.

20.6.2.1 Pathology

Gross Presentation: It is a soft, well-circumscribed, tan pink mass seen in any part of the breast, but the central/subareolar area is most commonly affected.

Microscopy: Solid papillary carcinomas are characterized by expansile nodules with a solid growth pattern and inconspicuous, delicate fibrovascular cores. The proliferation is composed of a monotonous population of round to spindle-shaped epithelial cells with (usually) mild-to-moderate nuclear atypia and a variable mitotic count. Extracellular mucin production can also be present and if it is prominent mucinous carcinoma must be excluded. Solid papillary carcinoma with invasion is diagnosed when solid papillary carcinoma is associated with areas featuring strands or large clusters of tumor cells. This is frequently seen within pools of extracellular mucin (typically infiltrating the surrounding tissue at the periphery of the lesion), corresponding to mucinous carcinoma. Fat infiltration by irregular solid papillary nests and vascular invasion may also be seen in these invasive cases.

Immunohistochemistry: The neoplastic cells lack the expression of high-molecular-weight cytokeratins. They are strongly and diffusely positive for ER and PR expression is variable. They do not show ERBB2 (HER2) overexpression. The Ki-67 proliferation index is usually low or intermediate. Neuroendocrine differentiation, which is demonstrated by synaptophysin and chromogranin expression, is frequent, in particular, when there is an associated mucinous component.

Differential Diagnosis: Papilloma with florid usual ductal hyperplasia that completely obliterates the spaces between papillae can be mistaken for solid papillary carcinoma. In such cases, the hyperplastic epithelial cells in papilloma express high-molecular-weight cytokeratins and show heterogeneous positivity for ER, whereas the neoplastic epithelial cells of solid papillary carcinoma lack expression of high-molecular-weight cytokeratins and typically show strong ER positivity.

20.6.3 Clinical Management

Management of Solid Papillary Carcinoma (SPC) varies from breast-conserving surgery to mastectomy. Most authors suggest complete excision of the mass or total/partial mastectomy. The role of sentinel lymph node biopsy is not clear. Some authors recommend sentinel lymph node biopsy, because SPC can be associated with an invasive component, and therefore, axillary lymph node metastasis could be present in approximately 3–5% of the cases [28].

Given the low incidence of local recurrence and metastasis, breast-conserving surgery is the optimal treatment. The role of postoperative radiotherapy and endocrine therapy in SPC remains controversial [29].

20.7 Invasive Papillary Carcinoma

This entity is extremely rare, and no specific epidemiological or clinical data are available. Most cases reported as invasive papillary carcinoma in the literature are in fact encapsulated papillary carcinoma or solid papillary carcinoma or metastases with primary from other sites, especially the ovary.

20.7.1 Imaging Features

On imaging distinguishing solid papillary carcinoma from invasive papillary carcinoma is difficult as both appear similar in all modalities (Fig. 20.11).

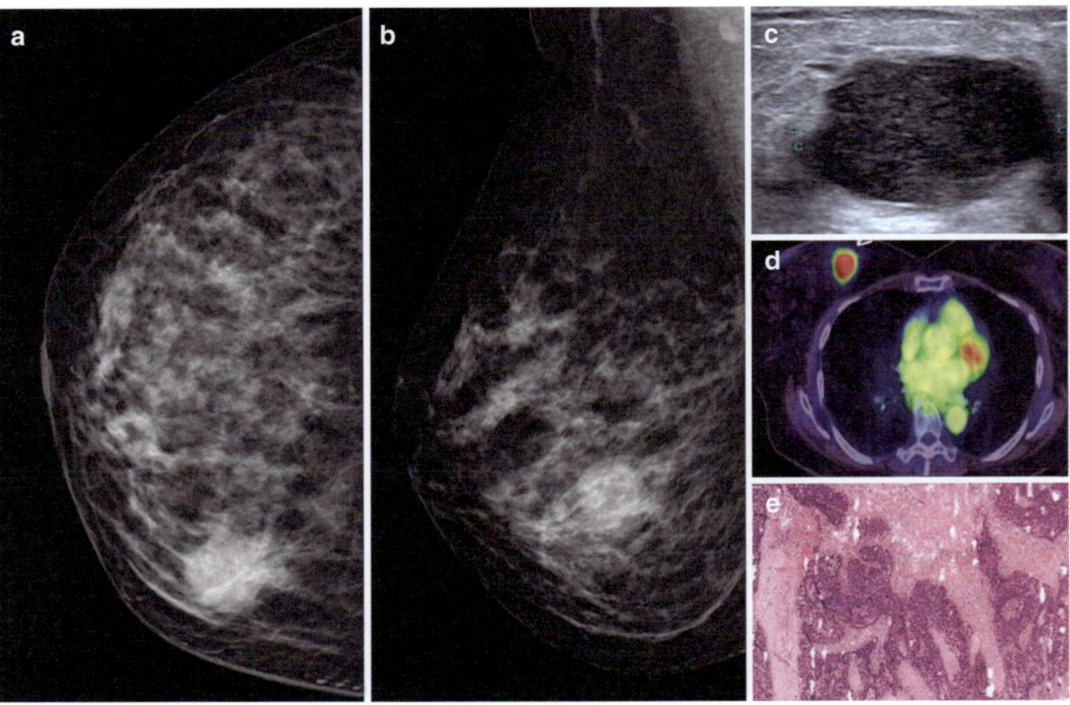

Fig. 20.11 Invasive papillary carcinoma. (**a**, **b**) X-ray mammogram reveals an irregular mass with indistinct posterior margins in the lower inner quadrant. (**c**) USG correlation reveals an irregular hypoechoic mass. (**d**) 18 FDG PET CT scan reveals increased uptake in the right breast mass. (**e**) Invasive growth pattern composed of mildly dilated ducts and microcysts containing papillary formations with adjacent areas of necrosis ×100

20.7.2 BI-RADS Category and Management

These lesions are categorized under **BI-RADS 4C/5**.

20.7.2.1 Pathology

Microscopy: Invasive papillary carcinomas display a frankly invasive growth pattern and are composed of mildly dilated ducts and microcysts containing papillary formations. Myoepithelial cells are absent at the periphery and along the papillary stalks.

Differential Diagnosis: These tumors should be differentiated from invasive micropapillary carcinoma and metastases to the breast from other organs. Invasive micropapillary carcinomas have a distinctive growth pattern characterized by clusters of cancer cells that lack fibrovascular cores and are surrounded by clear stromal spaces. Metastases of ovarian serous carcinoma, pulmonary papillary adenocarcinoma, and thyroid papillary carcinoma can be distinguished from breast carcinoma on the basis of careful morphological assessment and as needed, immunohistochemistry for site-of-origin markers. Invasive papillary carcinoma is distinct from encapsulated papillary carcinoma and solid papillary carcinoma, which are classified according to their specific morphological features. Additionally, the term should not be used for nonpapillary carcinomas arising in association with encapsulated papillary carcinoma or solid papillary carcinoma.

Myoepithelial marker staining on different papillary compartments [30]

ME marker staining	IDPC	EPC	SPC	DCIS involving papilloma
Periphery	Present	Absent	Absent/present	Present in papilloma
Around fibrovascular cores	Absent/scant	Absent/attenuated/retained	Absent/attenuated/retained	Present in papilloma

IDPC intraductal papillary carcinoma, *EPC* encapsulated papillary carcinoma, *SPC* solid papillary carcinoma, *DCIS* ductal carcinoma in situ

20.7.3 Molecular Alterations [30]

Both IDP and papillary carcinomas show Loss of Heterozygosity (LOH) on chromosome 16p13 in the TSC2 gene region, with similar frequencies (60–63%), while LOH at locus 16q23 is limited to papillary carcinomas. Also, IDPs with/without florid hyperplasia show higher frequency in PIK3CA or AKT mutation compared to papillary carcinomas, suggesting a potentially divergent molecular pathway in pathogenesis. Genomic profiling of papillary carcinomas (including EPCs and SPCs) shows a similar pattern of gene copy number aberrations as grade- and ER-matched infiltrating duct carcinomas, no special type (IDC-NSTs). However, papillary carcinomas display less genomic aberrations than IDC-NSTs and a higher mutation rate in PI3KCA. The genomic profiles of the three morphologic papillary carcinomas (EPC, SPC, and IPC) are remarkably similar.

20.7.4 Clinical Management

Fayanju et al. identified 45 females with papillary carcinoma. Twenty-one patients were identified with papillary in situ disease, 18 with papillary in situ disease associated with DCIS, and 6 with invasive papillary carcinoma. In this study, patients with invasive features were more likely to undergo an axillary staging procedure (100%) as compared to patients with in situ disease alone (29%) or in situ disease and associated DCIS (28%) ($p < 0.001$). Furthermore, patients with in situ disease alone were more likely to receive radiation therapy as compared to patients in the remaining categories ($p < 0.001$). Finally, endocrine therapy was more common in patients with invasive papillary carcinoma and in situ papillary carcinoma associated with DCIS. The rather discordant therapy of these three groups in the absence of definitive guidelines for management underscores the need for further treatment and outcome-related studies related to papillary carcinoma [26].

References

1. Markopoulos C, Mantas D, Kouskos E, Antonopoulou Z, Lambadariou K, Revenas K, Papachristodoulou A. Surgical management of nipple discharge. Eur J Gynaecol Oncol. 2006;27(3):275–8.
2. Fiorica JV. Breast diseases. In: DiSaia PJ, Creasman WT, editors. Clinical gynecologic oncology. 7th ed. Edinburgh: Mosby; 2007. p. 411–48. http://www.sciencedirect.com/science/article/pii/B9780323039789500174.
3. Muttarak M, Lerttumnongtum P, Chaiwun B, Peh WCG. Spectrum of papillary lesions of the breast: clinical, imaging, and pathologic correlation. Am J Roentgenol. 2008;191(3):700–7.
4. Tominaga J, Hama H, Kimura N, Takahashi S. Magnetic resonance imaging of intraductal papillomas of the breast. J Comput Assist Tomogr. 2011;35(1):153–7. https://journals.lww.com/jcat/Fulltext/2011/01000/Magnetic_Resonance_Imaging_of_Intraductal.28.aspx
5. WHO Classification of Tumours. 2020. https://whobluebooks.iarc.fr/publications/index.php.
6. MacGrogan G, Tavassoli FA. Central atypical papillomas of the breast: a clinicopathological study of 119 cases. Virchows Arch Int J Pathol. 2003;443(5):609–17.
7. Menes TS, Rosenberg R, Balch S, Jaffer S, Kerlikowske K, Miglioretti DL. Upgrade of high-risk breast lesions detected on mammography in the breast cancer surveillance consortium. Am J Surg. 2014;207(1):24–31.
8. Chang JM, Moon WK, Cho N, Han W, Noh D-Y, Park I-A, et al. Management of ultrasonographically detected benign papillomas of the breast at core needle biopsy. AJR Am J Roentgenol. 2011;196(3):723–9.
9. Wyss P, Varga Z, Rössle M, Rageth CJ. Papillary lesions of the breast: outcomes of 156 patients managed without excisional biopsy. Breast J. 2014;20(4):394–401.
10. Kuehner G, Darbinian J, Habel L, Axelsson K, Butler S, Chang S, et al. Benign papillary breast mass lesions: favorable outcomes with surgical excision or imaging surveillance. Ann Surg Oncol. 2019;26(6):1695–703.
11. Brookes MJ, Bourke AG. Radiological appearances of papillary breast lesions. Clin Radiol. 2008;63(11):1265–73.
12. Schell AM, Rosenkranz K, Lewis PJ. Role of breast MRI in the preoperative evaluation of patients with newly diagnosed breast cancer. Am J Roentgenol. 2009;192(5):1438–44.
13. Jorns JM. Papillary lesions of the breast: a practical approach to diagnosis. Arch Pathol Lab Med. 2016;140(10):1052–9.
14. Papillary lesions of the breast: what the radiologist should know. Contemp Diagn Radiol 2018;41(4). 7–8. https://journals.lww.com/cdronline/Fulltext/2018/02150/Papillary_Lesions_of_the_Breast__What_the.2.aspx.
15. Ciurea A, Calin A, Ciortea C, Dudea SM. Ultrasound in the diagnosis of papillary breast lesions. Med Ultrason. 2015;17(3):392.
16. Ni Y-B, Tse GM. Pathological criteria and practical issues in papillary lesions of the breast—a review. Histopathology. 2016;68(1):22–32.
17. Richter-Ehrenstein C, Tombokan F, Fallenberg E-M, Schneider A, Denkert C. Intraductal papillomas of the breast: diagnosis and management of 151 patients. Breast. 2011;20(6):501–4.
18. Youk JH, Kim E-K, Kwak JY, Son EJ, Park B-W, Kim S-I. Benign papilloma without atypia diagnosed at US-guided 14-gauge core-needle biopsy: clinical and US features predictive of upgrade to malignancy. Radiology. 2011;258(1):81–8.
19. Plantade R, Gerard F, Hammou JC. Management of non malignant papillary lesions diagnosed on percutaneous biopsy. J Radiol. 2006;87(3):299–305.
20. Kil W-H, Cho EY, Kim JH, Nam S-J, Yang J-H. Is surgical excision necessary in benign papillary lesions initially diagnosed at core biopsy? Breast. 2008;17(3):258–62.
21. Salem A, Mrad K, Driss M, Hamza R, Mnif N. Sénologie—carcinome papillaire mammaire intrakystique. J Radiol. 2009;90(4):515–8. /data/revues/02210363/00900004/515/. https://www.em-consulte.com/en/article/213327
22. Grabowski J, Salzstein SL, Sadler GR, Blair S. Intracystic papillary carcinoma: a review of 917 cases. Cancer. 2008;113(5):916–20.
23. Muttarak M, Somwangprasert A, Chaiwun B. Intracystic papillary carcinoma of the breast. Biomed Imaging Interv J. 2005;1(1):e5.
24. Rodríguez MCH, Secades AL, Angulo JM. Intracystic papillary carcinoma of the breast. Radiographics. 2010;30(7):2021–7.
25. Levêque J, Watier E, Lesimple T, Goyat F, Grall JY. Carcinome mammaire intrakystique. J Gynecol Obstet Biol Reprod. 1998;27(3):329–32. /data/revues/03682315/00270003/329/. https://www.em-consulte.com/en/article/113682.
26. Fayanju OM, Ritter J, Gillanders WE, Eberlein TJ, Dietz JR, Aft R, et al. Therapeutic management of intracystic papillary carcinoma of the breast: the roles of radiation and endocrine therapy. Am J Surg. 2007;194(4):497–500.
27. Solorzano CC, Middleton LP, Hunt KK, Mirza N, Meric F, Kuerer HM, et al. Treatment and outcome of patients with intracystic papillary carcinoma of the breast. Am J Surg. 2002;184(4):364–8.
28. Guo S, Wang Y, Rohr J, Fan C, Li Q, Li X, et al. Solid papillary carcinoma of the breast: a special entity needs to be distinguished from conventional invasive carcinoma avoiding over-treatment. Breast. 2016;26:67–72.
29. Inno A, Bogina G, Turazza M, Bortesi L, Duranti S, Massocco A, et al. Neuroendocrine carcinoma of the breast: current evidence and future perspectives. Oncologist. 2016;21(1):28–32.
30. Peng Y, Tang P. Practical breast pathology frequently asked questions. Cham: Springer; 2019.

Part VII

Premalignant and Malignant Lesions of the Breast

Premalignant Lesions

21

Bhawna Dev, Sandhya Sundaram, Leena Dennis Joseph, Mehak Garg, and Mohana Priya

Abstract

Ductal carcinoma in situ (DCIS) is a precursor lesion of invasive breast carcinoma accounting for 20–25% of the total breast carcinoma cases. As most of the patients with DCIS are usually asymptomatic, it is of utmost importance to pick these preinvasive lesions on imaging modalities—mammogram, ultrasound, and MRI breast—so that the appropriate timely management can be done. Lobular Carcinoma in Situ (LCIS) is a clinically occult tumor with vague imaging features radiologically. Thus, in a patient with strong suspicion, histopathology is the key to diagnose LCIS.

Keywords

Micro-calcifications · Asymmetry · Segmental distribution · Non-mass enhancement · LCIS · Occult imaging · Classical · Non-classical types · E-Cadherin · p120

21.1 DCIS

21.1.1 Introduction

Ductal Carcinoma In Situ (DCIS) as the name states is a proliferation of the neoplastic ductal epithelial cells confined to ducto-lobular system without stromal invasion (Fig. 21.1).DCIS accounts for a total of 20–25% of the breast cancers, which are detected on screening mammography. DCIS is classified predominantly on the basis of mammographic features and histologic characteristics like nuclear grade and presence or absence of necrosis. Several clinical studies have corroborated the hypothesis that DCIS is a precursor lesion of invasive breast cancer.

B. Dev (✉) · S. Sundaram · L. D. Joseph
Department of Pathology, Sri Ramachandra Institute of Higher Education and Research, Chennai, India
e-mail: bhawnadev@sriramachandra.edu.in; leenadennisj@sriramachandra.edu.in

M. Garg
Fellow in Breast Imaging, Department of Radiology, Sri Ramachandra Institute of Higher Education and Research, Chennai, India

M. Priya
Department of Surgery, Sri Ramachandra Institute of Higher Education and Research, Chennai, India
e-mail: mohanapriyadr@sriramachandra.edu.in

B. Dev, L. D. Joseph (eds.), *Holistic Approach to Breast Disease*,
https://doi.org/10.1007/978-981-99-0035-0_21

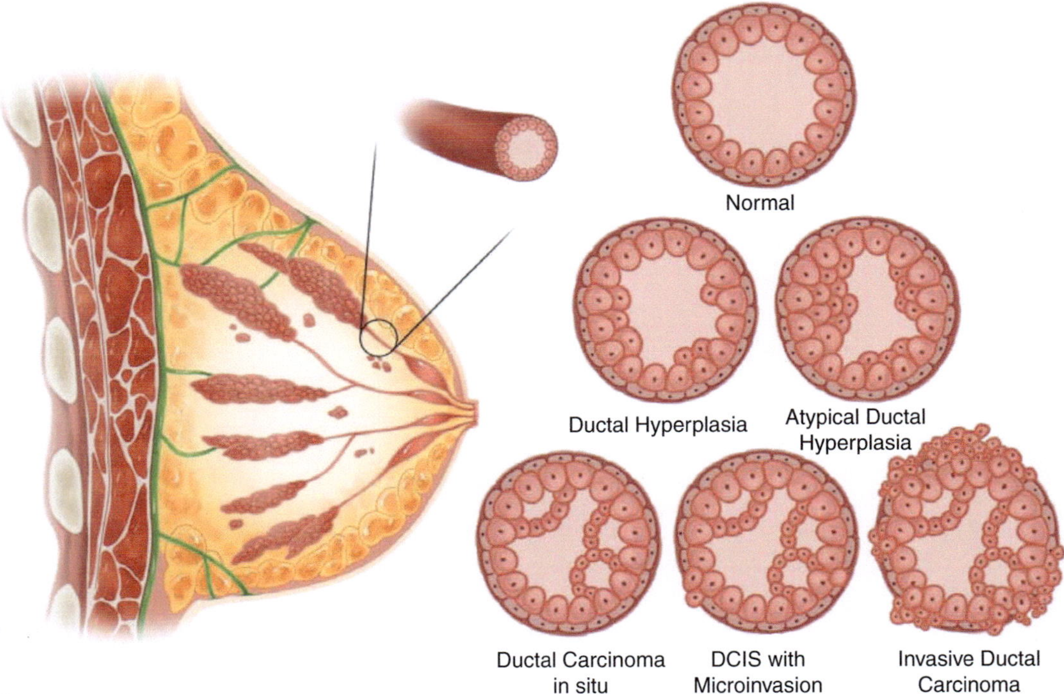

Fig. 21.1 Diagrammatic representation of DCIS

21.1.2 Clinical Presentation

The term DCIS was unheard of prior to breast screening era. DCIS is most often clinically occult, primarily diagnosed on imaging. Sometimes, a patient with DCIS may present as palpable lump or nipple discharge.

The relative risk for invasive carcinoma in patients with DCIS is 8–10 times compared to general population.

21.1.3 Radiology

X-ray mammogram—The hallmark of DCIS on mammograms is microcalcifications, but a low-grade DCIS, without necrosis, is less likely to present with microcalcifications. Majority of DCIS, around 75%, is present in varying forms of calcification on mammogram. Twenty three percent of DCIS may present as mass or asymmetry and approximately 12% are associated with palpable abnormality [1]. The reported sensitivity of mammography for detection of DCIS is 87–95%.

Three main patterns of calcifications are recognized with DCIS on mammogram:

1. Fine linear branching calcifications: These are also known as casting type of calcifications (as coined by Dr.Tabar), appear as V or Y shapes, and are highly suspicious of high-grade carcinoma (Fig. 21.2). It is important to differentiate the casting type fine linear branching calcifications from secretory calcifications. Secretory calcifications as seen in plasma cell mastitis are commonly bilateral and extensive. They appear smooth, linear, and rod shaped, pointing toward the nipple.
2. Irregular fine pleomorphic calcifications: These originate in TDLU and hence usually present in closely spaced groups formed either due to necrosis of the cells or secretory process. These have been described as crushed stone appearance by Dr. Tabar as they vary in their shape size and density. Segmental distribution of pleomorphic calcifications is highly suspicious of DCIS (Fig. 21.3). These can also be seen in early stage of involution of

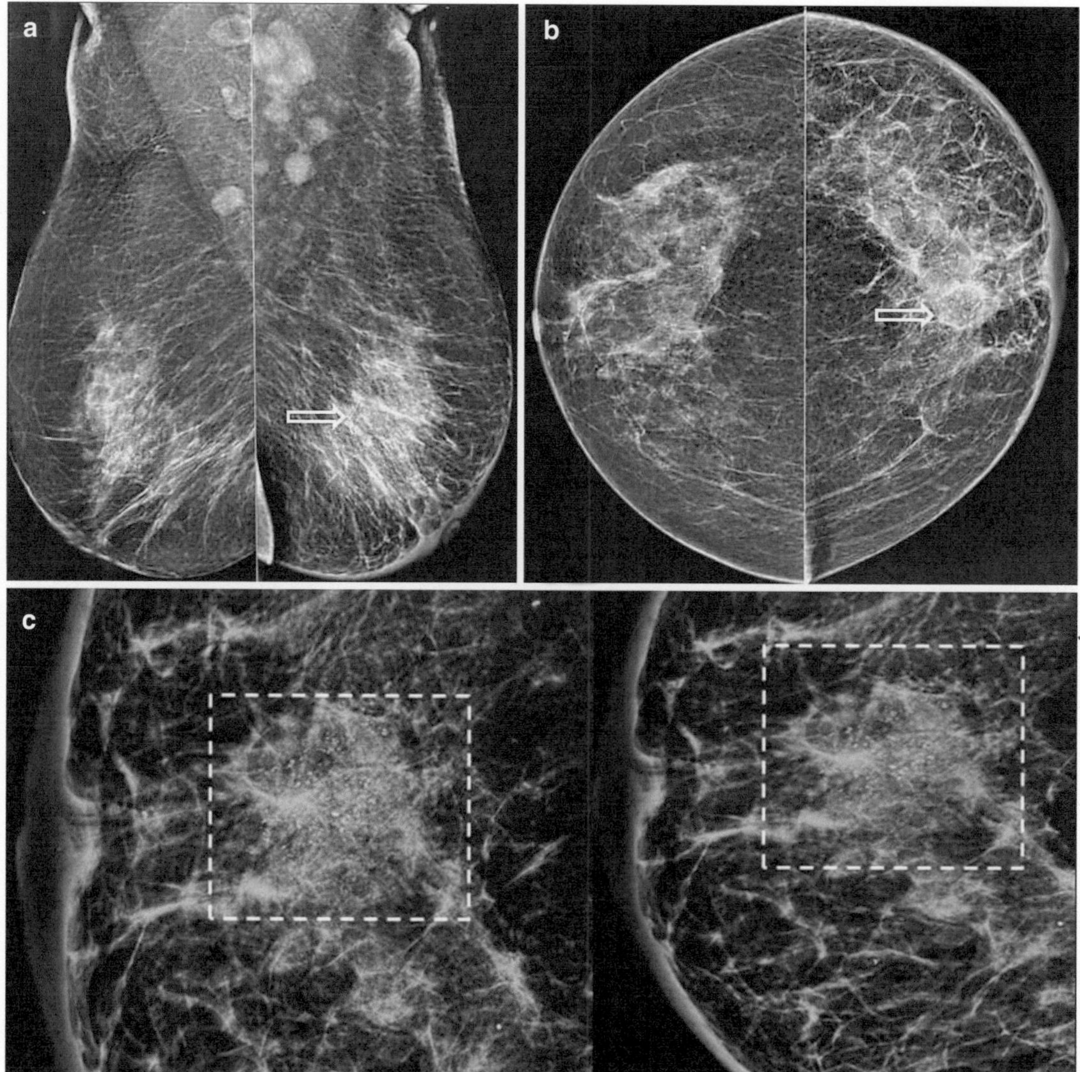

Fig 21.2 (**a**, **b**) MLO and CC views of both breasts, left breast showing fine linear branching type and pleomorphic calcifications in central quadrant of left breast. (**c**) Zoomed image of the CC view of left breast showing fine linear branching and pleomorphic calcifications—highly suspicious for malignancy

fibroadenomas and fibrocystic diseases. All grouped pleomorphic calcifications should be biopsied or put on 6-months short-term follow-up by X-ray mammogram at least for 18 months, if thought to be due to benign disease.

3. Indistinct, amorphous calcifications: As the name states these calcifications have no definite shape or form. They usually are very less dense and small in shape, appear hazy (powdered calcifications). Over 60% of these calcifications are found in benign breast diseases like fibrocystic disease and sclerosing adenosis. It is very essential to emphasize on the distribution and interval changes in the amorphous calcifications—grouped or segmental distribution of amorphous calcifications and interval changes in these calcifications are considered suspicious for malignancy and a biopsy is warranted.

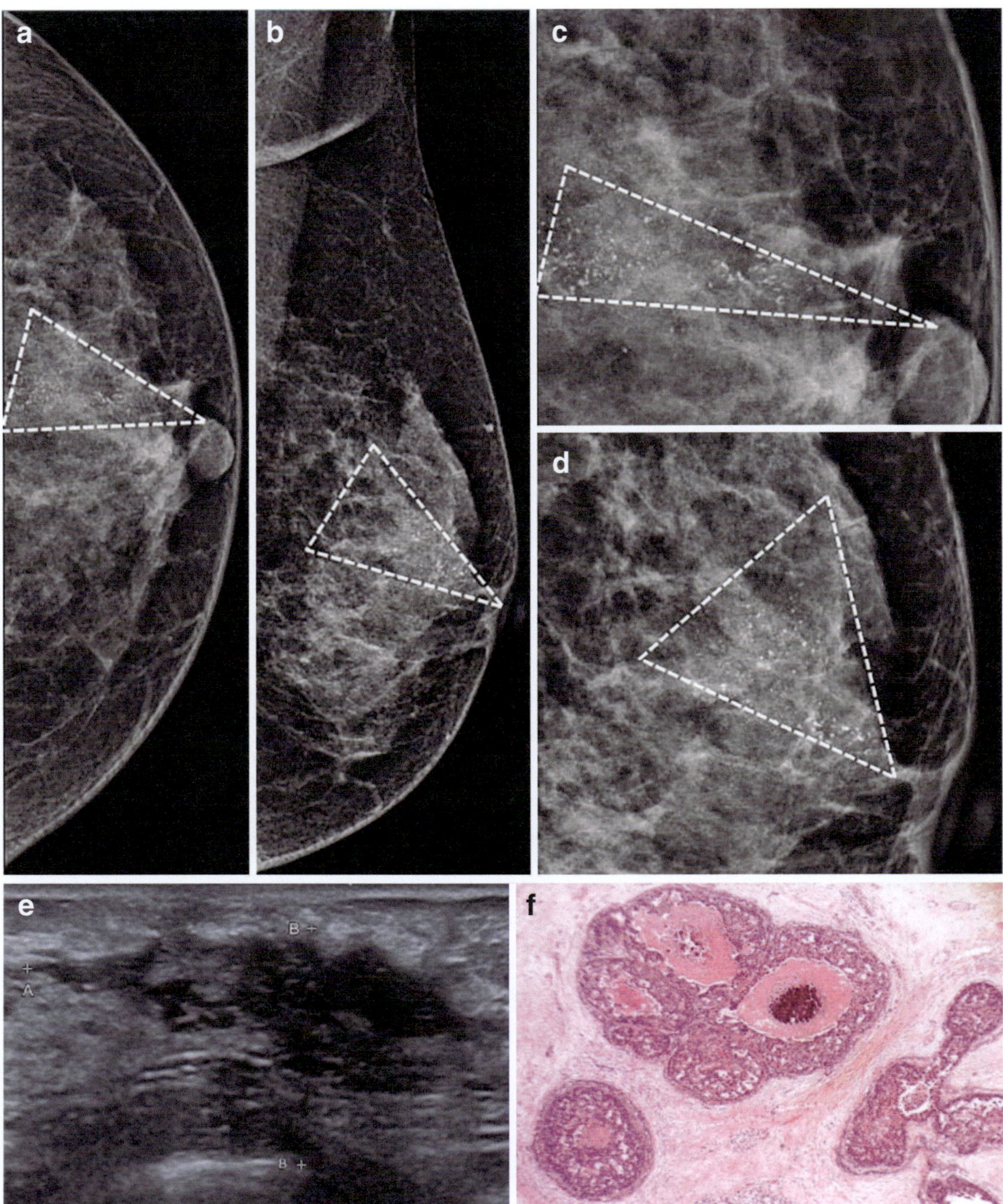

Fig. 21.3 (**a**, **b**) MLO and CC views of left breast showing pleomorphic calcifications in segmental distribution in upper outer quadrant pointing toward the nipple. (**c**, **d**) Zoomed images of the MLO and CC views depicting the same. (**e**) USG images showing irregular heterogenous parenchyma, area corresponding to the segmental distribution of pleomorphic calcifications on mammogram. (**f**) H&E stain shows high-grade DCIS with central comedo necrosis.

21.1.4 DCIS as Mass

In approximately 22–23% of the cases with DCIS, mass-like appearance or architectural distortion can be seen on mammogram, which is either a manifestation of existing soft tissue mass or it may be the result of periductal fibrosis producing irregular or spiculated margins around the nonmass lesion.

Low-grade DCIS without necrosis, usually are noncalcified in comparison to intermediate- or high-grade DCIS.

Ultrasound: It is usually considered to be an adjunct to screening mammogram in patients with incidentally detected DCIS. Breast ultrasound is superior to mammogram in detecting masses in patients with symptomatic DCIS [2].

Ultrasound is mainly helpful in detecting the solid invasive component of DCIS. The extent of the lesion is better appreciated on ultrasound as compared to mammogram (Fig. 21.3). The diseased area may show increased blood flow on color Doppler.

Calcifications on ultrasound are seen as echogenic foci either along the ducts, within the ducts, or in the mass. Microcalcifications, which are not associated with mass lesion, are usually associated with poor prognostic factors like high nuclear grade, comedo-necrosis, HER2 positivity, and an increased Ki-67 index [3]. In comparison to the benign calcifications seen in fibrocystic changes and sclersosing adenosis, the malignant calcifications of DCIS are visualized more easily on ultrasound.

21.1.5 MRI

MR imaging has the highest sensitivity in the detection of noncalcifying DCIS among all imaging studies and has higher accuracy in determining the extent of the disease [4].

Nonmass enhancement in form of clumped or cobblestone enhancement in segmental or ductal distribution is a hallmark of pure DCIS [4, 5] (Fig. 21.4). Most common MR imaging finding of DCIS is nonmass enhancement and is seen in 60–80% of cases. An enhancing mass on MRI can be seen in 14–34% of cases with DCIS. The least common finding is focal enhancement and seen only in 1–12% of cases [5–8].

There is no confirmed pathognomonic enhancement kinetic pattern on dynamic MR breast study for DCIS. Enhancement patterns are very variable especially in the delayed phase. In 49–68% of cases, initial phase is fast uptake, the delayed phase is more variable, with a plateau curve being the most common pattern, followed by washout and persistent enhancement [5–8].

Interventions: If the mass or the calcifications are seen on ultrasound, ultrasound-guided core biopsy or vacuum-assisted biopsy is performed. If calcifications are seen only on mammogram, stereotactic/tomosynthesis vac-

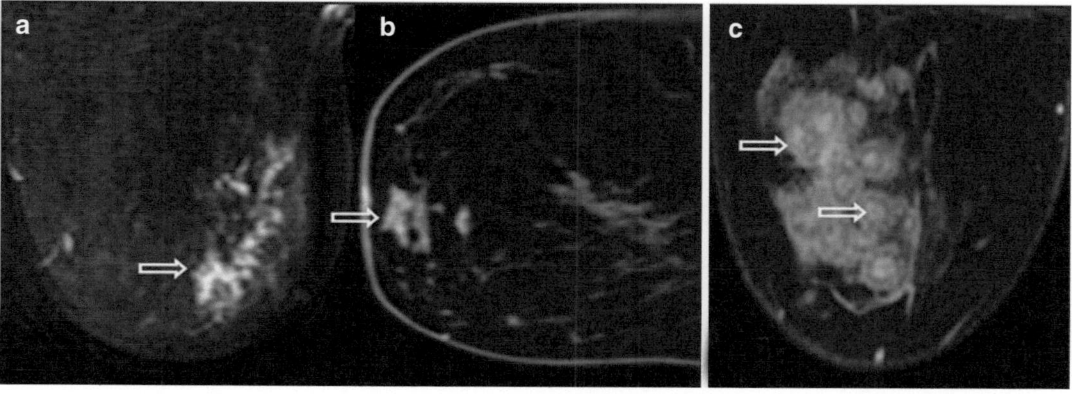

Fig. 21.4 MRI images in three different patients showing (**a**) clumped linear segmental nonmass enhancement (**b**) clumped and focal nonmass enhancement in retroareolar region (**c**) extensive clustered ring nonmass enhancement (highly suspicious of malignancy—91% of cases) involving both outer & central quadrant

uum-assisted biopsy is recommended. It is very important to confirm the calcifications in the sample obtained, by X-raying the sample before the patient is sent back. Sometimes, vacuum-assisted excision can be done for entire calcifications, in such cases, it is essential to leave a marker clip in order to localize the area of DCIS if the surgery is required later.

21.1.6 Pathology

Gross features Usually, DCIS shows no gross lesion, but rarely, high-grade DCIS may present as firm gritty mass with central area showing pale comedonecrosis (Fig. 21.5). Serial sequential sampling with mammographic correlation is useful to estimate the size of DCIS.

All suspected areas of DCIS must be carefully examined to exclude small foci of invasive carcinoma.

Microscopic appearance:

The Van Nuys classification system for DCIS is based primarily on the histologic nuclear grade and the presence of necrosis and is the simplest, most reproducible system for the histopathologic classification of DCIS into three groups.

Low-grade DCIS: shows round, regular to mildly irregular nuclei up to 2–3 times the size of a Red Blood Cell (RBC). Mitosis is infrequent in this category and comedo necrosis is absent.

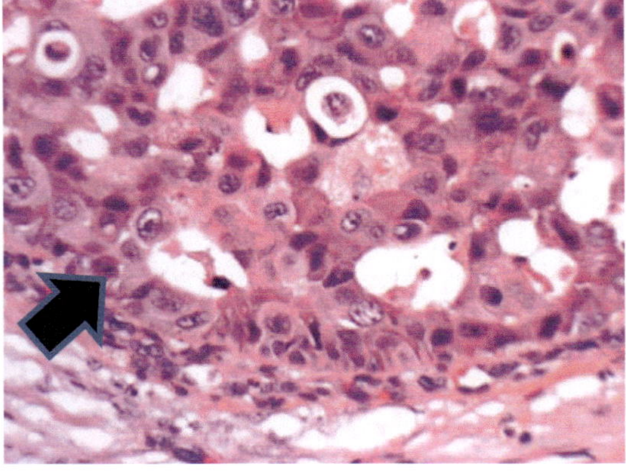

Fig. 21.5 The periphery of the ducts showing myoepithelial cells

Intermediate-grade DCIS: shows round, regular to mildly irregular nuclei up to 2–3 times the size of an RBC with presence of comedo necrosis.

High-grade DCIS: show highly pleomorphic nuclei greater than three times the size of RBC. Marked comedo necrosis usually present, hence is often diagnosed on mammogram as one of the pattern of DCIS calcifications.

When a lesion is in between low and high grade, they are usually graded as intermediate grade. It is essential to remember when different grades are found within the same lesion, the highest grade should be reported.

DCIS also shows several architectural patterns such as papillary, solid, cribriform, comedo and micropapillary. Roman bridges comprised of curvilinear trabecular bars connecting two portions of the epithelial lining is a classic feature of DCIS. Cells are comprised of rigid rows of cells with long axes perpendicular to the long axis of the bar.

According to the College of American Pathologists recommendations, necrosis should be reported as not present or present and, if present, must be differentiated as focal or comedo type. The pattern of myoepithelial expression helps in recognizing DCIS. Myoepithelial cell layer is usually intact in ducts with DCIS, but may be attenuated in some cases of high-grade DCIS. Presence of myoepithelial cells may be demonstrated by performing immunohistochemistry for myoepithelial markers like p63, p40, and calponin.

DCIS cannot be differentiated from invasive carcinoma by Fine Needle Aspiration Cytology (FNAC) and therefore, core needle biopsy is preferred to FNAC.

21.1.7 Treatment

Mammogram and core needle biopsy should be done to confirm the diagnosis. The main concern in the management of DCIS is to prevent the progression to invasive breast cancer. The treatment of DCIS depends on the size of the tumor. For nonpalpable masses, ultrasound-guided wire localization and wide local excision with 1 cm margin is done. After wide local excision, specimen mammogram is done to confirm the complete excision of the lesion. For breast lump less than 4 cm, breast conservation surgery with 1 cm margin is done and the margins are sent for frozen section to confirm negative margins. Axillary dissection is done if sentinel node biopsy is positive. This is followed by whole breast irradiation for high-risk patients. Hormone therapy is indicated for receptor positive patients. For tumors more than 4 cm, modified radical mastectomy is indicated. There is no role for chemotherapy, Hormone therapy is indicated in receptor positive patients [9, 10].

21.2 Premalignant Lesions: LCIS

21.2.1 Introduction

LCIS is a part of the spectrum of lobular intraepithelial neoplasms [11]. It is multicentric in 60–80% [12] patients and bilateral in 30–40% cases, and occurs predominantly in the premenopausal women [13]. LCIS is usually asymptomatic and are occult on imaging. These tumors are incidentally detected on histopathological examination [14]. Lobular carcinoma in situ is divided into two types, namely, classical and nonclassical types—pleomorphic and florid [15].

Imaging: Diagnosis of classic LCIS is usually an incidental finding in a breast biopsy performed for other indications, including screen detected calcifications or mass producing lesions. No specific features on imaging have been described for LCIS. However it can present in different forms on different imaging modalities.

Mammogram: LCIS usually presents as subtle focal asymmetry. LCIS may be associated with sclerosing adenosis, which presents as calcification, architectural distortion, or ill-defined mass [16]. Pleomorphic LCIS is a variant, which has necrosis and calcification due to its avid growth. Pleomorphic LCIS and LCIS with central necrosis presents as grouped pleomorphic or amorphous calcification or a mass with or without calcification on mammogram [17, 18].

Ultrasound: LCIS might mimic invasive mammary carcinoma presenting as an irregular mass lesion with indistinct margins [14]. They may present as solitary round or oval mass with smooth borders and are categorized as BI-RADS 4A. No posterior features are seen, which helps to distinguish them from other invasive carcinomas [19].

MRI: MRI features of LCIS tend to be more subtle than DCIS and other invasive cancers. LCIS tend to be multicentric and multifocal and are usually bilateral for which MRI is the most sensitive modality [20]. LCIS mostly presents as nonmass enhancement with heterogenous internal enhancement but sometimes a mass with irregular margins and homogenous internal enhancement. These lesions tend to display type 2 or type 3 kinetic curve on DCE images [16]. Associated sclerosing adenosis may be seen as a spiculated mass-like lesion.

Histopathology: Classically LCIS shows predominantly lobulocentric proliferation of monomorphic cells, which expands the acini (>50%) in the terminal duct lobular units. The lobules are distended and completely filled with neoplastic cells (Fig. 21.6a). Cells are uniform, round, small- to medium-sized neoplastic epithelial cells with lack of cohesiveness. The small central nucleus has a smooth nuclear membrane and inconspicuous nucleoli. Occasionally, intracytoplasmic vacuoles may be seen, mimicking signet ring cells. Necrosis, pleomorphism, and mitosis are minimal or absent.

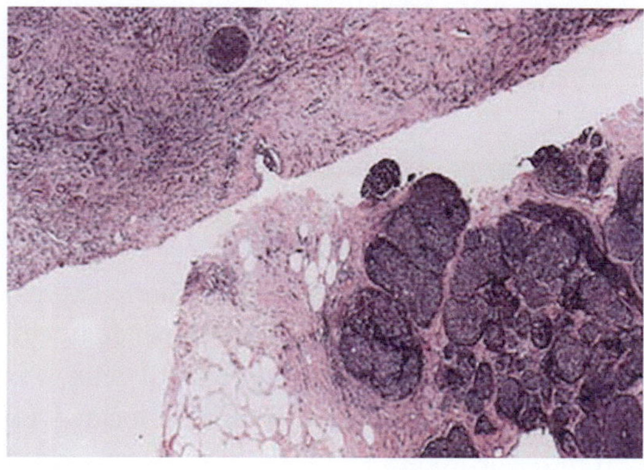

Fig. 21.6 H&E stain shows LCIS with distended lobules filled with neoplastic cells (lower right corner)

Usually, the cells are small cells, with scant cytoplasm (Type A cells). Larger cells with more cytoplasm are the Type B cells. These larger cells have bigger nuclei and more prominent nucleoli. Sometimes, cells can grow underneath the ductal epithelium from lobules into the terminal ducts—pagetoid extension. A characteristic "cloverleaf" pattern is seen on cross-section of a duct with pagetoid involvement by LCIS [15]. If the proliferative lesion is involving less than 50% of the acini of the TDLU, it is called Atypical Lobular Hyperplasia (ALH). The morphology and microscopy of ALH is similar to LCIS.

LCIS can show other architectural patterns nonclassical types: pleomorphic LCIS and florid LCIS.

Pleomorphic LCIS: This variant shows cells with marked nuclear pleomorphism and prominent nucleoli. This variant is usually seen in association with Pleomorphic-Invasive Lobular Carcinoma. However, isolated P-LCIS can also be seen. The cells in P-LCIS are larger cells with round to ovoid shape, abundant cytoplasm, and larger hyperchromatic nuclei, with prominent nucleoli. Mitotic activity is also evident in this variant of LCIS. Sometimes, there is the presence of central necrosis and calcification also. Based on the abundance of cytoplasm, they may be classified into apocrine and nonapocrine types. The solid growth pattern may be seen in some cases, which may mimic a DCIS. However, the cells of LCIS are dyshesive, lack two cell polarity, and do not form secondary lumina.

Florid LCIS: In this type, there is a massive expansion of the acini with neoplastic cells, which fill and expand the ducts in solid pattern. Comedo necrosis may be present.

21.2.2 Immunohistochemistry

21.2.2.1 E-Cadherin

LCIS and ILC show a loss of E cadherin expression. E cadherin is a calcium-dependent cell adhesion glycoprotein in the epithelial cells. It is encoded by CDH1 gene, which is located on chromosome 16q22.1 [21] LCIS is characterized by the complete loss or aberrant expression of E cadherin protein.

21.2.2.2 p120

This is a tyrosine kinase substrate, which interacts with E cadherin, which is important for Cadherin-mediated cell–cell adhesion. Cadherins are important to recruit p120 to the cell membrane. In absence of cadherin, there is increased cytoplasmic expression of p120 in all stages of lobular neoplasia. However, only a reduced membrane expression can be seen in ductal carcinoma.

21.2.2.3 ER, PR, Her 2Neu

Classic LCIS is usually positive for ER, PR and negative for Her 2 neu [22].

21.2.3 Management

LCIS represents both a risk factor and a nonobligate precursor of breast cancer. Classical LCIS confirmed on core needle biopsy, which is concordant on imaging and histopathology does not warrant surgical excision. Observation, active surveillance, and chemoprevention with tamoxifen or aromatase inhibitors is recommended in such cases [15]. The National Comprehensive Cancer Network (NCCN) guidelines recommend follow-up of patients with physical examinations every 6–12 months and annual diagnostic mammograms [23]. Variant or nonclassical LCIS diagnosed on needle core biopsy requires surgical excision [15].

References

1. Barreau B, de Mascarel I, Feuga C, et al. Mammography of ductal carcinoma in situ of the breast: review of 909 cases with radiographic–pathologic correlations. Eur J Radiol. 2005;54:55–61.
2. Scoggins ME, Fox PS, Kuerer HM, Rauch GM, Benveniste AP, Park YM, et al. Correlation between sonographic findings and clinicopathologic and biologic features of pure ductal carcinoma in situ in 691 patients. AJR Am J Roentgenol. 2015;204:878–88.
3. Cha H, Chang YW, Lee EJ, Hwang JY, Kim HJ, Lee EH, et al. Ultrasonographic features of pure ductal carcinoma in situ of the breast: correlations with pathologic features and biological markers. Ultrasonography. 2018;37(4):307–14.

4. Greenwood HI, Heller SL, Kim S, Sigmund EE, Shaylor SD, Moy L. Ductal carcinoma in situ of the breasts: review of MR imaging features. RadioGraphics. 2013;33:1569–88.
5. Jansen SA, Newstead GM, Abe H, Shimauchi A, Schmidt RA, Karczmar GS. Pure ductal carcinoma in situ: kinetic and morphologic MR characteristics compared with mammographic appearance and nuclear grade. Radiology. 2007;245(3):684–91.
6. Rosen EL, Smith-Foley SA, DeMartini WB, Eby PR, Peacock S, Lehman CD. BI-RADS MRI enhancement characteristics of ductal carcinoma in situ. Breast J. 2007;13(6):545–50.
7. Menell JH, Morris EA, Dershaw DD, Abramson AF, Brogi E, Liberman L. Determination of the presence and extent of pure ductal carcinoma in situ by mammography and magnetic resonance imaging. Breast J. 2005;11(6):382–90.
8. Vag T, Baltzer PA, Dietzel M, et al. Kinetic characteristics of ductal carcinoma in situ (DCIS) in dynamic breast MRI using computer-assisted analysis. Acta Radiol. 2010;51(9):955–61.
9. Wen HY, Brogi E. Lobular carcinoma in situ. Surg Pathol Clin. 2018;11(1):123–45. https://doi.org/10.1016/j.path.2017.09.009. Epub 2017 Dec 8.
10. Hanna WM, Parra-Herran C, Lu FI, Slodkowska E, Rakovitch E, Nofech-Mozes S. Ductal carcinoma in situ of the breast: an update for the pathologist in the era of individualized risk assessment and tailored therapies. Mod Pathol. 2019;32(7):896–915. https://doi.org/10.1038/s41379-019-0204-1. Epub 2019 Feb 13.
11. Jorns J, Sabel MS, Pang JC. Lobular neoplasia: morphology and management. Arch Pathol Lab Med. 2014;138(10):1344–9.
12. Powers RW, O'Brien PH, Kreutner A Jr. Lobular carcinoma in situ. J Surg Oncol. 1980;13:269–73.
13. Beute BJ, Kalisher L, Hutter RV. Lobular carcinoma in situ of the breast: clinical, pathologic, and mammographic features. AJR Am J Roentgenol. 1991;157:257–65.
14. Chaudhary S, Lawrence L, McGinty G, Kostroff K, Bhuiya T. Classic lobular neoplasia on core biopsy: a clinical and radio-pathologic correlation study with follow-up excision biopsy. Mod Pathol. 2013;26(6):762–71.
15. Wen HY, Brogi E. Lobular carcinoma in situ. Surg Pathol Clin. 2018;11(1):123–45.
16. Hande PC, Arneja SK, Desai SS. Imaging Spectrum of lobular carcinoma in situ and correlation with pathology findings. Indian J Radiol Imaging. 2021;31(3):551–9.
17. Stein LF, Zisman G, Rapelyea JA, Schwartz AM, Abell B, Brem RF. Lobular carcinoma in situ of the breast presenting as a mass. AJR Am J Roentgenol. 2005;184(6):1799–801.
18. Christiano JG, Duncan LD, Bell JL. Lobular carcinoma in situ of the breast presenting as a discrete mass. Am Surg. 2012;78(1):E38–40.
19. Choi BB, Kim SH, Park CS, Cha ES, Lee AW. Radiologic findings of lobular carcinoma in situ: mammography and ultrasonography. J Clin Ultrasound JCU. 2011;39(2):59–63.
20. Chu AJ, Cho N, Park IA, Cho SW. Features of pure lobular carcinoma in situ on magnetic resonance imaging associated with immediate re-excision after lumpectomy. J Breast Cancer. 2016;19(2):199–205.
21. Berx G, Staes K, van Hengel J, et al. Cloning and characterization of the human invasion suppressor gene E-cadherin (CDH1). Genomics. 1995;26:281–9.
22. Fisher ER, Costantino J, Fisher B, et al. Pathologic findings from the National Surgical Adjuvant Breast Project (NSABP) protocol B-17. Five-year observations concerning lobular carcinoma in situ. Cancer. 1996;78:1403–16.
23. National Comprehensive Cancer Network Version 2. 2017. https://www.nccn.org.

Carcinoma Breast

22

Harini Gnanavel, Bhawna Dev, Leena Dennis Joseph, Archana B, V. Pavithra, Sandhya Sundaram, and Ramya Ramakrishnan

Abstract

Breast cancer is the second leading cause of cancer death in women. Screening for breast cancer reduces breast cancer-related mortality, and earlier detection facilitates less aggressive treatment. Invasive breast carcinoma has a wide range of histological appearances. The major histological features that help to further characterize histological subtype are based on architecture, nuclear features and stromal features; Nottingham grading (detailed below); the presence or absence of tumour in the angiolymphatic spaces (only peritumoural lymphovascular invasion is assessed in breast cancer, and this should be differentiated from tissue retraction); and an associated in situ component.

H. Gnanavel (✉) · B. Dev
Department of Radiology, Sri Ramachandra Institute of Higher Education and Research, Chennai, India
e-mail: harini@sriramachandra.edu.in; bhawnadev@sriramachandra.edu.in

L. D. Joseph · A. B · V. Pavithra · S. Sundaram
Department of Pathology, Sri Ramachandra Institute of Higher Education and Research, Chennai, India
e-mail: leenadennisj@sriramachandra.edu.in; archanab@sriramachandra.edu.in; pavithrav@sriramachandra.edu.in

R. Ramakrishnan
Department of Surgery, Sri Ramachandra Institute of Higher Education and Research, Chennai, India
e-mail: ramya.r@sriramachandra.edu.in

Keywords

Breast malignancy · Pathology · Imaging · Treatment

22.1 Introduction

Breast cancer is the second leading cause of cancer death in women, exceeded only by lung cancer and the 5-year survival rate is largely dependent on disease stage. Imaging plays an important role in diagnosing and staging the disease [1].

The imaging findings in breast malignancy have overlapping findings in all suspicious masses requiring histopathological diagnosis for confirmation. Few subtypes like invasive lobular carcinoma and invasive mucinous carcinoma may present with possible unique imaging features.

B. Dev, L. D. Joseph (eds.), *Holistic Approach to Breast Disease*,
https://doi.org/10.1007/978-981-99-0035-0_22

Characteristics of Malignant Lesions on Mammogram [2, 3]

- Shape—irregular, round (Figs. 22.1, 22.2, and 22.3)
- Margins—not circumscribed—obscured, microlobulated, indistinct, spiculated and angulated (Figs. 22.1, 22.4, 22.5, 22.6 and 22.7)
- Calcification:
  - **Morphology**—amorphous, coarse heterogenous, fine pleomorphic, fine linear, fine linear branching type of suspicious calcifications
  - **Distribution**—grouped, linear, segmental
- Architectural distortion
- Asymmetry
- Associated features—skin and nipple retraction
  - Axillary adenopathy

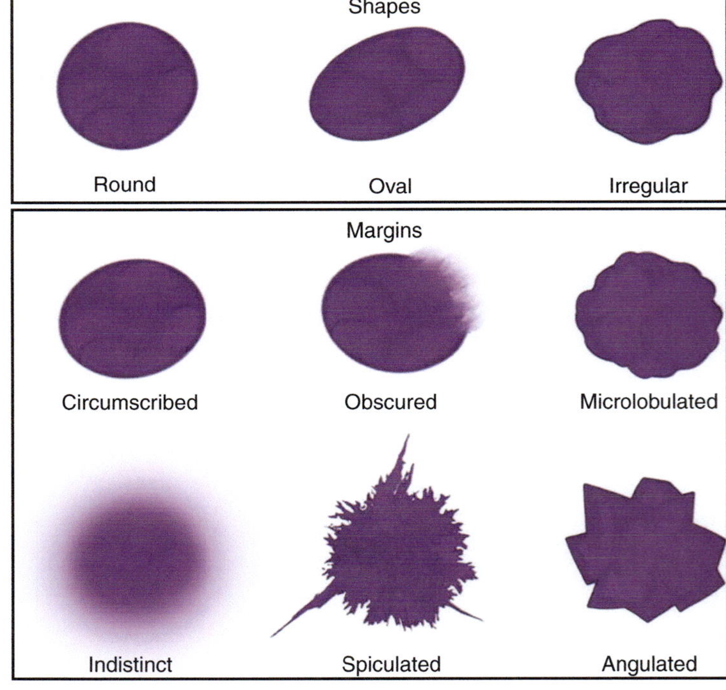

Fig. 22.1 Schematic representation of the various shapes and margins in suspicious mass

Shape:

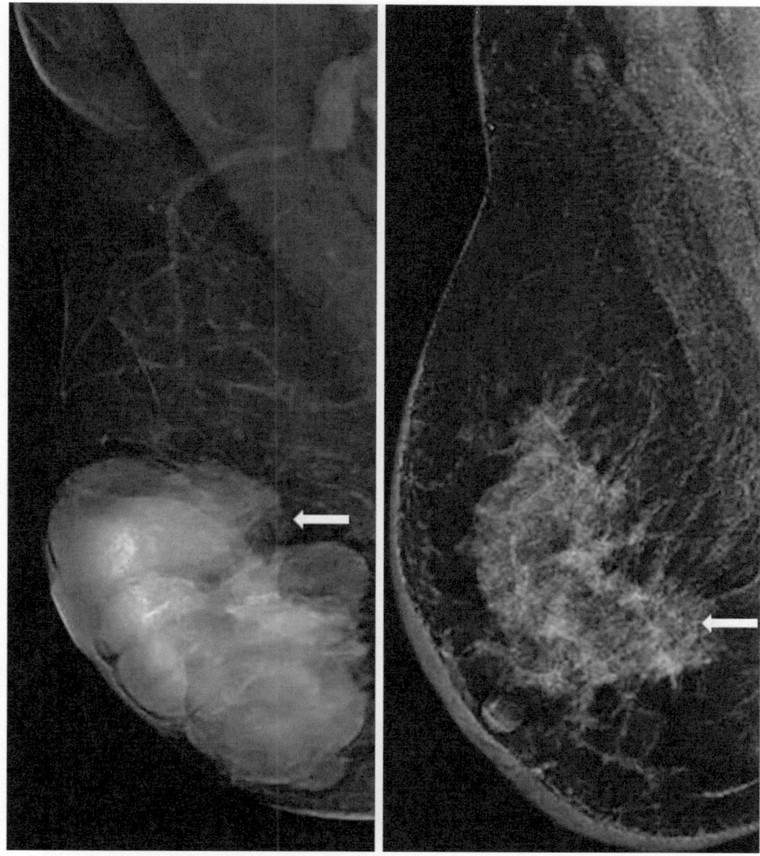

Fig. 22.2 X-ray mammogram mediolateral oblique (MLO) views showing irregular shaped mass in two different patients

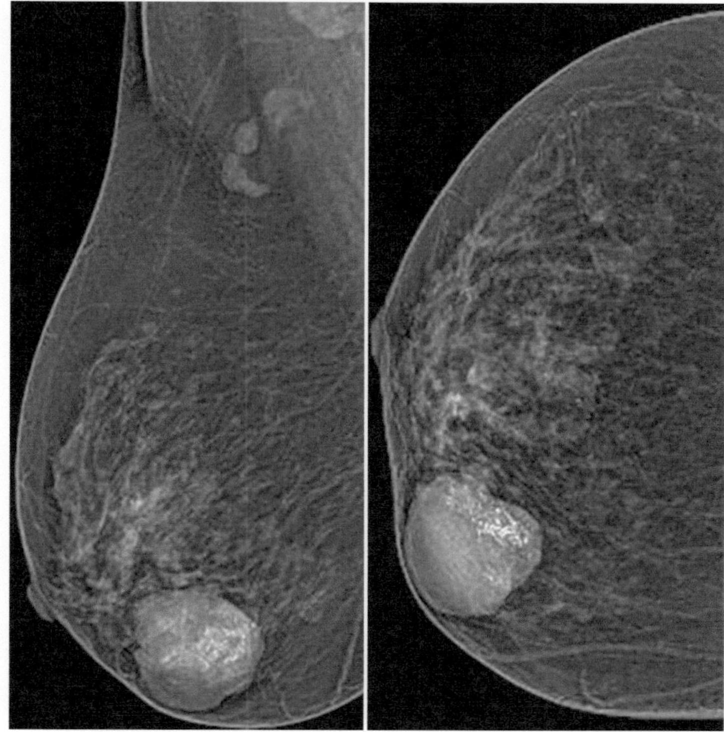

Fig. 22.3 X-ray mammogram showing round shaped mass in both MLO and craniocaudal (CC) views

Margins:

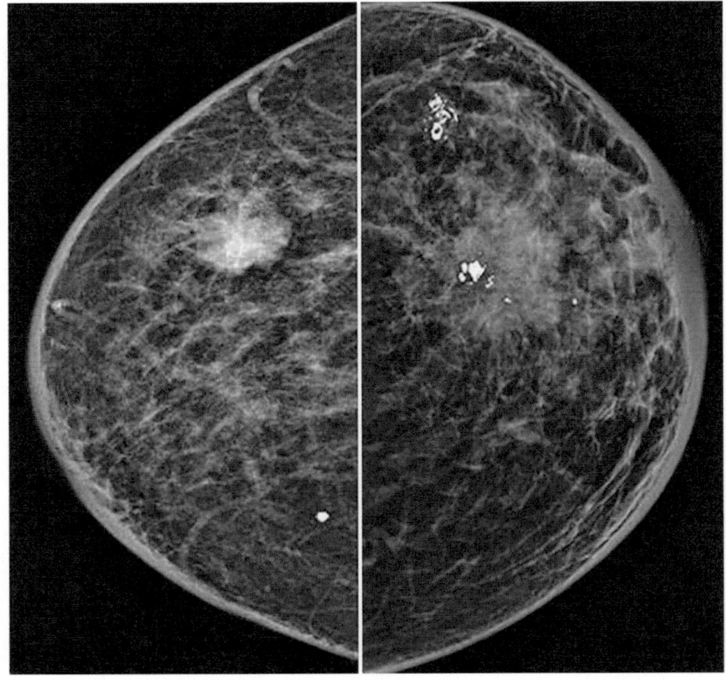

Fig. 22.4 X-ray mammogram of two different patients showing indistinct margins of the mass

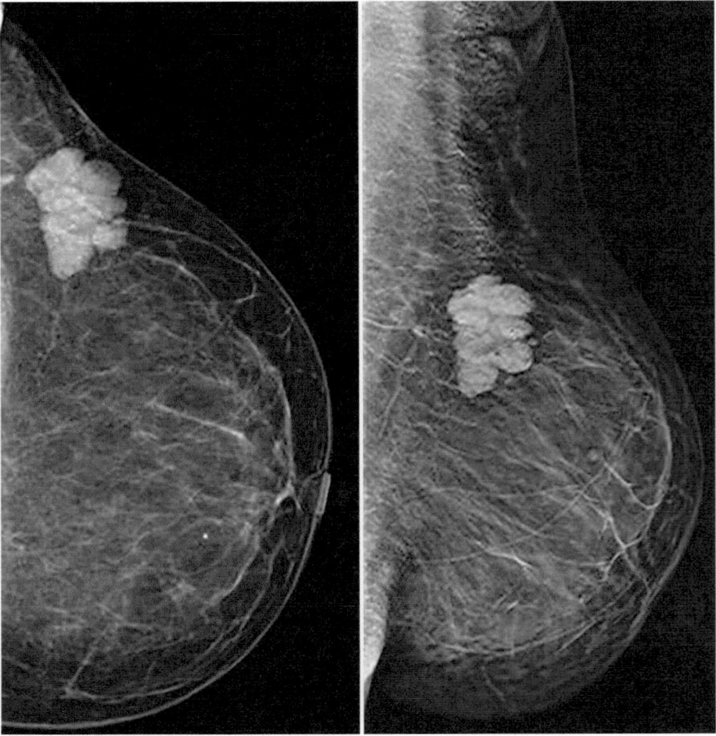

Fig. 22.5 X-ray mammogram showing microlobulated margins of a mass in extended CC and MLO views

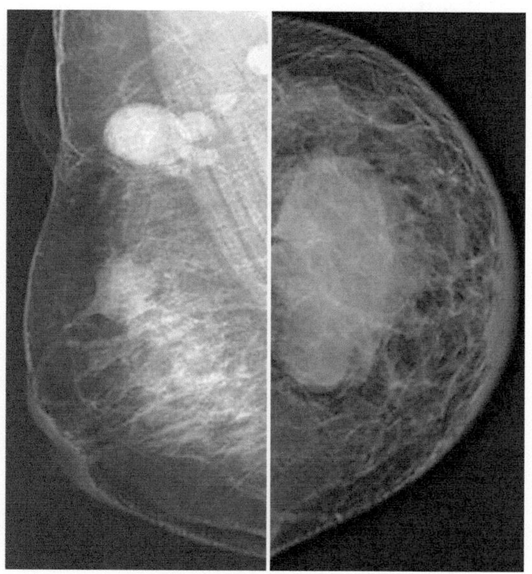

Fig. 22.6 X-ray mammogram showing partially obscured margins of the mass in two different patients

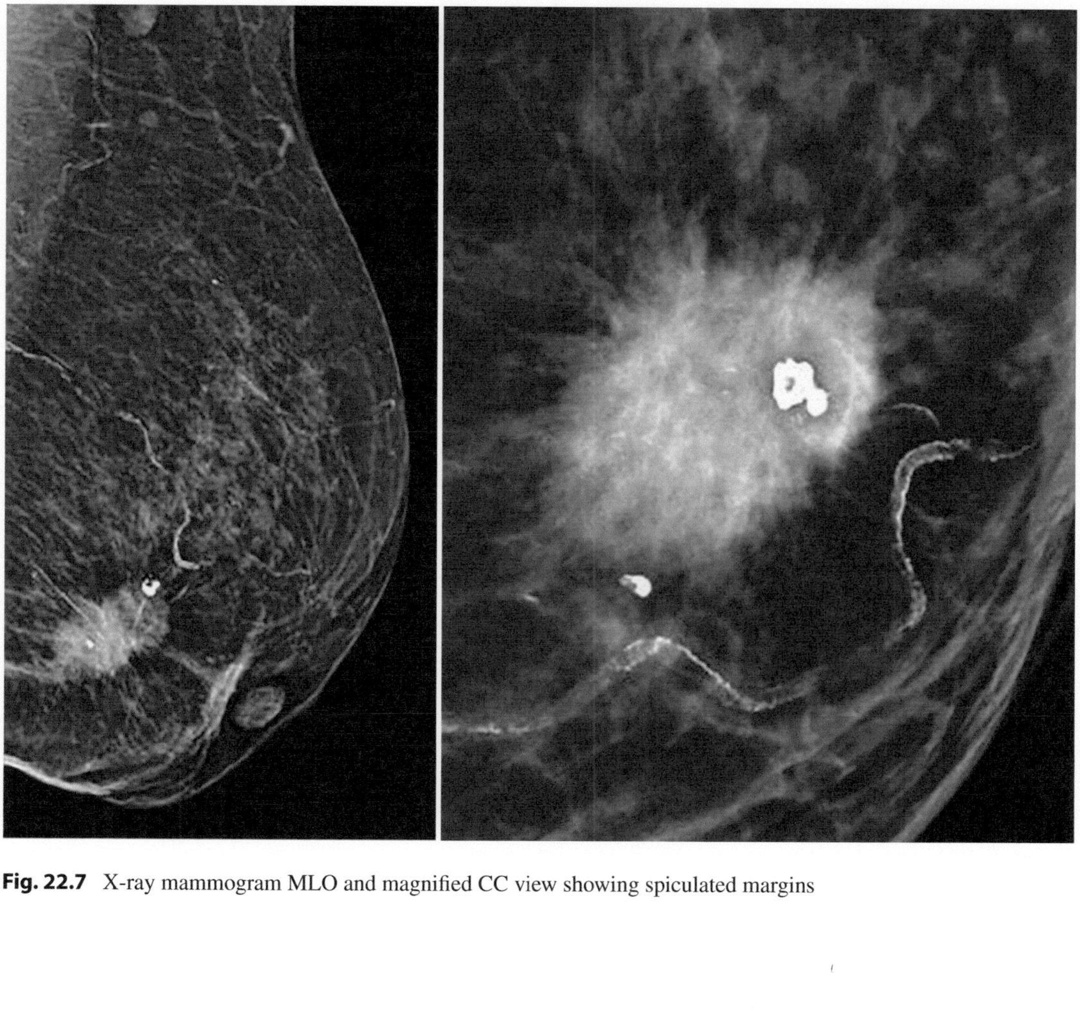

Fig. 22.7 X-ray mammogram MLO and magnified CC view showing spiculated margins

Characteristics of Malignant Lesions on Ultrasound [2, 4]

- Shape–irregular (Figs. 22.8 and 22.9)
- Margins–non-circumscribed (indistinct, angular, microlobulated, spiculated) (Figs. 22.10, 22.11, 22.12 and 22.13)
- Echoes–hypoechoic with ill-defined margins, heterogeneous, complex solid and cystic (Fig. 22.14)
- Calcification–microcalcification, intraductal
- Orientation–taller than wide (non-parallel)
- Posterior features–posterior acoustic shadowing
- Elasticity-hard
- Colour Doppler–significant vascularity within the mass (non-specific)
- Associated features
  - Axillary adenopathy with lost fatty hilum
  - Architectural distortion
  - Skin retraction
  - Skin thickening, edema

Shape:

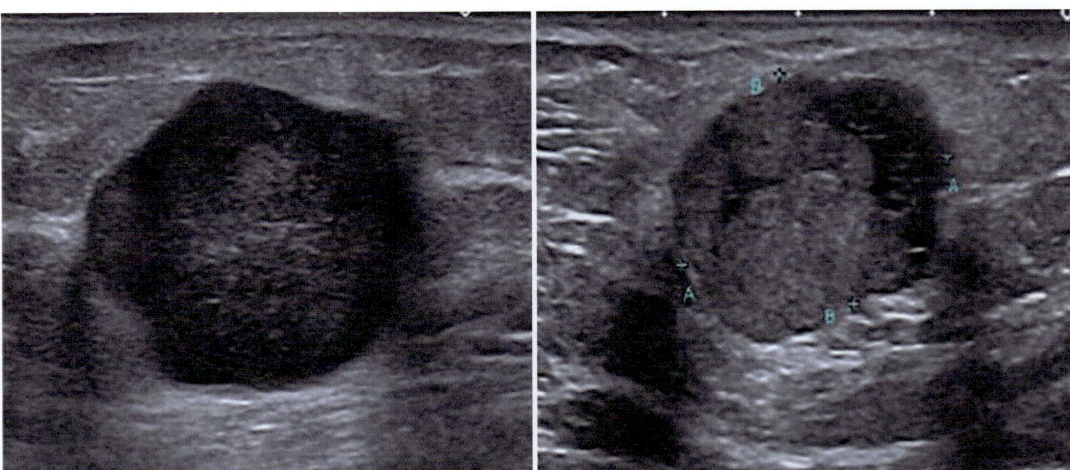

Fig. 22.8 Ultrasound showing round shape mass with multiple soft lobulations in two different patients

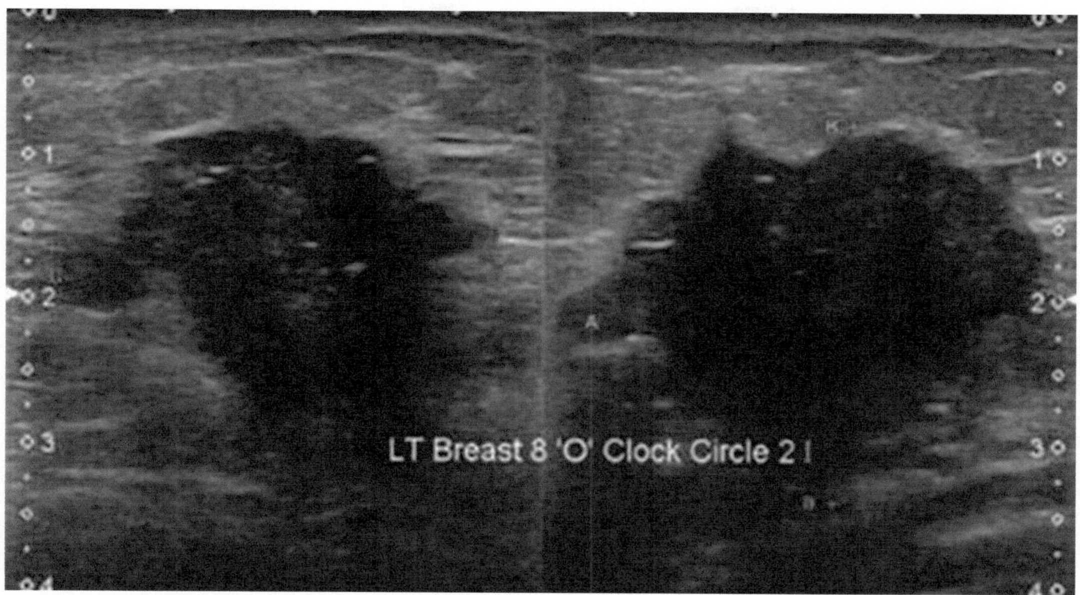

Fig. 22.9 Ultrasound showing irregular-shaped mass

Margins:

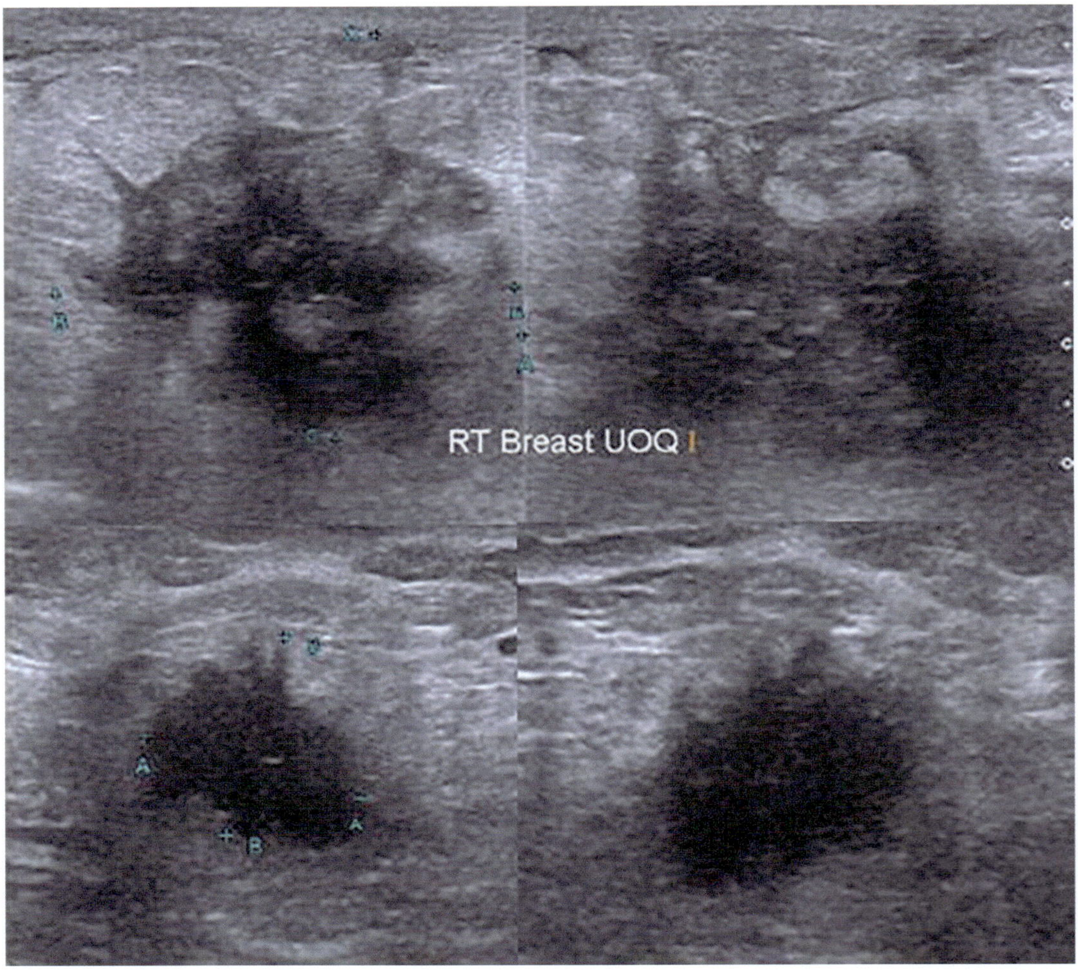

Fig. 22.10 Ultrasound showing mass with non-circumscribed, angular margins in different patients

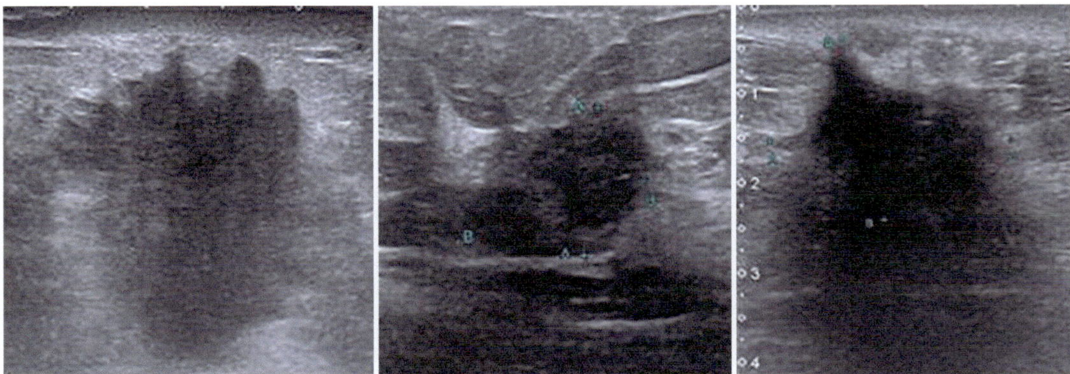

Fig. 22.11 Ultrasound depicting non-circumscribed, indistinct margins of mass in different patients

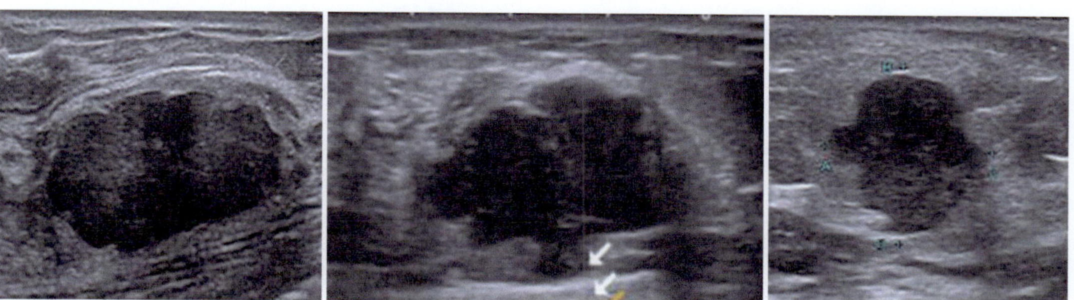

Fig. 22.12 Ultrasound showing non-circumscribed, microlobulated margins of mass in different patients

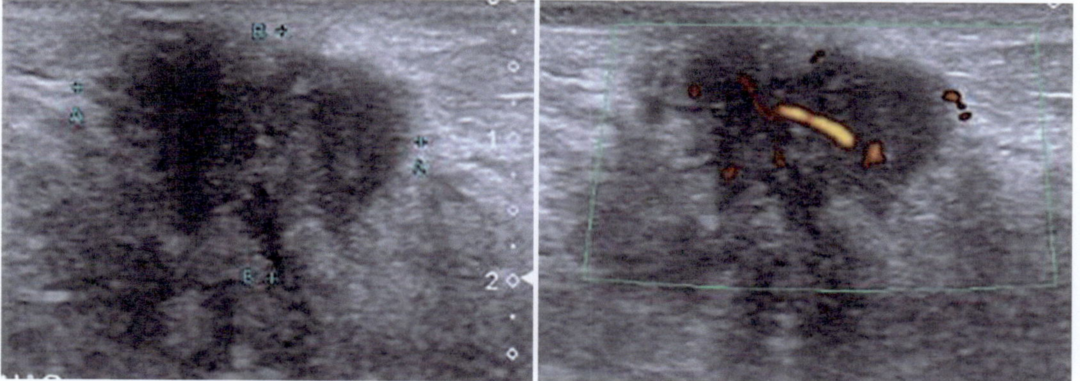

Fig. 22.13 Ultrasound showing non-circumscribed, spiculated margins of mass with increased vascularity

Echo pattern:

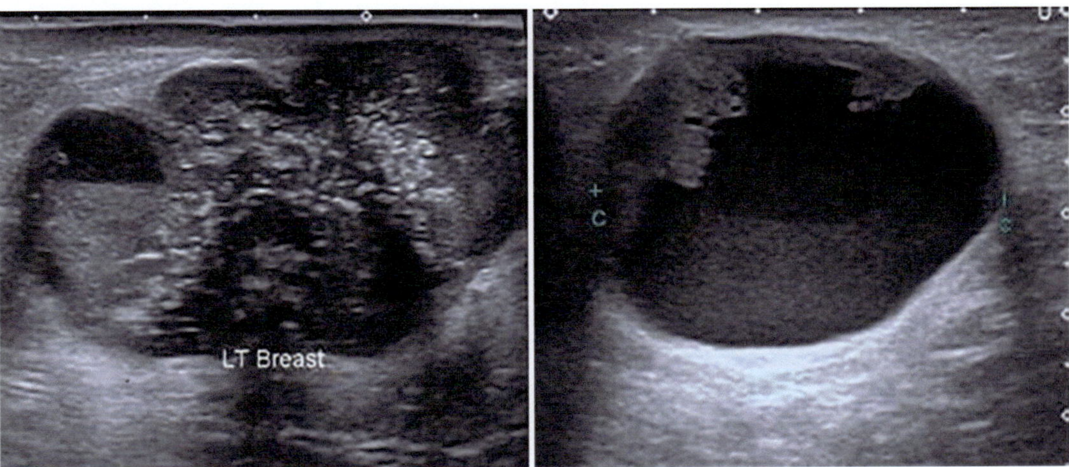

Fig. 22.14 USG showing solid cystic appearance of a mass in two different patients

Characteristics of Malignant Masses on Magnetic Resonance Imaging (MRI) [2]

- Shape—irregular.
- Margin—not circumscribed (irregular, spiculated).
- Enhancement pattern—rim enhancement, more suspicious if there is centripetal filling, heterogenous enhancement or enhancing internal septa
- Non mass enhancement—linear or segmental distribution
  - clumped or clustered ring pattern of internal enhancement.
- Kinetic curve—Type II and Type III kinetic curve/initial phase shows rapid uptake.
- Restricted diffusion with low apparent diffusion coefficient (ADC).
- Associated findings
  - Skin retraction, thickening, invasion
  - Nipple retraction, invasion
  - Axillary adenopathy
  - Pectoralis muscle, chest wall invasion
  - Architectural distortion

Note
Dynamic contrast enhanced MRI is part of the routine protocol in MRI Breast.

Below are the few differentiating points of various subtypes of carcinoma. Though these are common presentations of each subtype, they do not present always with the same features. Hence, imaging is not the modality to confirm the subtype, and histopathology remains gold standard.

22.2 Invasive Ductal Carcinoma (IDC)

- Usually presents as a palpable lump.
- Commonest age at presentation is 50–60 years.
- Presence of reversal/lack of diastolic flow is indicative of histologically high-grade IDC.

22.2.1 Pathogenesis

22.2.1.1 Molecular Aspects [5]

Estrogen Receptor positive (ER+) pathway can be characterised by gains of 1q, loss of 16q and may be amplification of 17q12. ER- pathway can be characterised by loss of 13q, gain of 11q13, amplification of 17q12. and are common with increased expression of genes associated with cell proliferation and are seen in many basal-like tumours. HER2 gene amplification is seen approximately in 15% of the cases. Gene expression profiling stratifies breast cancers into several intrinsic molecular subtypes (e.g. luminal A, luminal B, HER2 enriched, basal-like, etc.). Five to ten percent of breast cancers are hereditary as a result of mutations in various genes, such as BRCA1, BRCA2, TP53, STK11, CD1, PTEN, MDM2, RB and CHEK2. PI3KCA and ESR1 mutations are associated with resistance to endocrine therapy.

22.2.1.2 Imaging Findings

Ultrasound—narrow zone of transition, presence of suspicious calcifications located intraductally and within the mass are shown to have a mild to moderate association with histologically high grades of IDC [6].

MRI—usually present as irregularly shaped, spiculated mass, with rim or heterogeneous enhancement. These lesions often display Type-II or Type-III washout curves [7].

22.2.2 Pathology [5]

22.2.2.1 Gross Examination

Most of the invasive breast carcinomas are seen and palpated as a grossly evident mass with an irregular outline, at times with a stellate or a nodular configuration. The edge of the lesion is poorly defined and lacks circumscription (Fig. 22.15). They are firm to hard on palpation and may have a gritty feel, when cut with a knife (due to the calcification).

Post chemotherapy, the lesions may at times be grossly not easily identified. Careful correlation with imaging, at the time of grossing and extensive tissue sampling, is very useful. Radiography of large specimens may be helpful at times, to recognise the clips, the foci of calcification and so forth. The specimen should be adequately inked and serially sectioned at approximately 0.5 cm thick slices to ensure adequate fixation and identification of small lesions. Adequate sampling of the lesion is necessary for accurate T staging. Extensive sampling is needed for specimens, of post-neoadjuvant therapy and also for extensive ductal carcinoma in situ (DCIS).

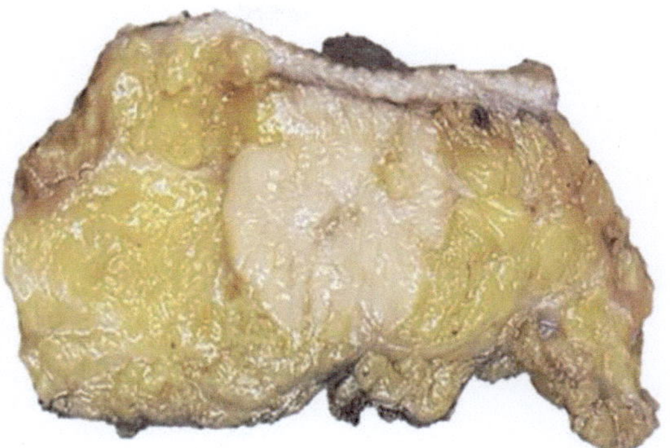

Fig. 22.15 Gross: Cut surface of a mastectomy specimen, showing an infiltrative grey white tumour, seen in the central quadrant, in close proximity to overlying nipple

Examination of skin ulceration, nipple changes and skin nodules should also be done and adequately sampled.

22.2.2.2 Histopathology

Invasive breast cancer (IBC) has a broad spectrum of histopathological features; the most common pattern is invasive ductal carcinoma (IDC). IBC showing a special histological pattern in more than 90% of the tumour are designated as a pure special tumour type, such as lobular, mucinous and tubular carcinoma.

However, if the tumour lacks such specific features with no myoepithelial cell lining (as seen in DCIS or benign lesions), it is designated as invasive carcinoma, NST, which accounts for the majority of the cases, including the mixed patterns. The tumour cells may be arranged in a glandular architecture with desmoplastic reaction (Fig. 22.16).

Nottingham Grade—Another very important parameter to be considered is the histological grading, which is based on three parameters: glandular differentiation, nuclear pleomorphism and mitotic count. A numerical score of 1–3 is used to categorise these three parameters.

For assessing a score for tubule formation, the whole tumour is assessed at low power magnifi-

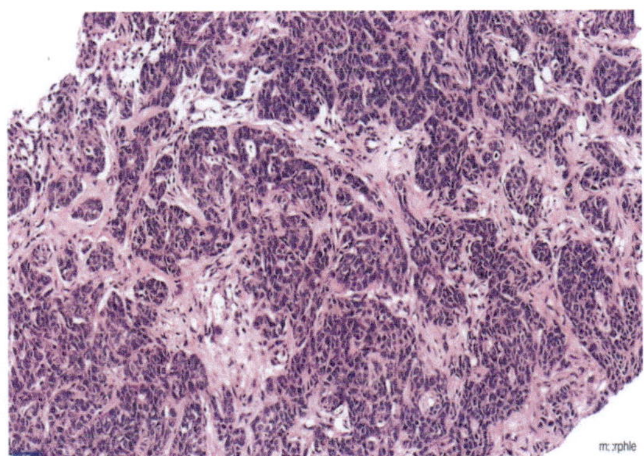

Fig. 22.16 H &E: Tumour cells arranged in a glandular pattern and eliciting a strong desmoplastic reaction (×200)

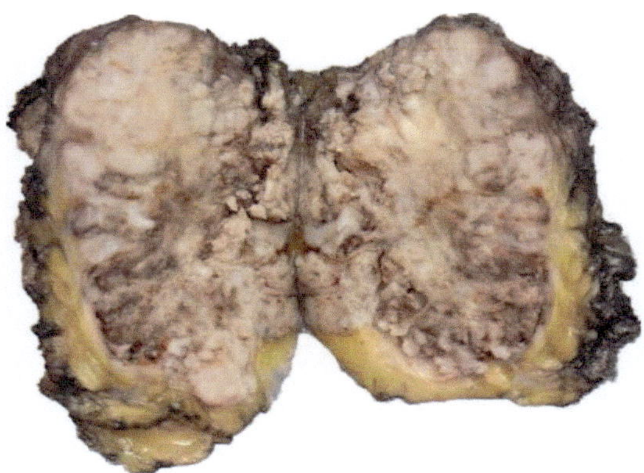

Fig. 22.17 Gross: fairly well-circumscribed moderately firm, fleshy and discrete tumour with a lobulated/nodular architecture and foci of haemorrhage (basal-like or medullary-like pattern)

cation; only structures exhibiting clear central lumina, surrounded by neoplastic cells are counted. The deciding cut-offs are 75% and 10%.

Nuclear pleomorphism scores are assessed in areas with the maximum pleomorphism, as compared to the normal adjacent breast tissue. Score 1 is assigned when the size of the nuclei are very similar to the size of the benign pre-existing epithelial cells (<1.5 times the size). The nuclei show minimal pleomorphism, an even chromatin and inconspicuous nucleoli. Score 2 nuclei are larger (1.5–2 times the size of benign epithelial cell nuclei) with mild to moderate pleomorphism and visible but small nucleoli. Score 3 are larger (more than 2 times the size of the benign epithelial cell nuclei), has a vesicular chromatin and there is a marked variation in size and shape with prominent nucleoli.

The evaluation of mitotic counts requires standardisation to a fixed field area, as the field areas vary between microscopes. The total number of mitosis per ten high-power fields is counted. The cut-off points for scoring depend on the field area size. The microscope used should be calibrated by measuring the diameter of the high-power field (40× objective). In the hot spot method, the scoring is performed in the areas exhibiting highest frequency of mitotic figures. Optimal tissue fixation and good quality sections are essential for counting mitotic figures.

These three values are added together to produce a score of 3–9 and based on that, grades are assigned. Three to five points is grade 1 (well differentiated), 6–7 points is grade 2 (moderately differentiated) and 8–9 points is grade 3 (poorly differentiated) tumours.

Other important parameters to be seen are angiolymphatic invasion, usually in the peritumoural lymphovascular spaces. The presence of associated in situ component is also important to be documented. The size of the tumour, distance to margins, stromal changes and tumour infiltrating lymphocytes are also relevant in the classification scheme.

There are various special histological patterns, which had been recently described under IBC. Current opinion is to consider such tumours as special morphologic patterns of IBC-NST to improve the diagnostic concordance of the classification system and to highlight the lack of prognostic and management implications. These patterns include:

- Basal-like or medullary-like patterns: These include breast carcinomas previously described as medullary-like carcinoma or carcinoma with medullary features, as well as basal-like carcinoma. Grossly, the tumour is fairly well circumscribed (Fig. 22.17). Microscopically, the tumour cells show a syncytial pattern with dense lymphocytic infiltrate (Fig. 22.18).
- A few other patterns include oncocytic, sebaceous, melanocytic, glycogen rich, lipid rich, carcinomas with osteoclast-like stromal giant

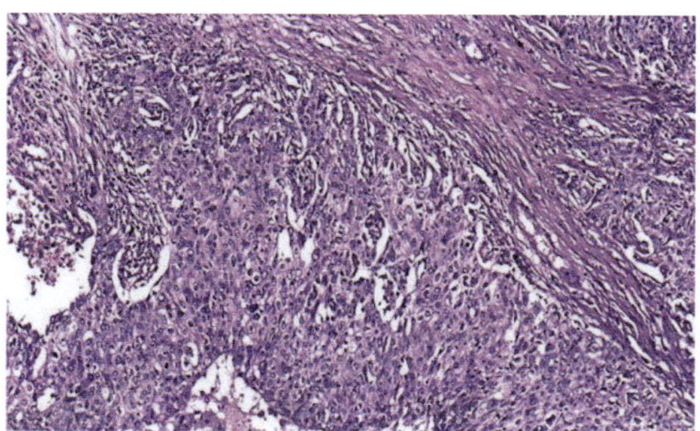

Fig. 22.18 H&E: Syncytial pattern of tumour cells, with surrounding lymphoplasmacytic infiltrate (×200) (basal-like or medullary-like pattern)

cells, pleomorphic and choriocarcinomatous carcinoma patterns.

– Invasive carcinoma with neuroendocrine differentiation: A proportion of IBC NST shows neuroendocrine differentiation of variable extent as determined by histological, histochemical and immunohistochemical analysis. However, it lacks histologic features to classify as large cell or small cell neuroendocrine carcinoma or neuroendocrine tumour of the breast.

22.3 Microinvasive Carcinoma [8]

Microinvasive carcinoma is ≤1 mm in size with exclusion of larger foci by deeper sections. The presence of pre-existing lesion, most often carcinoma in situ (usually high-grade ductal), should be a desirable criteria.

22.4 Invasive Lobular Carcinoma (ILC) [9]

- Invasive lobular carcinoma (ILC) is the second most common histological type of breast carcinoma with a higher rate of multiplicity, bilaterality and mortality. This lesion usually does not present as a palpable lump.
- ILC usually spreads diffusely through the breast stroma.
- Normal or benign mammographic findings are more frequently reported with ILC.
- The diffuse spread of neoplastic cells in ILC is also reflected by its unusual metastatic pattern to spread into the peritoneum-retroperitoneum, gastrointestinal tract, urogenital tract, leptomeninges and myocardium.

22.4.1 Pathogenesis

22.4.1.1 Molecular Aspects

ILCs display a characteristic pattern of somatic genetic mutations, including gains of 16q and 16p, losses of 16q, much encompass the CDH1 gene locus on 16q22.1. E-cadherin loss of function has now shown to be causative of the characteristic lack of cohesion and invasiveness pattern of lobular carcinoma cells.

22.4.1.2 Imaging Findings

Mammogram: Manifest as mass with an opacity equal to or less than that of normal fibroglandular tissue.

– Commonly, the mammograms are normal, if seen as an abnormality; the presentation is either as spiculated masses or architectural distortion. Microcalcifications are less frequently associated than with the usual type invasive ductal carcinoma [10].

Ultrasound: Can present as an irregular or angular mass with hypoechoic and heterogeneous echoes. It also can be seen as an ill-defined or spiculated lesion with posterior acoustic shadowing. It is sometimes sonographically invisible. Although the ultrasound (US) appearances of various subtypes of ILC overlap considerably, classic ILC tends to manifest as focal shadowing without a discrete mass, pleomorphic type ILC is more typically seen as a shadowing mass [10].

MRI: MRI has a higher sensitivity for lobular carcinoma and is a useful adjunct to detect additional ipsilateral and contralateral malignant findings not evident at mammography or US. It can accurately detect lesion size.

- The most common manifestation is a multicentric/multifocal, spiculated focus or mass with architectural distortion.
- Additional manifestations include a dominant lesion surrounded by multiple small enhancing foci, multiple small enhancing foci with interconnecting enhancing strands, architectural distortions, regional or focal heterogeneous enhancement and enhancing septa. Interestingly, histopathologic findings suggest that the enhancing strands and septa correlate with tumour cells streaming within the breast stroma.

Dynamic contrast-enhanced breast MRI demonstrate delayed maximum enhancement, with washout exhibited by only a minority of lesions. Enhancement can be asymmetric and non-mass like in a ductal, segmental, regional or diffuse pattern [10]

22.4.2 Pathology [9]

22.4.2.1 Gross Examination

Gross: ILCs frequently present as an irregular, grey-white and poorly delineated tumour that can be difficult to define macroscopically because of the diffuse growth pattern of the cell infiltrate. The size of ILC is also difficult to determine, although it has been reported to be slightly larger than that of IBC-NST in some series. Some tumours may present as hard nodules like pebbles or grains of sand.

22.4.2.2 Histopathology

Classic pattern of ILC shows proliferation of dyscohesive small cells dispersed throughout a fibrous connective tissue or arranged in single file linear cords that invade the stroma (Fig. 22.19). These infiltrating cords have a targetoid appearance (concentric pattern around normal ducts). There is little host reaction or disturbance of the background architecture. Tumour cells have round or notched ovoid nuclei, thin rim of cytoplasm and occasional intracytoplasmic lumen, which often harbour a central mucoid inclusion.

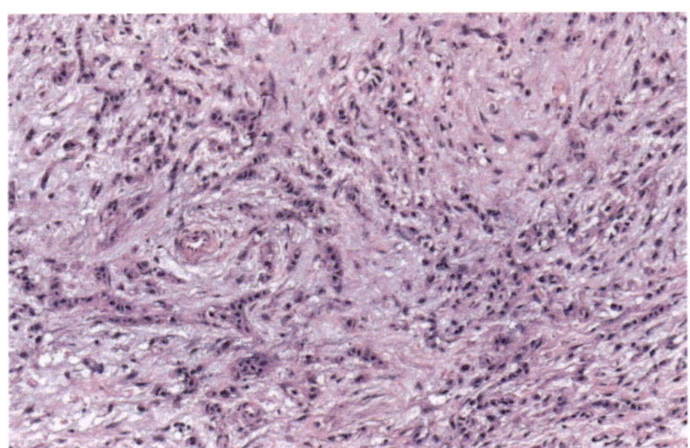

Fig. 22.19 H&E: Classic lobular pattern with tumour cells arranged in single file linear cords (40×)

Mitoses are typically infrequent and lymphovascular invasion is uncommon.

Other patterns of ILC include:

- **Solid pattern** is characterised by the typical non-cohesive and small cells of lobular morphology, but these cells grow in sheets and have a higher frequency of mitoses than in the classic type.
- **Alveolar pattern** are mainly arranged in globular aggregates of at least 20 cells (Fig. 22.20).
- **Pleomorphic lobular carcinoma (PLC)** retains the distinctive growth pattern of lobular carcinoma but exhibits a greater degree of pleomorphism (defined as larger cells with marked nuclear pleomorphism >4 times the size of lymphocytes/equivalent to that of high-grade ductal carcinoma in situ, with or without apocrine features) and a higher mitotic count than classic ILC. This pattern is frequently associated with lobular carcinoma in situ showing the same pleomorphic cytological features. PLC may show apocrine or histiocytoid differentiation and may be composed of signet-ring cells.
- The **tubulolobular pattern** is composed of the admixture of a tubular growth pattern and small uniform cells arranged in a linear pattern. Lobular carcinoma in situ is

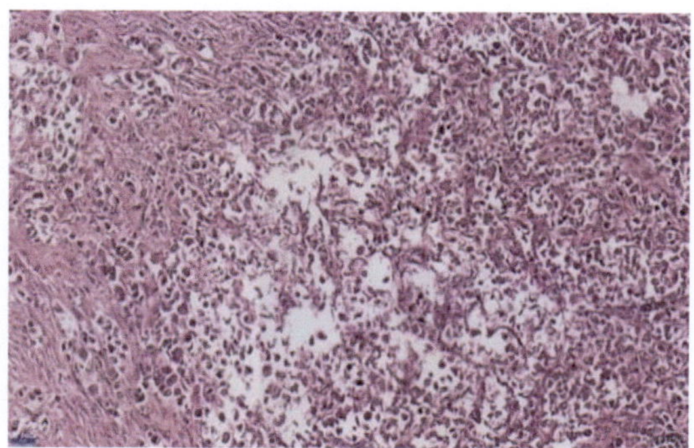

Fig. 22.20 H&E: Invasive lobular carcinoma—Alveolar type: Tumour cells are arranged in globular pattern (40×)

observed in about one-third of tubulolobular carcinomas.

- A **mixed group** is composed of cases showing an admixture of patterns (called invasive ductulolobular carcinomas)

22.4.3 Immunohistochemistry

Majority of the cases are positive for ER (80–95%) and PR (60–70%), thus belonging to luminal A or B. Very rarely Her2neu amplification/overexpression is noted. One of the most consistent molecular alterations in ILC is the loss of E-cadherin expression.

22.5 Invasive Mucinous Carcinoma

- Mucinous (colloid) carcinoma (MC) is a rare breast neoplasm, which presents over the age of 75 years.
- A mucin component >33–50% defines this type of tumour.
- It may be divided into pure mucinous and mixed entities.
- Pure mucinous carcinomas are associated with a better prognosis, a longer disease-free interval and a lower incidence of axillary node metastasis.
- Most mucinous carcinomas are readily detected on imaging.

22.5.1 Pathogenesis

22.5.1.1 Molecular Aspects: [11]

Categorised as luminal A with favourable prognosis. The tumour exhibits 1p gains and 16q losses with somatic mutations of PIK3CA and AKT1, which are common in other ER+, HER2- invasive breast carcinomas.

22.5.1.2 Imaging Findings

Mammogram: They appear as low-density, well-defined or microlobulated oval masses, and they generally belong to the category of “well-circumscribed” breast carcinomas.

- Microlobulated margins have been associated with higher mucin content, while irregular or spiculated margins correspond to lower percentages of mucin and infiltrating margins histologically.
- The irregular and infiltrating margins seen on mammography and histology have been attributed to greater degrees of fibrosis associated with the nonmucinous components.
- Calcifications are rare in these types of malignancies.

Ultrasound: These lesions typically present as complex mass of mixed echogenicity with solid and cystic-appearing components. If homogenous, they are seen as isoechoic or hypoechoic to subcutaneous fat, with posterior acoustic enhancement being a common finding. Microlobulated contour is often more readily demonstrated on ultrasound rather than mammogram.

MRI: Frequently these present as lobulated tumours on MRI.

- They classically demonstrate high signal intensity on T2-weighted images due to the intrinsic mucin component. Signal intensity on T1-weighted images vary from low to high, a feature that is largely dependent on the protein composition of the tumour.
- Dynamic time-signal intensity curves that exhibit a gradual contrast enhancement or

plateau-type pattern after the initial upstroke [12].
- Features vary depending on amount of mucin content and solid component.
- Typical invasive breast carcinomas display lower signal intensity on fat-saturated T2-weighted images than do benign masses [13].

22.5.2 Pathology [11]

22.5.2.1 Gross Examination

The mucinous carcinoma of the breast shows a glistening gelatinous lesion with pushing margins and a soft consistency that is readily recognisable. The tumours range in size from less than 1 cm to more than 20 cm (mean = 3 cm).

22.5.2.2 Histopathology

It is composed of at least 90% of abundant extracellular mucin admixed with invasive neoplastic epithelial cells (Fig. 22.21). The mucinous component of a mixed mucinous carcinoma will be less than 90% of the tumour. Extensive sampling may be needed to detect the neoplastic epithelium, when there is predominantly mucin. The neoplastic cells are arranged in a variety of patterns, including strands, alveolar nests, papillary and micropapillary clusters, and large cribriform sheets. Most of the mucinous carcinomas are well to moderately differentiated. Calcifications associated with these lesions tend to be coarse and irregular.

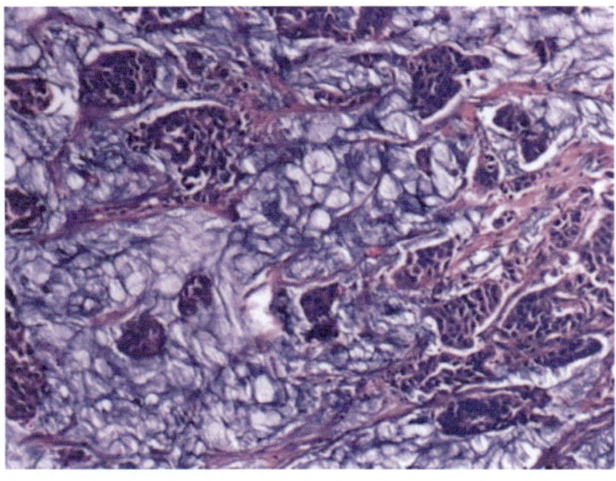

Fig. 22.21 H&E: Tumour cells are seen floating in pools of mucin (×200)

Histological subtypes of mucinous carcinoma: Capella et al. [14] classified mucinous carcinoma into two subtypes: Type A and B.

Type A is characterised by abundant extracellular mucin with epithelium seen in trabeculae and ribbons or festoons. Type B has less abundant extracellular mucin and consists of "clumps" of cells with intracytoplasmic mucin and often granular cytoplasm. Some authors consider Type B to be having endocrine differentiation.

Micropapillary variant of mucinous carcinoma [15]: This variant of MC is characterised by micropapillae arranged in small and tightly cohesive clusters or in ring like structures in a space filled with mucin. It may have psammomatous calcifications. Rarely, the tumour cells can have a signet ring cell morphology, within the pools of mucin. The signet ring cells may be arranged in large solid clusters or as single cells and are more common in Type B MC with neuroendocrine features.

Mucinous carcinoma associated with solid and papillary carcinoma—MC can also arise in association with solid papillary carcinoma. These tumours usually are Type B MCs with neuroendocrine morphology, and some may also express neuroendocrine markers.

Ductal Carcinoma: In situ DCIS may be associated with MC; however, the nuclear grade is low in most of the cases. High nuclear grade is more common with subtype B and mixed MC.

22.5.3 Immunohistochemistry

Typically, mucinous carcinoma shows positive expression for estrogen and progesterone receptors, while androgen receptors are expressed at a low level, and HER2 is not amplified. Pure and mixed mucinous carcinomas are reported to express WT1 [7]. Mucinous breast carcinoma expresses predominantly MUC2 and MUC6 among the family of MUC genes [16].

22.6 Tubular Carcinoma

- Tubular carcinoma of the breast is a well-differentiated type of invasive ductal carcinoma. They present as a non-palpable lesion, often first detected on screening mammography. This tumour affects younger population and has an excellent prognosis [17].

22.6.1 Pathogenesis

22.6.1.1 Molecular Aspects

Low frequency of genetic alteration with most frequent being are 16q loss (78–86%) and 1q gain (50–62%). In mRNA (Gene Expression Profiling), the tubular carcinoma are members of luminal A molecular class of breast cancer, which should show low recurrence score by Oncotype DX test. There is a strong expression of hormone receptors and related proteins with low expression of proliferation markers.

22.6.1.2 Imaging Findings

Mammogram: The lesions are usually less than 1 cm and present as architectural distortion or as an irregularly shaped mass with spiculated margins, with or without calcifications. The appearance mimics invasive ductal carcinoma (IDC-NOS). The spicules are often longer than the central mass.

Ultrasound: The appearance also mimics IDC-NOS, manifesting as a hypoechoic solid mass with ill-defined margins and posterior acoustic shadowing.

MRI: shows characteristics of a malignant tumour, more commonly an irregular mass with a Type 3 enhancement curve [17].

> **Note**
> Tubular carcinoma should be considered in the differential diagnosis of a small spiculated mass, especially if it has long spicules.

Differential diagnosis: Radiologically, it closely mimics a radial scar.

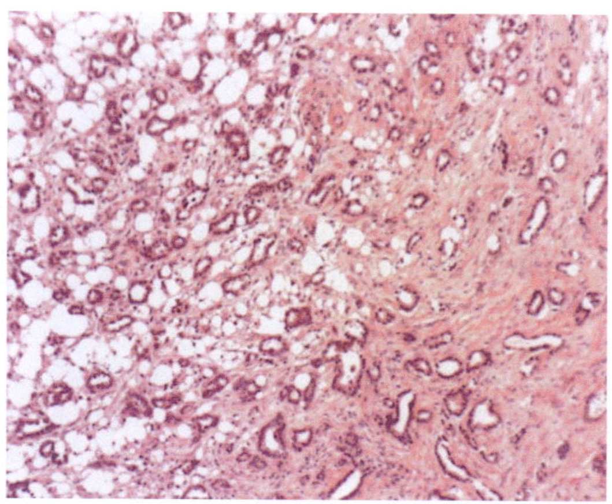

Fig. 22.22 H & E: angulated glands lacking myoepithelial cells and infiltrating the stroma (×200)

22.6.2 Pathology

Gross: Majority of tubular carcinomas are ≤1 cm, and they appear as irregular grey-white mass with retraction of surrounding tissue.

Microscopy: This tumour shows a haphazard infiltrative proliferation of well-formed glands with single layer of low-grade epithelial cells and no myoepithelial cell layer. Tubules have open lumina and angulated contours with tapering ends (Fig. 22.22). More than 90% of tumour demonstrates a characteristic tubular morphology. Calcifications may be associated with secretory material in lumina. Lymphovascular invasion is highly unusual. Tubular carcinoma is frequently associated with low-grade DCIS (cribriform and micropapillary patterns) and is also frequently associated with columnar cell changes, flat epithelial atypia, atypical lobular hyperplasia and lobular carcinoma in situ.

22.6.3 Immunohistochemistry

This tumour is strongly positive for ER (>95%), PR (>75%) expression and negative for Her2Neu in vast majority of cases with Ki 67 showing low proliferative index and myoepithelial markers are absent [18].

22.7 Metaplastic Carcinoma Breast (MCB)

This tumour is a rare and aggressive form with a rapid growth. It usually presents as a palpable lump and seen in postmenopausal women. Pathologically, this malignancy has both epithelial (carcinoma) and mesenchymal (sarcomas) subtypes. Haematogenous spread is more frequent than lymphatic spread, reflecting the sarcomatoid behaviour. Lung and bone are the most common metastatic sites. It should be distinguished from invasive ductal carcinoma, because MCB has a worse prognosis, and from breast sarcoma, because the treatment approach is different [19].

22.7.1 Pathogenesis

22.7.1.1 Molecular Aspects

It is predominantly basal-like molecular subtype. It may affect *TP53*, *RB1*, *TERT* promoter genes, chromatin remodelling genes (i.e. *ARID1A*, *KMT2C*), genes related to PI3K pathway (i.e. *PIK3CA*, *PIK3R1*, *PTEN*), MAPK pathway (*NF1*, *KRAS*, *NRAS*) or WNT pathway (*FAT1*, *APC*, *CCN6*) [20].

22.7.1.2 Imaging Findings

Mammogram: A dense mass is the most frequent feature with more benign appearance than invasive ductal carcinoma, with round, lobular or oval shape and predominantly circumscribed margins. Calcifications are often absent. Associated features, such as architectural distortion, is uncommon.

Ultrasound: Usually seen as oval, round and lobular in shape with circumscribed margins.

Possibly due to the cystic component or due to the mass hypercellularity, there is frequent posterior acoustic enhancement, creating greater confusion in the distinction with benign lesions. This is in clear contrast to invasive ductal carcinoma, generally displaying posterior acoustic shadowing.

MRI: Often seen as a round or lobular mass with relatively smooth margins. It is similar to other types of breast cancer as it is T1 iso- or hypointense. On the other hand, T2 sequences are important for the differential diagnosis, because MCB is generally heterogeneously T2 hyperintense. There are T2 iso- or hypo intense solid components and hyperintense portions, frequently attributed to necrosis, but also due to cystic degeneration, myxoid matrix, intratumoural haemorrhagic changes and loose oedematous stroma. For the same reasons, the enhancement pattern is frequently heterogeneous or ring-like [19].

22.7.2 Pathology

Gross: These tumours grossly can present as well-circumscribed mass, or it can have indistinct, irregular borders. Cystic degeneration is not unusual if associated with squamous cell carcinoma. Pearly white-to-grey white and glistening cut surfaces can represent areas of cartilage, whereas the cut surface of areas of osteoid can be gritty and hard. Metaplastic carcinomas tend to be larger, ranging from 2 to >10 cm. Thorough sampling of the lesion is strongly advised.

Microscopy: It can be a monophasic (epithelial carcinoma/sarcomatoid) or biphasic with a combination of both components. Epithelial only carcinomas may predominantly include low or high-grade adenosquamous carcinoma and squamous cell carcinoma. Pure (monophasic) sarcoma includes fibromatosis-like metaplastic carcinoma and spindle cell carcinoma. Heterologous mesenchymal components include chondroid, osseous, rhabdomyosarcomatous, angiosarcomatous, liposarcomatous and neuroglial differentiation or in combination (Fig. 22.23).

Mesenchymal component can show a wide spectrum of atypia, from minimal to frankly malignant (Fig. 22.24) Extensive sampling or performing immunohistochemistry for identification of epithelial component is mandatory [20].

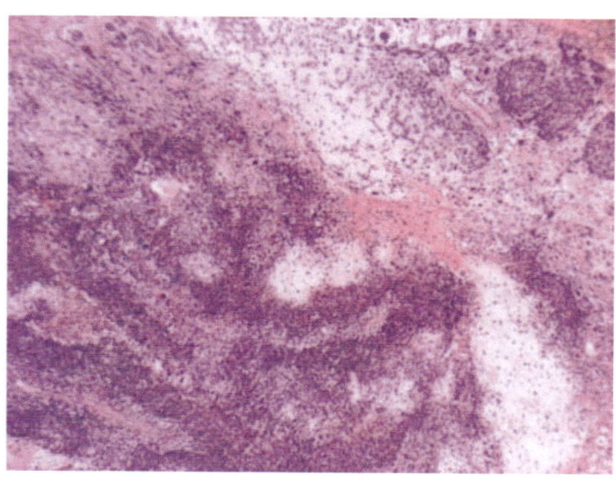

Fig. 22.23 H & E: Foci of cartilaginous component in metaplastic carcinoma (×200)

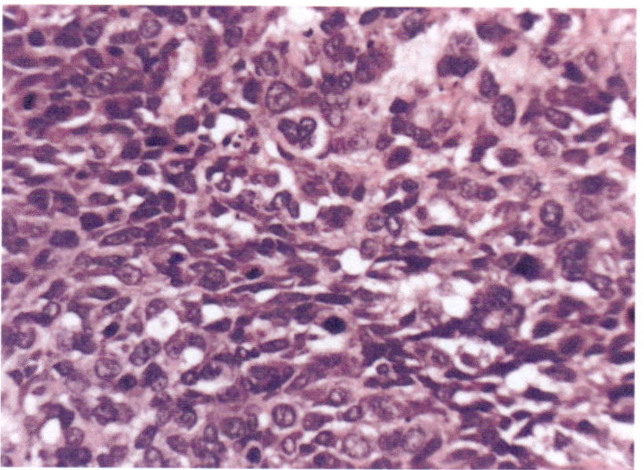

Fig. 22.24 H & E: mitosis with pleomorphic tumour cells (×400)

22.8 Invasive Micropapillary Carcinoma

- Invasive micropapillary carcinoma can affect any quadrant, and axillary lymph nodes are usually involved at diagnosis. These tumours are rare, accounting for 0.9–2% of all IBCs. Mixed forms are more common, usually in association with IBCs. In view of its higher nodal metastasis, prognosis is worse than classic IBC.

22.8.1 Pathogenesis: [21]

22.8.1.1 Molecular Aspects

These tumours are luminal A or B carcinomas by gene expression profiling. Array comparative genomic hybridisation has detected recurrent gains of 8q, 17q and 20q with deletions of 6q and 13q.

22.8.2 Pathology

Gross: Tumours with >50% of micropapillary growth tend to be larger than those with lesser amount of this pattern, and they might have a lobulated outline.

Microscopy: This tumour shows groups of cells that are arranged around pseudopapillae, hollow tubules and morula that are surrounded by empty clear spaces formed by fibrocollagenous stroma (Fig. 22.25). Cells show characteristic reverse polarity with apical surface abutting the epithelial stromal interface. Nuclei around the periphery bulge with serrated appearance. Angiolymphatic invasion is extensively seen. Uncommon variant features include psammoma bodies, microcystic dilation of lumina with cell clusters, apocrine differentiation, multinucleated

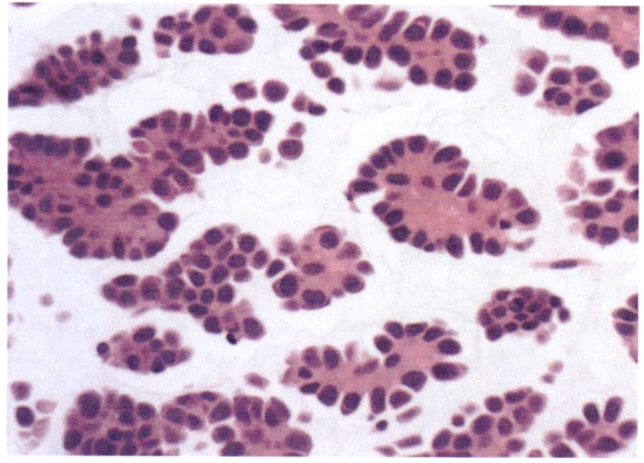

Fig. 22.25 H & E: structures with a characteristic inside-out pattern (×400)

giant cells (e.g. osteoclast). Invasive mucinous carcinoma may contain micropapillary component, also called mucinous micropapillary carcinoma.

22.8.3 Immunohistochemistry

Most of these carcinomas are ER and PR positive, a triple negative phenotype may be seen in 15–20% of cases. The Epithelial Membrane Antigen (EMA) or MUC1 expression is seen on the stroma facing surface of the membrane, in contrast to IBC, where it is seen on the luminal aspect of the membrane.

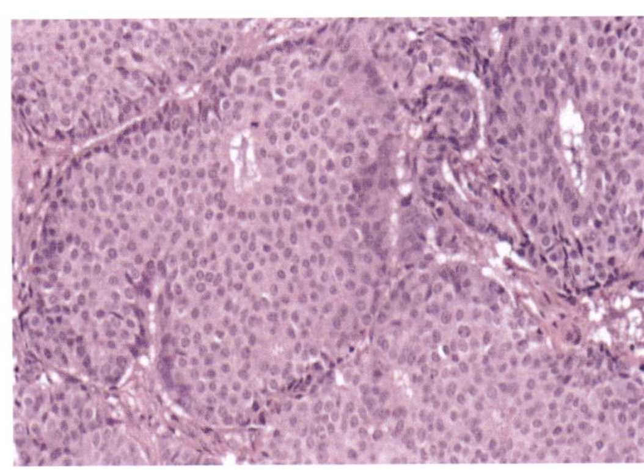

Fig. 22.26 H & E: Tumour cells with abundant cytoplasm, eosinophilic granules and central to eccentric vesicular nuclei (×400)

22.9 Carcinoma with Apocrine Differentiation

Rare, 1–4% of all breast carcinomas.

22.9.1 Pathogenesis

22.9.1.1 Molecular Aspects

Abnormalities at 7q (codes for GCDFP-15 and prolactin inducible protein). Also loss of heterozygosity for p53 gene, VHL (3p25) gene, NB gene (1p35–36) and PKD1/TSC2 gene at 16p1.

22.9.2 Pathology [22]

Gross: Indistinguishable from infiltrating ductal carcinoma.

Microscopy: Tumour cells will have distinct cell margins, abundant cytoplasm with eosinophilic granules and central to eccentric vesicular nuclei with prominent nucleoli (Fig. 22.26). Other subtypes including tubular, lobular, mucinous, invasive micropapillary or medullary should be excluded.

22.9.3 Immunohistochemsitry

Carcinomas with apocrine differentiation express GCDFP-15. They also have a characteristic receptor profile that is ER-negative, PR-negative, and AR-positive. GATA3 is expressed in 90% of carcinomas with apocrine morphology and in >70% of AR-positive triple-negative carcinomas.

The above spectrum of histological patterns is considered to be seen very frequently in our clinical settings. There are also few other patterns, which can occur rarely such as: [5].

- Cribriform carcinoma
- Mucinous cystadenocarcinoma
- Rare and salivary gland-type tumours: Acinic cell carcinoma, Adenoid cystic carcinoma, Secretory carcinoma, Mucoepidermoid carcinoma, Polymorphous adenocarcinoma and Tall cell carcinoma with reversed polarity.
- Neuroendocrine neoplasms: Neuroendocrine tumour, Neuroendocrine carcinoma

22.10 Multiple Lesion/Calcification

Synchronous cancer is defined as two distinct breast cancer lesions detected at the same time or within 6 months from the first diagnosis (Fig. 22.27).

Metachronous cancer are two breast cancer lesions, with the second primary lesion diagnosed after 6 months from the first breast cancer lesion with different histology. Such lesions are most commonly seen with invasive lobular carcinoma [23].

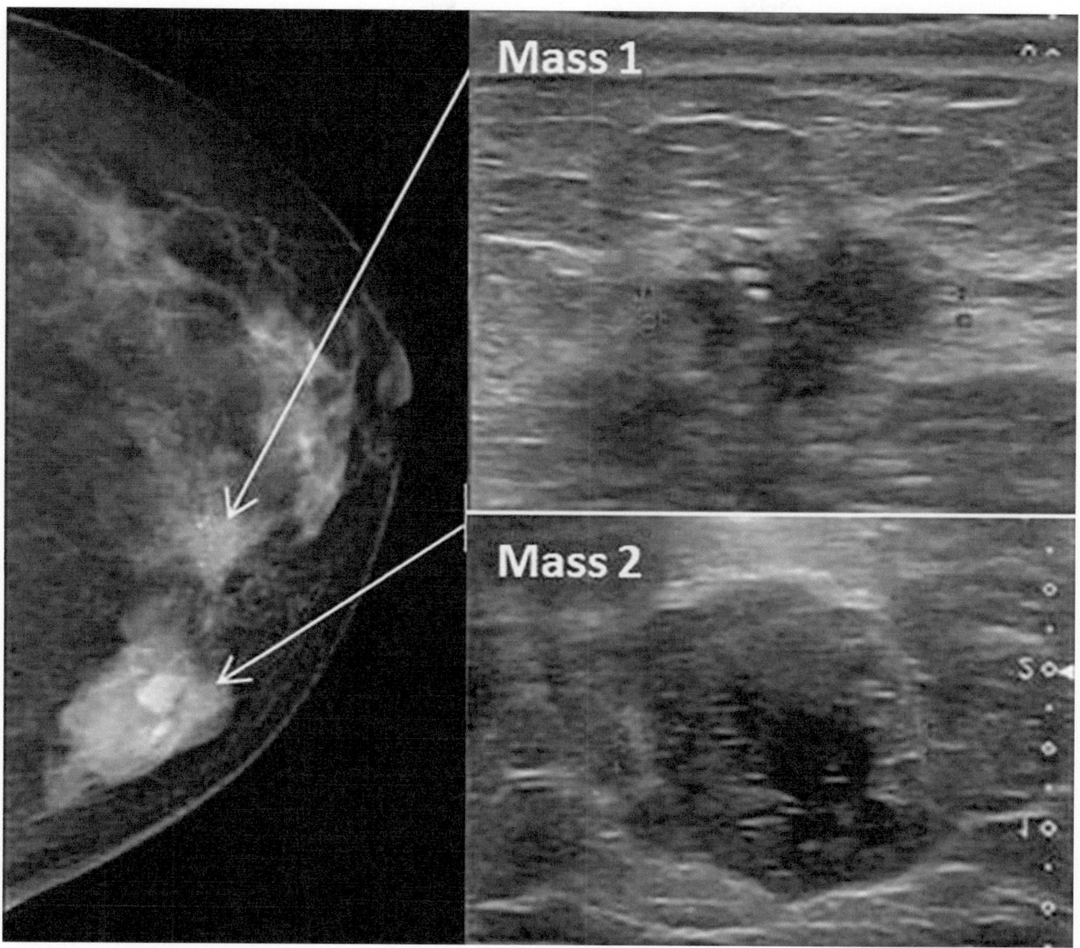

Fig. 22.27 X-ray mammogram and ultrasound showing synchronous cancer-2 different malignant lesions at the same visit. (lesion 1 and lesion 2)

Multifocal-multicentric tumours of the breast are defined by the presence of two or more physically separate neoplasms in the same breast (Fig. 22.28). Pathologists describe it as multiple (two or more foci), primary lesions that occur simultaneously without intervening neoplastic tissue. It is termed as multifocal when the tumour is present in one breast quadrant and multicentric when two or more quadrants are involved (Fig. 22.29). Although radiologicaly there is no exact definition, tumours are considered as multifocal when the distance is less than or equal to 5 cm and multicentric when the distance is more than 5 cm between lesions [24].

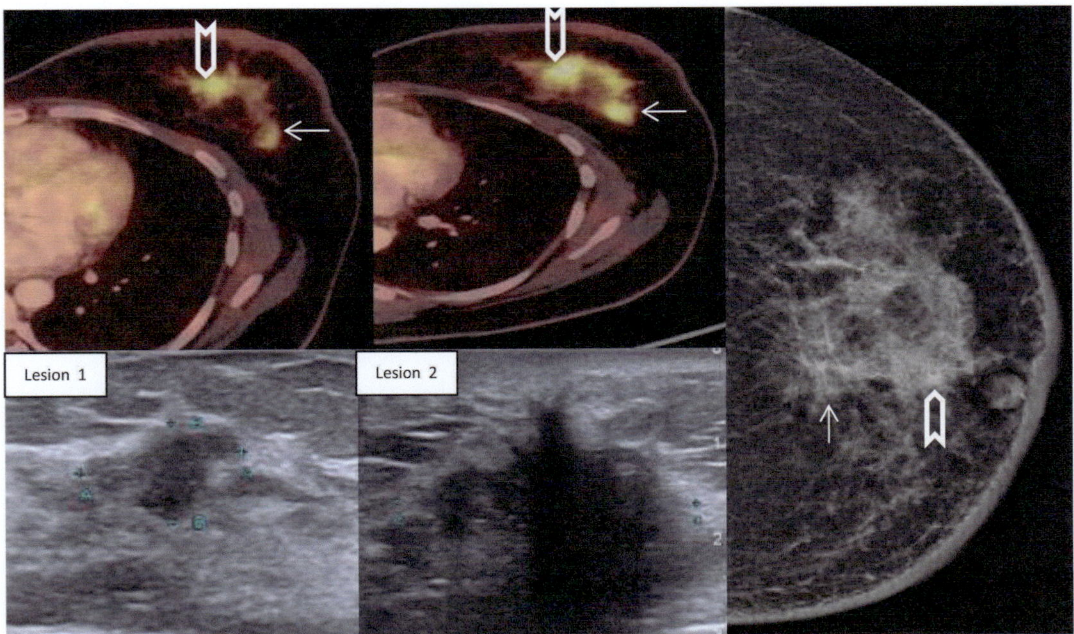

Fig. 22.28 X-ray mammogram, PET CT and ultrasound showing multifocal cancer—involving one quadrant (lesion 1 in central quadrant marked with thin arrow and lesion 2 in central quadrant marked with arrowhead)

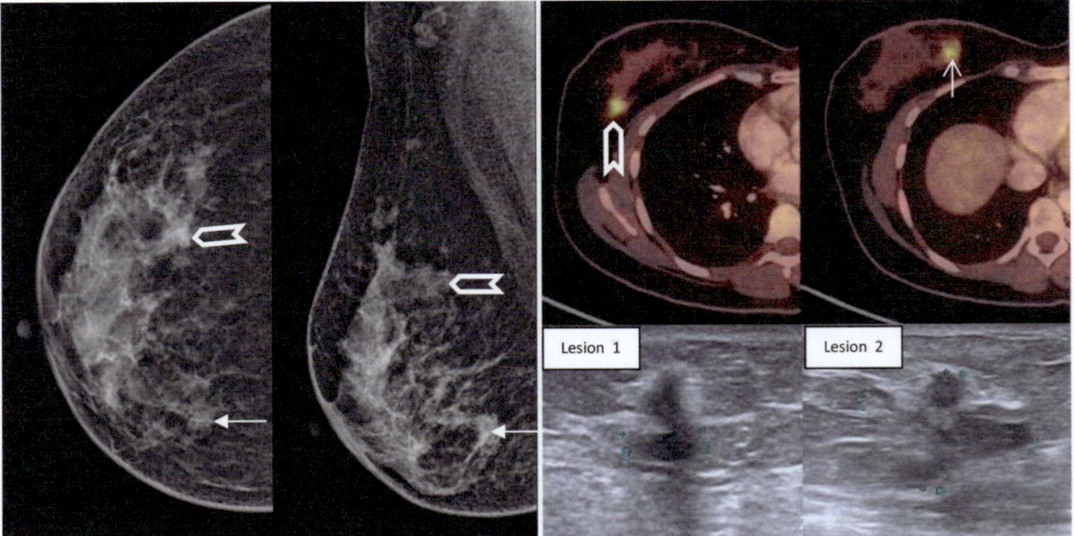

Fig. 22.29 X-ray mammogram, PET CT and ultrasound showing multicentric cancer—seen involving 2 quadrants. (lesion 1 in outer quadrant marked with arrowhead and lesion 2 in inner quadrant marked with thin arrow)

References

1. Lee SC, Jain PA, Jethwa SC, Tripathy D, Yamashita MW. Radiologist's role in breast cancer staging: providing key information for clinicians. Radiographics. 2014;34(2):330–42.
2. ACR BIRADS atlas 5th edition.
3. Popli MB. Pictorial essay: mammographic features of breast cancer. Ind J Radiol Imaging. 2001;11(4):175.
4. Gokhale S. Ultrasound characterization of breast masses. Ind J Radiol Imaging. 2009;19(3):242.
5. WHO Classification of Tumours Editorial Board. WHO classification of tumours: breast tumours. 5th ed. Lyon: International Agency for Research on Cancer; 2019.
6. Gupta K, Kumaresan M, Venkatesan B, Chandra T, Patil A, Menon M. Sonographic features of invasive ductal breast carcinomas predictive of malignancy grade. Ind J Radiol Imaging. 2018;28(1):123.
7. Macura KJ, Ouwerkerk R, Jacobs MA, Bluemke DA. Patterns of enhancement on breast MR images: interpretation and imaging pitfalls. Radiographics. 2006;26(6):1719–34.
8. American Joint Committee on Cancer. In: Edge SB, Byrd DR, Compton CC, et al. (editors), Cancer staging manual, 7th ed. New York: Springer; 2010.
9. Moller Talman ML, Jensen MB, Rank F. Invasive lobular breast cancer. Prognostic significance of histological malignancy grading. Acta Oncologica. 2007;46(6):803–9.
10. Lopez JK, Bassett LW. Invasive lobular carcinoma of the breast: spectrum of mammographic, US, and MR imaging findings. Radiographics. 2009;29(1):165–76.
11. Marrazzo E, Frusone F, Milana F, Sagona A, Gatzemeier W, Barbieri E, Bottini A, Canavese G, Rubino AO, Eboli MG, Rossetti CM, Testori A, Errico V, De Luca A, Tinterri C. Mucinous breast cancer: a narrative review of the literature and a retrospective tertiary single-Centre analysis. Breast. 2020;49:87–92. https://doi.org/10.1016/j.breast.2019.11.002. Epub 2019 Nov 11.
12. Jeong SJ, Lim HS, Lee JS, Park MH, Yoon JH, Park JG, Kang HK. Medullary carcinoma of the breast: MRI findings. Am J Roentgenol. 2012;198(5):W482–7.
13. Ha KY, DeLeon P, DeLeon W. Invasive mucinous carcinoma of the breast. Proc (Bayl Univ Med Cent). 2013;26(3):295–7.
14. Capella C, Eusebi V, Mann B, et al. Endocrine differentiation in mucoid carcinoma of the breast. Histopathology. 1980;4:613–30.
15. Pareja F, Selenica P, Brown DN, Sebastiao APM, da Silva EM, Da Cruz PA, Del A, Fu L, Weigelt B, Brogi E, Reis-Filho JS, Wen HY. Micropapillary variant of mucinous carcinoma of the breast shows genetic alterations intermediate between those of mucinous carcinoma and micropapillary carcinoma. Histopathology. 2019;75(1):139–45. https://doi.org/10.1111/his.13853. Epub 2019 Jun 13.
16. Bitencourt AG, Graziano L, Osório CA, Guatelli CS, Souza JA, Mendonça MH, Marques EF. MRI features of mucinous cancer of the breast: correlation with pathologic findings and other imaging methods. Am J Roentgenol. 2016;206(2):238–46.
17. Vilaverde F, Rocha A, Reis A. Tubular carcinoma of the breast: advantages and limitations of breast tomosynthesis. Case Rep Radiol. 2016;2016:3906195.
18. Fernández-Aguilar S, et al. Tubular carcinoma of the breast and associated intra-epithelial lesions: a comparative study with invasive low-grade ductal carcinomas. Virchows Arch. 2005;447(4):683–7.
19. Donato H, Candelária I, Oliveira P, Gonçalo M, Caseiro-Alves F. Imaging findings of metaplastic carcinoma of the breast with pathologic correlation. J Belg Soc Radiol. 2018;102(1):46.
20. McMullen ER, Zoumberos NA, Kleer CG. Metaplastic breast carcinoma: update on histopathology and molecular alterations. Arch Pathol Lab Med. 2019;143(12):1492–6. https://doi.org/10.5858/arpa.2019-0396-RA.
21. Yang YL, Liu BB, Zhang X, Fu L. Invasive micropapillary carcinoma of the breast: an update. Arch Pathol Lab Med. 2016;140(8):799–805. https://doi.org/10.5858/arpa.2016-0040-RA.
22. Matsuo K, Fukutomi T, Hasegawa T, Akashi-Tanaka S, Nanasawa T, Tsuda H. Histological and immunohistochemical analysis of apocrine breast carcinoma. Breast Cancer. 2002;9(1):43–9. https://doi.org/10.1007/BF02967546.
23. Londero AP, Bernardi S, Bertozzi S, Angione V, Gentile G, Dri C, Minucci A, Caponnetto F, Petri R. Synchronous and metachronous breast malignancies: a cross-sectional retrospective study and review of the literature. Biomed Res Int. 2014;2014:250727.
24. Bozzini A, Renne G, Meneghetti L, Bandi G, Santos G, Vento AR, Menna S, Andrighetto S, Viale G, Cassano E, Bellomi M. Sensitivity of imaging for multifocal-multicentric breast carcinoma. BMC Cancer. 2008;8(1):275.

Part VIII

Non-epithelial Lesion of the Breast

Mesenchymal Lesions of the Breast

23

Priya K. Palanisamy, V. Pavithra, Sandhya Sundaram, and Bhawna Dev

Abstract

Mesenchymal lesions of the breast though not very common in clinical practice, knowledge about these relatively rare pathologies is essential. In this chapter, we have briefly discussed the clinical presentation, imaging and histopathological features and management aspects of the mesenchymal lesions of the breast. Most of the lesion requires tissue biopsy for diagnosis due to their variable imaging features.

Keywords

Mesenchymal lesions · Lipoma · Angiosarcoma · Hemangioma · Angiolipoma

23.1 Introduction

Mesenchymal lesions of the breast essentially arise from the stromal tissue of the breast. Since majority of breast neoplasms occur in the epithelial tissue, mesenchymal neoplasms of the breast are rarely encountered. These range from benign to highly malignant variants as described in Table 23.1.

P. K. Palanisamy (✉) · S. Sundaram · B. Dev
Department of Radiology, Maidstone and Tunbridge Wells NHS Trust, Kent, UK
e-mail: bhawnadev@sriramachandra.edu.in

V. Pavithra
Department of Pathology, Sri Ramachandra Institute of Higher Education and Research, Chennai, India

B. Dev, L. D. Joseph (eds.), *Holistic Approach to Breast Disease*,
https://doi.org/10.1007/978-981-99-0035-0_23

Table 23.1 Mesenchymal lesions of the breast

Benign (common)	Malignant	Miscellaneous (benign)
• Lipoma • Hamartoma • Angiolipoma • Hemangioma • Pseudo angiomatous stromal hyperplasia	• Primary breast sarcomas • Secondary breast sarcoma • Metastatic sarcoma	• Granular cell tumor • Myofibroblastoma • Fibromatosis • Neurofibroma • Schwannoma • Leiomyoma • Inflammatory myofibroblast tumors • Myxoma

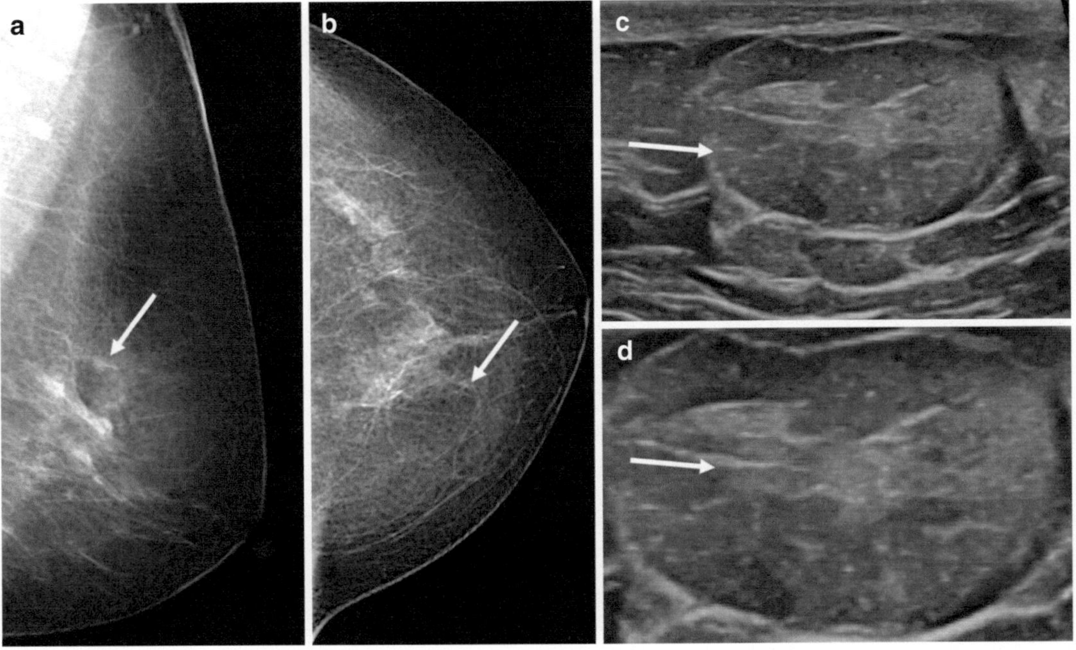

Fig. 23.1 A 38-year woman with palpable mobile lump in the left breast. MLO and CC view mammogram of left breast (**a**, **b**) shows a well-defined oval subtle low-density mass in the upper inner quadrant (arrow) with no associated suspicious features. High-resolution transverse USG of left breast (**c**) confirms a subcutaneous lipoma isoechoic to surrounding fat with echogenic capsule along the margins (arrow) and (**d**) echogenic internal septations (arrow)

23.2 Benign Mesenchymal Lesions

23.2.1 Lipoma

It is the commonest benign mesenchymal lesion of the breast containing mature adipocytes.

23.2.1.1 Clinical Presentation

It is frequently seen in perimenopausal women and presentsl circumscribed soft non-tender mass.

23.2.1.2 Imaging Features

- **Mammogram**: Well circumscribed fat containing (low density) mass (Fig. 23.1a, b).
- **Ultrasound**: On ultrasound (USG), lipoma can be isoechoic (to surrounding fat), hypoechoic, or hyperechoic with no associated internal vascularity. Echogenic capsule can be seen surrounding the periphery (Fig. 23.1c) and has multiple echogenic striation within, parallel to the skin surface, which helps in distinguishing lipoma from hamartoma (Fig. 23.1d).

- **Magnetic Resonance Imaging (MRI)**: Appears as a well-circumscribed, T1 hyperintense non-enhancing mass, which gets suppressed in T1 fat suppression sequences.

BI-RADS category: **2 (Benign)**

23.2.1.3 Histopathology

Gross
These tumors are typically well-circumscribed masses of mature adipose tissue with or without areas of necrosis and hemorrhage.

Microscopy [1]
Lipoma is a well-circumscribed and encapsulated mass consisting of mature adipocytes and pushing adjacent fibro glandular breast elements. The nuclei of adipocytes are small, uniform, and located at periphery of cell. They may show varying degrees of fibrosis, myxoid change, lipogranulomas or calcification.

23.2.1.4 Differential Diagnosis

1. *Myofibroblastoma (MFB)*: Consist of admixtures of benign spindle cell, dense hyalinized collagen and varying degrees of myxoid changes.
2. *Hamartoma*: Consist of normal-appearing ducts and lobules in addition to minor component of fat.
3. *Hibernoma*: Composed of brown fat (coarsely multi-vacuolated fat cells that lack atypia).
4. *Liposarcoma*: Extremely rare in breast and most seen as component of high-grade phyllodes tumor, which presents as large palpable mass with irregular or ill-defined borders. Microscopically, there is variation in size of adipocytes with atypia, lipoblasts, and fibrous septa, which are good diagnostic clues for malignancy.

Management: Usually does not require surgery unless for cosmetic reasons. In case of rapidly enlarging masses or diagnostic uncertain masses, biopsy can be performed.

23.2.2 Angiolipoma

Contains mature adipocytes admixed with capillaries. These usually account for about 5–17% of all lipomas. Breast angiolipomas are relatively rare and are more commonly seen in males.

23.2.2.1 Clinical Presentation

Non-tender, smooth solitary palpable masses.

23.2.2.2 Imaging Features

Angiolipoma are usually well-circumscribed masses with nonspecific imaging features

- **Mammogram**: The masses may vary in density and margin characteristics.
- **Ultrasound**: Commonly seen as well-circumscribed oval or round hyperechoic masses with increased vascularity on color Doppler study.
- **MRI**: appears hypointense on T1 and hyperintense on T2 sequences and shows enhancement after IV contrast administration.

BI-RADS category: **BI-RADS—3/4** (probably benign/mildly suspicious). Requires tissue biopsy.

23.2.2.3 Histopathology

Gross
Well-circumscribed lesions consisting of mature adipose tissue with areas of hemorrhage.

Microscopy [1]
A well-circumscribed mass composed of an admixture of mature adipose tissue and non-infiltrative small vascular spaces. The vascular spaces may be compressed and slit-like lined by bland endothelial cells containing intravascular hyaline microthrombi.

23.2.2.4 Differential Diagnosis

1. *Angiosarcoma*: Large palpable mass with irregular or ill-defined borders. Microscopic features show malignant irregularly shaped blood vessels, which dissection surrounds tis-

sue with nuclear atypia and tufting. Foci of solid areas and blood lakes are also common.

Management: Generally kept under follow-up. If imaging features and histopathology are equivocal, then surgical excision is recommended.

23.2.3 Hemangiomas

These are the commonest vascular lesions of the breast that can be located within the breast parenchyma as well as superficially in the skin and subcutaneous tissue of the breast.

23.2.3.1 Etiopathogenesis

Estrogen plays role in development of hemangiomas. Expression of estrogen and progesterone receptors has been reported in some vascular masses.

Genetic syndrome: Hemangioma is a part of Kasabach-Merritt syndrome, which occurs most commonly in extremities but can involve any anatomic site, including breast.

23.2.3.2 Clinical Presentation

Usually seen in all age groups and present as superficial palpable masses with overlying skin discoloration.

23.2.3.3 Imaging Features

Nonspecific imaging features mostly presenting as well-circumscribed mass

- **Mammogram**: round or oval, hypodense or isodense mass with macro-lobulated margins and associated calcifications in few cases (Fig. 23.2).
- **USG**: Often seen as superficial hyper/hypoechoic mass, which are hypovascular on color Doppler (Fig. 23.3).
- **MRI**: They are typically T1 isointense and T2 hyperintense showing slow progressive enhancement pattern on dynamic contrast-enhanced MRI.

BI-RADS category: **BI-RADS—2/3**. May require tissue biopsy if clinically and radiologically equivocal.

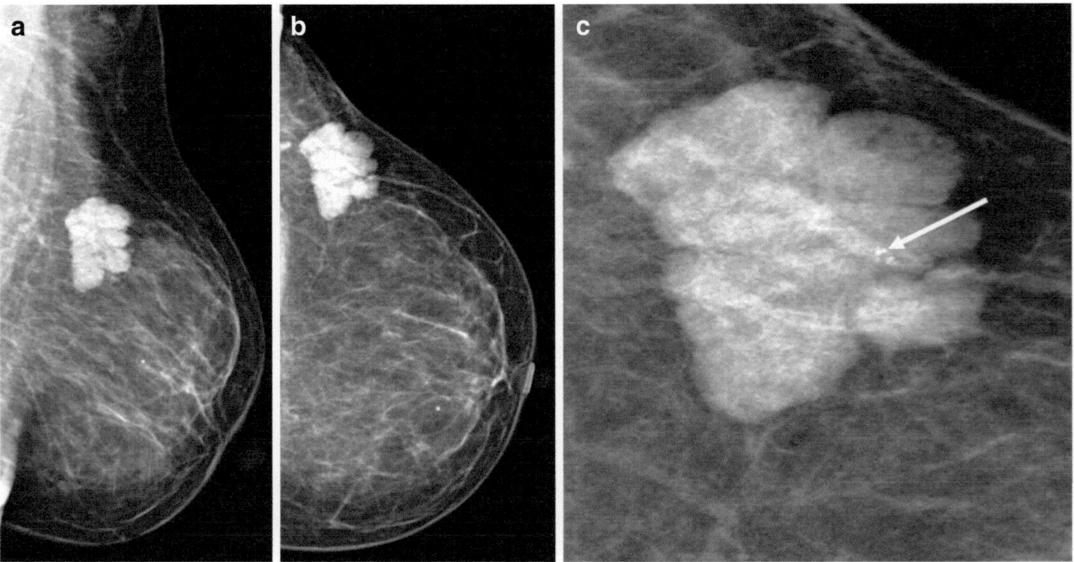

Fig. 23.2 Mammogram appearance of biopsy proven hemangioma in a 68-year-old woman with palpable lump. MLO and CC view mammogram of left breast (**a**, **b**) shows a high-density lobulated mass in the upper outer quadrant. (**c**) on magnification, there are few benign punctate calcifications within this mass as shown by an arrow

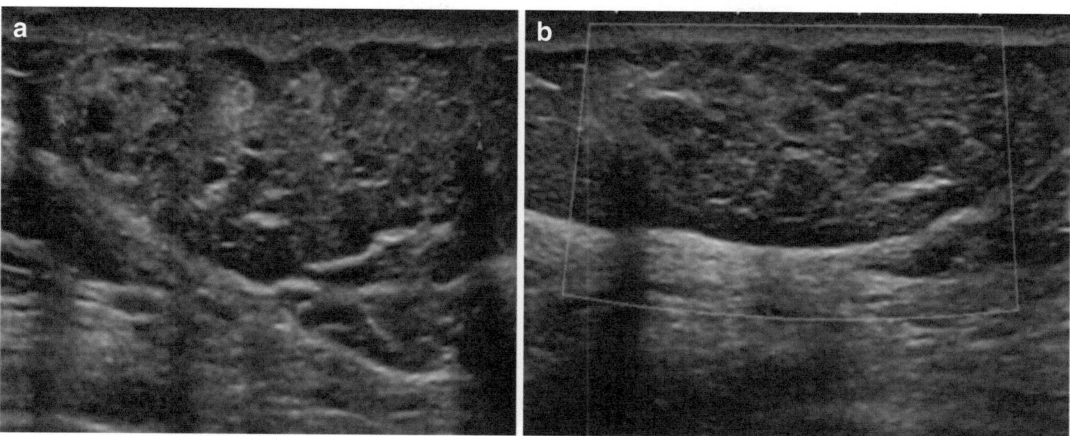

Fig. 23.3 High-resolution transverse Ultrasound appearance of hamartoma—(**a**) shows an oval lobulated superficial hypoechoic mass with no significant vascularity (**b**)

23.2.3.4 Histopathology

Gross

Hemangiomas are well-circumscribed, soft, spongy masses usually less than 2 cm in size. They are reddish brown in color due to blood and hemosiderin.

Microscopic Variants [2]

- **Perilobular hemangioma**: Most common vascular lesion. Typically small and are often intermingled with lobular and terminal duct epithelium. Vascular spaces are lined by flattened endothelium, and the vessels are small and rounded with little or no muscular coat.
- **Cavernous hemangioma**: Composed of large, cavernous vascular channels with dilated thin-walled vessels lined by flattened endothelium, congested with blood. Thrombosis may be present with papillary endothelial hyperplasia (Masson lesion).
- **Capillary hemangioma**: Composed of capillary-sized, well-formed blood vessels. Usually forms a circumscribed or lobulated mass, and some may have irregular margins.
- **Complex hemangioma**: Composed of variably sized small blood vessels, sometimes forming irregular anastomosing channels. No nuclear pleomorphism or atypia and are usually small (<1 cm) with circumscribed borders.
- **Venous hemangioma**: Composed largely of venous channels with disorderly vascular proliferation with smooth muscle walls of varying thickness. The vascular spaces may appear empty or filled with blood.
- **Atypical hemangiomas**: These lesions show features of complex anastomosing vessels, central infarction, thrombosis with papillary endothelial hyperplasia, pseudo-papillary areas, and focal endothelial hyperplasia.
- **Dermal hemangiomas**: Cutaneous lesions are usually benign capillary hemangiomas and must be distinguished from atypical vascular lesions occurring in skin after radiation treatment.

23.2.3.5 Immunohistochemistry

Endothelial cells express vascular markers like CD31, CD34, and factor VIII. Smooth muscle actin can be used to identify muscle coat. Ki-67 may be absent or low.

23.2.3.6 Differential Diagnosis

1. *Pseudoangiomatous Stromal Hyperplasia* (PASH): Pseudo vascular spaces in pseudoangiomatous stromal hyperplasia are not lined by true endothelial cells. May mimic vascular lesions due to anastomosing slit-like spaces in collagen.
2. *Angiolipoma*: Benign mass consisting of adipose tissue and small round blood vessels.

3. *Angiomatosis*: Very rare vascular lesion consisting of both blood and lymphatic vessels and presents as large palpable mass, typically >9 cm.
4. *Angiosarcoma*: Usually present as clinically apparent palpable mass with irregular border with majority >2 cm and often >5 cm in size. Low-grade masses consist of thin-walled vessels lined by flattened epithelium, and high-grade masses consist of solid sheets of epithelioid or spindle-shaped cells with marked nuclear pleomorphism.

23.2.3.7 Management

Annual follow up for 2 years is usually recommended to establish stability. In case of patients with atypical or suspicious imaging findings, image guided core biopsy is recommended to exclude the possibility of angiosarcoma.

23.2.4 Hamartoma and Pseudoangiomatous Stromal Hyperplasia: *Discussed in Detail in Chap.* 18

23.3 Malignant Mesenchymal Lesions

23.3.1 Sarcomas of the Breast

These are heterogenous group of malignant tumors of mesenchymal origin accounting for 1% of malignant breast tumors and < 5% of all sarcomas [3]. They can be either

- **Primary sarcomas** (Spontaneous)—occurring sporadically.
- **Secondary sarcomas**—Occurs as a sequalae to breast cancer treatments like external beam radiation and chronic lymphedema.

Angiosarcomas are the most common subtype of sarcomas, estimated at 20–30% of primary breast sarcomas and 50–70% of secondary breast sarcomas [4]. Other common subtypes include **malignant fibrous histiocytoma** and **fibrosarcoma**. These are aggressive tumors with poor prognosis because of local recurrence and early development of hematogenous distant metastasis.

23.3.1.1 Clinical Presentation

Primary angiosarcoma of the breast (PAB) are much rarer variant of the two. PAB occurs sporadically among young women in their third and fourth decade with no known risk factors [5]. Secondary angiosarcomas of the breast on the contrary, occurs frequently in elderly women in their sixth and seventh decade, associated with the risk factor of radiation therapy post-breast conservation surgery. An average latency period of about 7–10 years is observed between the radiation therapy and the development of secondary angiosarcoma [5].

Primary and secondary breast sarcomas usually present as a solitary, rapidly enlarging breast lump, with pain reported in 7–21% [6]. Associated skin thickening and nipple retraction can be seen, especially with angiosarcomas, which are more infiltrative. Sarcomas tend to grow larger than primary carcinomas with a median size of approximately 5 cm [7].

23.3.1.2 Imaging Features

Imaging findings in sarcoma vary and may depend on histologic subtype.

- **Mammogram**: Iso- to hyperdense mass with well-defined or ill-defined margins or architectural distortion without associated calcifications. About 19% of the angiosarcomas have negative mammogram [6].
- **USG**: Hypoechoic, round to oval mass with indistinct margins, internal vascularity, and variable posterior features (Fig. 23.4a–c).
- **MRI**: A heterogeneous mass that is hypointense on T1-weighted and intermediate to hyperintense on T2-weighted images. High-grade tumors show more rapid enhancement with washout kinetics in dynamic contrast enhanced MRI (Fig. 23.5).

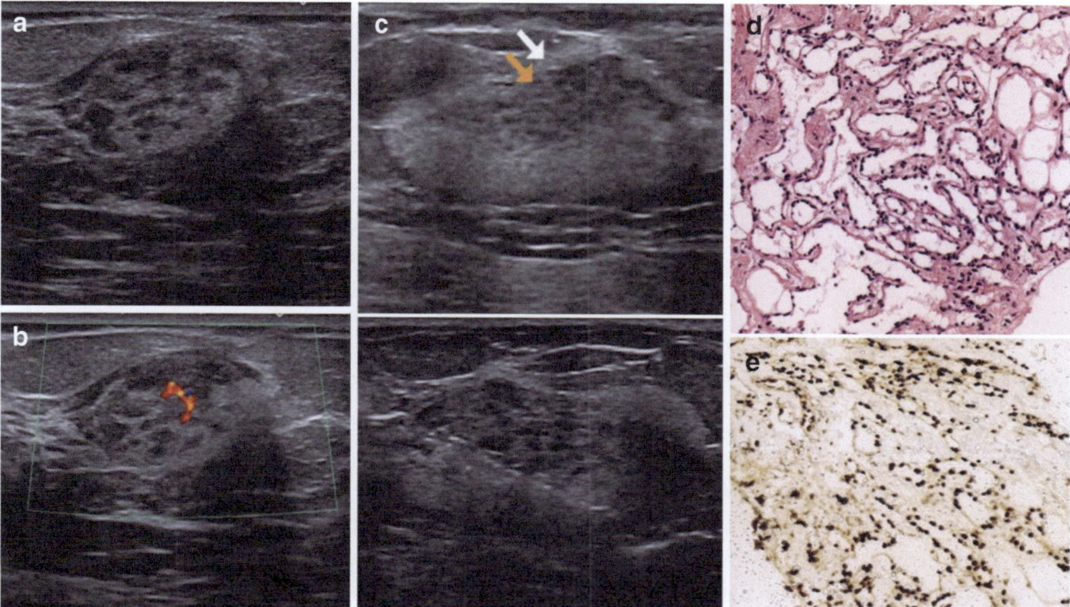

Fig. 23.4 A 38-year-old lactating women with biopsy proven primary angiosarcoma. High-resolution transverse ultrasound image of the right breast shows a well-circumscribed mixed echogenic lesion (**a**) with hypoechoic areas within (arrows). On color Doppler, lesion shows minimal internal vascularity (**b**). USG-guided core needle biopsy (CNB) image shows needle within the right breast lesion in (**c**). H&E: Shows multiple vascular channels with plump endothelial cells showing nuclear atypia (×100) (**d**). Immunohistochemistry of the sample shows ERG-1 positive nuclear staining along the endothelial cells (**e**)

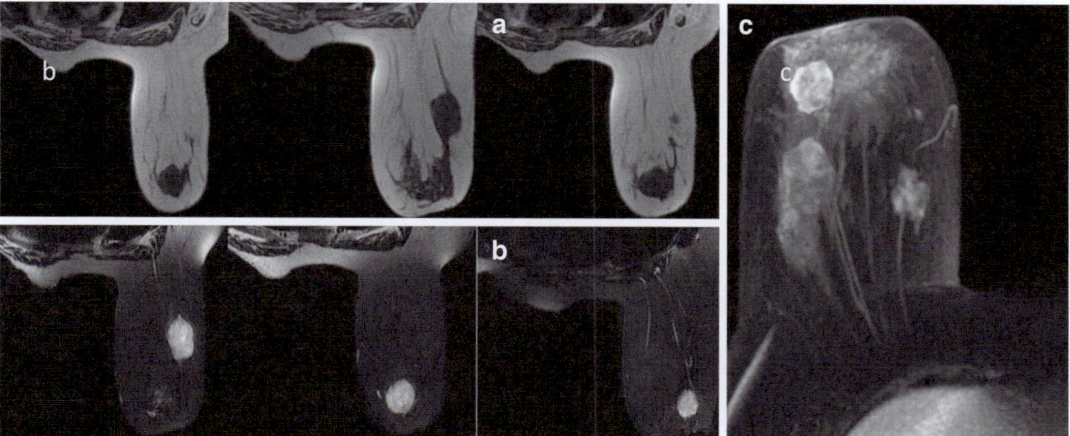

Fig. 23.5 MRI breast with contrast of the 35-year-old lactating woman with biopsy proven primary angiosarcoma. Axial MRI sections of right breast shows three discrete masses which are homogenously T1 hypointense (**a**) and T2 hyperintense (**b**) and shows rapid marked post-contrast enhancement with neovascularization in the firm of multiple feeding arteries from the chest wall in the Molecular Inversion Probe (MIP) sequence (**c**)

Table 23.2 Histological grading of angiosarcoma

Feature	Low grade	Intermediate grade	High grade
Nuclear Pleomorphism	Minimal	Intermediate	Marked
Blood lakes	Absent	Absent	Present
Necrosis	Absent	Absent	Present
Mitosis	Absent	Absent	Frequent
Solid foci	Absent or rare	Present focally	Present

23.3.1.3 Histopathology

Gross

Most of the sarcoma tumors range in size from 1 to 20 cm with majority are >2 cm; average size is 5 cm. Central portion of tumor may be hemorrhagic, myxoid, calcified, or may show lipomatous changes with firm to hard on palpation. Infiltrative periphery of tumor can blend into surrounding tissue and may not be visible. Necrosis may or may not be present depending on the pathological kind of sarcoma.

Microscopy

1. **Angiosarcoma** [8]: Abnormal, anastomosing vascular channels with infiltrative borders and not well circumscribed (Fig. 23.4d, e).In poorly differentiated tumors, solid areas without evident of vessel formation may be present. Blood lakes due to massive extravasation from tumor vessels are helpful diagnostic feature. Tumor cells are abnormal in appearance with pleomorphic nuclei, and frequent mitotic figures may be seen. The histological grading of angiosarcoma are briefed in Table 23.2.
2. **Liposarcoma** [9]: All grades of liposarcoma have been reported arising in breast as primary tumor. Low-grade tumors and myxoid variant more common than pleomorphic variant in most series, and the low-grade tumors have more favorable outcome compared with pleomorphic variants. The tumor cells include lipoblasts and other atypical appearing adipocytic cells. Liposarcomatous heterologous differentiation can be seen more often in phyllodes tumor rather than in primary sarcomas. Diagnosis of primary liposarcoma of breast is one of exclusion and must be distinguished from lipomas.
3. **Leiomyosarcoma (LMS)** [10]: Intersecting bundles of spindle cells with eosinophilic cytoplasm and elongated nuclei with blunt ends and varying degrees of pleomorphism with mitotic activity. Morphologic and immune histochemical findings are like LMS arising in other sites. Immunohistochemistry shows positivity for keratin in some tumors.
4. **Extra skeletal osteogenic sarcoma (OGS)** [11]: Extra skeletal OGS rarely arises in breast. All histologic variants, including fibroblastic, osteoblastic, chondroblast, and telangiectatic, have been reported. It is a high-grade, mitotically active tumor, which tends to have worse outcome. Extra skeletal OGS of breast is a diagnosis of exclusion. Osteogenic differentiation can be seen in metaplastic carcinoma and phyllodes tumor and may be prominent.
5. **Pleomorphic spindle cell sarcoma** [12]: Some tumors in this category have been classified as fibrosarcomas or malignant fibrous histiocytoma. It is a malignant spindle cell proliferation arranged in herringbone or storiform pattern. These tumors tend to be high grade with frequent mitotic activity and areas of necrosis. These may arise at site of prior breast radiation. It is important to exclude metaplastic carcinoma and malignant phyllodes tumor. Tumor cells should be cytokeratin (−) (including high molecular weight keratins) and p63 (−).
6. **Sarcomas in adolescents and children** [12]: Rarely, rhabdomyosarcomas and synovial sarcomas can involve breast in younger patients. It may represent primary or metastatic disease. Primary tumors are usually alveolar rhabdomyosarcoma.

23.3.1.4 Immunohistochemistry

Lineage-specific markers are helpful to identify the specific types of sarcomas: for angiosarcoma, the vascular markers; leiomyosarcoma, the smooth muscle markers (smooth muscle actin, desmin, caldesmon); rhabdomyosarcoma, the skeletal muscle markers (desmin, myogenin, myoglobin); and malignant peripheral nerve sheath tumors (S100). Keratins are used to exclude carcinoma.

23.3.1.5 Differential Diagnosis

1. *Metaplastic carcinoma*: Subsets of these carcinomas show features characteristic of myoepithelial cells. Spindle cell morphology ± squamous differentiation is presented with matrix (basement membrane) formation. The matrix can resemble cartilage or osteoid. Extensive sampling to detect areas of epithelial differentiation and/or ductal carcinoma in situ (DCIS) can help exclude sarcoma. Carcinomas are important to be distinguished from sarcoma. Nodes are evaluated for carcinomas. Panel of immune stains for cytokeratin (particularly high molecular weight) and p63 are important to help confirm diagnosis.
2. *Phyllodes tumor*: High-grade phyllodes tumors can have areas of heterologous differentiation like liposarcoma, rhabdomyosarcoma, or osteogenic sarcoma, which may be seen. Extensive sampling looking for biphasic pattern can help to identify phyllodes tumor.
3. *Fibromatosis*: More common in breast than sarcomas. Can invade into normal tissue, into skeletal muscle, and around nerves. Minimal nuclear pleomorphism and absence of mitoses distinguish fibromatosis from sarcoma.
4. *Nodular fasciitis*: Usually in superficial location or in muscle fascia. Cells have haphazard arrangement, whereas malignant spindle cell tumors usually grow in organized fascicular patterns. Minimal to no nuclear pleomorphism with fine chromatin and atypical mitotic figures should not be seen.
5. *Dermatofibrosarcoma protuberans*: Spindle cell neoplasm arise in dermis and infiltrate into subcutaneous tissue. Dermal-based lesions can invade into breast. Spindle cells are arranged in storiform pattern with minimal pleomorphism and rare mitoses.
6. *Myofibroblastoma*: It is a benign neoplastic proliferation of myofibroblasts with minimal nuclear pleomorphism and does not infiltrate around normal breast epithelium.

23.4 Secondary Sarcoma [13]

This arises after radiation. The most common is angiosarcoma followed by undifferentiated sarcomas. Postradiation angiosarcomas occur primarily in skin. The criteria for defining postradiation sarcoma is histological confirmation of sarcoma and prior history of RT in setting of chronic lymphedema. Chronic edema increases risk of sarcoma at multiple sites (Fig. 23.6). For Stewart-Treves syndromes, one of the components is angiosarcoma of edematous arm. Lymphedema-associated lymphangiosarcoma can also occur very rarely.

Management of breast sarcomas: The management of sarcoma in the breast is similar to any other sarcomas elsewhere in the body. Computed tomography (CT) whole body/ Positron emission tomography (PET)-CT is recommended to rule out distant metastasis as they commonly metastasize to lungs. Though primary sarcomas have better prognosis than secondary, management of these are essentially the same. Breast conserving surgery is recommended in all variants except angiosarcoma in which achieving negative margins is difficult. Surgery is usually followed by chemotherapy and radiotherapy. Axillary clearance is not recommended as sarcomas have hematogenous metastasis, and lymphadenopathy usually are reactive in nature on sentinel node biopsies. Prognosis of sarcoma depend on histological grade, tumor size (<5 cm good prognosis), and surgical margins. Angiosarcoma, overall, has poor prognosis.

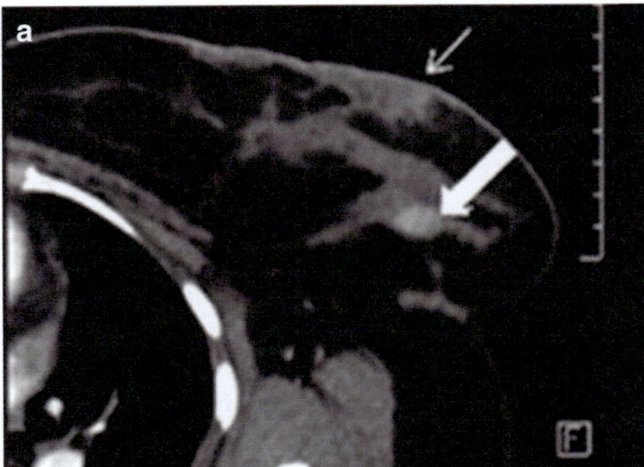

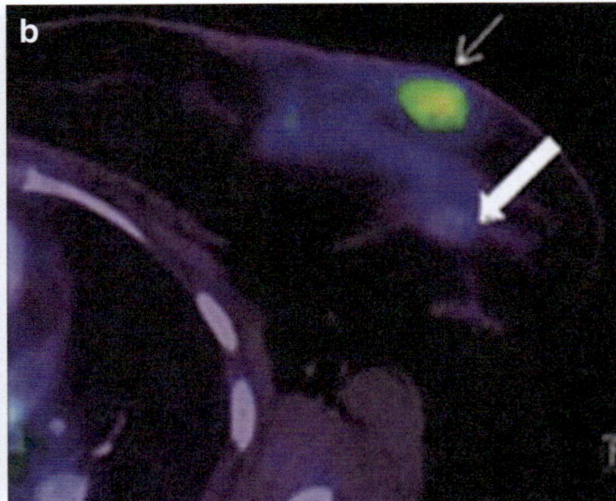

Fig. 23.6 Fluorodeoxyglucose (FDG) PET-CT in the 68 year who had postradiation-associated secondary angiosarcoma after wide local excision and RT for angiosarcoma 5 years back. (**a**, **b**) shows the focal thickening and soft tissue edema with stranding (thin arrow), which is FDG avid. The prominent axillary nodes are non-avid (thick arrow)

23.4.1 Sarcomatous Metastasis to Breast

Metastasis to the breast is rare and accounts for about 1–2% of all breast malignancies [14]. Though sarcomatous metastasis make the most of the breast metastasis, it is extremely rare. The most common extramammary sarcoma that metastasize to breast is rhabdomyosarcoma (often in adolescents). Other sarcomas that metastasize to breast are osteosarcoma, leiomyosarcoma, and liposarcoma.

23.4.1.1 Clinical Presentation

Sarcomatous metastasis to breast is mostly seen in young women (due to abundant blood supply). It presents as painless solitary mass, most times discovered incidentally on staging imaging. It can be bilateral, multiple, and most commonly, in the upper outer quadrant. Prior history of sarcoma at another site is generally available.

23.4.1.2 Imaging Features

Though they have distinct imaging features, they can be mistaken for benign entities like fibroadenoma.

- **Mammogram**: Circumscribed, round to oval, iso- to hyper- dense mass without associated calcifications.
- **USG**: Presents as hypoechoic masses with micro-lobulated to circumscribed margins and posterior acoustic enhancement. On color Doppler, they appear hypervascular.
- **MRI**: They are often isointense to normal breast tissue on both T1- and T2-weighted. They show rapid homogeneous early enhancement and variable delayed kinetics with contrast administration.

> **NOTE**: Coarse calcifications are specific for metastasis from osteosarcoma.

Management: Poor prognosis and the treatment depends on the extent of metastasis in the breast and primary sarcoma histological grade.

23.5 Miscellaneous Benign Mesenchymal Masses of the Breast

23.5.1 Granular Cell Tumors (GCT)

These are neoplastic proliferations, likely from Schwann cells, which can occur throughout the body and often in oropharynx, skin and subcutaneous tissue, and gastrointestinal tissues. Approximately 5–6% of cases are found in the breast, predominantly among premenopausal women with women-to-men ratio of 9:1 and more commonly among African-Americans [15]. GCTs comprise 0.1% of breast cancers [16].

23.5.1.1 Clinical Presentation

They present as palpable, often superficial lumps with associated skin thickening and retraction, mimicking breast cancers.

23.5.1.2 Imaging Features

They have nonspecific and frequently appear suspicious on imaging requiring core biopsy for tissue characterization.

- **Mammogram**: This can present as noncalcified high-density masses, often with indistinct margins.
- **USG**: It has variable appearance as in mammogram, can present as hypoechoic mass with variable posterior features, and may demonstrate increased vascularity on Doppler.
- **MRI**: Homogeneous masses, low to intermediate intensity on T1W and peripheral high signal on T2W images with peripheral enhancement.

BI-RADS Category: BI-RADS 4 (Suspicious) and requires USG guided core biopsy.

23.5.1.3 Histopathology

Gross: Presents as palpable, white to yellow, firm to hard mass closely resembling invasive carcinoma with borders that may be circumscribed, ill-defined, or irregular.

Microscopy

Solid proliferation of tumor cells infiltrating as cohesive sheets or small nests. Infiltration into adjacent connective tissue creates spiculated margins. Cells are rounded or spindle-shaped with abundant eosinophilic granular cytoplasm (Fig. 23.7). Granules are PAS (+) and diastase resistant. Nuclei are uniform in size and shape, small and oval with minimal pleomorphism. Majority are benign; however, 1–3% of lesions are malignant.

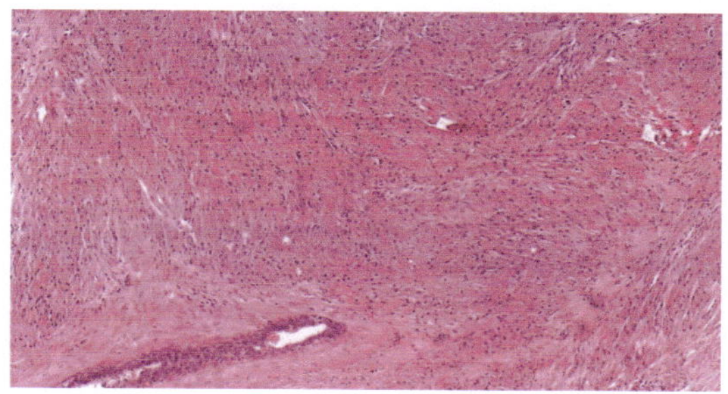

Fig. 23.7 H&E: Tumor cells are spindle-shaped with abundant eosinophilic granular cytoplasm (×200)

Immunohistochemistry

It has strong positive immunoreactivity of S100 in nucleus and cytoplasm, which supports peripheral nerve sheath origin. Calretinin may be positive.

CD68 will be positive in the intracytoplasmic phagolysosomes. Inhibin-α/Neuron specific enolase may also be positive. Hormone receptors will be negative.

Electron Microscopy

Granules seen by light microscopy correspond to numerous lysosomes.

23.5.1.4 Differential Diagnosis

1. *Benign inflammatory lesions*: Histiocytes and granular cells can be similar in appearance. The cause of histiocytic infiltrate is usually apparent and most seen in ruptured cysts or fat necrosis.
2. *Invasive carcinoma*: Carcinomas with apocrine or histiocytoid features can resemble GCT.
3. *Metastatic tumors*: Melanomas are most common type of metastasis to breast. Renal cell carcinoma may also have granular cytoplasm, but metastasis to the breast is very rare.
4. *Alveolar soft part sarcoma*: Originally named malignant granular cell myoblastoma, as it was thought to be malignant counterpart to GCT. Rare type of sarcoma that would be highly unusual in breast. Cells are dyscohesive in clustered pseudo- alveolar pattern and have distinct PAS (+) crystalline structures in cytoplasm. It is negative for cytokeratin, HMB-45, and S100 in majority of cases.

23.5.1.5 Management

Wide local excision is recommended because of its infiltrative nature. Recurrence may occur if the mass is not completely excised.

23.5.2 Myofibroblastoma

These are rare, benign stromal tumors containing myofibroblasts with genetic alteration in chromosome 13q [17].

23.5.2.1 Clinical Presentation

Most commonly present in the fifth to sixth decade with slight male predominance. This presents as unilateral painless, well-defined, mobile mass. It can exhibit rapid growth pattern.

23.5.2.2 Imaging Features

It has nonspecific imaging features.

- **Mammogram**: well-circumscribed, round or ovoid, non-calcified masses.
- **USG**: well- circumscribed, solid, heterogeneously or homogeneously hypoechoic masses with variable posterior features (Fig. 23.8). At times, they may exhibit hypervascularity in color doppler with ill-defined margins.
- **MRI**: show low signal intensity on T1-weighted and high signal intensity on T2-weighted images, with homogeneous enhancement, internal septations, and washout kinetics.

BI-RADS Category: BI-RADS 3 or 4, depending on the margin characteristics and warrants biopsy.

23.5.2.3 Histopathology

Gross

Well-circumscribed, most are <4 cm lobulated mass with firm or rubbery consistency. Surface is pink-tan, homogeneous whorled or nodular appearance.

Microscopy [18]

It has well-circumscribed borders tending to compress normal breast parenchyma at periphery with no true capsule and no entrapment of ducts and/or lobules within tumor with haphazardly arranged intersecting fascicles of spindle cells interrupted by thick bands of brightly eosinophilic hyalinized collagen (Fig. 23.9). There is

Fig. 23.8 High-resolution transverse USG image of right breast shows round heterogeneously hypoechoic mass with posterior acoustic enhancement. Biopsy confirmed myofibroblastoma

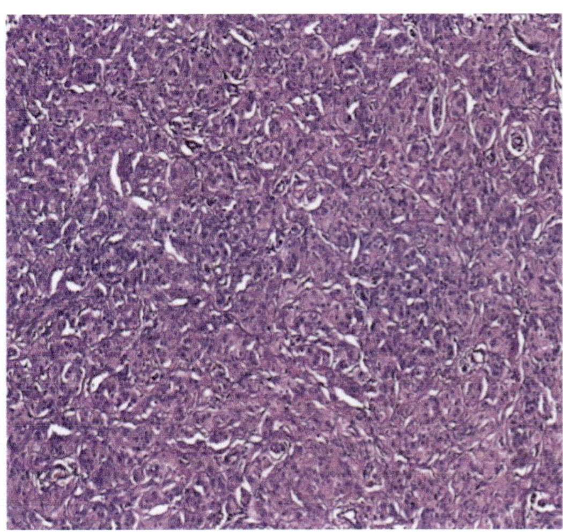

Fig. 23.9 H&E: Haphazardly arranged intersecting fascicles of spindle cells interrupted by thick bands of brightly eosinophilic hyalinized collagen (×400)

uniform spindle cell proliferation with scant pale cytoplasm and ovoid uniform nuclei with inconspicuous/absent nucleoli. Necrosis is not present.

Immunohistochemistry

CD34, Smooth Muscle Actin, Bcl2, Desmin, hormone receptors (ER, PR, Her2neu), and STAT6 shows positivity. There is variable positivity for CD99 and CD10. S100 (−ve) and there will also be loss of Rb in these lesions.

23.5.2.4 Differential Diagnosis

1. *Spindle cell lipoma*: More abundant adipose tissue compared to MFB generally negative for muscle markers and shares the loss of same region at 13q14 with loss of expression of Rb.
2. *Solitary fibrous tumor*: Clinical and morphologic overlap with MFB. Typically, positive for STAT 6 and negative for muscle markers and hormone receptors. Has characteristic NAB2-STAT6 gene fusion (12q13).
3. *Leiomyoma*: May arise from smooth muscle of areola or from blood vessels. CD34 is generally negative in leiomyoma and positive in MFB.
4. *Fibromatosis*: Highly infiltrative lesions with lymphocytic infiltrate at border of lesion. CD34 and hormone receptors are negative with nuclear β-catenin positivity, which is supportive but not entirely specific for fibromatosis.
5. *Nodular fasciitis*: Infiltrative borders and like fibromatosis, nodular fasciitis is negative for CD34. There should be diagnosis of exclusion after other spindle cell lesions have been ruled out.
6. *Spindle cell sarcoma*: Sarcomas of breast are very rare and are usually high-grade invasive tumor with infiltrating borders.
7. *Spindle cell metaplastic carcinoma*: Invasive carcinoma consisting entirely or predominantly of spindle cells. DCIS may be present but is typically absent or scant. Immunohistochemistry is helpful for diagnosis.
8. *Invasive lobular carcinoma*: Circumscribed borders with spindle tumor cells with absence of LCIS and tumor cells which do not invade around normal structures should raise the possibility of myofibroblastoma.

23.5.2.5 Management

Requires fine needle aspiration/core biopsy for tissue diagnosis. Interval follow up with imaging is preferred over surgical excision [19].

23.5.3 Fibromatosis

Also known as **Desmoid tumor**, it is a rare benign infiltrating spindle cell tumor accounting for <0.2% of all breast tumors [20]. Most often occurs sporadically, but it may occur in association with prior trauma or surgery and sometimes associated with Gardner's syndrome. Sporadic cases are also associated with mutations in APC gene (20%) or β-catenin gene (50%).

23.5.3.1 Clinical Presentation

Frequently seen in women of age 37–50 years. Clinically, they present like malignant lesion as firm palpable mass with skin retraction, dimpling with invasion into pectoralis muscle sometimes.

23.5.3.2 Imaging Features

- **Mammogram**: They appear as irregular, speculated noncalcified mass.
- **USG**: irregular hypoechoic mass with no significant vascularity on color doppler.
- **MRI**: appears isointense on T1-weighted images and heterogeneously hyperintense on T2-weighted images. Based on tumor cellularity and myxoid component, shows variable enhancement kinetics in dynamic contrast sequences.

BI-RADS Category: BI-RADS 4 (suspicious) and warrants tissue biopsy.

23.5.3.3 Histopathology

Gross [21]

Firm to rubbery white mass with circumscribed or irregular borders and size ranging from 1 to >10 cm.

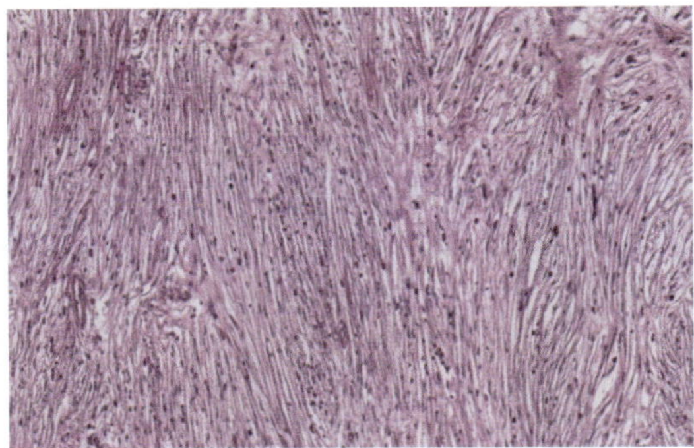

Fig. 23.10 H&E Long fascicles of spindle cells with bland nuclei (×400)

Microscopy

Long fascicles of spindle cells that infiltrate around normal ducts and lobules and may infiltrate into muscle (Fig. 23.10). Cells are bland, and mitoses are absent or rare with lymphocytic aggregates at periphery of tumor.

Immunohistochemistry: There is aberrant nuclear β-catenin positivity and absence of CD34 in majority.

23.5.3.4 Differential Diagnosis

1. *Myofibroblastoma*: Benign neoplasm of myofibroblasts. Cells are positive for CD34, muscle markers, and estrogen and progesterone receptors.
2. *Nodular Fasciitis*: Clinical history should be of rapidly growing painful mass. Tumor cells are usually haphazardly arranged and not in long fascicles. Like fibromatosis, cells are negative for CD34 and can be positive for muscle markers, and unlike fibromatosis, cells are negative for nuclear β-catenin.
3. *Pseudoangiomatous stromal hyperplasia*: Reactive lesion of myofibroblasts. Cells are short and rarely form well-defined fascicles.
4. *Phyllodes tumor*: Tumors with stromal overgrowth and infiltration into surrounding breast tissue can closely resemble fibromatosis with nuclear pleomorphism, and mitoses are usually present. The lesion is positive for CD34.
5. *Spindle cell carcinoma*: Fibromatosis-like metaplastic carcinoma can closely resemble fibromatosis.
6. *Sarcoma*: Most sarcomas are highly cellular and generally have markedly pleomorphic nuclei. Mitoses are usually present and may be atypical. Histologic features of specific sarcoma types may be present (e.g., liposarcoma, rhabdomyosarcoma, osteosarcoma).

23.5.3.5 Management

Due to their suspicious imaging features, core biopsy is required with wide local excision with negative margins. Recurrence occurs in about 27% of cases [20].

23.5.4 Schwannoma

Breast schwannomas are more common in woman.

23.5.4.1 Clinical Presentation

Presents as benign appearing smooth mobile palpable masses or incidentally found on imaging.

23.5.4.2 Imaging Features

Shows benign imaging features; appearing as well-circumscribed oval or round high-density mass on **mammogram** (Fig. 23.11a); on **USG**, they appear as circumscribed hypoechoic solid mass with cystic spaces within (Fig. 23.11b); on **MRI**, these are heterogeneously hyperintense on T2-weighted images and isointense on T1-weighted images with intense contrast enhancement.

23.5.4.3 Histopathology

Gross

The circumscribed tumor consists of dense, firm gray or white tissue, which may have soft mucoid regions.

Microscopy

Microscopic examination of a schwannoma reveals the typical histological features of a benign nerve sheath tumor, consisting of spindle cells in bundles, sometimes with nuclei arranged in a palisading pattern (Antoni type A). The

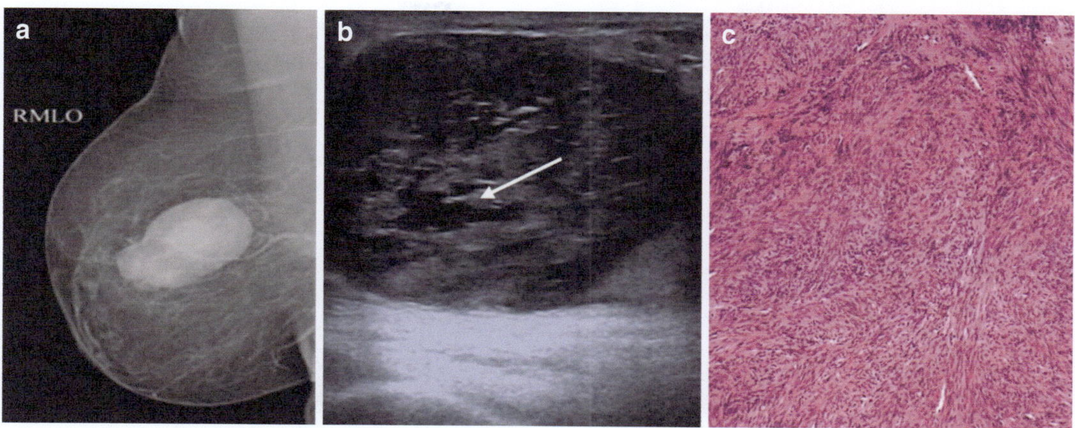

Fig. 23.11 A 55-year-old woman with schwannoma. MLO view mammogram of the right breast shows a oval high-density mass in the upper breast (**a**). On ultrasound, it appears as Oval complex lesion with cystic space within (**b**) H&E: Spindle cells in bundles, with nuclei arranged in a palisading pattern (×200) (**c**)

Antoni B pattern may be present as well (Fig. 23.11c). Vascular thrombi, hyalinized blood vessels, cells with atypical nuclei, and xanthomatous areas can also be seen.

Immunohistochemistry

Schwannomas tend to demonstrate more diffuse expression of S100 protein.

23.5.4.4 Differential Diagnosis

1. *Neurofibroma*: It demonstrates delicate spindle cells with wavy, dark nuclei. Set within a background of ropy collagen. Myxoid change may be present.
2. *Fibroadenoma,* phyllodes tumor, fibromatosis, and metaplastic carcinoma: These lesions are usually readily distinguished in histologic sections. The nuclei of cells seeing the aspirate from a benign neural tumor are typically spindly or oval with homogeneous fine chromatin. The diagnosis of a benign peripheral nerve sheath tumors supported by a positive immune-histochemical stain for S-\100 protein, a negative immunostain for actin, and the absence of mitotic activity.

Management: It is usually treated conservatively.

23.5.5 Neurofibroma

These are benign peripheral nerve sheath tumors, commonly associated with Nneurofibromatosis (NF-I) especially if located in the breast.

23.5.5.1 Etiopathogenesis

Mutations in neurofibromin (NF1) lead to loss of function of the NF1 protein, which regulates cell proliferation via mTOR and via inactivation of p21 (ras), a proto-oncogene protein. The majority of neurofibromas involving the breast occur in patients with NF1, which is due to autosomal dominant mutations in the NF1 gene, which encodes the protein neurofibromin (NF1). CDKIV2A/CDKIV2B losses are found in tumors diagnosed as atypical neurofibromas in patients with NF1, suggesting that such tumors may be pre-malignant lesions.

23.5.5.2 Clinical Presentation

Multiple cutaneous, painless, frequently peri-areolar, or parenchymal masses that may be palpable or incidental on imaging.

23.5.5.3 Imaging Features

On **mammogram**—circumscribed, homogeneously dense masses with a surrounding rim of air density if cutaneous. On **USG**—hypoechoic with posterior acoustic enhancement, similar to fibroadenomas. On **MRI**—low to intermediate signal intensity on T1-weighted and high signal intensity on T2-weighted images with internal heterogeneity.

23.5.5.4 Histopathology

Gross

Neurofibromas of the breast have a variable appearance; they can be solitary and well circumscribed or multinodular and poorly defined.

Microscopy [22]

Neurofibromas are composed in large part of neoplastic Schwann cells with thin, curved to fusiform nuclei and scant cytoplasm, as well as fibroblasts in a variably collagenous and myxoid matrix. Prominent mast cells with laminated, round, eosinophilic structures (pseudo-Meissner corpuscles) are also seen.

Atypical neurofibroma is a subtype defined with high cellularity, scattered mitotic figures, and/or fascicular growth in addition to cytological atypia, and it is difficult to distinguish from low-grade malignant peripheral nerve sheath tumor.

Immunohistochemistry

A proportion of spindled cells express S100 and SO × 10, in contrast to the diffuse labeling seen in schwannomas. Scattered cells, presumably of perineurial origin may show GLUTl and claudin positivity. EMA typically highlights the residual perineurium. CD34 stains a subset of stromal cells, whereas KIT (CD117) highlights mast cells. Loss of pl6 (CDKN2A) expression in cytologically atypical nuclei is an important finding for atypical neurofibroma and distinguishes it from ancient-type change. Neurofibromas are negative for cytokeratins, EP, actin, and desmin.

23.5.5.5 Differential Diagnosis

1. Schwannoma
2. Low grade malignant peripheral sheath tumor

Management: Usually treated conservatively. However, it may require serial imaging follow-up since sarcomatous transformation have been reported when associated with NF-I.

23.5.6 Leiomyoma

Benign tumors of smooth muscle origin, rarely present in the breast but are more commonly seen in nipple-areolar complex than in the parenchyma. If present in breast parenchyma its only seen in females, whereas leiomyomas of nipple are seen in both sexes.

23.5.6.1 Clinical Presentation

Parenchymal lesions—as palpable masses which are tender sometimes. Nipple lesions—presents with skin changes and pruritis.

23.5.6.2 Imaging Features

Shows benign imaging features mostly. On **mammogram**—well-circumscribed non-calcified lesion; on **USG**—appear as circumscribed, homogeneously hypoechoic mass. On **MRI**—low signal intensity on T1-weighted images, low to intermediate intensity on T2-weighted images, and homogeneous enhancement.

23.5.6.3 Gross

In contrast to the poorly defined superficial lesions, deep (parenchymal) lesions are well circumscribed. The neoplasm is firm, rubbery, and grey to tan, with a whorled cut surface. Superficial lesions are commonly smaller than deep-seated ones.

23.5.6.4 Microscopy [23]

The histopathology and immune phenotype of these lesions are identical to those of smooth muscle tumors elsewhere in the body. The spindle cells have elongated cigar-shaped nuclei and eosinophilic cytoplasm. Focal degenerative cytological atypia may be seen, but mitotic figures are absent. Lesions within the parenchyma are (multi) nodular and well circumscribed. This consist of intersecting fascicles of elongated smooth muscle cells with or without slight degenerative atypia. Mitotic activity is usually absent or low.

23.5.6.5 Immunohistochemistry

Immunohistochemical markers (SMA and desmin) may be used to confirm a smooth muscle phenotype.

Differential diagnosis: Myoid hamartoma, Fibromatosis, Fibroadenoma, Benign phyllodes tumors, Myofibroblastoma, Leiomyosarcoma.

Management: Local recurrence and malignant transformation is very rare in breast. Hence, managed conservatively with serial imaging follow up.

23.5.7 Inflammatory Myofibroblastic Tumor: (IMT)

Considered as subset of **inflammatory pseudotumor (IPT)**. These are extremely rare lesions in the breast.

Pathogenesis: About two-thirds of inflammatory myofibroblastic tumors harbor receptor tyrosine kinase gene rearrangements, most often involving the ALK (anaplastic lymphoma kinase) locus at 2p23, with diverse fusion partners pointing toward the cancerous behavior.

Clinical feature: Unlike IMT/IPT of other organs (like lungs) which most commonly occurs in young patients, IMT of breast occurs in relatively old patients >40 years of age as palpable masses.

Imaging Features [24]: Nonspecific imaging features and may present as suspicious lesion.

- **Mammography**: It can present as irregular soft tissue mass with obscured boundaries.
- **USG**: It presents solid irregular hypoechoic mass with unclear boundaries showing marginal vascularity on color Doppler.
- **MRI**: It presents irregular soft tissue mass, which shows rapid uneven enhancement curve in dynamic contrast MRI.

23.5.7.1 Histopathology

Gross [25]

Most tumors are <5 cm in size, with white to grey, and sometimes yellow cut surfaces.

Microscopy

Loose fascicles of uniform, plump spindle cells with vesicular chromatin, small nucleoli, and pale eosinophilic to amphophilic cytoplasm are typically observed. The stroma may be myxoid or collagenous, usually containing an inflammatory infiltrate dominated by lymphocytes and plasma cells, with fewer eosinophils and neutrophils. Mitotic activity is low, and necrosis is usually absent.

Immunohistochemistry

Inflammatory myofibroblastic tumors are nearly always positive for SMA, and more than half of cases are also positive for desmin. About 60% of inflammatory myofibroblastic tumors express ALK (usually with a diffuse cytoplasmic pattern).

BI-RADS category: **BI-RADS 4a**.

Management: Since an IMT of the breast can mimic or even behave as true malignancy, wide excision with negative margins is highly recommended as local recurrence and metastasis has been reported in few cases.

23.5.8 Myxoma

Myxomas are benign tumors, with very few cases described in the breast. Few have been reported as sporadic or in association with Carney complex, a rare autosomal-dominant syndrome defined by cardiac and extracardiac myxomas and skin pigmentation.

Clinical Features: presents as palpable, nontender masses found incidentally on mammogram.

Imaging findings: nonspecific and not well documented.

23.5.8.1 Histopathology

Gross

Tumors range in size from 1.5 to 8 cm. They are well circumscribed with gray-white, gelatinous cut surfaces. Occasional tumors are multinodular.

Microscopy [26]
Microscopic examination reveals hypocellular myxoid neoplastic tissue containing bland stellate and spindle-shaped undifferentiated mesenchymal cells without mitotic activity. The myxoid material is positive with Alcian blue at pH 2.5, and positivity is lost after hyaluronidase digestion. The myxoid stroma is also positive for colloidal iron and negative with the PAS stain.

Immunohistochemistry: The tumor cells are positive for vimentin. They may demonstrate focal immunoreactivity for actin and calponin. The tumor cells are negative for CD34, CD99, CD117, CD10, alpha 1 antitrypsin, desmin, myogenin, EMA, CK, p63, ER, and PR.

Management: Tissue diagnosis is necessary. Considering reports of local recurrence, malignant transformation, and challenges in differentiation from malignant lesions on core histology, wide local excision is recommended for definitive management.

Differential diagnosis: Myxoid fibroadenoma, Myxoid stromal change (myxomatosis), myxoid neurofibromas, myxoid myofibroblastoma, mucinosis.

References

1. Kryvenko ON, Chitale DA, Van Egmond EM, Gupta NS, Schultz D, Lee MW. Angiolipoma of the female breast: clinicomorphological correlation of 52 cases. Int J Surg Pathol. 2011;19(1):35–43.
2. Brodie C, Provenzano E. Vascular proliferations of the breast. Histopathology. 2008;52(1):30–44.
3. Smith TB, Gilcrease MZ, Santiago L, Hunt KK, Yang WT. Imaging features of primary breast sarcoma. Am J Roentgenol. 2012;198(4):W386–93.
4. Yin M, Wang W, Drabick JJ, Harold HA. Prognosis and treatment of non-metastatic primary and secondary breast angiosarcoma: a comparative study. BMC Cancer. 2017;17(1):295.
5. Arora TK, Terracina KP, Soong J, Idowu MO, Takabe K. Primary and secondary angiosarcoma of the breast. Gland Surg. 2014;3(1):28–34.
6. Yang WT, Hennessy BTJ, Dryden MJ, Valero V, Hunt KK, Krishnamurthy S. Mammary Angiosarcomas: imaging findings in 24 patients. Radiology. 2007;242(3):725–34.
7. Wienbeck S, Meyer HJ, Herzog A, Nemat S, Teifke A, Heindel W, et al. Imaging findings of primary breast sarcoma: results of a first multicenter study. Eur J Radiol. 2017;88:1–7.
8. Frey JD, Levine PG, Darvishian F, Shapiro RL. Angiosarcoma of the breast masquerading as Hemangioma: exploring clinical and pathological diagnostic challenges. Arch Plast Surg. 2015;42(2):261–3.
9. Mazaki T, Tanak T, Suenaga Y, Tomioka K, Takayama T. Liposarcoma of the breast: a case report and review of the literature. Int Surg. 1981;87:164–70.
10. Cameron HM, Hamperl H, Warambo W. Leiomyosarcoma of the breast originating from myothelium (myoepithelium). J Pathol. 1974;114(2):89–92.
11. Trihia H, Valavanis C, Markidou S, Condylis D, Poulianou E, Arapantoni-Dadioti P. Primary osteogenic sarcoma of the breast: cytomorphologic study of 3 cases with histologic correlation. Acta Cytol. 2007;51(3):443–50.
12. Adem C, Reynolds C, Ingle JN, Nascimento AG. Primary breast sarcoma: clinicopathologic series from the mayo clinic and review of the literature. Br J Cancer. 2004;91(2):237–41.
13. des Guetz G, Chapelier A, Mosseri V, Dorval T, Asselain B, Pouillart P. Postirradiation sarcoma: clinicopathologic features and role of chemotherapy in the treatment strategy. Sarcoma. 2009;2009:764379. https://www.ncbi.nlm.nih.gov/pmc/articles/PMC2790134/.
14. Sippo DA, Kulkarni K, Carlo PD, Lee B, Eisner D, Cimino-Mathews A, et al. Metastatic disease to the breast from extramammary malignancies: a multimodality pictorial review. Curr Probl Diagn Radiol. 2016;45(3):225–32.
15. Irshad A, Pope TL, Ackerman SJ, Panzegrau B. Characterization of sonographic and mammographic features of granular cell tumors of the breast and estimation of their incidence. J Ultrasound Med. 2008;27(3):467.
16. Al-Balas M, De Leo A, Serra M, Santini D, Taffurelli M. Granular cell tumour of the breast: a rare presentation of a breast mass in an elderly female with a subsequent breast cancer diagnosis. SAGE Open Med Case Rep. 2019;7:2050313X19841154. https://www.ncbi.nlm.nih.gov/pmc/articles/PMC6457014/.
17. Howitt BE, Fletcher CDM. Mammary-type myofibroblastoma: clinicopathologic characterization in a series of 143 cases. Am J Surg Pathol. 2016;40(3):361–7.
18. Salomão DR, Crotty TB, Nascimento AG. Myofibroblastoma and solitary fibrous tumour of the breast: histopathologic and immunohistochemical studies. Breast. 2001;10(1):49–54.
19. Dockery WD, Singh HR, Wilentz RE. Myofibroblastoma of the male breast: imaging appearance and ultrasound-guided core biopsy diagnosis. Breast J. 2001;7(3):192–4.
20. Glazebrook KN, Reynolds CA. Mammary fibromatosis. AJR Am J Roentgenol. 2009;193(3):856–60.
21. Abdelwahab K, Hamdy O, Zaky M, Megahed N, Elbalka S, Elmetwally M, et al. Breast fibromatosis, an unusual breast disease. J Surg Case Rep. 2017;2017(12):rjx248.

22. Murat A, Kansiz F, Kabakus N, Kazez A, Ozercan R. Neurofibroma of the breast in a boy with neurofibromatosis type 1. Clin Imaging. 2004;28(6):415–7.
23. Boscaino A, Ferrara G, Orabona P, Donofrio V, Staibano S, De Rosa G. Smooth muscle tumors of the breast: clinicopathologic features of two cases. Tumori. 1994;80(3):241–5. https://core.ac.uk/display/55072504.
24. Mao X, Liu H, Du J, Yu N, Chen L, Zhang L. Imaging findings of inflammatory myofibroblastic tumor in breast: a case report. Medicine. 2018;97(32):e11804.
25. Zhao HD, Wu T, Wang JQ, Zhang WD, He XL, Bao GQ, et al. Primary inflammatory myofibroblastic tumor of the breast with rapid recurrence and metastasis: a case report. Oncol Lett. 2013;5(1):97–100.
26. Balci P, Kabakci N, Topcu I, Canda T, Güray M, Özfıdan S. Breast myxoma: radiologic and histopathologic features. Breast J. 2007;13(1):88–90.

24 Haematolymphoid Neoplasms of Breast

Sanjivanee Ingole, Leena Dennis Joseph, Bhawna Dev, and Harini Gnanavel

Abstract

Breast is a rare site for haematological malignancies, of which lymphomas account for the majority of cases. Breast lymphomas may be either primary or secondary to systemic involvement. The low prevalence, non-specific radiological imaging findings and overlap of the radiological features with benign lesions make their diagnosis difficult. However, it is vital to recognise these tumours as the treatment is mainly non-surgical in contrast to the other breast cancers.

Keywords

Breast cancer · Haematological malignancy · Lymphoma · Breast implant-associated anaplastic large cell carcinoma

S. Ingole (✉) · B. Dev · H. Gnanavel
Department of Radiology, Sri Ramachandra Institute of Higher Education and Research, Chennai, India
e-mail: bhawnadev@sriramachandra.edu.in

L. D. Joseph
Department of Pathology, Sri Ramachandra Institute of Higher Education and Research, Chennai, India

24.1 Haematological Malignancies

World Health Organization (WHO) classifies haematological malignancies as myeloid, lymphoid and histocytic/dendritic neoplasms with its various subtypes in each category according to the fourth revised edition 2016 [1]. Lymphomas, although rare, account for majority of the breast haematological malignancies with prevalence of 0.04–0.7% [2]. The low prevalence of lymphomas in breast is probably because of the sparsity of lymphoid tissue in breast [3]. These may be either Primary Breast Lymphomas (PBL), where there is no evidence of concurrent extramammary disease apart from the ipsilateral axillary lymph nodes, or secondary to systemic involvement. Secondary breast lymphoma (SBL) is the most common metastatic breast cancer accounting for 17% of all breast metastasis [4]. The low prevalence, non-specific radiological imaging findings and overlap of the radiological features with the benign lesions make their diagnosis difficult [4, 5]. However, it is vital to recognise these tumours as the treatment is non-surgical in contrast to the other breast cancers. In addition, haematolymphoid malignancies might mimic benign lesions such as fibroadenoma and hamartomas.

B. Dev, L. D. Joseph (eds.), *Holistic Approach to Breast Disease*,
https://doi.org/10.1007/978-981-99-0035-0_24

24.1.1 Clinical Features

Primary and secondary breast lymphomas exhibit similar clinical features to other breast malignancies. The median age for PBL is 60–65 years and that for SBL is 60–70 years [6, 7] with considerably higher prevalence in women. They most commonly present as palpable lump with progressive enlargement. Few of the lymphomas are associated with pain. High-grade lymphomas with diffuse parenchymal involvement show skin retraction, *peau d' orange* appearance and erythema. Palpable ipsilateral axillary lymph nodes are seen in about 40% of the patients [4]. Nipple involvement in the form of nipple retraction or discharge is uncommon. About 10% cases are bilateral, and <10% presents as multiple tumours. Bilaterality and multiplicity is more common with secondary breast lymphomas [6, 8]. Screening mammograms identify around 10% of clinically occult cases.

As a consequence of the widespread disease in secondary breast lymphoma, systemic symptoms such as night sweats, fever and weight loss are more common.

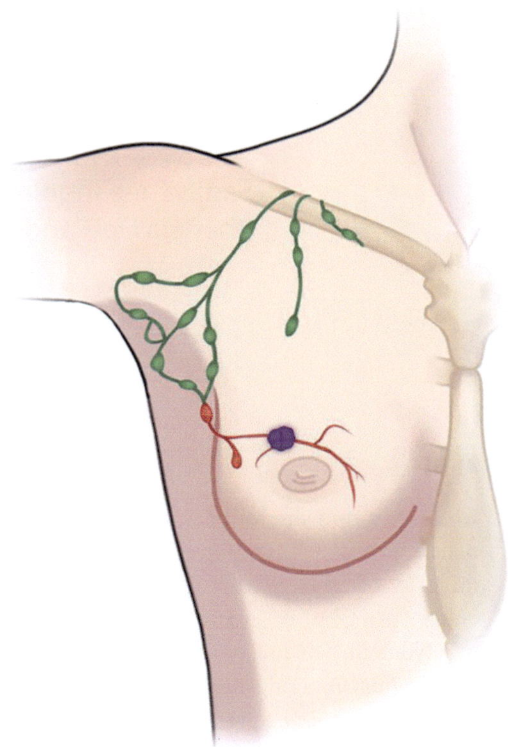

Fig. 24.1 Pictorial representation of primary breast lymphoma with ipsilateral axillary lymphadenopathy

24.1.2 Primary Breast Lymphoma

This is defined as the lymphoma in breast without any other concurrent involvement in the body apart from the ipsilateral axillary lymph nodes (Fig. 24.1).

The diagnostic criteria commonly used for PBL was coined by Wiseman and Liao, which mainly includes anatomic proximity to breast parenchyma and/or lymphomatous infiltrate for histopathological evaluation, no previous diagnosis of extramammary lymphoma, no concurrent widespread disease, except for ipsilateral axillary lymph node enlargement [9].

It was updated later, to add on ipsilateral supraclavicular lymphadenopathy stating regional disease [10].

In addition to this, reclassification on the basis of isolated or multiple extra nodal disease is proposed to show differences in prognosis and biologic behaviour (Fig. 24.2) [11].

24.1.3 Histopathology

Various histological types are seen with majority of them being B-cell lymphomas [12].

Among the non-Hodgkin's lymphoma, Diffuse Large B Cell Lymphoma (DLBCL) is the most common histological subtype, followed by follicular lymphoma and Mucosa Associated lymphoid tissue (MALT) (Fig. 24.3). The occurrence of a Hodgkin's lymphoma or a T cell lymphoma is rare.

The microscopic appearance is quite characteristic with a monotonous appearance of tumour cells, which are small round blue cells, with no epithelial connections. The nuclear cytoplasmic ratio is also higher, distinguishing them from epithelial cells. The nuclear chromatin is finer in lymphomas. Further a panel of immunohistochemical markers is needed to categorise the lymphomas (Figs. 24.4e, f and 24.5e, f). These tumour cells pose a close differential diagnosis

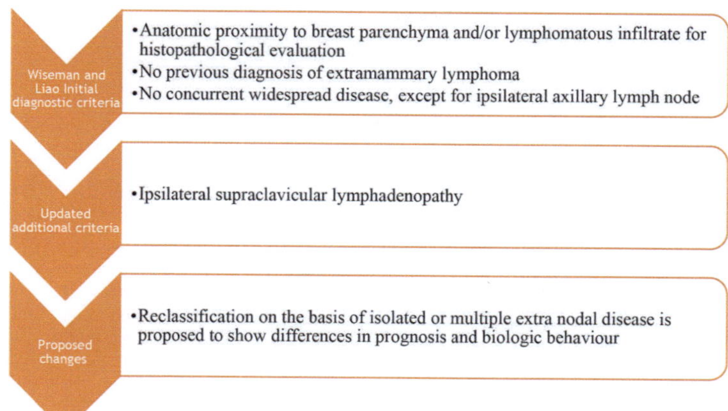

Fig. 24.2 Wiseman and Liao diagnostic criterion for primary breast lymphoma

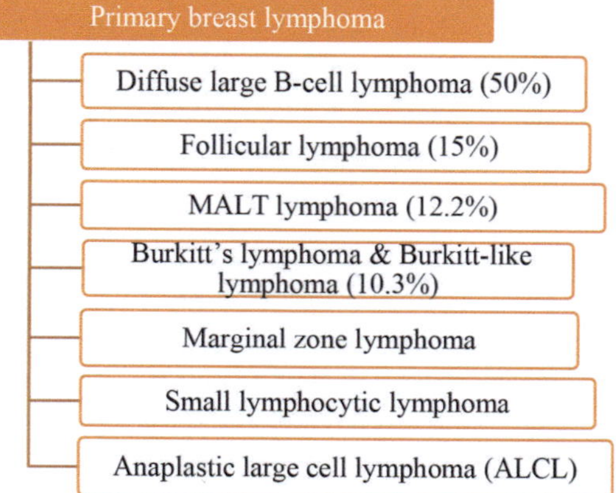

Fig. 24.3 Histological variants of primary breast lymphoma

with epithelial malignancies of the breast-like solid invasive ductal carcinoma and lobular carcinoma; however, the negative immunohistochemical markers rule out the same [13].

24.1.4 Secondary Breast Lymphoma

This is lymphoma secondary to systemic disease. It is the most common metastasis in breast. Although multiplicity and bilaterality are a feature of SBL, it commonly presents as a solitary metastasis to breast [6, 8, 14]. On contrary to PBL, subtyping is not uniform throughout the literature, with rare documentation of follicular and mucosa-associated lymphoid tissue subtypes [2, 6, 15].

24.1.5 Radiological Features

Primary and secondary breast lymphomas share few common imaging features.

Mammogram: Around 69–76% of lymphomas present as a solitary mass most of them being round or oval [16, 17]. Margins can be circumscribed, indistinct or rarely spiculated (Fig. 24.4a, b). On rare occasion asymmetries (20%) [16], architectural distortions (8%) [18], skin thickening and lymphedema (9%) [16] are seen, but these are more common features of other breast malignancies. Calcifications are conspicuously absent [2, 4].

Ultrasound: Lymphomas are round, oval or irregular with variable echo pattern on ultrasound. They may be heteroechoic or hypoechoic. Margins are either circumscribed (Fig. 24.4c) or indistinct (Fig. 24.5a, b). Posterior acoustic enhancement is commonly present, which makes it difficult to distinguish from the benign mimics [16, 18]. Sometimes, surrounding lymphedema is seen as echogenic rim around the mass giving it an onion peel appearance. Fifty-five to sixty-four percent of lymphoma exhibits avid vascularity [4, 16, 18].

T-cell lymphomas may involve skin and appear as indistinct irregular hyperechoic masses in the subcutaneous layer with hypoechoic branching within. The hyper echogenicity may represent the high cellularity of the tumour [2].

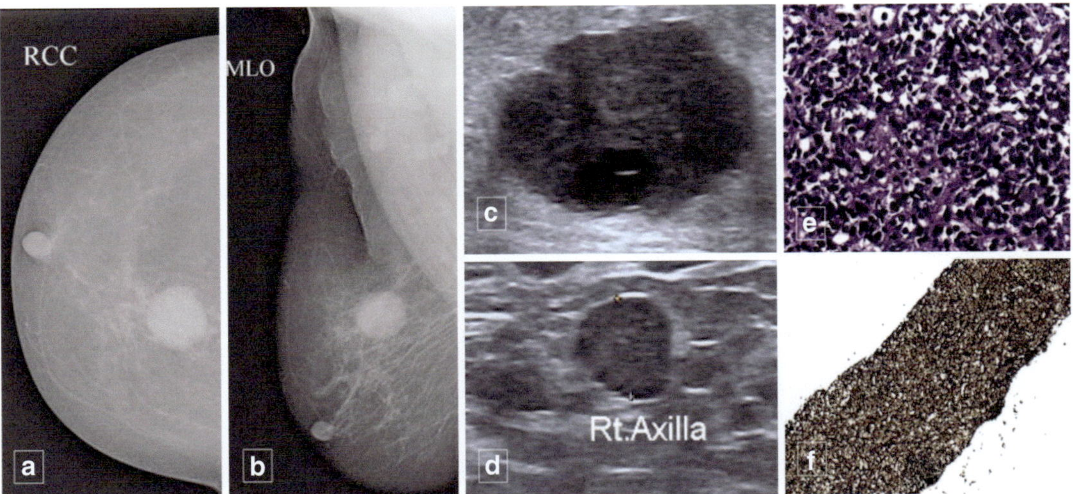

Fig. 24.4 A 66-year-old woman with complaints of lump in right breast (**a**, **b**), craniocaudal (CC) and mediolateral oblique (MLO) views on mammography showed a circumscribed round mass (**c**), ultrasonography (USG) showed an irregular hypoechoic microlobulated mass. (**d**) USG of right axilla showed an enlarged round lymph node with loss of fatty hilum. (**e**) Light microscopy showing a monotonous population of atypical cells in a diffuse pattern (**f**). Immunohistochemistry showing diffuse positivity for CD 20, suggesting B cell lineage)

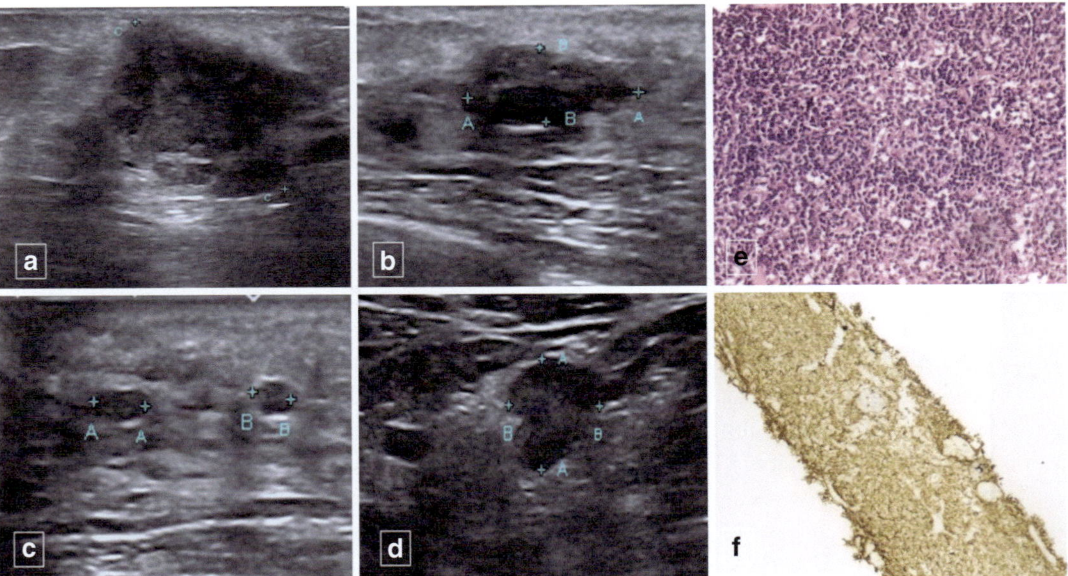

Fig. 24.5 (**a**, **b**) Ultrasound breast in a 62-year-old woman with irregular, non-circumscribed hypoechoic masses with no posterior features and (**c**) few sub-centimetric nodules in subareolar region. (**d**) Ultrasound of axilla shows an enlarged lymph node with loss of fatty hilum (**e**), light microscopy showing small round blue cell tumour, (**f**) immunohistochemistry showing diffuse CD45 positivity suggesting a lymphoid origin)

Axilla usually shows suspicious enlarged round lymph nodes with loss of fatty hilum (Figs. 24.4d and 24.5d).

24.1.5.1 Elastography

Limited literature is available on breast elastography of lymphomas. Lymphomas appear hard on elastography with mean elasticity ranging from 72.2 to 182.2 Kpa. This is lesser than the mean elasticity of the invasive breast cancers. This may be due to less desmoplastic reaction in the surrounding tissue in breast lymphomas [19].

Magnetic resonance imaging (MRI): MRI is the modality of choice to evaluate multicentricity, multifocality, treatment response, residual disease and recurrence in expected cases of lymphoma [20, 21]. Lymphoma presents as a mass similar to the other breast cancers [2, 16, 18]. Typically seen as a round to oval mass with intervening areas, which are hypo to isointense on T1weighted images and hyperintense on T2 weighted images. On dynamic contrast, they commonly exhibit Type II curve with rapid enhancement in early phase and plateau in delayed phase kinetics. Less often Type III curves are seen with rapid enhancement and rapid washout. Diffuse infiltration causes skin thickening and is observed in 9–30% of cases of combined primary and secondary breast lymphomas [2, 17, 21, 22].

Positron emission tomography (**PET**): Lymphoma is indistinguishable from other breast cancers and shows high fluorodeoxyglucose (FDG) uptake. FDG PET has high sensitivity for lymphoma and thus can be used for tumour staging, distant metastasis and treatment response [16, 23, 24].

24.1.6 Differentiating Features of Primary and Secondary Lymphoma

Features of primary and secondary lymphomas are fairly overlapping, but certain characteristics favour one over the other.

Primary breast lymphoma: Solitary mass with or without ipsilateral axillary lymphadenopathy favours PBL over SBL. PBL tends to be larger with average diameter of 2.3–4.6 cm in comparison to their secondary counterparts with average diameter of 1.2–2.8 cm [11, 16, 18]. Some studies have showed higher prevalence of cystic component in primary breast lymphoma, but its statistical significance is yet to be proven [25, 26].

Secondary breast lymphoma: SBL more commonly features multifocality, multicentricity and bilaterality (Fig. 24.5a–c). Ipsilateral axillary lymphadenopathy may or may not be present in addition to extramammary disease. SBL may also present as trabecular and skin thickening without any mass [16, 27]. Oval or round shape with circumscribed margins favour the diagnosis of SBL, although these features may also be present in PBL.

24.2 Breast Implant Associated Anaplastic Large Cell Lymphoma (BIA-ALCL)

BIA-ALCL is a rare disease with incidence ranging from 1 in 1000 to 1 in 10,000 patients with bilateral breast implants [28]. These patients present either with effusion after 1 year or even more (late onset) or infrequently as a mass forming lesion after 10 years of exposure to implants [29, 30]. Majority of the cases are unilateral and seen in patients with textured implants rather than smooth implants [31]. Unlike their other counterparts BIA-ALCL require surgery and have a better prognosis [32].

24.2.1 Clinical Features

Clinically 85% of the patients present as progressive swelling owing to the periprosthesis effusion or as a palpable mass adjoining the prosthesis (Fig. 24.6). Some patients present with pain and few with skin involvement in the form of subcu-

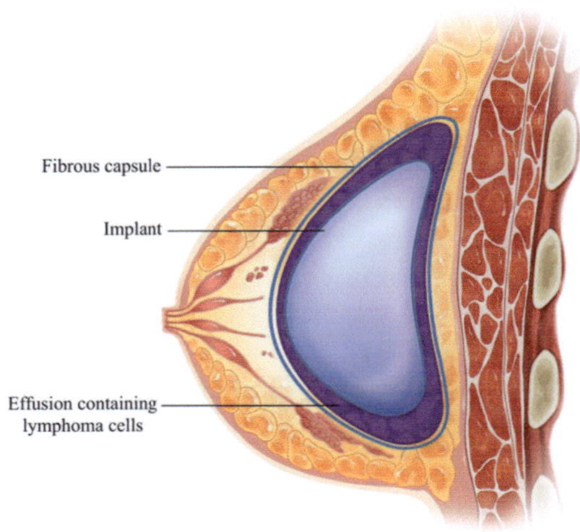

Fig. 24.6 Pictorial representation of periprosthetic effusion containing lymphoma cells in BIA-ALCL

taneous nodules, erythema, erosions and ulcer [29, 30]. Grade III to grade IV implant contracture may be seen. Two to fourteen percent of patients have nodal involvement in the form of ipsilateral axillary lymphadenopathy (most common), supraclavicular, internal mammary and mediastinal lymphadenopathy [32]. Distant metastasis and systemic symptoms such as fever, weight loss and night sweats are rare.

24.2.2 Radiological Features

Mammogram: In comparison to other breast cancers, X-ray mammogram is proven to be less accurate in diagnosis of BIA-ALCL. Non-specific circumferential peri-implant asymmetry, capsular thickening or irregular mass-like changes are seen. Similar to other lymphoma subtypes calcification are absent [4, 33].

Ultrasound: BIA-ALCL presents as a homogenous peri-implant effusion associated with inflammatory changes in the surrounding parenchyma. Irregular contour of the capsule can be observed in some cases. Although ultrasound has a high sensitivity in detection of malignant peri-implant effusion, other causes of homogenous peri-implant effusion such as implant rupture, gel bleed, haematoma, seroma, inflammation and infection must be contemplated [33, 34].

Similar to the other breast lymphomas, a circumscribed oval hypoechoic mass may be observed but hypervascularity is noticeably absent [29]. Rarely, it may present as a complex solid cystic mass, which has also been demonstrated in some cases [33].

MRI: MRI is useful in lesions that are undetectable or equivocal on ultrasound. Peri-implant effusions and mass lesions can be characterised in addition to evaluation of implant capsule contractures, implant integrity and tissue edema [35].

PET: PET has low (38%) sensitivity for malignant peri-implant effusion and 64% sensitivity for BIA-ALCL mass [33]. This is due to the low cell density in the peri-implant effusion fluid, which is inadequate to produce measurable positron signal thus giving a false negative result. In addition to this inflammatory reaction, granulation tissue surrounding the implant and the loco regional reactive lymphadenopathy can result in false positive interpretation [29]. However, FDG-PET is valuable in evaluation of distant metastasis before surgical resection.

24.3 Summary

- Breast lymphoma can be differentiated from breast carcinomas based on certain imaging characteristics (Fig. 24.7).
- It is also possible to discern types of breast lymphoma based on clinical and imaging characteristics (Fig. 24.8).

Lymphoma	Other breast carcinomas
Local pain	Nipple retraction
Edema	Nipple discharge
Subcutaneous/skin nodules	Skin edema (Inflammatory carcinoma)
Oval/ round	Irregular
Circumscribed	Spiculated/microlobulated
No calcification	Suspicious calcification

Fig. 24.7 Imaging features differentiating breast lymphomas from other breast malignancies

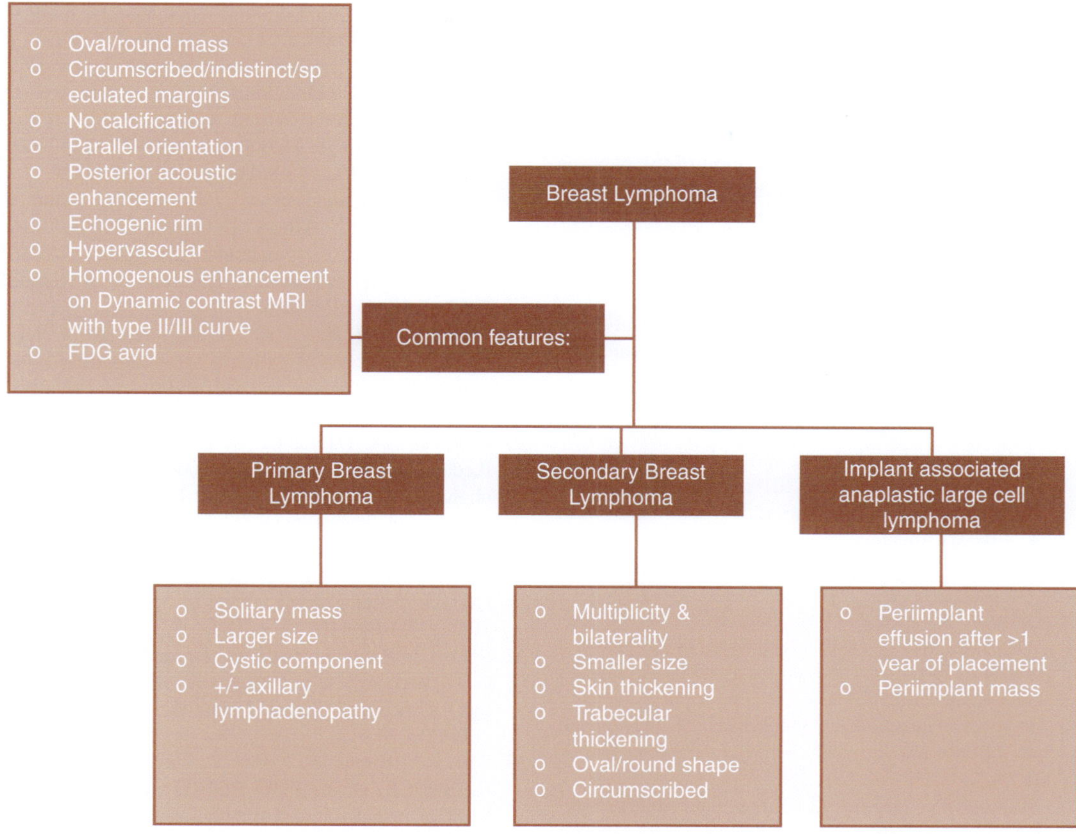

Fig. 24.8 Imaging features of subtypes of breast lymphoma

24.4 Treatment and Prognosis

Universally accepted standard protocol for treatment of breast lymphoma is yet to be established. At present, treatment includes a combination of surgery, chemotherapy (anthacyclin based) and radiotherapy. In low-grade disease, lumpectomy with radiation is performed similar to other early breast cancers. Mastectomy does not offer any additional benefit in regards to the survival rate or risk of recurrence and on the contrary can lead to delay in chemotherapy [4]. Axillary lymph nodal dissection for the purpose of staging is still considered controversial [36, 37]. Radiation therapy as a sole treatment is proven to be ineffective. The combination of radiotherapy and anthracycline is still controversial [38]. The risk for secondary breast malignancy persists in these cases. The research for improved methods of treatment is still underway.

Immunotherapy has proven to be effective in extra-mammary diffuse B cell lymphoma, but no improvement has been documented in 5 year survival rate of PBL. Thus, the role of immunotherapy remains ambiguous [39].

Prognosis depends on the type of lymphoma, its grade and stage. Due to the advanced stage of the disease in SBL, poor prognosis is anticipated. As regards local control and survival rate, low-grade PBL has better prognosis than high grade PBL. Diffuse large cell subtype, which is more common, has poorer prognosis than its rarer counterparts such as small, cleaved subtype and mixed small-and-large cell subtypes. Tumour size does not affect prognosis. Systemic recurrence is more often seen than local recurrence and is observed to occur within 2 years [10–12].

BIA ALCL follows a more indolent course with over 91% 5 year survival rate. These usually do not have disseminated disease [32].

References

1. Gaillard F. WHO classification of tumours of haematopoietic and lymphoid tissues. Radiology. Radiopaedia.org Radiopaedia. 2022. https://radiopaedia.org/articles/who-classification-of-tumours-of-haematopoietic-and-lymphoid-tissues-1.
2. Shim E, Song SE, Seo BK, Kim YS, Son GS. Lymphoma affecting the breast: a pictorial review of multimodal imaging findings. J Breast Cancer. 2013;16(3):254–65.
3. Dao AH, Adkins RJ, Glick AD. Malignant lymphoma of the breast: a review of 13 cases. Am Surg. 1992;58(12):792–6.
4. Raj SD, Shurafa M, Shah Z, Raj KM, Fishman MDC, Dialani VM. Primary and secondary breast lymphoma: clinical, pathologic, and multimodality imaging review. Radiographics. 2019;39(3):610–25.
5. Gomaa W, Ghanim A, Emam E, Bayoumi K, Ghanim A. Primary myeloid sarcoma of the breast: a case report and review of literature. J Microsc Ultrastruct. 2018;6(4):212–4.
6. Duncan VE, Reddy VVB, Jhala NC, Chhieng DC, Jhala DN. Non-Hodgkin's lymphoma of the breast: a review of 18 primary and secondary cases. Ann Diagn Pathol. 2006;10(3):144–8.
7. Brogi E, Harris NL. Lymphomas of the breast: pathology and clinical behavior. Semin Oncol. 1999;26(3):357–64.
8. Giardini R, Piccolo C, Rilke F. Primary non-Hodgkin's lymphomas of the female breast. Cancer. 1992;69(3):725–35.
9. Wiseman C, Liao KT. Primary lymphoma of the breast. Cancer. 1972;29(6):1705–12.
10. Kuan JW, Lau NS, Wong LL, Lau LG, Chang KM. Case series of primary breast diffuse large B-CLL lymphoma in Ampang Hospital, Malaysia. Blood. 2012;120(21):5113.
11. Sabaté JM, Gómez A, Torrubia S, Camins A, Roson N, De Las HP, et al. Lymphoma of the breast: clinical and radiologic features with pathologic correlation in 28 patients. Breast J. 2002;8(5):294–304.
12. Joks M, Myśliwiec K, Lewandowski K. Primary breast lymphoma—a review of the literature and report of three cases. Arch Med Sci. 2011;7(1):27–33.
13. Yoneyama K, Nakagawa M, Hara A. Primary lymphoma of the breast: a case report and review of the literature. Radiol Case Rep. 2021;16(1):55–61.
14. Vizcaíno I, Torregrosa A, Higueras V, Morote V, Cremades A, Torres V, et al. Metastasis to the breast from extramammary malignancies: a report of four cases and a review of literature. Eur Radiol. 2001;11(9):1659–65.
15. Domchek SM, Hecht JL, Fleming MD, Pinkus GS, Canellos GP. Lymphomas of the breast. Cancer. 2002;94(1):6–13.
16. Yang WT, Lane DL, Le-Petross HT, Abruzzo LV, Macapinlac HA. Breast lymphoma: imaging findings of 32 tumors in 27 patients. Radiology. 2007;245(3):692–702.
17. Liberman L, Giess CS, Dershaw DD, Louie DC, Deutch BM. Non-Hodgkin lymphoma of the breast: imaging characteristics and correlation with histopathologic findings. Radiology. 1994;192(1):157–60. https://doi.org/10.1148/radiology.192.1.8208929.
18. Surov A, Holzhausen HJ, Wienke A, Schmidt J, Thomssen C, Arnold D, et al. Primary and secondary breast lymphoma: prevalence, clinical signs and radiological features. Br J Radiol. 2012;85(1014):e195–205.
19. Kim Y, Ko KH, Jung HK, Lee HJ. Shear-wave elastography features of primary non-Hodgkin's lymphoma of the breast: a case report and literature review. J Clin Diagn Res. 2016;10(12):TD01–3.
20. Espinosa LA, Daniel BL, Jeffrey SS, Nowels KW, Ikeda DM. MRI features of mucosa-associated lymphoid tissue lymphoma in the breast. AJR Am J Roentgenol. 2005;185(1):199–202.
21. Kiresi DA, Kivrak AS, Ecirli S, Toy H. Secondary breast, pancreatic, and renal involvement with non-Hodgkin's lymphoma: imaging findings. Breast. 2006;15(1):106–10.
22. Rizzo S, Preda L, Villa G, Brambilla S, Pruneri G, Alietti A, et al. Magnetic resonance imaging of primary breast lymphoma. Radiol Med. 2009;114(6):915.
23. Santra A, Kumar R, Reddy R, Halanaik D, Kumar R, Bal CS, et al. FDG PET-CT in the management of primary breast lymphoma. Clin Nucl Med. 2009;34(12):848–53.
24. Kyoung Jung H, Kim EK, Yun M, Jung Kim M, Young KJ. Bilateral breasts involvement in Burkitt's lymphoma detected only by FDG-PET. Clin Imaging. 2006;30(1):57–9.
25. Gal-Gombos EC, Esserman LE, Poniecka AW, Poppiti RJ. Is a pseudocystic serpentine mass a sonographic indicator of breast lymphoma? Radiologic-histologic correlation of an unusual finding. Am J Roentgenol. 2001;176(3):734–6.
26. Mason HS, Johari V, March DE, Crisi GM. Primary breast lymphoma: radiologic and pathologic findings. Breast J. 2005;11(6):495–6.
27. Jackson FI, Lalani ZH. Breast lymphoma: radiologic imaging and clinical appearances. Can Assoc Radiol J. 1991;42(1):48–54.
28. Fleming D, Stone J, Tansley P. Spontaneous regression and resolution of breast implant-associated anaplastic large cell lymphoma: implications for research, diagnosis and clinical management. Aesthet Plast Surg. 2018;42(3):672–8.
29. Sharma B, Jurgensen-Rauch A, Pace E, Attygalle AD, Sharma R, Bommier C, et al. Breast implant–associated anaplastic large cell lymphoma: review and multiparametric imaging paradigms. Radiographics. 2020;40(3):609–28.
30. Miranda RN, Aladily TN, Prince HM, Kanagal-Shamanna R, de Jong D, Fayad LE, et al. Breast implant–associated anaplastic large-cell lymphoma:

long-term follow-up of 60 patients. J Clin Oncol. 2014;32(2):114–20.

31. McCarthy CM, Loyo-Berríos N, Qureshi AA, Mullen E, Gordillo G, Pusic AL, et al. Patient registry and outcomes for breast implants and anaplastic large cell lymphoma etiology and epidemiology (profile): initial report of findings 2012–2018. Plast Reconstr Surg. 2019;143(3):65S–73S.
32. Clemens MW, Medeiros LJ, Butler CE, Hunt KK, Fanale MA, Horwitz S, et al. Complete surgical excision is essential for the management of patients with breast implant–associated anaplastic large-cell lymphoma. J Clin Oncol. 2016;34(2):160–8.
33. Adrada BE, Miranda RN, Rauch GM, Arribas E, Kanagal-Shamanna R, Clemens MW, et al. Breast implant-associated anaplastic large cell lymphoma: sensitivity, specificity, and findings of imaging studies in 44 patients. Breast Cancer Res Treat. 2014;147(1):1–14.
34. Taylor KO, Webster HR, Prince HM. Anaplastic large cell lymphoma and breast implants: five Australian cases. Plast Reconstr Surg. 2012;129(4):610e.
35. Lourenco AP, Moy L, Baron P, Didwania AD, di Florio RM, Heller SL, et al. ACR appropriateness criteria® breast implant evaluation. J Am Coll Radiol. 2018;15(5, Supplement):S13–25.
36. Jennings WC, Baker RS, Murray SS, Howard CA, Parker DE, Peabody LF, et al. Primary breast lymphoma. Ann Surg. 2007;245(5):784–9.
37. Durodola JI. Burkitt's lymphoma presenting during lactation. Int J Gynecol Obstet. 1976;14(3):225–31.
38. Babovic N, Jelic S, Jovanovic V. Primary non-Hodgkin lymphoma of the breast. Is it possible to avoid mastectomy. J Exp Clin Cancer Res. 2000;19(2):149–54.
39. Ryan G, Martinelli G, Kuper-Hommel M, Tsang R, Pruneri G, Yuen K, et al. Primary diffuse large B-cell lymphoma of the breast: prognostic factors and outcomes of a study by the international extranodal lymphoma study group. Ann Oncol. 2008;19(2):233–41.

Part IX

Management of Breast Cancer

Staging and Surgical Management of Breast Cancer

25

Ramya Ramakrishnan

Abstract

The diagnosis of breast cancer is made using the principles of triple assessment. Staging of the disease is imperative in order to prognosticate and plan the management of the patient. The treatment should be given by a multidisciplinary team specialised in breast cancer management. Surgery forms a very important part of the treatment strategy. The breast lesion and the axilla have to be addressed by surgery. There are two main types of surgery done for the breast lesion—breast conserving surgery (BCS) or mastectomy. Axillary surgery would be a sentinel lymph node biopsy for the clinical N0 stage and axillary dissection for those patients with palpable nodes. Surgery is done either upfront or following neoadjuvant chemotherapy. Adjuvant therapy options include chemotherapy, hormonal therapy, radiotherapy and targeted therapy.

Keywords

Triple assessment · Staging · Multidisciplinary team · Breast conserving surgery · Mastectomy · Sentinel lymph node biopsy · Adjuvant therapy

R. Ramakrishnan (✉)
Sri Ramachandra Institute of Higher Education and Research (Deemed University), Chennai, India
e-mail: ramya.r@sriramachandra.edu.in

The diagnosis of breast cancer is based on clinical examination and imaging and confirmed by pathological assessment. Clinical examination includes inspection and palpation of the breasts and regional lymph nodes and assessment for distant metastases (bones, liver and lungs and a neurological examination if required). Bilateral mammography and ultrasound of the breast and regional lymph nodes should be done. A magnetic resonance imaging (MRI) of the breast should be considered only in the following situations:

- BRCA mutations associated familial breast cancer
- Lobular carcinoma
- Dense breasts
- When multifocality/multicentricity is suspected (particularly in lobular carcinoma)
- Significant discordance between conventional imaging and clinical examination
- To evaluate the response to neoadjuvant systemic therapy
- When the findings of conventional imaging are inconclusive (such as a positive axillary lymph node status with an occult primary tumour in the breast) [1]
- In case of breast implants

Pathological diagnosis should be based on a core needle biopsy, preferably obtained by ultrasound or stereotactic guidance. A core needle

B. Dev, L. D. Joseph (eds.), *Holistic Approach to Breast Disease*,
https://doi.org/10.1007/978-981-99-0035-0_25

biopsy (if this is not possible, at least a fine-needle aspiration) must be obtained before any type of treatment is initiated. Core needle biopsy is mandatory if preoperative systemic therapy is planned. This is to ensure a diagnosis of invasive disease and also to assess biomarkers. The recommendation is that at least two to three cores should be obtained. All lesions should be biopsied in case of multifocal and multicentric tumours. A marker in the form of a surgical clip or carbon should be placed into the tumour at biopsy. This is done to ensure resection of the correct site and to enable pathological assessment of the surgical specimen. Ultrasound-guided fine-needle aspiration or core biopsy of suspicious lymph nodes should be carried out, preferably followed by clip or carbon marking of biopsied lymph nodes. Rarely, repeated negative core biopsies warrant an excisional biopsy.

The pathological diagnosis should be made according to the World Health Organisation (WHO) classification [2]. The two most frequent subtypes are invasive carcinoma of the breast, not otherwise specified (NOS, previously named ductal carcinoma) (70–75%) and lobular carcinoma (12–15%). Each of these specific subtypes has a different prognosis. The pathological report should include presence/absence of ductal carcinoma in situ (DCIS); the histological type, grade and immunohistochemistry (IHC) evaluation of ER status; and, for invasive cancer, IHC evaluation of PgR and HER2 expression or HER2 gene amplification. Proliferation markers such as the Ki67 labelling index may give useful information regarding the biologic behaviour of the tumour. In case of negativity of ER/PgR and HER2 in the biopsy specimen, it is advisable to retest for them in the surgical specimen, and this result will be taken as the definite one. In case of a HER2-positive test on biopsy, retesting for HER2 on the surgical specimen is mandatory for invasive carcinoma NOS grade I, ER- and PgR-positive or adenoid cystic carcinoma or secretory carcinoma (which are both usually triple negative).

In order to help us prognosticate and devise the correct treatment protocol, the tumours should be grouped into surrogate intrinsic subtypes, defined by routine histology and IHC data (Table 25.1). Typical Luminal A-like tumours are low grade, strongly ER-positive/PgR-positive, HER2-negative and have low proliferative index. Luminal B-like tumours are ER-positive but may exhibit variable degrees of ER/PgR expression, are of higher grade and have higher proliferative fraction [3].

Table 25.1 Intrinsic subtypes of breast cancer

Intrinsic subtype	Clinicopathological surrogate definition
Luminal A	'Luminal A-like' ER-positive HER2-negative Ki67 low PgR high Low-risk molecular signature (if available)
Luminal B	Luminal B-like (HER2-negative)' ER-positive HER2-negative And either Ki67 high or PgR low High-risk molecular signature (if available) 'Luminal B-like (HER2-positive)' ER-positive HER2-positive Any Ki67 Any PgR
HER2	'HER2-positive (non-luminal)' HER2-positive ER and PgR absent
"Basal-like"	'Triple-negative' ER and PgR absent HER2-negative

ER oestrogen receptor, *HER2* human epidermal growth factor receptor 2, *PgR* progesterone receptor

25.1 Staging

Once a diagnosis of carcinoma breast is made, it is imperative to stage the disease before formulating a treatment plan. Clinical staging is done using the TNM classification (American Joint Committee on Cancer staging system—AJCC staging) [4]. Histological confirmation of the malignancy is followed by appropriate staging investigations.

The AJCC eighth edition includes two staging systems—the anatomic stage, which includes the size of the primary tumour, nodal status and distant metastasis; and the prognostic stage, which includes tumour grade, hormone receptor and oncogene expression and the results of multigene panel testing—to accurately predict a patient's outcome.

1. The anatomic stage group table is based solely on anatomic extent of cancer as defined by the T, N and M categories.
2. The prognostic stage group table is based on populations of persons with breast cancer that have been offered—and mostly treated with—appropriate endocrine and/or systemic chemotherapy, which includes anatomic T, N and M plus tumour grade and the status of the biomarkers human epidermal growth factor receptor 2 (HER2), estrogen receptor (ER) and progesterone receptor (PR).

The **AJCC eighth edition clinical anatomic staging** groups patients based on the tumour size (T), lymph node status (N) and distant metastasis (M) into four stages.

The categories of clinical anatomic staging of the primary tumour (T categories) range from Tis to T4 and are identical to those of pathologic anatomic staging of the primary tumour [5]. DCIS and Paget disease without underlying invasive carcinoma or DCIS are both considered to be category Tis, regardless of the size of the tumour. One of the changes for breast cancer staging in the eighth edition of the AJCC manual is that lobular carcinoma in situ is no longer included as a Tis category but rather is considered a benign entity that confers a higher risk of future breast cancer.

- **Primary tumour (T)**
  - Tx: Primary tumour cannot be assessed
  - T0: No evidence of primary tumour
  - Tis (DCIS): Ductal Carcinoma in situ
  - Tis (Paget): Paget disease of the nipple NOT associated with invasive carcinoma and/or carcinoma in situ (DCIS) in the underlying breast parenchyma. Carcinomas in the breast parenchyma associated with Paget disease are categorised based on the size and characteristics of the parenchymal disease, although the presence of Paget disease should still be noted
  - T1 Tumour ≤ 20 mm in greatest dimension.
  - T1mi Tumour ≤ 1 mm in greatest dimension.
  - T1a Tumour > 1 mm but ≤ 5 mm in greatest dimension (round any measurement from >1.0–1.9 mm to 2 mm).
  - T1b Tumour > 5 mm but ≤ 10 mm in greatest dimension.
  - T1c Tumour > 10 mm but ≤ 20 mm in greatest dimension.
  - T2 Tumour > 20 mm but ≤ 50 mm in greatest dimension.
  - T3 Tumour > 50 mm in greatest dimension.
  - T4 Tumour of any size with direct extension to the chest wall and/or to the skin (ulceration or macroscopic nodules); invasion of the dermis alone does not qualify as T4.
  - T4a Extension to the chest wall; invasion or adherence to pectoralis muscle in the absence of invasion of chest wall structures does not qualify as T4.
  - T4b Ulceration and/or ipsilateral macroscopic satellite nodules and/or edema (including *peau d'orange*) of the skin that does not meet the criteria for inflammatory carcinoma.
  - T4c Both T4a and T4b are present.
- T4d Inflammatory carcinoma

Axillary lymph node levels are defined by the relationship of the lymph node to the pectoralis minor muscle. Level I axillary nodes are located lateral to the lateral border of the pectoralis minor muscle. Level II axillary nodes are located between the medial and lateral borders of the pectoralis minor muscle and also include the interpectoral (Rotter's) lymph nodes. Level III axillary nodes are located medial to the medial margin of the pectoralis minor muscle and inferior to the clavicle.

- **Regional lymph nodes (N)**
  - cNx: Regional lymph nodes cannot be assessed (e.g, previously removed).
  - cN0: No regional lymph node metastasis.
  - cN1: Metastasis to movable ipsilateral level I and/or level II axillary lymph node(s).
  - cN2: Metastasis to ipsilateral level I and/or level II axillary lymph node(s) fixed or matted, or in clinically apparent ipsilateral internal mammary nodes in the absence of clinically evident axillary lymph node metastasis.

    cN2a: Metastasis to fixed or matted ipsilateral level I and/or level II axillary lymph nodes.

    cN2b: Metastasis to ipsilateral internal mammary nodes without axillary metastases.
  - cN3: Metastases to ipsilateral level III axillary nodes with or without level I and/or level II axillary metastases; or metastases to ipsilateral internal mammary nodes with level I and/or level II axillary metastases; or metastases to ipsilateral supraclavicular nodes.

    cN3a: Metastases to ipsilateral level III axillary nodes with or without level I and/or level II axillary metastases.

    cN3b Metastases to ipsilateral internal mammary nodes with level I and/or level II axillary metastases.

    cN3c Metastases to ipsilateral supraclavicular node.
- **Distant metastasis**
  - M0 No clinical or imaging evidence of distant metastases. cM0(i+) No clinical or imaging evidence of distant metastases but with tumour cells or deposits measuring ≤0.2 mm detected in circulating blood, bone marrow or other non-regional nodal tissue in the absence of clinical signs and symptoms of metastases
  - M1: Distant metastasis on the basis of clinical or imaging findings

Table 25.2 TNM stage grouping

T	N	M	Stage
Tis	N0	M0	0
T1	N0	M0	IA
T0	N1mi	M0	IB
T1	N1mi	M0	IB
T0	N1	M0	IIA
T1	N1	M0	IIA
T2	N0	M0	IIA
T2	N1	M0	IIB
T3	N0	M0	IIB
T1	N2	M0	IIIA
T2	N2	M0	IIIA
T3	N1	M0	IIIA
T3	N2	M0	IIIA
T4	N0	M0	IIIB
T4	N1	M0	IIIB
T4	N2	M0	IIIB
Any T	N3	M0	IIIC
Any T	Any N	M1	IV

Anatomic stage grouping: The TNM classification is used to stage the patient into different stage groups as follows (Table 25.2):

25.2 Prognostic Staging

The prognostication is more accurate with the addition of the tumour grade, hormone receptor, oncogene expression (including ER, PR and HER2) and multigene panel results to the anatomic information. According to the eighth edition of the AJCC manual [5], the tumour grade defined by the histologic grading system of Scarff, Bloom and Richardson is now a recommended component for assigning the stage of breast cancer. (For DCIS, however, the assigned grade should be nuclear grade.) According to the eighth edition of the AJCC manual, all invasive carcinomas should have the ER, PR and HER2 status determined by using appropriate assays.

It is very well known that the progression of ER-positive and PR-positive tumours is slowed down as a result of tamoxifen therapy and other endocrine therapies [6]. The amplification or overexpression of HER2, which is an oncogene, is associated with a worse prognosis regardless of nodal status. HER2 expression is more commonly seen in invasive ductal carcinoma, rather than invasive lobular carcinoma, but is associated with a poor prognosis when found in the latter. The prognosis of patients with HER2 positive tumours is improved with the use of anti-HER2 therapies, including that with the monoclonal antibody trastuzumab [7].

Prognostic gene profiling is based on patterns of expression of combinations of up to thousands of genes in tumour cells. Several multigene panels have developed as a consequence of the advances in gene expression profiling. Many of these panels have been validated as prognostic tools. The most validated multigene panel is the Oncotype DX Breast Recurrence Score (Genomic Health, Redwood City, Calif). This panel is currently incorporated into prognostic staging of the eighth edition of the AJCC manual. Oncotype DX recurrence scores are currently used for hormone-positive node-negative tumours to evaluate whether the addition of adjuvant chemotherapy to hormonal therapy gives any additional benefit. This panel is used to evaluate 16 genes and 5 reference genes, in order to predict the likelihood of recurrence in patients undergoing endocrine therapy alone. It categorises an individual patient into those having a low, intermediate or high risk of recurrence [8]. The model predicts no additional benefit of chemotherapy for patients with a low-risk recurrence score (<18). The eighth edition of the AJCC manual now incorporates Oncotype DX recurrence scores to potentially downstage tumours.

25.3 Stage Migration

The inclusion of biomarkers in the prognostic staging system results in stage migration for some patients (Table 25.3). For example, a patient with a T2N1M0 cancer that is grade 2–3 and triple negative would be placed in the category of stage IIB according to AJCC anatomic staging and as stage IIIB according to the clinical prognostic staging. A patient with a T3N0M0 cancer that is grade 1–3 and ER, PR and HER2 positive would be classified as stage IIB according to AJCC anatomic staging and as stage IB according to the clinical prognostic staging. Generally, triple-negative tumours are "upstaged" in their prognostic stage, and HER2 expression is considered as a "downstaging" factor. The downstaging is due to the success of anti-HER2 therapies [9].

Table 25.3 Stage migration

TNM	Biomarkers	Anatomic staging	Prognostic staging
T2N0M0	Grade 1–3, ER positive, PR positive or negative, HER2 negative, Oncotype DX score < 11	IIA	IA[a]
T2N1M0	Grade 1–3, ER positive, PR positive, HER2 positive	IIB	IB[b]
T2N1M0	Grade 2–3, ER negative, PR negative, HER2 negative	IIB	IIIB[b]
T3N0M0	Grade 1–3, ER positive, PR positive, HER2 positive	IIB	IB[b]
T3N0M0	Grade 2–3, ER negative, PR negative, HER2 negative	IIB	IIIB[b]
T3N2M0	Grade 1–2, ER positive, PR positive, HER2 positive or negative	IIIA	IIA[b]

[a] Pathologic prognostic stage
[b] Clinical prognostic stage

25.4 Staging Investigations

In patients with early breast cancer, routine staging investigations are done to rule out locoregional spread. Asymptomatic distant metastases are rare, and most patients do not benefit from comprehensive laboratory tests and radiological staging. A complete blood count, liver, renal function tests, alkaline phosphatase and calcium levels is recommended before surgery.

A CT scan of the chest, USG, CT or MRI scan of the abdomen and a bone scan can be considered for patients with:

- Clinically positive axillary nodes
- Large tumours (e.g. >5 cm)
- Aggressive biology
- Presence of metastases as suggested by clinical signs, symptoms or laboratory reports

When conventional methods of staging are inconclusive, a fluorodeoxyglucose (FDG) positron emission tomography (PET)-CT may be useful. PET-CT scanning can also replace traditional imaging for staging in high-risk patients, although in cases of lobular cancers and low-grade tumours, PET-CT may be less sensitive [10]. There is no evidence currently to advocate the use of FDG-PET-CT in the staging of locoregional disease. This is due to its low sensitivity when compared with the gold standard, sentinel lymph node biopsy (SLNB) and axillary lymph node dissection (ALND). In patients planned for neoadjuvant systemic treatment with anthracyclines and/or trastuzumab, cardiac function has to be evaluated either with a cardiac USG or a multi-gated acquisition (MUGA) scan.

Prognostic and predictive factors for invasive breast cancer

Tumour factors	Host factors
Nodal status	Age
Tumour size	Menopausal status
Histologic/nuclear grade	Family history
Lymphatic/vascular invasion	Previous breast cancer
Pathologic stage	Immunosuppression
Hormone receptor status	Nutrition
DNA content	Prior radiation therapy
Extensive intraductal component	

The most important prognostic factors in early breast cancer are as follows:

- The presence of ER/PgR, HER2 receptors,
- Proliferative index (Ki67).
- The number of involved regional lymph nodes,
- Tumour histology,
- The size, grade of the tumour,
- Presence of peritumoural vascular invasion.
- The status of the surgical margins and the presence of DCIS, in patients who have undergone breast conservation therapy.

The validated predictive factors that help in the selection of patients for endocrine therapy (ET) and anti-HER2 therapies, are ER/PgR and HER2, respectively. Chemotherapy has less absolute benefit in patients with high ER expression.

MammaPrint, Oncotype DX Recurrence Score, Prosigna, Endopredict and Breast Cancer Index are all Gene expression profiles that may be used to gain additional prognostic and/or predictive information about the benefit of adjuvant chemotherapy. All tests except the first one (MammaPrint) were developed for patients with ER-positive early breast cancer only.

25.5 Overview of Treatment

The treatment should be given by a multidisciplinary team specialised in breast cancer working in a specialised breast centre, consisting of breast radiologists, breast pathologists, breast surgeons, medical oncologists, radiation oncologists and breast nurses [11, 12].

- The breast centre should have other specialists like plastic/reconstructive surgeons, psychologists, physiotherapists and geneticists or should be able to refer appropriate patients to these specialists.
- A breast nurse or a similarly trained health care practitioner should be available to act as a patient navigator.
- Verbal or written details about the diagnosis of breast cancer and the treatment options should be given to the patients and their relatives

repeatedly, in a thorough and easily understandable form.

- All management decisions should be taken with the active involvement of the patients.
- Factors like size and location of primary tumour, number of lesions, extent of lymph node involvement and pathology (including receptor status), as well as the age, menopausal status, general health condition and preferences of the patient should form the basis of the treatment strategy.
- Age should not be the sole determinant for withholding or recommending a treatment.
- Fertility issues and fertility-preservation techniques should be discussed in younger premenopausal patients before the initiation of any systemic treatment [13].

25.6 Local Treatment

25.6.1 Surgery

Surgery forms a very important part of the treatment strategy. The breast lesion and the axilla have to be addressed by surgery. There are two main types of surgery done for the breast lesion—breast conserving surgery (BCS) or mastectomy. Axillary surgery would be a sentinel lymph node biopsy for the clinical N0 stage and axillary dissection for those patients with palpable nodes.

In situ breast cancer (stage 0). Bilateral mammography is done to determine the extent of the in situ cancer and to exclude a second cancer. As lobular carcinoma in situ (LCIS) is considered a marker for increased risk rather than a precursor of invasive cancer, the current treatment of LCIS is observation with or without tamoxifen. The goal of treatment is to prevent or detect at an early stage, the invasive cancer that subsequently develops in 25–35% of these patients.

Mastectomy is required for women with DCIS involving two or more quadrants. For women with limited disease, breast conservative surgery is recommended. Tamoxifen as an adjuvant therapy is advised for all patients with DCIS.

Axillary node evaluation with SLNB is not required with in situ malignancy but may be required in large and/or high-grade tumours, especially when mastectomy is required (in anticipation of an incidental invasive cancer in the resected surgical specimen).

25.6.2 Recommendations

- BCS followed by whole breast radiotherapy (WBRT) or total mastectomy are acceptable treatment options for DCIS.
- A 2-mm margin is considered adequate while doing BCS in a patient with DCIS (as the remaining breast will be subsequently treated with WBRT) [14].
- Patients with DCIS should not be routinely subjected to SLNB, unless they have large and/or high-grade tumours, and when mastectomy is required.

Early invasive breast cancer (stage I, IIa or II b). There has been a major shift towards breast conservation procedures in the surgical treatment of primary breast cancer. Currently, mastectomy with assessment of axillary lymph nodal status and breast conservation (lumpectomy with assessment of axillary lymph nodal status and radiation therapy) are considered equivalent treatments for stages I and II cancer. Several large population-based studies reported a possible improved outcome after breast conserving therapy compared to radical surgery, after all the adjustments [15].

Relative contraindications for breast conservative therapy include:

- Prior radiation therapy to the breast or chest wall.
- Multicentric disease.
- Involved surgical margins or unknown margin status following re-excision.
- Scleroderma or other connective tissue disorders.
- First or second trimester pregnancy.

Mastectomy may still be the treatment of choice due to:

- Large tumour in relation to the breast size
- Multicentric tumour
- Persistent positive surgical margins after multiple resection
- Contraindications to RT
- History of previous radiation to the chest wall/breast
- Not suitable for oncoplastic breast conservation
- Patient choice

Breast-conserving surgery: This is the primary surgical choice for patients with breast cancer. For patients undergoing wide local excision, breast surgeons are trained to undertake oncoplastic approaches to reduce the impact of local tumour excision on cosmesis, often using tissue displacement techniques. Oncoplastic surgery is the seamless joining of extirpative and reconstructive breast surgery performed by a single surgeon.

The techniques utilised in oncoplastic breast surgery can be classified into two levels.

Level 1: This involves excision of less than 20% of the breast volume without any skin excision. Reconstruction is by way of simple reshaping techniques. The surgeon does not require any training in plastic surgery.

Level II: This involves excision of 20–50% of breast volume with some amount of skin excision. Reshaping of the breast is done by using mammoplasty techniques. The surgeon needs training in plastic surgery.

Oncoplastic procedures result in good cosmetic outcomes, especially in patients with a less favourable tumour/breast size ratio, large breasts or a central or inferior location of the tumour within the breast.

Margin status should be reported according to the recommendations of the College of American Pathologists (CAP); for example, a margin is positive, when there is ink touching invasive cancer or DCIS; the exact anatomic location of the positive margin should be highlighted in oriented specimens. For negative margins, the distance of invasive cancer and/or DCIS from the margin (s) should be reported. There should be no tumour at the inked margin for invasive cancer and distance of tumour from the inked margin should be >2 mm for in situ disease [14].

The tumour bed should be marked with clips in a standardised way. This facilitates accurate planning of the radiation boost if indicated. Currently achievable low local recurrence rates (<0.5% per year (with a target of <0.25%) and 10% overall at very long term follow-up) should be maintained. All patients are subjected to WBRT following the breast conservative surgery.

Mastectomy: The most common type of mastectomy done is the modified radical mastectomy where the nipple areola complex with the entire breast and the skin over it and axillary pad of fat with all the lymph nodes up to Level II are removed. The pectoralis major muscle is preserved, but the fascia over this muscle is removed along with the breast. In the original radical mastectomy advocated by Halstead, both pectoralis major and minor muscles are removed, resulting in greater morbidity. The modification can be that of Patey, Scanlon or Auchincloss. Patey's technique involves removal of the pectoralis minor muscle; Scanlon detaches the pectoralis minor tendon from its insertion and re-sutures it to the lower fibres of pectoralis major and in Auchincloss method, the pectoralis minor is retracted to ensure adequate axillary node dissection [16].

The other types of mastectomy that are being used nowadays are simple mastectomy, skin-sparing mastectomy (SSM) that preserves the skin envelope and nipple sparing mastectomy (NSM). NSM has been shown to be safe from an oncological point of view in selected patients. It improves cosmetic outcomes for therapeutic and prophylactic surgeries [17].

Breast reconstruction can be done following a mastectomy, either immediately or later. The only contraindication for immediate reconstruction is inflammatory carcinoma. Radiotherapy is no longer a contraindication for immediate autologous tissue reconstruction.

There are many surgical options available for women who want to undergo breast reconstruction. Silicone gel implants are safe and acceptable components of the reconstructive armamentarium. Autologous tissue flaps can replace relatively large volumes of breast tissue. Tissue can be taken from the latissimus dorsi muscle, transverse rectus abdominis muscle or deep inferior epigastric perforator flap, among others. The optimal reconstruction technique for each patient should be discussed individually taking into account anatomic, treatment- and patient-related factors and preferences.

Advances in axillary management: Regional lymph node involvement remains one of the strongest predictors of long-term prognosis in primary breast cancer.

Traditionally, dissection of axillary lymph node levels I and II has been performed in early invasive cancer (Figs. 25.1 and 25.2). ALND is associated with lymphoedema affecting the upper limb in up to 25% of women following surgery (up to 15% following axillary radiotherapy (RT) without surgical clearance and below 10% following SLNB) [18]. The incidence of lymphoedema rises significantly (to 40%) when axillary clearance is combined with RT to the axilla.

On the other hand, Sentinel lymph node biopsy (SLNB) results in less morbidity in terms of shoulder stiffness and arm swelling and allows for a reduced hospital stay. Sentinel lymph node biopsy is now being performed for assessment of lymph nodal involvement. The sentinel node is the first draining lymph node on the direct lymphatic pathway from the primary tumour site, and so it is the first node to harbour cancer cells detached from the primary tumour (Fig. 25.3). Candidates for this procedure have clinically uninvolved nodes, a T1, T2 or T3 primary cancer. The technique is done using either dyes (Isosulfan blue/patent blue/methylene blue) or radiocolloids. The dye or the radiocolloid is injected either peritumourally or in the peri-areolar or sub-areolar site (Figs. 25.4, 25.5 and 25.6). The depth of the injection has to be intradermal as well as sub- dermal. If the sentinel

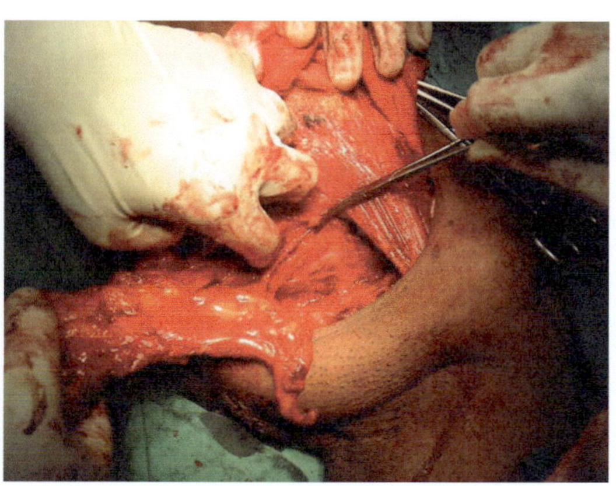

Fig. 25.1 Axillary lymph node dissection

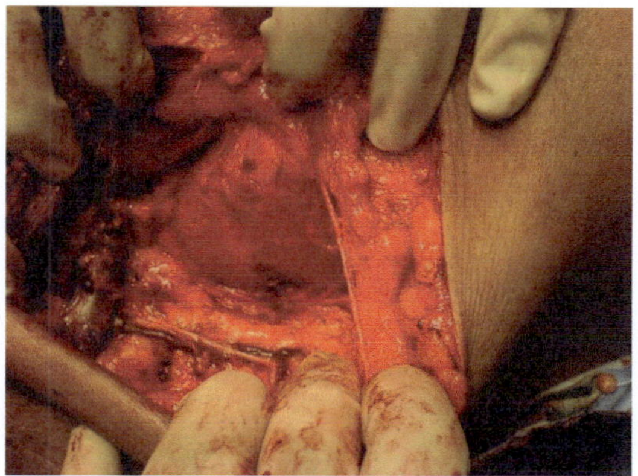

Fig. 25.2 Axillary lymph node dissection—completed

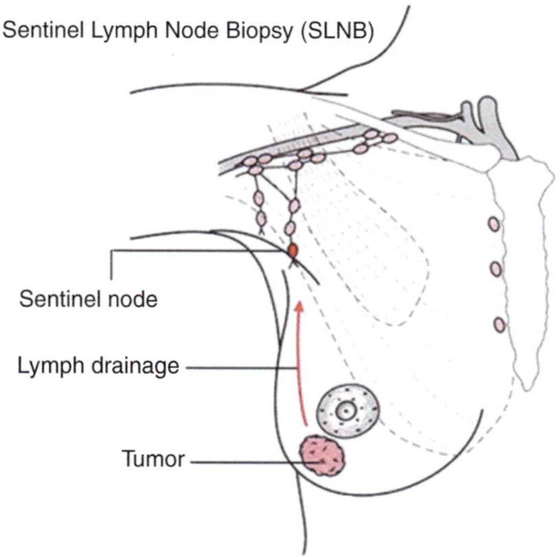

Fig. 25.3 Sentinel lymph node biopsy

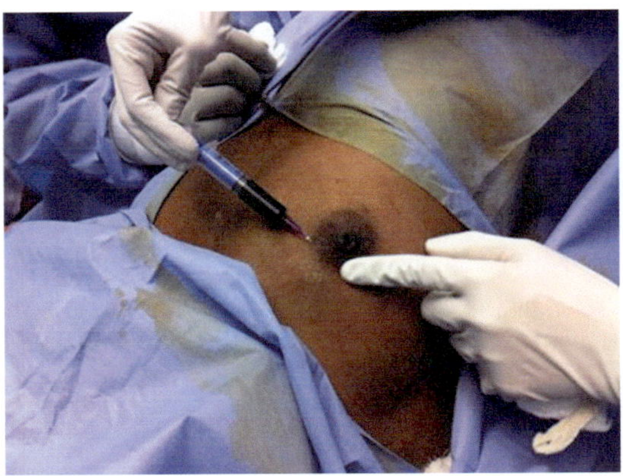

Fig. 25.4 Peri-areolar injection of methylene blue in Sentinel lymph node biopsy

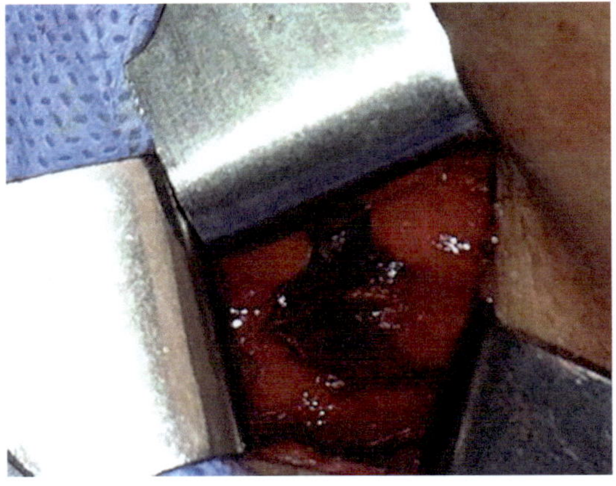

Fig. 25.5 Sentinel node with the blue dye uptake identified in the axilla

node cannot be identified or is found to harbour metastatic disease, then an axillary dissection is performed.

Mapping using blue dye results in 83.1% accuracy. Mapping using radioisotopes results in 89.2% accuracy. Combining both techniques results in 91.9% accuracy. It is possible to achieve high identification rates (over 97%), low false-negative rates and low axillary recurrence rates following SLNB with appropriate training in the dual radiocolloid/blue dye technique [19].

There is no clear cut consensus for the pathological assessment of SLNB. There is no significant effect of occult micro-metastases on the surgical management and patient outcome. Thus, routine immunohistochemistry (IHC) or polymerase chain reaction (PCR) for the evaluation of sentinel lymph nodes (SLNs) in patients unexposed to preoperative systemic therapy is not recommended [20].

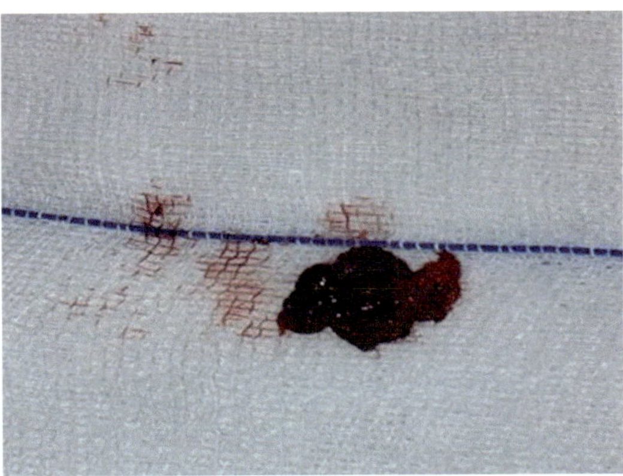

Fig. 25.6 The excised sentinel lymph node

25.6.3 Recommendations

- SLNB, rather than axillary clearance, is the standard of care for axillary staging in early, clinically node-negative breast cancer.
- A positive SLNB with low axillary disease burden in the form of micro-metastases or 1–2 SLNs that are positive for metastatic deposits does not warrant further axillary surgery, provided these patients will be treated with post-operative tangential breast RT.
- Irrespective of the type of breast surgery done, axillary radiation is a good alternative in patients with positive SLNB.

Adjuvant chemotherapy for early invasive breast cancer is considered for all node-positive cancers, all cancers that are larger than 1 cm in size, and node-negative cancers larger than 0.5 cm in size when adverse prognostic features are present. Adverse factors include blood or lymph vessel invasion, high nuclear grade, high histologic grade, HER-2/neu over expression and negative hormone receptor status.

Adjuvant endocrine therapy consisting of tamoxifen or an aromatase inhibitor is considered for hormone receptor positive women with cancers that are larger than 1 cm in size.

Advanced locoregional breast cancer (stage IIIa or IIIb): These women have advanced locoregional disease but no clinically detected distant metastases. Surgery is an integral part along with radiation therapy and chemotherapy (Fig. 25.7).

Stage IIIb patients undergo neo-adjuvant chemotherapy and then after three to four cycles, tumour response is assessed and then the surgery is planned. The molecular type of the cancer will determine the type of neo-adjuvant therapy—whether it is chemotherapy, hormonal therapy or therapy with trastuzumab. Tumour response is assessed both clinically and radiologically. MR mammography is the preferred imaging to assess the tumour response. Ideally a baseline MR mammogram should be done prior to starting the neo-adjuvant therapy.

Stage IIIa patients are divided into those that have operable disease and those who have inoperable disease. In practice, neoadjuvant chemotherapy and hormonal therapy is used routinely for patients with inoperable locally advanced cancer. This neoadjuvant regimen allows for assessment of therapy response, which is of well-established prognostic value and may guide choice of postoperative treatment. Most of these patients will undergo mastectomy, radiation therapy, and additional systemic therapy.

The operable group undergo mastectomy followed by radiation therapy and further systemic therapy. The neoadjuvant approach is also used

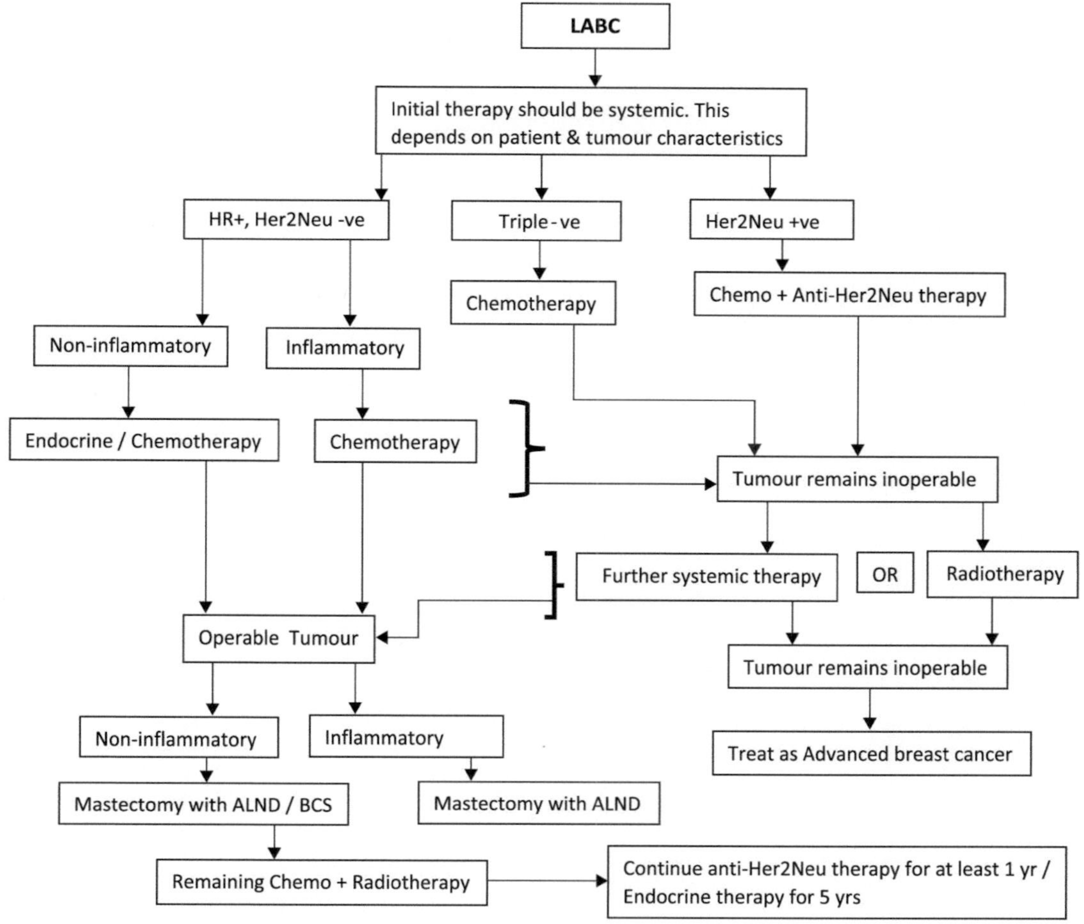

Fig. 25.7 Algorithm for management of locally advanced breast cancer (LABC)

for operable patients who would require mastectomy due to the tumour size. These women could become candidates for breast conservation if their primary tumour size could be reduced before surgery.

The algorithm below outlines the basic steps of management of a locally advanced breast cancer.

Distant metastases (stage IV): Treatment for this group of patients is not curative but may prolong the survival and enhance the quality of life.

Appropriate candidates for initial hormonal therapy include women with (1) hormone receptor positive cancers (2) bone or soft tissue metastases only (3) limited and asymptomatic visceral metastases.

Systemic chemotherapy is considered for women with (1) hormone receptor negative tumours (2) symptomatic visceral metastases and (3) hormone refractory metastases.

These women may develop anatomically localised problems, which will benefit from individualised surgical treatment such as brain metastases, fungating tumours of the breast, pathological fractures of long bones, spinal cord compression and so forth. Biphosphonates, which may be given in addition to chemotherapy or hormonal therapy, should be considered in women with bone metastases.

References

1. Sardanelli F, Boetes C, Borisch B, et al. Magnetic resonance imaging of the breast: recommendations from the EUSOMA working group. Eur J Cancer. 2010;46(8):1296–316.
2. Lakhani SR, Ellis IO, Schnitt SJ, et al. WHO classification of tumours of the breast. WHO classification of tumours, Vol. 4. 4th ed. Geneva: IARC Press; 2012.
3. Goldhirsch A, Winer EP, Coates AS, et al. Personalizing the treatment of women with early breast cancer: highlights of the St Gallen international expert consensus on the primary therapy of early breast cancer 2013. Ann Oncol. 2013;24(9):2206–23.
4. Giuliano AE, Connolly JL, Edge SB, et al. Breast cancer-major changes in the American joint committee on cancer eighth edition cancer staging manual. CA Cancer J Clin. 2017;67(4):290–303.
5. Hortobagyi GN, Connolly JL, D'Orsi CJ, et al. Breast. In: Amin MB, Edge S, Greene F, et al., editors. American joint committee on cancer. AJCC cancer staging manual. 8th ed. New York, NY: Springer; 2017. p. 589–636.
6. Davies C, Godwin J, Gray R, et al. Early breast cancer trialists' collaborative group. Relevance of breast cancer hormone receptors and other factors to the efficacy of adjuvant tamoxifen: patient-level meta-analysis of randomised trials. Lancet. 2011;378(9793):771–84.
7. Slamon D, Eiermann W, Robert N, et al. Adjuvant trastuzumab in HER2-positive breast cancer. N Engl J Med. 2011;365(14):1273–83.
8. Sparano JA, Gray RJ, Makower DF, et al. Prospective validation of a 21-gene expression assay in breast cancer. N Engl J Med. 2015;373(21):2005–14.
9. Cserni G, Chmielik E, Cserni B, Tot T. The new TNM-based staging of breast cancer. Virchows Arch. 2018;472(5):697–703.
10. Koolen BB, Vrancken Peeters MJ, Aukema TS, et al. 18F-FDG PET/CT as a staging procedure in primary stage II and III breast cancer: comparison with conventional imaging techniques. Breast Cancer Res Treat. 2012;131(1):117–26.
11. Cardoso F, Cataliotti L, Costa A, et al. European breast cancer conference manifesto on breast centres/units. Eur J Cancer. 2017;72:244–50.
12. Wilson AR, Marotti L, Bianchi S, et al. The requirements of a specialist breast centre. Eur J Cancer. 2013;49(17):3579–87.
13. Peccatori FA, Azim HA Jr, Orecchia R, et al. Cancer, pregnancy and fertility: ESMO clinical practice guidelines for diagnosis, treatment and follow-up. Ann Oncol. 2013;24(6):vi160–70.
14. Morrow M, Van Zee KJ, Solin LJ, et al. Society of Surgical Oncology-American Society for Radiation Oncology-American Society of Clinical Oncology consensus guideline on margins for breast-conserving surgery with whole-breast irradiation in ductal carcinoma in situ. J Clin Oncol. 2016;34(33):4040–6.
15. Gentilini OD, Cardoso MJ, Poortmans P. Less is more. Breast conservation might be even better than mastectomy in early breast cancer patients. Breast. 2017;35:32–3.
16. Scanlon EF, Caprini JA. Modified radical mastectomy. Cancer. 1975;35(3):710–3.
17. De La Cruz L, Moody AM, Tappy EE, et al. Overall survival, disease-free survival, local recurrence, and nipple-areolar recurrence in the setting of nipple-sparing mastectomy: a meta-analysis and systematic review. Ann Surg Oncol. 2015;22(10):3241–9.
18. Donker M, van Tienhoven G, Straver ME, et al. Radiotherapy or surgery of the axilla after a posi-

tive sentinel node in breast cancer (EORTC 10981-22023 AMAROS): a randomised, multicentre, open-label, phase 3 non-inferiority trial. Lancet Oncol. 2014;15(12):1303–10.
19. Krag DN, Anderson SJ, Julian TB, et al. Sentinel-lymph-node resection compared with conventional axillary-lymph-node dissection in clinically node-negative patients with breast cancer: overall survival findings from the NSABP B-32 randomised phase 3 trial. Lancet Oncol. 2010;11(10):927–33.
20. Lyman GH, Somerfield MR, Bosserman LD, et al. Sentinel lymph node biopsy for patients with early-stage breast cancer: American Society of Clinical Oncology clinical practice guideline update. J Clin Oncol. 2017;35(5):561–4.

Chemotherapy, Hormonal and Targeted Therapy in Breast Cancer

26

P. Jovita M. Martin Daniel

Abstract

The prevention of breast cancer, diagnostic workup, genetic tests, and the recent guidelines in management in the management of early, locally advanced, and metastatic breast cancer are mentioned in this chapter.

Keywords

Genetics in cancer · Chemotherapy · Radiation · Anti-HER2 treatment · Targeted therapy

26.1 Epidemiology

The Globocon 2020 data have suggested that the rate of breast cancers has increased to 2,261,419 (24.5%) of all cancers. Breast cancer currently is one in four cancers diagnosed in women worldwide. With better diagnostics, the detection rate of early cancers is better [1].

P. J. M. M. Daniel (✉)
Sri Ramachandra Institute of Higher Education and Research, Chennai, India
e-mail: drjovitamartin@sriramachandra.edu.in

26.2 Breast Cancer Risk and Prevention

Collectively, the rare genes found to date account for 30% of the heritability, which is the proportion of the phenotypic variance that can be attributed to genetic variation (Table 26.1). Despite the huge amount of work undertaken thus far, ~70% of the disease heritability remains unexplained (signifying missing genes). The common, low-penetrance variants identified through genome-wide association studies (GWAS) have contributed only a small proportion of this missing heritability. The test is done via GWAS uses panels of up to a million or more single nucleotide polymorphisms (SNPs) to identify common genetic variants in large case and control samples [2, 3].

However, about 95% of the patients do not any family history of breast cancer. The risk prediction of breast cancer is not very clear and is far less well established. There is a 12% population lifetime risk of breast cancer (Table 26.2). Deleterious common mutations contribute a 24–36% lifetime risk. This may be high enough to investigate with earlier and more intensive screening for common genetic forms of the disease. Gulcher and Stefansson pointed out that some women classified as average risk were reclassified as at higher risk; likewise, some women might be reclassified as having lower-than-average risk based on their common gene profile. The multi-

B. Dev, L. D. Joseph (eds.), *Holistic Approach to Breast Disease*,
https://doi.org/10.1007/978-981-99-0035-0_26

Table 26.1 Primary breast cancer prevention

RISK FACTORS			
MODIFIABLE	NON-MODIFIABLE	INSUFFICIENT DATA	NOT ASSOCIATED
Relevant lifestyle, obesity, alcohol consumption, physical inactivity, fiber-containing foods, smoking, and exposition to ionizing radiation. Mediterranean diet with consumption of extra virgin olive oil, nuts (>10 g/day), and reduced consumption of fat and red meat can decrease the incidence of breast cancer.	Genetics collectively, the breast cancer genes identified to date contribute only ~30% of the familial risk. [Andrew Collins]	Supplementation of vitamin D, vegetarian or vegan diet, vegetables, fruits, or phytoestrogens.	Oral contraception does not increase the risk of mortality from breast cancer.

Table 26.2 Genes in breast cancer

Genes in Breast Cancer - 30 Identified		
Low Penetrance	Moderate Penetrance	High Penetrance
(Relative risk is 1.5 times the normal population) 10 SNPs in the genes COMT, CYP1A1,CYP1B1, GSTM1 and GSTT1, FGFR2 gene, CASP8 (caspase 8), TOX3 gene, formerly called TNRC9 in which varriant ra3803662 contributes a 1.64-fold homozygote risk, Mitoses-activated protein kinase (MAP3K1) breast cancer gene, LSPI gene, Signals on 3p24, potentially relating to the genes SLC4A7 or NEK10, and on 17q22, perhaps related to COX11, MRPS30 on 5p12 was found to confer higher risk of ER+ disease, SNP in the pericentromeric part of chromosome 1, within a region containing NOTCH2 and FCGR1B, and a signal associated with another double-strand break repair gene (RAD51IL1) on 14q24.1. There is evidence that the chromosome 1 locus is more strongly associated with ER+ disease.	*(2–3 fold increased risk for cancer 2–3% show inherited cancer)* PTEN12 and STK1113 genes cause Cowden and Peutz-Jeghers syndromes, The E-cadherin gene (CDH1), RAD51C is another gene involved in the recombinational repair of dsDNA breaks Ataxia-telangiectasia (ATM) gene, increased risk (~2.2-fold) in carriers of heterozygous mutations, below the age of 50 years. BRIP1 (encoding a BRCA1-interacting protein), PALB2 gene interacts with BRCA2, and mono-allelic mutations are involved in familial breast cancer, conferring a 2.3-fold risk. Checkpoint kinase 2 (CHEK2) gene are known to underlie an approximately twofold increase.	*(8-10 fold increased risk for cancer)* BRCA1 BRCA2 TP53 gene causing Li Fraumeni.

plication of risks from the genetic profiles with independent risks from conventional measures, such as family history, age at menarche, and pregnancy history, could yield a reliable estimate of the risk. Astute application of common breast cancer gene profiles in our day-to-day clinical practice would have several potential benefits such as facilitating earlier diagnosis, reduced costs, less intensive therapeutic intervention, and disease management in the longer term [4].

26.3 Recommendation for Genetic Counseling and Testing

Germline *BRCA1* and *BRCA2* mutations tests must be offered to breast cancer patients in the high-risk groups, that is, those with a strong family history of breast, ovarian, pancreatic, and/or high grade/metastatic prostate cancer, as well as breast cancer diagnosed before the age of 50, triple-negative breast cancer (TNBC) diagnosed before the age of 60, and personal history of ovarian cancer or second breast cancer or male sex.

26.4 Lesions of Uncertain Malignant Potential (B3)

The group of lesions of uncertain malignant potential classified as B3 are detected typically in core or vacuum-assisted biopsy in asymptomatic women. The risk associated with these B3 lesions cannot be strictly categorized according to the type of lesions. These are

- Atypical ductal hyperplasia [ADH] (should be excised in most instances)
- Flat epithelial atypia [FEA]
- Lobular intraepithelial neoplasia
- Papilloma and
- Radial scar

According to Christiane Richter-Ehrenstein et al, additional clinical and pathological factors must be taken into consideration in the diagnosis. Further excision of B3 lesions aims to detect more severe lesions such as (DCIS) and minimize the risk of progression of a lesion of low malignant potential to an in situ or invasive carcinoma. In these cases, an open biopsy is needed with careful radiological-pathological correlation [5].

Clinical features of early breast cancer (EBC)

- Swelling of all or part of a breast (even if no lump is felt);
- Skin dimpling (sometimes looking like an orange peel).
- Axillary lymph node (LN) may be palpable (non-matted, single, mobile).

Clinical features of locally advanced breast cancer (LABC)

- Skin: ulceration, dermal infiltration, erythema over the tumor, satellite nodules, *peau d'orange*
- Chest wall tumor fixation to ribs, serratus anterior, intercostal muscles
- Axillary nodes: Nodes fixed to one another (matted) or other structures

Clinical features of inflammatory breast cancer

- Inflammatory breast cancer is defined as erythema or *peau d'orange* of >1/3 of the skin of the breast with the edema having a defined border.
- Generally Stage 3a or 3b or Stage 4 depending on the nodal involvement.
- The primary tumor is always T4d.
- Inflammatory tumors have dermal lymphatics clogged with tumor emboli.

Diagnostic workup for breast cancer

- Complete history, including menopausal status
- Comorbidities (e.g., cardiac diseases, diabetes mellitus, thromboembolic diseases, renal, or liver disease)

Early breast cancer

- Assessment of general health: Physical examination, complete blood count, liver, renal, and cardiac (in patients planned for anthracycline and/or trastuzumab treatment) function tests, alkaline phosphatase, and calcium.

- Assessment of tumor: Physical examination (including primary tumor, regional lymph nodes), mammography, breast ultrasonography (USG), breast magnetic resonance imaging (MRI) in selected cases, core biopsy with the pathological determination of histology, grade, ER, PR, HER2 neu, Ki6, (AR, EGFR optional).
- Assessment of LN: Physical examination of, ultrasound (US)-guided biopsy if suspicious.
- Assessment of metastasis: Other tests are not routinely recommended, a disease with less high tumor burden, aggressive biology, or when symptoms suggestive of metastases are present.

Locally advanced or metastatic breast cancer

- A detailed history of the primary tumor and its biology, management, and status at the last follow-up.
- History of recurrent/metastatic disease, including duration, with the previous sites of involvement, previous treatments given, and their effects current symptoms, performance status, socioeconomic background, and preferences are needed.

Assessment of visceral disease

- Chest: preferably CT; chest X-ray has low sensitivity and should be replaced by chest computed tomography (CT) whenever possible. Abdomen: ultrasound, CT (preferably), or MRI.
- Bone scan, with confirmation of lesions and further workup (i.e., fracture risk, etc.) if needed by X-ray/CT/MRI.
- CT and/or MRI of the CNS should be symptom driven.
- Positron emission tomography (PET)/PET-CT should not be used routinely as part of the initial workup in early breast cancer but can be useful for identifying metastasis in symptomatic patients in early/locally advanced breast cancer (a situation where patients may benefit from a more aggressive multidisciplinary approach) and to identify the site of relapse when traditional imaging methods are conflicting.
- Estrogen, progesterone, and HER2 receptors of the metastatic lesion should be obtained at least once in the evolution of the disease, if technically possible, and particularly if not available from the primary tumor.
- Circulating tumor cells are still an experimental technique and should not be used outside a clinical trial.
- In case of lesions inaccessible for biopsy, functional imaging such as PET–CT, DCE-MRI, or MR-DWI may be helpful to confirm their malignant character.

26.5 Management of Early Breast Cancer (EBC)

26.5.1 Guidelines for the Management of Early Breast Cancer (EBC)

DCIS:

- Total mastectomy is done then only tamoxifen or AI is given for 5 years. Adjuvant hormonal therapy 5 years of tamoxifen (NSABP B 24) /AI (NSABP B35) is recommended.
- If lumpectomy is done, Adjuvant radiation (NSABP B17), substantially reduced the incidence of ipsilateral breast tumor recurrence from 35.0% in the lumpectomy only group to 19.8% in the lumpectomy followed by the radiotherapy group.
- When treated with breast-conserving surgery (BCS), a 2-mm margin is adequate in DCIS treated with whole breast radiotherapy (WBRT).

The tumor is <5 mm (T1a)

- It carries an excellent prognosis. However, controversy exists over the extent of treatment.
- Chemo and anti-Her2 therapy can be skipped if low-grade and complete surgery have been done.
- If estrogen receptor (ER), progesterone receptor (PR) positive aromatase inhibitor is the option in older women.

- In younger women, TNBC or HER2 positive or higher grade better not to compromise on the treatment. Kiel et al. [6].

Tumor is 5–10 mm (T1b), >T1c

- Chemotherapy is mandatory; anti-HER2 treatment, and hormonal treatment are a must as per the receptor positivity [7].
- pT1micN0; pT1aN0; <pT2N0 and Luminal A (Ki 67 < 20%) low risk: No adjuvant chemotherapy (NSABP B20/DBCG77B—San Antonio).

26.5.2 Mastectomy a Mandatory in (Flow Chart 26.1)

- Tumor size large (relative to breast size).
- Tumor multicentricity.
- If there is the inability to achieve negative surgical margins after multiple resections.
- If there was prior radiation to the chest wall/breast or other contraindications to RT.
- If the patient has unsuitability for oncoplastic breast conservation and patient choice,
- BCS is the preferred local treatment option for the majority of early breast cancer patients, with the use of oncoplastic techniques, to maintain good cosmetic outcomes in technically challenging cases, when needed.
- Careful histological assessment of resection margins is essential. No tumor at the inked margin is required and >2 mm for in situ disease is preferred.

Types of Mastectomy*:* Besides simple mastectomy and skin-sparing mastectomy (SSM) that preserves the skin envelope, nipple-sparing mastectomy (NSM) has been increasingly been used in the last decade.

26.5.3 Reconstruction (Flow Chart 26.4)

Breast reconstruction should be available and proposed to all women requiring mastectomy.

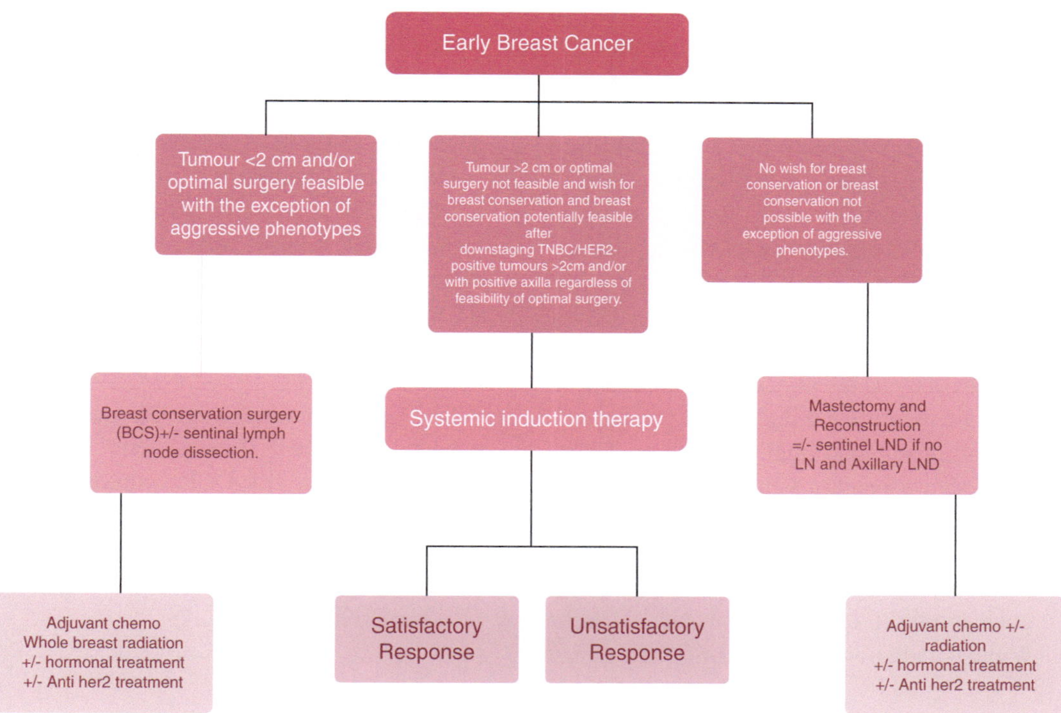

Flow Chart 26.1 EBC surgical management

Immediate breast reconstruction should be offered to the vast majority of patients, except for those presenting with inflammatory cancer. The optimal reconstruction technique for each patient should be discussed individually taking into account anatomic, treatment, and patient-related factors and preference.

26.5.4 Sentinal Lymphnode Biopsy (SLNB)

SLNB, rather than full nodal clearance, is the standard of care for axillary staging in early, clinically node-negative breast cancer. Further axillary surgery following positive SLNB is not required in case of low axillary disease burden (micrometastases or 1–2 SLNs containing metastases, treated with postoperative tangential breast RT. Axillary radiation is a valid alternative in patients with positive SLNB, irrespective of the type of breast surgery.

26.5.5 Radiation

- Radiation is a very important adjuvant treatment in breast cancer. With developments in the newer technologies from 3dCRT 3-dimensional conformal radiotherapy, intensity-modulated radiotherapy (IMRT), image-guided radiotherapy (IGRT), volumetric modulated arc therapy (VMAT), postmastectomy radiation (PMRT), accelerated partial breast radiation (APBI), and brachytherapy (Mammosite therapy/Interstitial brachy) there are means by which the radiation dose to heart and lung has been minimized to a great extent. Dimensional conformal treatment. RTOG 9804, shows benefits with adjuvant radiation.
- EBCTCG (The Early Breast Cancer Trialists' Collaborative Group) meta-analysis has concluded that radiation can be avoided in low-grade tumors, tumor >2 mm, negative margin. Without radiation 10 years Ipsilateral breast recurrence is 30%, and with radiation, it is 18%.
- BCS followed by WBRT, whole breast radiation or total mastectomy, are acceptable treatment options for DCIS.
- In occult breast cancer with axillary lymph node dissection (ALND), the patient is offered WBRT.
- Postoperative radiation is strongly advised after BCS.
- Boost radiotherapy (RT) is recommended to reduce the risk of in-breast field relapse in patients at higher risk of local recurrence.
- APBI is an acceptable treatment option in patients with a low risk for local recurrence.
- PMRT is recommended for high-risk patients, including those with involved resection margins, involved axillary lymph nodes, and T3–T4 tumors; it should also be considered in patients with 1–3 positive axillary lymph nodes.
- Comprehensive nodal RT is recommended for patients with involved lymph nodes (the role of irradiating particular nodal volumes is poorly defined).
- Postoperative RT, if indicated, can be administered after immediate breast reconstruction have traditionally been 45–50 Gy in 25–28 fractions of 1.8–2.0 Gy with a typical boost dose of 10–16 Gy in 2 Gy single doses. Shorter fractionation schemes (e.g., 15–16 fractions with 2.5–2.67 Gy single dose) have shown similar effectiveness and comparable side effects.
- RT may be delivered safely during anti-HER2 therapy, ET and non-anthracycline, and non-taxane-based ChT.
- WBRT is recommended for the majority of women with DCIS treated with BCS. In patients with low-risk DCIS, omitting radiation is an option. Tumor bed boost can be considered for patients at higher risk for local failure. PMRT is not recommended for DCIS. ESMO 2021 [8].

26.6 **Systemic Therapy** (Flow Charts 26.2 and 26.3) (Table 26.3)

- In the evolution of primary systemic therapy (PST) (chemotherapy, chemo, ChT) in breast cancer, a 30-year follow-up study by Bonnadona et al. showed that six cycles of cyclophosphamide, methotrexate, and fluorouracil (CMF regimen) in patients with operable breast cancer significantly reduced the relative risk of relapse of disease and death at a median follow up of 20 years.
- MILAN Trial showed four cycles of Adriamycin Cyclophosphamide (AC)/ Epirubicin Cyclophosphamide (EC) was superior to standard six cycles CMF.
- CALGB 9344 showed the benefit of using taxane in node-positive breast cancer, which increased the overall survival (OS) and disease-free survival (DFS).
- CALGB 9741 used ACx4 followed by Taxane × 4 every 3 weeks. Dose-dense chemo 2 weekly did show an advantage in overall survival at the expense of toxicity.
- Trials have proven the equivalent results with the use of Paclitaxel or Docetaxel.
- The sequencing of AC followed by taxol is better than the Taxol, Adriamycin, and Cyclophosphamide (TAC) regimen, which carries a higher toxicity rate.
- Adjuvant systemic treatment should preferably start within 3–6 weeks postsurgery, and neoadjuvant systemic therapy should start as soon as diagnosis and staging are completed (ideally within 2–4 weeks).
- The decision on adjuvant systemic therapies should be based on the patient's biological age; performance status; an individual's risk of relapse (tumor burden and tumor biology); the predicted sensitivity to particular types of treatment; the benefit from their use; and their associated short- and long-term toxicities, comorbidities, preferences, and financial status.
- In Luminal A, patients are treated with endocrine therapy. However, Luminal A-like tumors with a high disease burden do require chemotherapy.

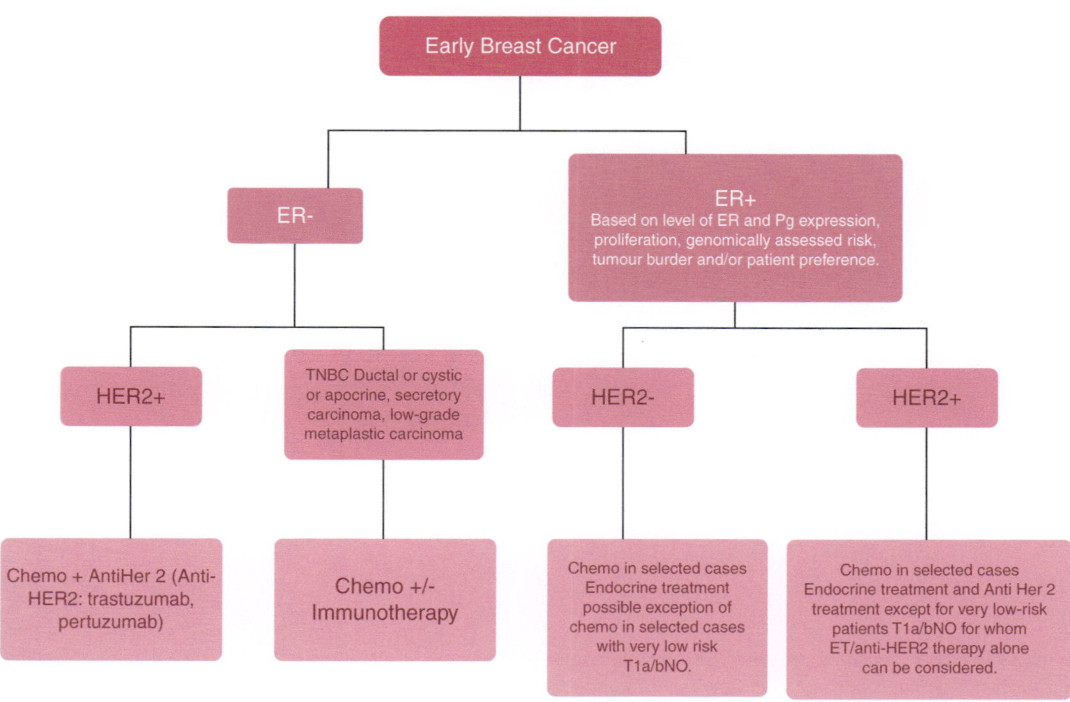

Flow Chart 26.2 EBC systemic treatment with chemotherapy, hormones, and anti-HER2 neu therapy

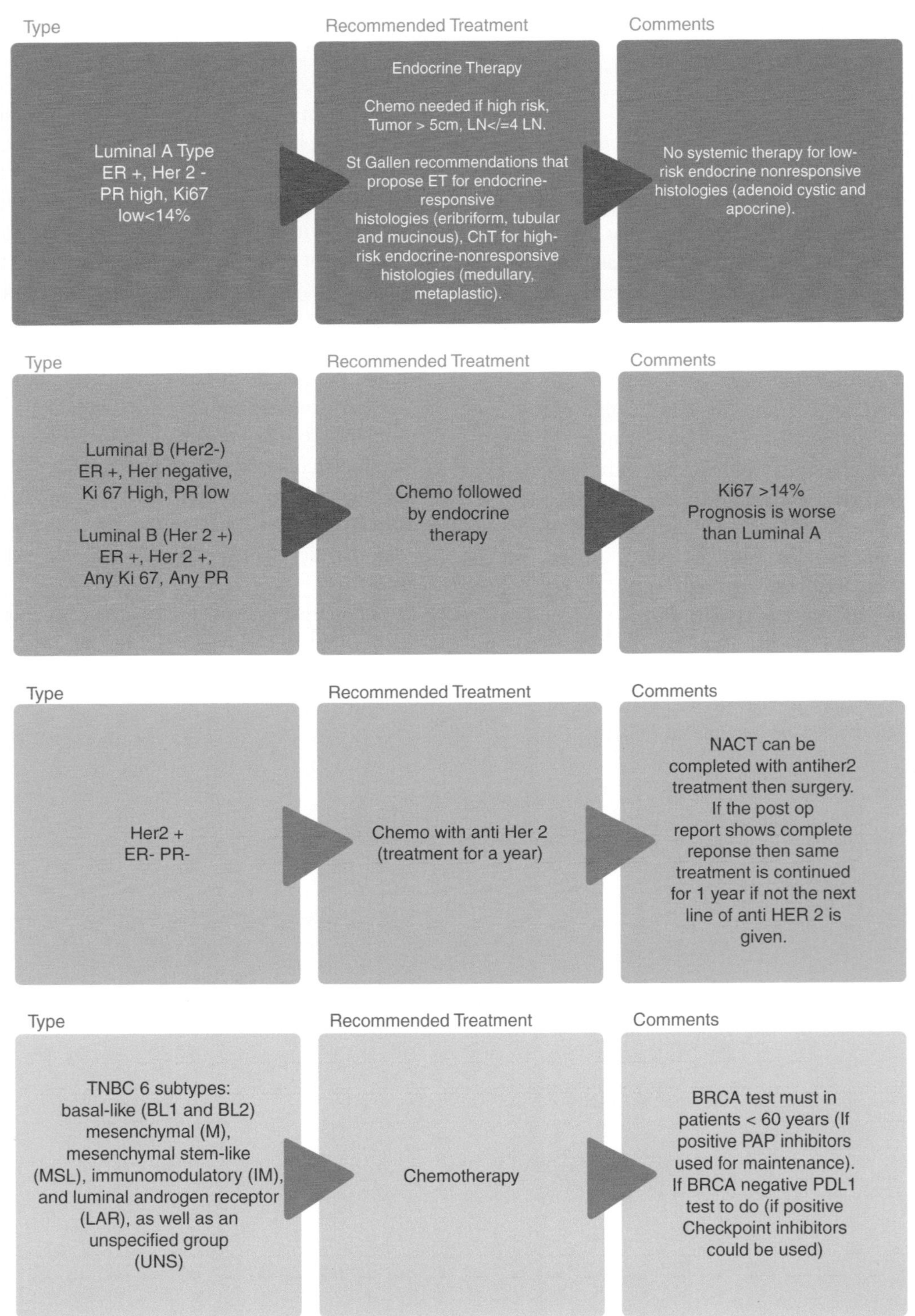

Flow Chart 26.3 Systemic treatment recommendations for early breast cancer based on subtypes. *ER* estrogen receptor, *HER2* human epidermal growth factor receptor 2, *MRI* magnetic resonance imaging, *PR* progesterone receptor, *US* ultrasound, *ET* endocrine therapy, *HER2* human epidermal growth factor receptor 2, *RT* radiotherapy, *TNBC* triple-negative breast cancer, *TPBC* triple-positive breast cancer, *LN* lymph node, *ChT*/Chemo chemotherapy, *OFS* ovarian function suppression, *AI* aromatase inhibitor

Table 26.3 Common chemotherapy regimens are used in different subtypes of breast cancers. NCCN 2021 [9] (Flow Chart 26.3)

Luminal A Common chemo regimens Neoadjuvant/ Adjuvant	Luminal B Common chemo regimens Neoadjuvant/ Adjuvant	Luminal B with HER 2 positive Neoadjuvant/ Adjuvant	HER 2 positive Neoadjuvant/ Adjuvant	TNBC Neoadjuvant/ Adjuvant
• AC 4 cycles (T1/T2 N0 M0) • AC 4 cycles + Taxol 4 cycles (Node positive, T>5cm, high risk) • Oder patients EC 4 cycles • FAC regimen	• AC 4 cycles (T1/T2 N0 M0) • AC 4 cycles +Taxol 4 cycles (Node positive, T>5cm, high risk) • Dose Dense AC Plus weekly Paclitaxel or 3 weekly Paclitaxel • Docetaxol / Paclitaxol + Carboplatin • T regimen	• AC 4 cycles + Taxol + Trastuzumab 4 cycles Followed by trastuzumab for one year • AC 4 cycles + Taxol + Trastuzumab + Pertuzumab 4 cycles Followed by trastuzumab + pertuzumab for one year • TCH regimen • TCH + Pertuzumab	• AC 4 cycles + Taxol + Trastuzumab 4 cycles Followed by trastuzumab for one year • AC 4 cycles + Taxol + Trastuzumab + Pertuzumab 4 cycles Followed by trastuzumab + pertuzumab for one year • TCH regimen • TCH + Pertuzumab Post-chemo Neratinib as extended anti-HER2 treatment	• AC 4 cycles +Taxol +/- Carboplatin 4 cycles • Taxol + Carboplatin 6 cycles

A/T Adriamycin-Taxol, *AC* Adriamycin + cyclophosphamide, *EC* Epirubicin + cyclophosphamide, *TCH* Taxol Carbo trastuzumab

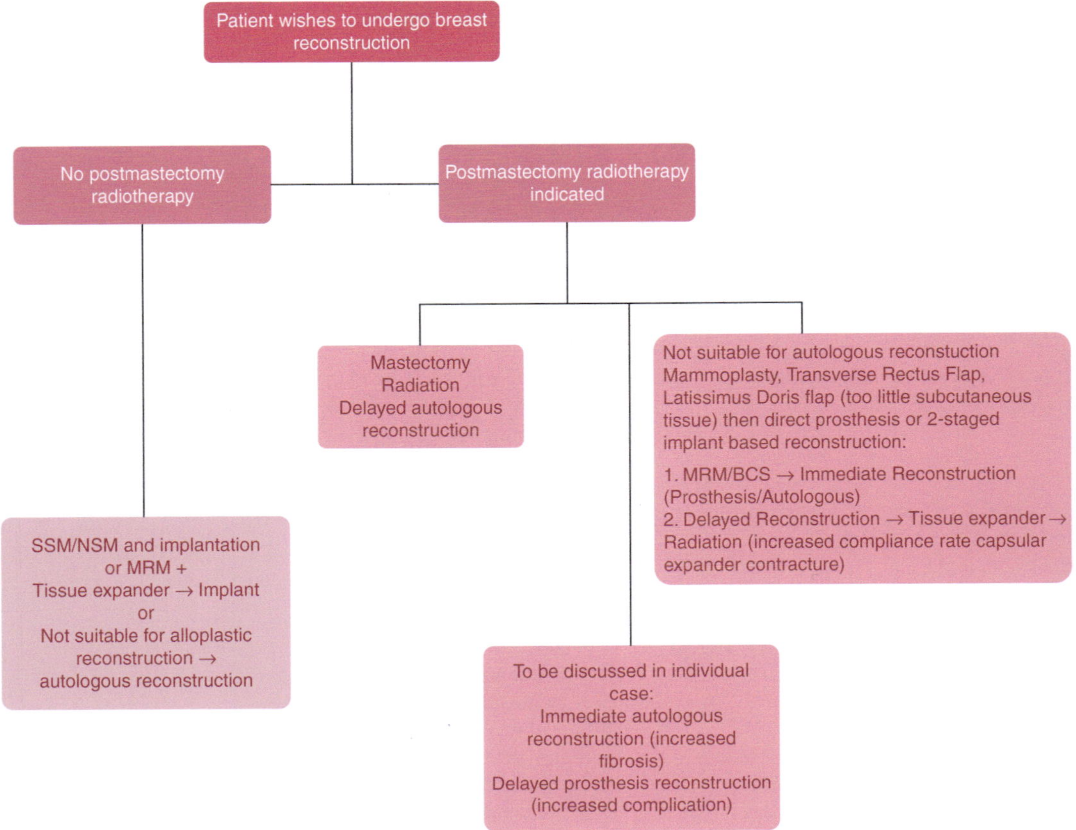

Flow Chart 26.4 On the choice of breast surgery

- The decision on the appropriate use of adjuvant Chemo (after consideration of all clinical and pathological factors) is done with the gene expression assays, such as MammaPrint, Oncotype DX, Prosigna, Endopredict, or Breast Cancer Index, or expression of uPA-PAI1 can be used.
- Chemo use in Luminal B-like HER2-negative patients depends on individual risk of recurrence, presumed responsiveness to ET, and patient preferences as well, for example, pT1b—T2N0 and Luminal B (Ki 67 > 20%). An informed decision regarding benefits and risks after gene expression assays and treatment TC (Docetaxel Cyclophosphamide) × 4 cycles (US Oncology Research Trial 9735 trial).
- Luminal B-like HER2-positive tumors should be treated with chemo, and anti-HER2 therapy followed by adjuvant ET postsurgery and radiation (as and when needed).
- In selected low-risk patients (T1abN0), the combination of anti-HER2 therapy and ET alone may be used without chemotherapy.
- TNBC patients should receive chemo, with the possible exception of low-risk "special histological subtypes" such as secretory or adenoid cystic carcinomas or very early (T1aN0) tumors. ESMO 2021 [8].
- In patients with LN+, >T3, Age< 35 years Dose Dense AC (Adriamycin Cyclophosphamide) × 4 cycles → Dose Dense Paclitaxel × 4 cycles (CALGB 9741 trial).
- Ischemic heart disease TC (Docetaxel Cyclophosphamide) × 6 cycles in the first cycle 75% of the dose of chemo used followed by escalation based on tolerance (US Oncology Research Trial 9735 trial); or CMF 6 cycles.

- GnRH analog administration with chemo shows a 16.8% absolute reduction in chemo-induced premature ovarian insufficiency (POI) for those who might plan for future pregnancy (Lambertien et al. ASCO, PROSPERO trial). However, the factors that might be looked into for fertility posttreatment would be younger age < 40 years and baseline levels of anti-Müllerian hormone (patient-related factors), co-administration of GnRHa, the addition of taxanes to anthracycline-based chemotherapy, and addition of endocrine therapy to chemotherapy.

26.6.1 Anti-HER2 Treatment (Table 26.3)

- HER2-positive cancers should be treated with chemo and anti-HER2 therapy, with the possible exception of selected cases with very low risk, such as T1aN0 tumors.
- Chemo should not be used concomitantly with ET, except gonadotropin-releasing hormone (GnRH) analogs used for ovarian protection. Anti-HER2 therapy may routinely be combined with non-anthracycline-based chemo ET and radiation.
- HR+/HER2− and high-risk conventional dosed Adriamycin-Taxol (A/T) based chemo q3 weeks, Dose-dense chemotherapy (include the weekly schedule), and Endocrine treatment.
- HER2 + Trastuzumab + Pertuzumab neoadjuvant at high risk (APHINITY trial), Sequential A/T based regimen with concurrent T (Taxol) and Anti-HER2 therapy (HERA, NSABP B 37, NCCTGN 9831, BCIRG006).
- Her 2 positive: Size > T1c or T1b with high-risk factors (High Grade, ER/PR negative, Node +) TCH (Docetaxel Carboplatin Trastuz umab) × 6 cycles → Trastuzumab total 1 year (BCIRG 006).
- Unwilling for 1 year of adjuvant Trastuzumab → Dose Dense AC × 4 cycles→ Dose Dense Paclitaxel × 4 cycles with Short Course Trastuzumab (BCIRG 006/FINHER trials).

26.7 TNBC (Table 26.3)

- Conventionally dosed A/T based chemo, dose-dense chemotherapy, NACT platin containing chemo
- If ChT and RT are to be used in the adjuvant setting, ChT should usually precede RT
- Triple Negative Breast Cancer Dose Dense AC × 4 cycles → Dose Dense Paclitaxel × 4 cycles (CALGB 9741 trial).\
- High-risk LN positive TNBC: Neoadjuvant use of AC × 4 cycles→ Paclitaxel + Carboplat in increases the Pathological Response rate. (GeparSixto trial, GEICAM, I-SPY 2 study, CALGB 40603).
- If post-surgery there is a residual disease after completion of neoadjuvant chemotherapy/ neoadjuvant chemo-radiation Capecitabine × 6 cycles (Create X trial, SYSUCC-002 trial).

26.7.1 Endocrine Therapy

- EBCTCG a meta-analysis of 60 trials with a follow-up of 15 years with the use of Tamoxifen for 5 years showed a 41% decrease in annual recurrence rate.
- For premenopausal women, tamoxifen for 5–10 years is a standard of care (ATLAS, aTTOM trials). As ER positive patients have a long latency period for relapse. Ten-year use of Tamoxifen showed increased DFS, OS, with LN positive, High-grade tumors with high Oncotype DX score.
- In patients becoming postmenopausal during the first 5 years of tamoxifen, a switch to letrozole should be considered, depending on the predicted risk of late recurrence.
- In patients requiring chemo and who recover menses (in particular in the first year but acceptable within the first 2 years), the addition of ovarian function suppression (OFS) to ET should be strongly considered (TEXT and ABCSG-12 trial). SOFT Trial LHRH agonist + AI (Aromatase Inhibitor) was used in high risk, LN positive, Ki 67 high, which showed superior results.

- The role of replacing tamoxifen with an AI can be considered in high-risk patients; if used, it mandates effective OFS, with regular biochemical control of estrogen levels.
- The role of OFS in patients <35 years not requiring chemo is not clear, but inferior outcomes of young luminal early breast cancer patients suggest the use of the most effective ET (i.e., combination with OFS).
- OFS during chemo provides some protection of ovarian function and has no negative impact on oncological outcomes; thus, it should be proposed to patients. It should not, however, be the sole fertility preservation method used, in case of a desired pregnancy (POEMS/S0230 trial).
- For postmenopausal women, AIs (both nonsteroidal and steroidal) and tamoxifen are considered standard treatments (BIG 1–98, NSABP B-42).
- AIs can be used upfront (nonsteroidal AI or steroidal AI—exemestane), after 2–3 years of tamoxifen or as extended adjuvant therapy, after 5 years of tamoxifen (letrozole and anastrozole) (Arimidex-Nolvadex (ARNO 95) and Austrian Breast and Colorectal Cancer Study Group (ABCSG 8) trials).
- Switch therapy for a prolonged period in high-risk patients with LN +, high Ki 67 and figh grade, high oncotype Dx with 5 years of Tamoxifen and 5 years of Letrozole showed increased DFS but no benefit in OS (MA17R, NSABP B42).
- Extended adjuvant therapy should be discussed with all patients, except those with a very low risk of relapse, but the optimal duration and regimen of adjuvant ET are currently unknown. There is only a minimal benefit for the use of AIs for more than 5 years.

26.7.2 Chemotherapy

- Chemo should be administered for 12–24 weeks (four to eight cycles).
- Sequential anthracycline/taxane-based regimen is the standard for the majority of patients.
- In selected lower risk patients, four cycles of anthracycline- or taxane-based chemo or CMF may be used.
- Non-anthracycline regimens may be used in patients at risk of cardiac complications.
- Anthracycline-based regimens should not include 5-FU (EC or AC is standard).
- Platinum compounds should not be used routinely in the adjuvant setting. The use of dose-dense schedules [with granulocyte colony-stimulating factor (G-CSF) support] should be considered, particularly in the highly proliferative tumor. ESMO 2021 [8].

26.7.3 Anti-HER2 Therapy (Flow Chart 26.2)

- Neoadjuvant trastuzumab is highly effective and should be given to all HER2-positive early breast cancer patients who do not have contraindications (cardiac issues) for its use, with the possible exception of selected cases with very low risk, such as T1aN0 tumors. One year of neoadjuvant trastuzumab remains a standard for the vast majority of HER2-positive patients. (NOAH trial-Trastuzumab) (NeoSphere trial-Trastuzumab + Pertuzumab in high-risk patients)
- In highly selected, low-risk patients who receive anthracycline/taxane-based chemo, shortening trastuzumab duration to 6 months may be discussed.
- Trastuzumab should usually not be given concomitantly with anthracycline-based ChT; it can be safely combined with non-anthracycline-based chemo (i.e., taxanes) and its concomitant use is more effective than sequential treatment. Regular cardiac monitoring is essential before and during trastuzumab treatment.
- Dual blockade with trastuzumab/lapatinib has not led to improved long-term outcomes and cannot, therefore, be recommended.
- Dual blockade with trastuzumab/pertuzumab can be considered in high-risk patients, defined as N-positive or ER-negative, for 1 year, starting before or after surgery.

- In the neoadjuvant setting patients who have the residual invasive disease after completion of chemo combined with anti-HER2 therapy, adjuvant trastuzumab should be replaced by adjuvant T-DM1.
- Extended anti-HER2 therapy with neratinib may be considered in selected high-risk patients but not in patients previously treated with the dual blockade. Neratinib requires appropriate diarrhea prophylaxis and management (ExteNET trial).
- Primary systemic therapy (PST) should be used to reduce the extent of surgery in locally advanced and large operable cancers, in particular when mastectomy is required due to tumor size. It should also be considered in all patients with tumors >2 cm for which chemo is deemed necessary, in particular with triple-negative and HER2-positive subtypes.
- Drugs and drug regimens used in the preoperative setting should be selected according to rules identical to those in the postoperative setting. A sequential regimen of anthracyclines and taxanes is recommended for the vast majority of patients.
- The addition of a platinum compound may be considered in triple-negative tumors and/or in patients with deleterious *BRCA1/2* mutations.
- If PST is used, all chemo should be delivered preoperatively.
- In high-risk, triple-negative patients not achieving PCR after standard neoadjuvant ChT, the addition of metronomic chemo as extended adjuvant chemo with capecitabine for 1 year postoperatively should be considered.
- In postmenopausal patients with ER-positive/HER2-negative cancers requiring PST and without a clear indication for chemo, preoperative ET (4–8 months or until maximum response) should be considered and continued postoperatively,
- Bisphosphonates for early breast cancer are recommended in women with low-estrogen status (undergoing OFS or postmenopausal), especially if at high risk of relapse.
- Bisphosphonates are also recommended in patients with treatment-related bone loss.

26.7.4 Male Breast Cancer

- Tamoxifen is the standard adjuvant ET for male breast cancer patients.
- If a strong contraindication exists for the use of tamoxifen, a combination of an AI plus a luteinizing hormone-releasing hormone (LHRH) agonist may be considered, but its higher toxicity must be discussed with the patient to avoid compliance issues.
- An AI alone should not be used as adjuvant ET in male breast cancer patients.
- Chemo and anti-HER2 therapy indications and regimens should follow the same recommendations as those for breast cancer in female patients.

26.7.5 Bone Health

- In patients especially at high risk of relapse, bisphosphonates for early breast cancer are recommended in women with low-estrogen status (undergoing OFS or postmenopausal).
- Bisphosphonates are also recommended in patients with treatment-related bone loss (osteoporosis). ESMO 2021 EBC [8].

26.7.6 Ongoing Trials

There are many trials in the pipeline trying to use CDK 4/6 inhibitors in the neoadjuvant setting in Luminal A patients in early or LABC. Some of them are

- PALLAS,PENELOPE-B, (Palbociclib)
- PALTAN, PATRICIA, (Palbociclib + Trastuzumab)
- PATINA, NA-PHER-2 (Palbociclib + Trastuzumab+Pertuzumab)
- EARLEE-1, NATALIE (Ribociclib)
- MONARCH E, Neo MONARCH (Abemaciclib)
- Monarc HER2 (Abemaciclib + trastuzumab)

26.7.7 Guidelines for the Management of Locally Advanced Breast Cancer (LABC)

Locoregional recurrence is a harbinger of systemic recurrence; hence, one needs to address the local disease and the systemic disease.

26.7.8 Available Chemotherapy Agents/Regimens for LABC (Flow Charts 26.5 and 26.6)

Commonly used regimens in LABC.

Anthracycline-containing

- Doxorubicin or epirubicin monotherapy (weekly or tri-weekly) Doxorubicin/cyclophosphamide or Epirubicin/cyclophosphamide Liposomal doxorubicin ± cyclophosphamide Fluorouracil/doxorubicin/cyclophosphamide or fluorouracil/epirubicin/cyclophosphamide
- Taxane-containing Paclitaxel monotherapy weekly
- Docetaxel monotherapy tri-weekly or weekly Abraxane (nab-paclitaxel)
- Anthracycline (doxorubicin or epirubicin)/taxane (paclitaxel or docetaxel)
- Docetaxel/capecitabine Paclitaxel/gemcitabine Paclitaxel/vinorelbine Paclitaxel/carboplatin

The treatment plan in LABC (Flow Charts 26.5 and 26.6)

- In selected LABC patients: Dose-dense AC (Adriamycin Cyclophosphamide) × 4 cycles dose-dense Paclitaxel × 4 cycles → Surgery → Radiation (CALGB 9741 trial) can be used as well.
- In LABC patients with HER2 neu overexpression or TPBC: TCH (Docetaxel Carboplatin Trastuzumab) × 6 cycles → Surgery → Radiation with adjuvant Trastuzumab × 1 year. If the patient is unwilling for 1 year of Trastuzumab → AC × 4 cycles → Paclitaxel + Short

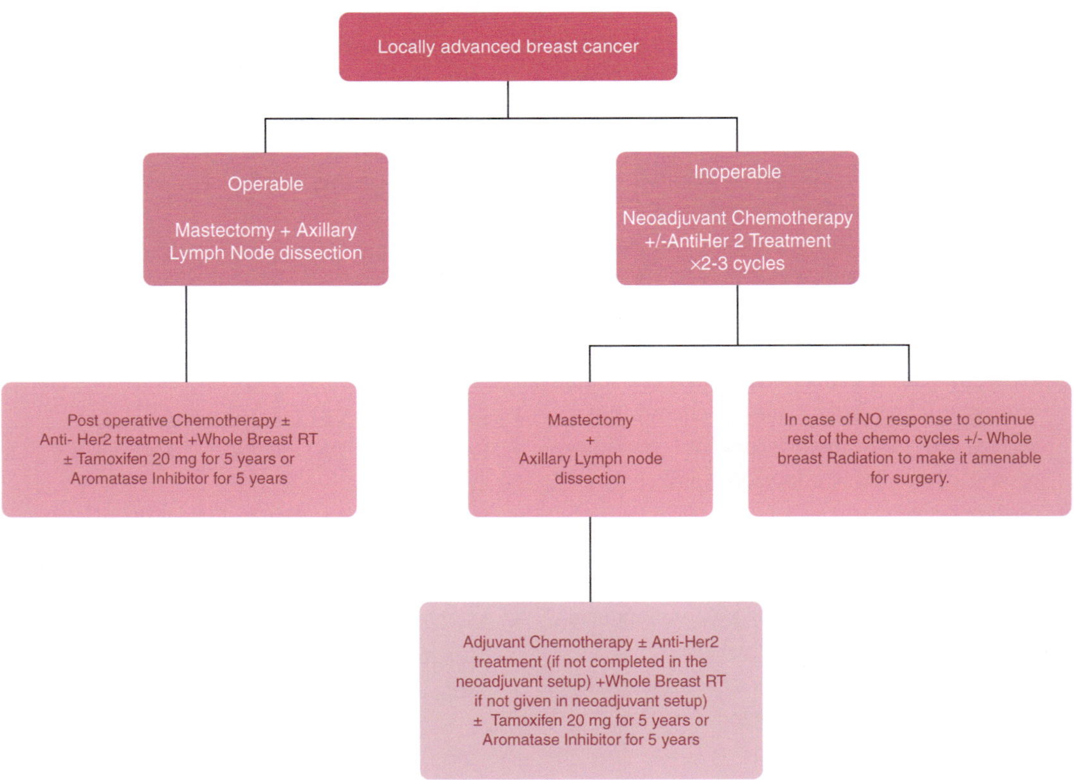

Flow Chart 26.5 Management of LABC is a flowchart

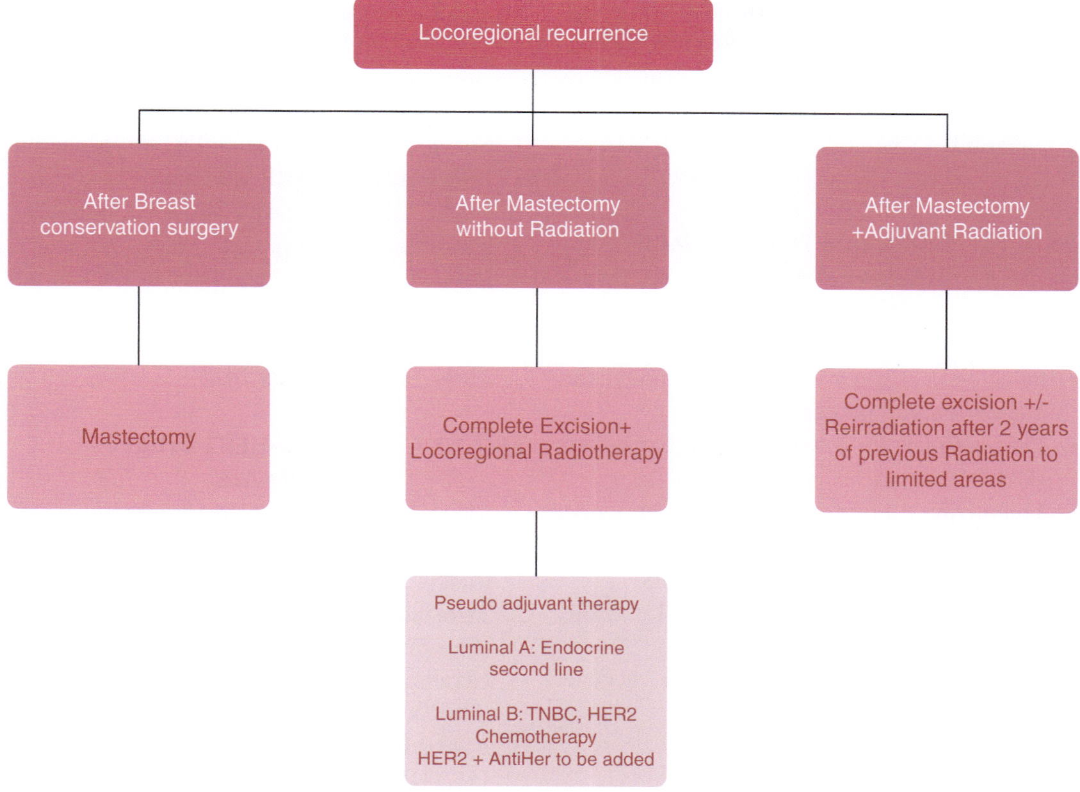

Flow Chart 26.6 Management of locoregional recurrence in breast cancer in a flow chart

course Trastuzumab → Surgery (BCIRG 006, FINHER trials).

- Ischemic heart disease TC (Docetaxel Cyclop hosphamide) × 6 cycles → Surgery → Radiati on (US Oncology Research trial 9735).
- If post-surgery there is a residual disease after completion of neoadjuvant chemotherapy/neoadjuvant chemo-radiation Capecitabine × 6 cycles (Create X trial, SYSUCC-002 trial).

26.7.9 Guidelines for the Management of Metastatic Breast Cancer (MBC)

26.7.9.1 Available Chemotherapy Agents/Regimens for MBC

Regimens used for LABC are also used for MBC. There are other single agents used as follows

- Eribulin
- Ixabepilone (not approved by EMA) non-anthracycline-containing cyclophosphamide/methotrexate/fluorouracil (CMF)
- Platinum-based combinations (TNT Trial in TNBC) (e.g., cisplatinum + 5-fluorouracil; carboplatin + gemcitabine)
- Capecitabine Vinorelbine
- Capecitabine + vinorelbine Vinorelbine ± gemcitabine
- Oral cyclophosphamide with or without methotrexate (metronomic chemotherapy)

26.7.9.2 Brain Metastasis

- In active brain metastasis (BM): 1–10 BM with favorable prognostic factors resection or stereotactic radiation is offered (SRT); >10 BM with unfavorable BM then whole brain radiation.
- In active metastasis without local intervention, options would be Tucatinib + Capecitabi ne + Trastuzumab or Trastuzumab deruxtecan.

- If unknown or stable BM Tucatinib + Capecit abine + Trastuzumab or Trastuzumab deruxtecan, Lapatinib + Trastuzumab, Margetuximab + Chemotherapy, Neratinib + Chemothearapy. ESMO 2022.

26.7.10 Endocrine Therapy Used in Luminal A MBC Is as Follows

- Selective estrogen response modulator: Tamoxifen, Raloxifene
- Estrogen receptor down-regulator: Fulvestrant (FALCON trial)
- Luteinizing hormone-releasing hormone: Goserelin, leuprorelin analogs, triptorelin
- Third-generation aromatase inhibitors
- Nonsteroidal: Anastrazole, Letrozole, Exemestane
- Steroidal: Medroxy progesterone acetate, megestrol acetate
- Progestins: Nandrolone decanoat
- Anabolic steroids
- Estrogen
- CDK 4/6 Inhibitors:
  - Palbociclib: PALOMA 2, PALOMA 3 (Postmenopausal) Trials)
  - Ribociclib: MONALESSA 2,MONALESSA 3 (Postmenopausal), MONALESSA 7 (premenopausal) trials
  - Abemaciclib: MONARCH 2 trial (pre-, peri-, and postmenopausal)
- MTOR Inhibitors: Everolimus (BOLERO 2 trials)
- PIK3CA inhibitors: Alpelisib (SOLAR-1 trial)

26.7.11 First Line in HR + MBC

- Any ER + MBC without imminent organ failure: ET + CDK4/6 inhibitors till progression
- Any ER + MBC with imminent organ failure: ChT

26.7.12 Second Line in HR + MBC

On progression, the tests offered to do would be

1. Somatic BRCA mutation/PALB1 Mutation/ESR Mutation: PARP Inhibitor
2. PIK3CA Mutation: Alpelisib + Fulvestrant
3. Everolimus + Fulvestrant
4. Progression after several lines of ET and targeted therapy: Chemotherapy (We may check for a low HER2 neu expression by IHC, MSI, TMB, NTRK) ESMO 2022

26.7.12.1 The Anti-HER2 Drugs Available Are

1. Monoclonal antibodies (MAbs); Trastuzumab, Pertuzumab (CLEOPATRA, MARIANNE trials)
2. Tyrosine Kinase Inhibitors: Lapatinib (Capecitabine + Lapatinib EGF100151), Neratinib (NALA trial), Tucatinib (HER2CLIMB trial)
3. Antibody-drug conjugates (ADCs)
   (a) TDM 1 ado-trastuzumab emtansine (EMILIA, TH3RESA trials)
   (b) Margituximab (SOPHIA trial)
   (c) Trastuzumab deruxtecan (two phase III trials are investigating trastuzumab deruxtecan in patients with HER2-low MBC (DESTINY-Breast04)
   (d) Trastuzumab duocarmazine (SYD985) (TULIP trial).

26.7.13 First Line MBC HER2 Enriched

HR+

- If Chemo contraindicated:
  - Trastuzumab ± Pertuzumab + ET
- If no ChT contraindications:
  - Taxol + Trastuzumab-Pertuzumab >/= 6 cycles followed by Trastuzumab Pertuzumab ET maintenance

HR–

- If chemo contraindicated:
  - Trastuzumab ± Pertuzumab until progression
- If no ChT contraindications:
  - Taxol + Trastuzumab-Pertuzumab >/= 6 cycles followed by Trastuzumab Pertuzumab maintenance

On further progression, we may check for MSI, TMB, NTRK. ESMO 2022.

26.7.13.1 Newer Drugs in TNBC (Table 26.4)

- PARP inhibitors (BRCA Mutation Positive):
  - Olaparib (Olympia, Neo-Olympia and Olympiad)
  - Talazoparib (EMBRACA trial)
- Checkpoint Inhibitors (PDL1 Positive)
  - Nivolumab (TONIC Trial)
  - Pembrolizumab (Anti-PD-1 Antibodies) (KEYNOTE-355 Trial)
  - Atezolizumab (PD-L1 Inhibitor) (IMpassion130 Trial)

Table 26.4 TNBC and its therapeutic targets (Lehmann et al., Yin et al.)

Subtypes	Genetic abnormalities	Therapeutic targets
BL1	Cell cycle gene expression DNA repair gene (ATR-BRCA pathway) Proliferation genes	Mitosis inhibitors Cytostatics PARP inhibitors DNA synthetic inhibitors
BL2	Inhibit TP63, EGFR, and MET signaling	Cytostatics PARP inhibitors Growth factor inhibitors mTOR inhibitors
IM (immunomodulatory)	Inhibit immune signaling	Cytostatics PARP inhibitors Immune checkpoint inhibitors
M (mesenchymal)	Inhibit EMT, Wnt, PI3K, mTOR, Scr, TGFβ, IGF1R, notch	Growth factor inhibitors mTOR inhibitors Scr inhibitors PI3K inhibitors
MSL (mesenchymal stem-like)	Inhibit EMT, Wnt, TGFβ, MAPK, Rac, PI3K, mTOR, Scr, PDGF	Growth factor inhibitors mTOR inhibitors PI3K inhibitors MAPK inhibitors Scr inhibitors
LAR (luminal androgen receptor)	Inhibit AR signaling, FOXA1, and ERBB4 signaling	Nonsteroidal antiandrogens mTOR inhibitors PI3K inhibitors

Mitosis inhibitors (Paclitaxel, Docetaxel, Ixabepilone, Nab-Paclitaxel, Vinorelbine)
Cytostatics (Cisplatin, Carboplatin, Nedaplatin, Eptaplatin, Oxaliplatin, Lobaplatin, Satraplatin, Mercaptopurine)
PARP inhibitors (Olaparib, Rucaparib, Talazoparib, Niraparib)
DNA Synthetic inhibitors (Topotecan, Irinotecan, Camptothecin, Doxorubicin, Daunorubicin, Mitomycin)
Growth Factor inhibitors (Erlotinib, Gefitinib, Afatinib, Osimertinib, Olmutinib, Nazartinib, Avitinib, Lapatinib, Cetuximab, Panitumumab, Vandetanib, Bevacizumab, Pertuzumab, Ramucirumab, Trastuzumab, Axitinib, Cabozantinib, Ceritinib, Crizotinib, Lenvatinib, Nilotinib, Pazopanib, Regorafenib, Sorafenib, Sunitinib)
mTOR inhibitors (Rapamycin, Everolimus, RapaLink-1)
Scr Inhibitors (Bosutinib, Dasatinib)
PI3K Inhibitors (Idelalisib)
MAPK Inhibitors (Trametinib, Dabrafenib)
Nonsteroidal Antiandrogens (Bicalutamide)
Immune Checkpoint Inhibitors (Ipilimumab, Nivolumab)

- PDL1–
  - Imminent Organ Failure: AC + Taxol, Taxol+Bevacizumab, Capecitabine +Trastuzumab
  - No Imminent Organ Failure: Anthracycline Monotherapy (ESMO2022)
- Sacituzumab Govitecan (ASCENT, IMMU-132)
- Any Further Progression ChT: Eribulin, Capecitabine, Vinorelbine

26.8 Summary of Recommendations for the Management of Metastatic Breast Cancer

26.8.1 Advanced Breast Cancer ESMO 2021 ABC [10]

- The management of metastatic breast cancer should involve all appropriate specialties in a multi/interdisciplinary team.
- From the start of the diagnosis of metastatic breast cancer, patients should be offered personalized appropriate psychosocial, supportive, and symptom-related interventions as a routine part of their care. Due to the recent advancements and improvements in the options in the armamentarium of drugs, there is increased overall survival, progression-free survival, and disease-free survival.
- Patients with oligometastatic have improved survival to the point of conversion of intent from palliative to curative.
- Whether oligometastasis or polymetastasis timely incorporation of different modalities is imperative, such as radiation (EBRT/SBRT) and surgery.
- Following a thorough assessment and confirmation of metastatic breast cancer, the realistic treatment goals must be specified and discussed. Patients and caregivers (if the patient prefers to) should be invited to participate in decision-making.
- An aggressive multidisciplinary approach including local therapy may be warranted in selected patients with limited metastatic disease.
- The clinical value of tumor markers is not well established for diagnosis or follow-up; however, their use for monitoring response to treatment, particularly in patients with the nonmeasurable disease, is useful.
- Treatment choice should take into account tumor biology and disease burden, previous therapies and responses obtained, patient preferences, performance status, comorbidities, socioeconomic, psychological factors, and therapies available in the patient's country.
- Endocrine therapy is the preferred option for hormone receptor-positive disease unless the rapid response is warranted or endocrine resistance is suspected.
- HER2-directed therapy should be offered early to all HER2-positive metastatic breast cancer patients, either as a single agent, combined with chemo-, or with endocrine therapy. Patients progressing on an anti-HER2 therapy combined with a cytotoxic agent should be offered a second line of anti-HER2 therapy.
- Sequential single-agent chemotherapy is the preferred option in metastatic breast cancer in the absence of rapid clinical progression, life-threatening visceral metastases, or the need for rapid symptom and/or disease control.
- If the patient has a visceral crisis, hormone negative and hormone resistance (>3 lines exposed) first line can be Paclitaxel; second line can be Adriamycin based (if previously not exposed), third line can be Capecitabine (Cochrane review).
- Prior exposure to Anthracycline and Taxane first line would be Capecitabine; second line would be Eribulin/Vinorelbine/rechallenge with Paclitaxel (DFS > 1 year).
- In cases with HER2 positive first line—TH (Docetaxel + Trastuzumab)/THP (Docetaxel + Trastuzumab + Pertuzumab). If the patient is unwilling to anti-HER2 therapy → Single-agent chemotherapy can opt. (CLEOPATRA trial). For a second Line—Trastuzumab Emtansine (TDM1)/Lapatinib + Capecitabine can be used (EMILIA trial).

- In postmenopausal, hormone receptor positive, HER2 negative: Letrozole + Palbociclib; if unwilling for Palbociclib: Letrozole alone (PALOMA 2 Trial).
- In premenopausal, hormone receptor-positive, HER2 negative Oophorectomy/Radio-castration → Letrozole + Palbociclib. If unwilling for ovarian suppression therapy: Tamoxifen (PALOMA 2 Trial).
- In postmenopausal, hormone receptor-positive, prior exposed to Letrozole to use Exemestane or Fulvestrant (EFECT trial).
- Bone metastasis Zoledronic Acid Q 3 monthly × 2 years (CALGB trial).
- Patients with metastatic disease might be exposed to several lines of treatment on a sequential basis until the time of progression (with no more agents that can be tried due to exhaustion of all drugs possible) or intolerance or financial exhaustion.
- There are only a few proven standards of care in metastatic breast cancer management, and inclusion of patients in well-designed, independent, prospective randomized trials must be a priority.
- Given the rising costs of metastatic breast cancer treatment, balanced decisions should be made, but patient well-being, length, and quality of life must always be the main decision factors.
- Validated patient-reported outcome measures to provide useful information about symptom severity and the burden and impact of these symptoms on the overall quality of life and should be collected and integrated with other clinical assessments, to form part of the treatment decision making.

References

1. Globocon data 2021.
2. UICC.GLOBOCAN 2020: new global cancer data. 2020. https://www.uicc.org/news/globocan-2020-new-global-cancer-data.
3. Collins A. The genetics of breast cancer: risk factors for disease. Appl Clin Genet. 2011;4:11–9.
4. Gulcher J, Stefansson K. Genetic risk information for common diseases may indeed be already useful for prevention and early detection. Eur J Clin Investig. 2010;40(1):56–63.
5. Richter-Ehrenstein C. Lesions of "uncertain malignant potential" in the breast (B3) were identified with mammography screening. BMC Cancer. 2018;18:829.
6. Kiel KD. Management of T1a breast cancer. Clin Breast Cancer. 2004;5(1):43–51.
7. Ditsch N, Untch M, Thill M, Müller V, Janni W, Albert US, et al. AGO recommendations for the diagnosis and treatment of patients with early breast cancer: update 2019. Breast Care (Basel). 2019;14(4):224–45.
8. Cardoso F, et al. Early breast cancer: ESMO clinical practice guidelines for diagnosis, treatment, and follow-up. Ann Oncol. 2019;30:1194–220.
9. NCCN. Guideline V. 2021.
10. Gennari A, André F, Barrios CH, ESMO Guidelines Committee, et al. ESMO clinical practice guideline for the diagnosis, staging, and treatment of patients with metastatic breast cancer. Ann Oncol. 2021;32(12):1475–95.

27 Imaging Surveillance of Treated Breast

M. C. Sheela, Bhawna Dev,
and Anupama Chandrasekharan

Abstract

There are various surgical procedures of the breast ranging from simple lumpectomy to radical mastectomy and similarly reconstructing techniques. The role of imaging in postoperative breast is to identify the possible complications and most importantly to rule out recurrence.

Keywords

Postoperative imaging · Seroma · Fat necrosis · Abscess · Recurrence

27.1 Introduction

The common surgical techniques are [1].

- **Oncological:**
  - Modified Radical Mastectomy (MRM)
  - Breast Conservation Surgery (BCS)
  - Skin sparing mastectomy
  - Nipple sparing mastectomy
- **Reconstructive breast surgery:**
  - Synthetic implants (Discussed elsewhere in the book)
  - Autologous tissue transfer (flaps)

    Common pedicled flaps: Transverse Rectus Abdominus muscle flap (TRAM), Latissmusdorsi muscle flap (LDM)

    Common free flaps: TRAM, deep inferior epigastric perforator flap (DIEP), superior gluteal artery perforator flap (SGAP), inferior gluteal artery perforator flap (IGAP)
  - Autologous fat grafting—filling of lumpectomy/excisional biopsy defect
  - Neoadjuvant chemotherapy (NAC) reconstruction, primary augmentation, and augmentation in conjunction with flaps
- **Cosmetic:**
  - Augmentation mammoplasty
  - Reduction mammoplasty

27.1.1 Few Facts About Role of Imaging in Postoperative Breast

- Regular follow-up imaging is indispensable in women treated for breast cancer.
- There is no definite consensus regarding follow-up imaging in carcinoma breast.
- Recurrence can be an ipsilateral recurrence, a contralateral breast cancer, an axillary recurrence, or distant metastases.

M. C. Sheela (✉) · B. Dev · A. Chandrasekharan
Department of Radiology, Sri Ramachandra Institute of Higher Education and Research, Chennai, India
e-mail: sheelamc@sriramachandra.edu.in; bhawnadev@sriramachandra.edu.in

B. Dev, L. D. Joseph (eds.), *Holistic Approach to Breast Disease*,
https://doi.org/10.1007/978-981-99-0035-0_27

- Annual follow up mammography is considered standard practice. Imaging surveillance should not commence earlier than 12 months after diagnosis or 6 months after completion of radiation therapy.
- Routine ultrasound surveillance is not recommended by most guidelines. However, optional surveillance is recommended for young women or women with dense breasts.
- Routine breast magnetic resonance imaging (MRI) surveillance is also not recommended, unless women carry additional risk factors, indicating a lifetime recurrence risk >20% [2].

27.1.1.1 Mammogram

Mammogram of the conservatively treated breast is performed for several reasons [3], mainly

- To confirm complete removal of the biopsy-proven malignancy
- To identify post procedural fluid collections, microcalcifications, fat necrosis, scarring, and architectural distortion
- To detect residual or recurrent tumor
- To screen for metachronous cancers in the affected breast and contralateral breast

27.1.1.2 Ultrasound

- To diagnose seromas/abscess
- Axilla screening
- Guided interventions like aspirations in abscess/seroma/biopsy of suspicious recurrent lesions

27.1.1.3 MRI

- Problem solving in tool in indeterminate lesions in mammogram and ultrasound
  - For example, scar versus recurrence, fat necrosis versus recurrence
- For guided interventions when lesions are conclusively seen only on MRI

27.2 A Chronology of the Common Postoperative Changes

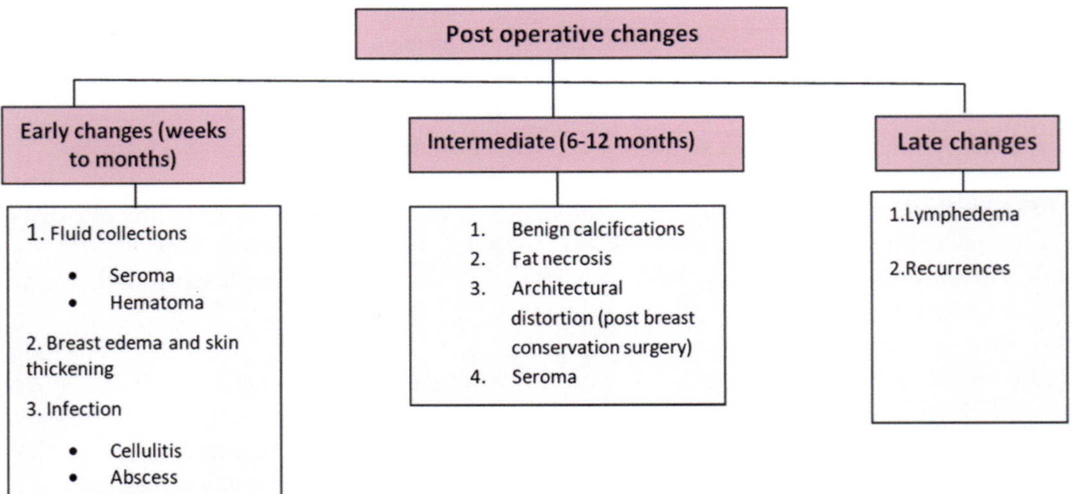

27.2.1 Early Postoperative Changes

27.2.1.1 Fluid Collection—Seroma and Hematomas

The most common postoperative finding is seroma.

Etiopathogenesis: The rich lymphatic drainage patterns of the breast, potential space intentionally created by surgical excision for better cosmesis, and low fibrinogen levels within lymph fluid are thought to contribute to seroma formation [4].

Clinical Presentation: Swelling in the postoperative site, usually painless. More common in older, obese women and following MRM than lumpectomy.

Imaging Features

Usually ultrasound is done as first-line imaging to map seroma postsurgically.

Mammogram: Appears as well-defined oval or round equal or high-density lesion at the postoperative site/axilla (if axillary clearance is performed).

Ultrasound: Seromas appear as well-defined anechoic fluid (Fig. 27.1) or a complex fluid collection, showing, mild internal echoes and septations (Fig. 27.2) with posterior acoustic enhancement. On color Doppler study, there is no significant internal or peripheral vascularity. Hematomas appear as fluid collection with internal echoes (Fig. 27.3).

MRI: Seroma appears as a T1W hypointense and T2W hyperintense signal intensity (Fig. 27.2) with no/mild uniform peripheral enhancement. Hematoma has variable appearances depending on the age of the hematoma.

BI-RADS category: **BI-RADS 2**

Clinical Management: Usually managed conservatively. If symptomatic, ultrasonography (USG)-guided aspiration of the seroma is performed.

Follow up: Approximately half of breast cancer patients had fluid collections at the surgical site at 4 weeks after surgery and about 25% at 6 months and generally completely resolved by 12–18 months [3, 5].

27.2.1.2 Breast Edema and Skin Thickening

Normal breast skin thickness is about 1–2 mm. Skin thickening (more than 2 mm) is the most common finding after breast-conserving therapy (BCT), reported in up to 90% of patients [6].

Etiopathogenesis: Prominent periareolar edema is occasionally present as a result of surgical disruption of the lymphatics. Skin thickening during the period after radiation is secondary to breast edema from the damage of small vessels.

Clinical Presentation: In postlumpectomy patients, edema is limited to the postoperative site in contrast to radiation therapy where it involves the entire breast.

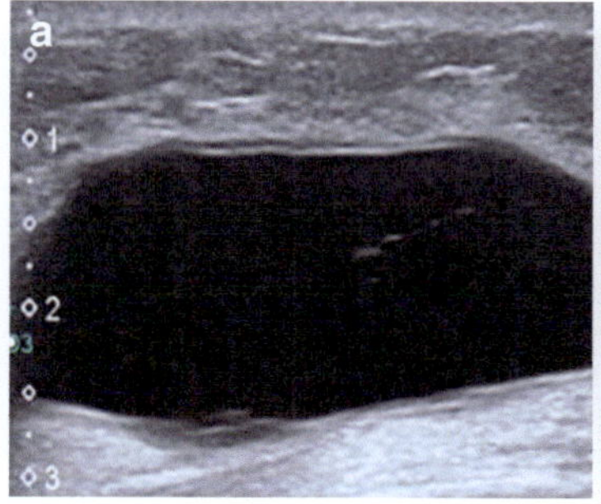

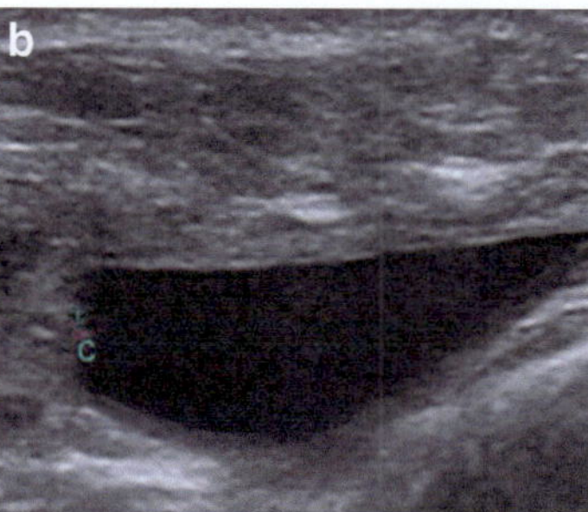

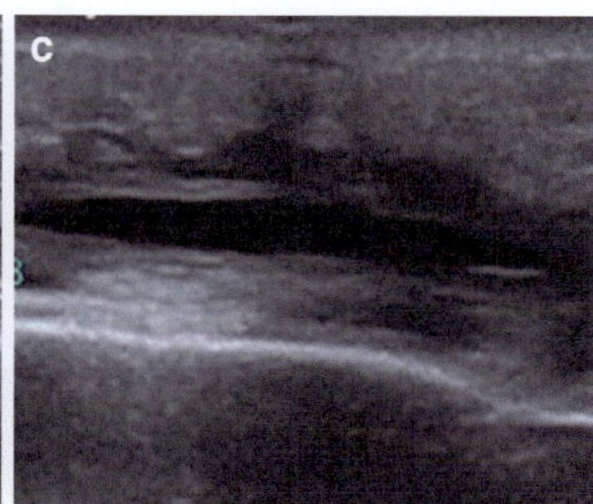

Fig. 27.1 Seroma. (**a**) USG of post mastectomy scar area reveals a well defined thin walled anechoic collection along the scar site, representing seroma. (**b**) Follow up ultrasound after 5 months and at 1 year. (**c**) reveal gradual reduction in the size of the seroma

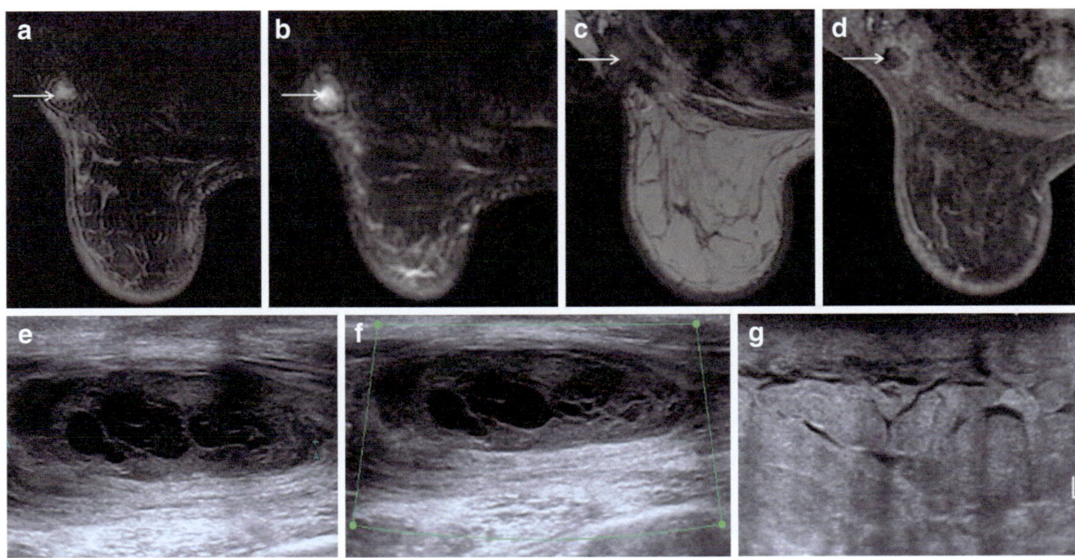

Fig. 27.2 Organized seroma—post BCS (1 year. postoperative status) on follow up. (**a**, **b**) STIR and T2W fat-saturated sequence reveals a thick-walled cystic mass (arrow) in the left axilla, appearing hypointense on T1W (**c**) with no significant enhancement (**d**). (**e**) Ultrasound reveals a complex heteroechoic collection in the left axilla with no significant vascularity (**f**). Ultrasound showing edema of the adjacent subcutaneous tissue (**g**)

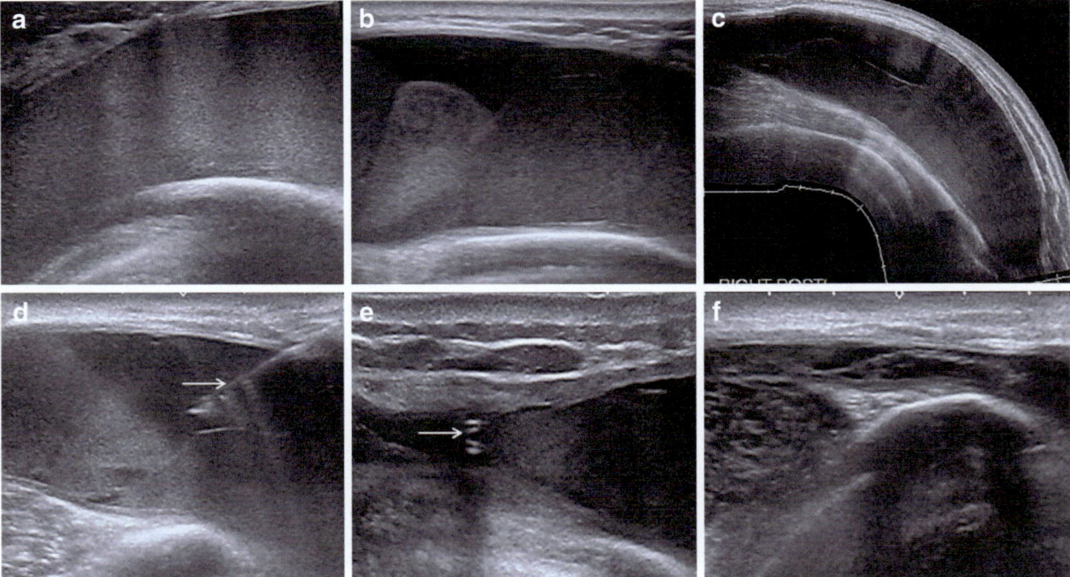

Fig. 27.3 Hematoma. (**a**, **b**) USG reveals a collection with mobile internal echoes along the post-MRM scar site—s/o hematoma. (**c**) Panoramic view of the same showing complete extent of collection. (**d**) USG-guided aspiration done with needle in situ (arrow). (**e**) Follow-up ultrasound after 2 days showed reaccumulation of hematoma, hence pig tail catheter placement done (arrow). (**f**) Follow up after 2 weeks revealed complete resolution of the hematoma

Imaging Features

Mammogram: Breast edema presents as more of an accentuated trabecular pattern when the degree of edema is moderately severe or as overall increased breast density when the degree of edema is marked (Fig. 27.4a, c), in contrast to contralateral normal breast (Fig. 27.4b, d). The perceived increased density in the irradiated breast may also be by suboptimal exposure at the time of imaging, as treated breast often is swollen and less compressible.

On ultrasound (Fig. 27.4e, f) and **MRI** (Fig. 27.5): It reveals decrease in skin thickness as compared to the prior imaging.

The differential diagnoses of recurrent or worsening breast edema include the lymphatic spread of cancer, obstructed venous drainage, congestive heart failure, and infection.

> Edema or skin thickening that increases after stability has been achieved is an alarming sign necessitating further investigation.

BI-RADS category: **BI-RADS 2** in usual postoperative cases. In suspicious increase in skin thickening on follow up cases, *BI-RADS 0 with further assessment/BI-RADS 4*, if a frank mass is visualized.

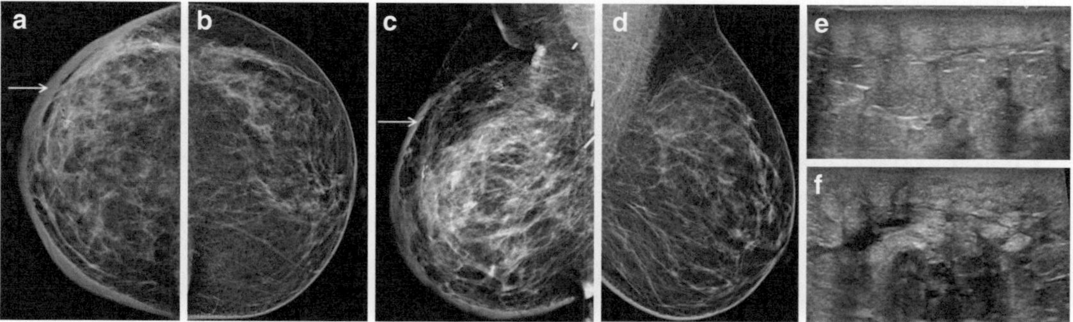

Fig. 27.4 Skin thickening. CC (**a**, **c**) and MLO (**b**, **d**) views of both the breasts shows asymmetric diffuse thickening of the skin and subcutaneous tissue in the right breast (arrows). (**e**, **f**) USG shows edema of the skin, subcutaneous tissue, and breast parenchyma

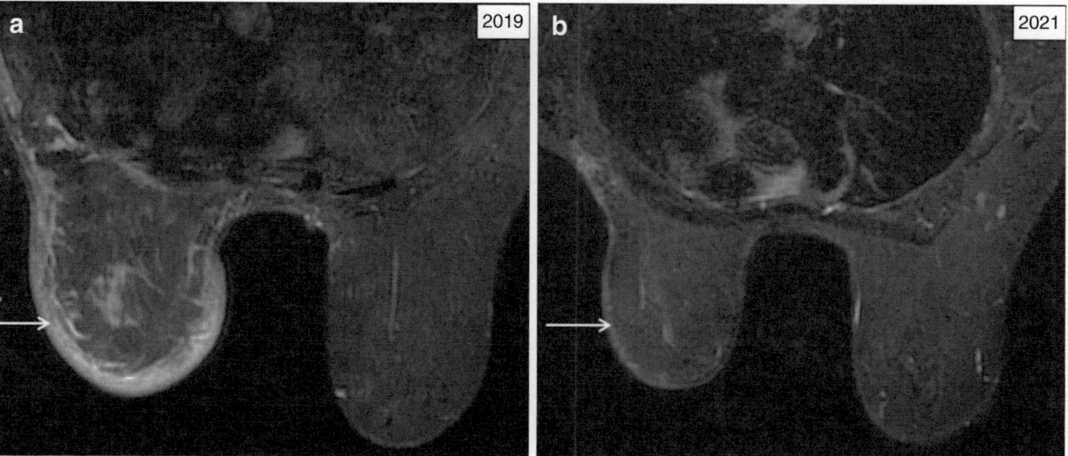

Fig. 27.5 (**a**) MRI-STIR sequence reveals diffuse thickening of the skin (arrow) with intra parenchymal edema involving the left breast. (**b**) Follow up MRI after 2 years show complete regression of the skin thickening and edema—resolving skin thickness

Clinical Management

Conservative management for benign postoperative/postradiotherapy-induced edema.

Prognosis: Maximum breast edema and skin thickening are usually seen during the first 6 months after completion of radiation therapy and then diminish and attain stability for many patients by 2–3 years [3].

27.2.1.3 Infection

The rate of postoperative infection is variable, ranging from 1% to 20% [5]. It is usually cellulitis or abscess.

Cellulitis

Etiopathogenesis: The presence of a large seroma increases the likelihood of associated postoperative infection due to lymph stasis or percutaneous aspiration (during which skin bacteria may be introduced into the seroma). Delayed cellulitis is usually due to lymph stasis.

Clinical Presentation: Cellulitis usually appears within 1 month of surgery. It present as painful tender and swollen breast. It may be associated with systemic features like fever and malaise.

Imaging Features

On **Mammogram**—It appears as increased skin thickening (>3 mm) with thickened trabeculae (Fig. 27.6a, b).

On ultrasound—It appears as thickened skin with fluid insinuating between the fat, which is indistinguishable from a postoperative change (Fig. 27.6c).

On MRI—The usual findings are increased skin thickening with T2W hyperintensities along the trabeculae.

Abscess

Clinical Presentation: This occurs usually within 1–2 weeks after surgery, presenting as a fluctuant tender mass at the surgical site.

Imaging Features

Ultrasound evaluation is the usual investigation of choice and reveals a complex hypoechoic (Fig. 27.6d) or isoechoic fluid collection. Mobile

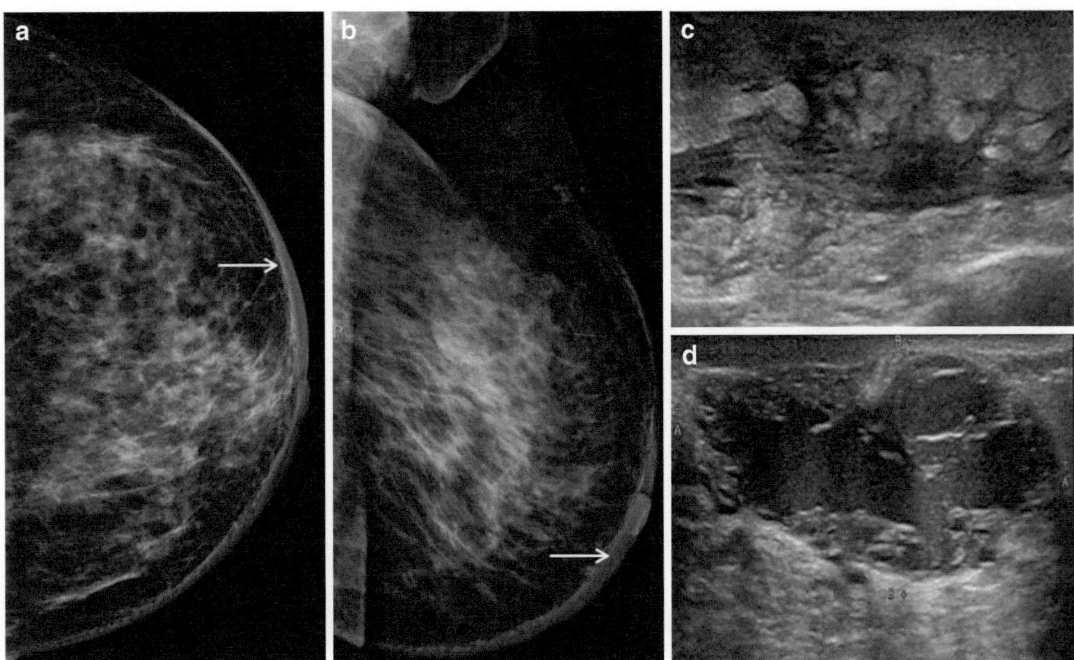

Fig. 27.6 Post-BCS patient, presenting with pain in left breast and fever. (**a**, **b**) CC and MLO view shows diffuse increase in skin thickening. (**c**) USG showed thickened skin with fluid insinuating between the fat. (**d**) Follow-up ultrasound after 4 days showed heteroechoic collection suggestive of abscess formation

debris within the fluid collection and hypervascularity of the adjacent breast tissue may also be seen. There may be associated probe tenderness.

BI-RADS CATEGORY: **BI-RADS 2.**

Management

Definitive abscess management usually requires surgical or percutaneous drainage depending on the size of the abscess.

27.3 Intermediate Postoperative Changes

27.3.1 Fat Necrosis

Etiopathogenesis: Fat necrosis is a sterile inflammation of fat in the breast resulting from loss of vascular supply. It is commonly seen in a reconstructed autologous flap. It is also secondary to radiotherapy.

Lipolysis, inflammatory cell infiltration, and hemorrhage occur acutely followed by the formation of fibrous scar or a calcified cystic mass as the lesion evolves resulting in a variable imaging appearance (1).

Clinical Presentation: It is a common complication of myocutaneous flaps usually seen after 6–12 months of treatment and clinically present as a palpable mass that is firm or hard [6].

27.3.1.1 Imaging Features

It has a variable imaging appearance.

Mammogram: Fat necrosis most commonly appears as an irregular (Fig. 27.8a, b) or spiculated mass, microcalcifications, coarse calcifications, or lucent oil cysts (Fig. 27.7a, b). The calcifications are characteristically oval or round

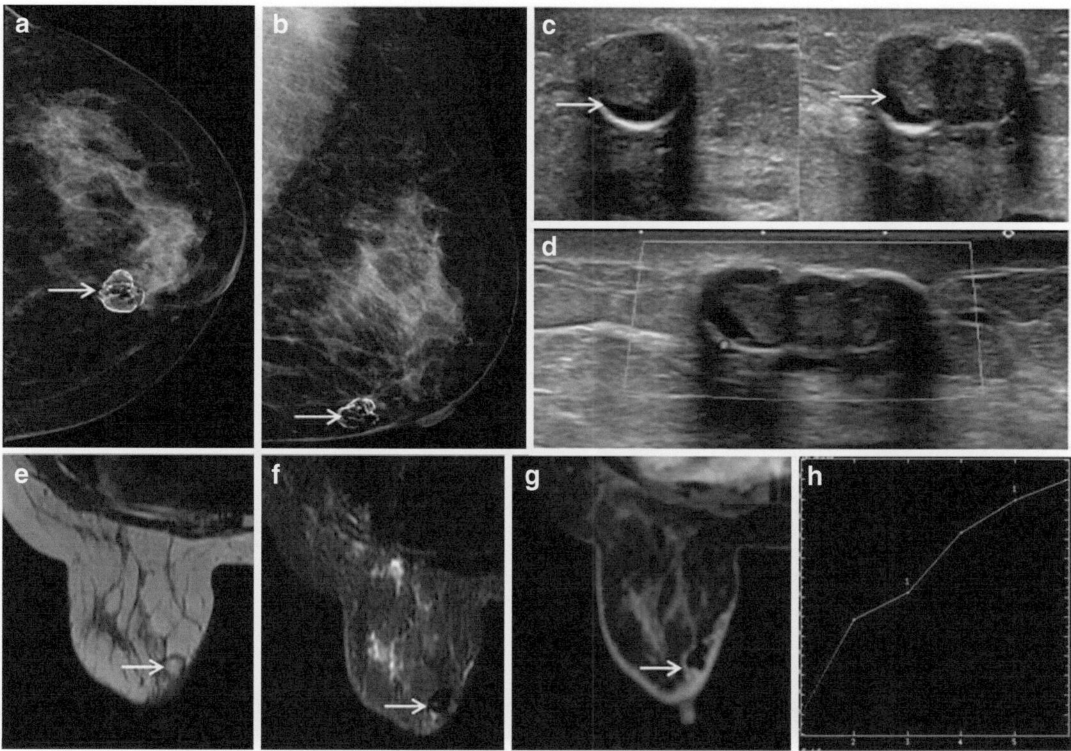

Fig. 27.7 Fat necrosis. (**a**, **b**) CC and MLO view of x-ray mammogram reveals a calcified mass (arrow) in the lower inner quadrant. (**c**) USG showing a well-circumscribed oval isoehoic mass with fat—fluid layer (arrow) and no significant vascularity (**d**). (**e**) T1W image shows the mass (arrow) isointense to fat, suppressed on fat sat images (**f**) with mild peripheral contrast enhancement (**g**). (**h**) Mass shows type I kinetic curve—suggestive of benign mass

lucency with curvilinear or arc-like peripheral calcifications (oil cysts).

Ultrasound: Fat necrosis appears as a complex mass or an anechoic round mass with hyperechoic walls with posterior acoustic shadowing (Fig. 27.7c). On Doppler study, fat necrosis usually shows no significant vascularity (Fig. 27.7d).

MRI: It follows the fat signal in all the sequences (Figs. 27.7e, h and 27.8c–f). On the contrast-enhanced dynamic sequence, fat necrosis may manifest as a mass with rim enhancement or variable non mass like enhancement.

Computed tomography (CT): The mass will have fat attenuation centrally, and there may be adjacent soft-tissue fat stranding and enhancement.

Positron emission tomography (PET) CT: The fat necrosis can have increased 18F-fluorodeoxyglucose (FDG) uptake in an acute stage and therefore mimic disease recurrence.

The imaging appearance of fat necrosis on all imaging modalities can be sometimes indistinguishable from malignancy, necessitating biopsy correlation.

BI-RADS category: **BI RADS 2** in classical cases with furnished history. In complicated cases, BI-RADS 3 with short-term follow-up or BI-RADS 4 with biopsy correlation depending on the findings and the clinical scenario. Palpable mass with atypical appearance on mammogram, ultrasound followed by biopsy may become requisite to confirm the diagnosis.

27.3.1.2 Management

No active surgical management required.

27.3.2 Calcifications

Benign calcifications are seen on mammogram in about 28% within 6–12 months after radiation therapy [3].

Etiopathogenesis: Usually in association with fat necrosis and secondary to radiotherapy.

Morphologically, these calcifications (Fig. 27.9) are large (>5 mm) and irregular in outline with central lucencies, with no associated mass/density and always occur at the site of surgery [6].

Early rim calcification of evolving fat necrosis may produce an appearance that is mammographically indeterminate.

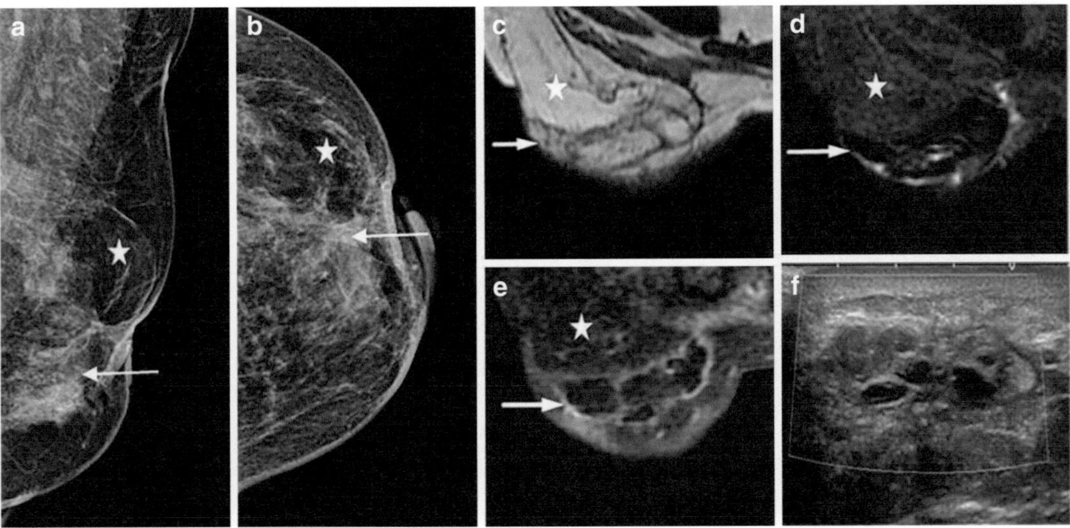

Fig. 27.8 Post-BCS with LD flap. CC view (**a**) and MLO view (**b**) shows LD flap (Asterix) in the upper and outer quadrant of left breast with an architectural distortion inferior to the flap (arrow). (**c**) T1W sequence reveals a fat containing mass (arrow) anterior to the flap, showing fat suppression on STIR sequence (**d**) with mild peripheral enhancement (**e**). (**f**) USG reveals a heteroechoic mass, consistent with fat necrosis

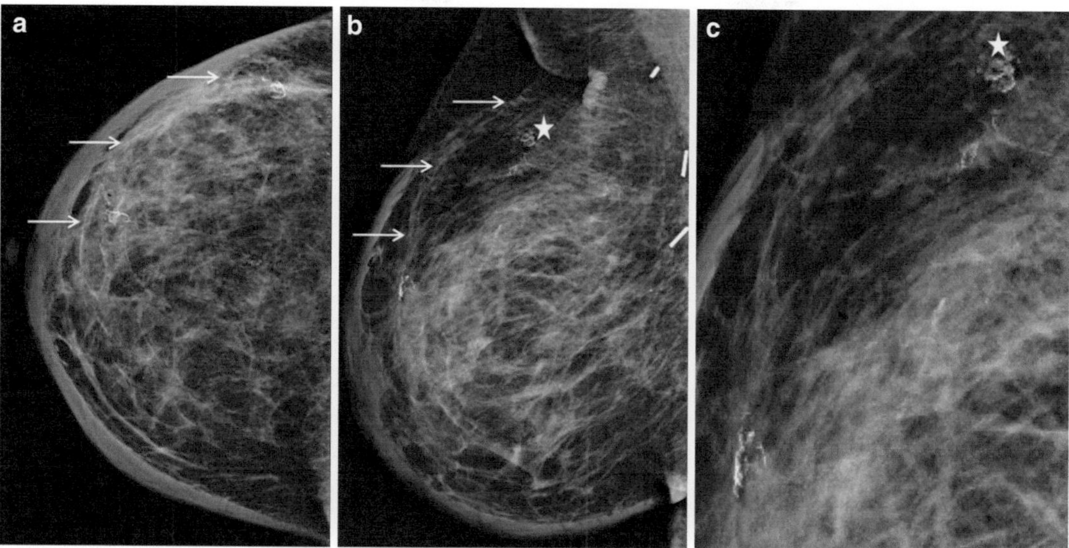

Fig. 27.9 Dystrophic calcifications. (**a**, **b**) CC and MLO views show diffuse skin thickening with few scattered dystrophic calcifications along the scar site (arrow). (**c**) Magnified view of dystrophic calcification (asterisks). Surgical clips are seen posteriorly in MLO view

Use of spot magnification view and comparison with prior mammogram is mandatory. If calcifications cannot be distinguished from a possible malignant process on mammogram, biopsy should be considered.

BI-RADS category: **BI RADS 2**

27.3.2.1 Management

No active intervention needed in benign calcifications. If inconclusive, stereotactic biopsy/VAB/excision biopsy indicated.

27.3.3 Postsurgical Scar

Imaging Features: A postsurgical scar appears as an area of architectural distortion contiguous with contour deformity of surgery.

Mammogram: It appears as a spiculated or irregular, poorly marginated, soft-tissue density associated with skin retraction that mimics recurrent malignancy (Fig. 27.10).

A true recurrence appears the same on all mammographic views and has a dense center, whereas a scar has varied appearances on different projections with fat lucencies within [6]. These features may be better imaged on spot compression or magnification views [3].

The scar usually decreases in density and/or size on serial imaging or remains stable by 2 years. An increase in size or density on follow-up imaging is suspicious for recurrence.

BI-RADS category: **BI RADS 2**

27.3.3.1 Management

Annual follow-up mammograms are necessary to show the sequential decrease in the size and prominence of the density (Fig. 27.11a–c). If ominous features develop, it is essential to do biopsy.

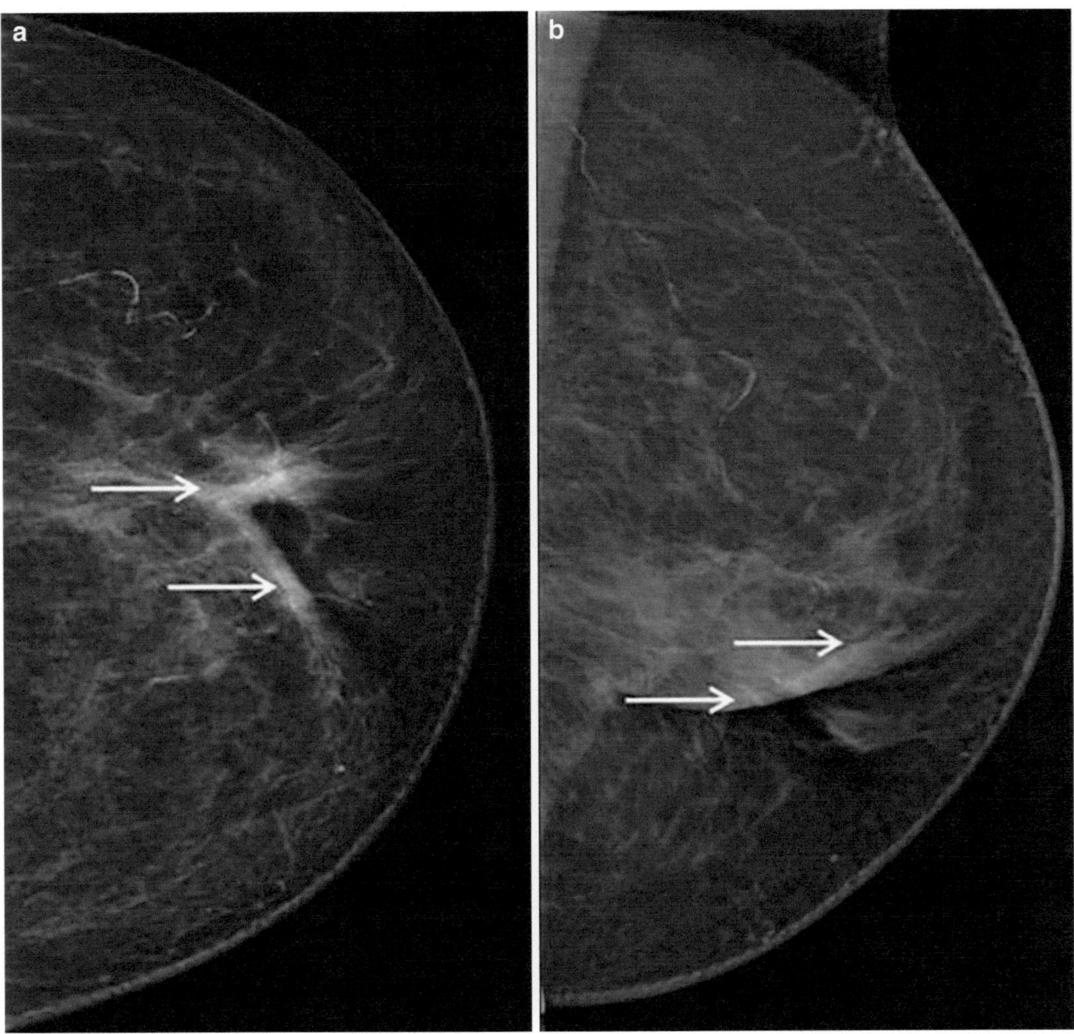

Fig. 27.10 Postsurgical scar. (**a**, **b**) Architectural distortion (arrow) noted in the upper outer and central region of the left breast with associated nipple retraction—post-BCS changes

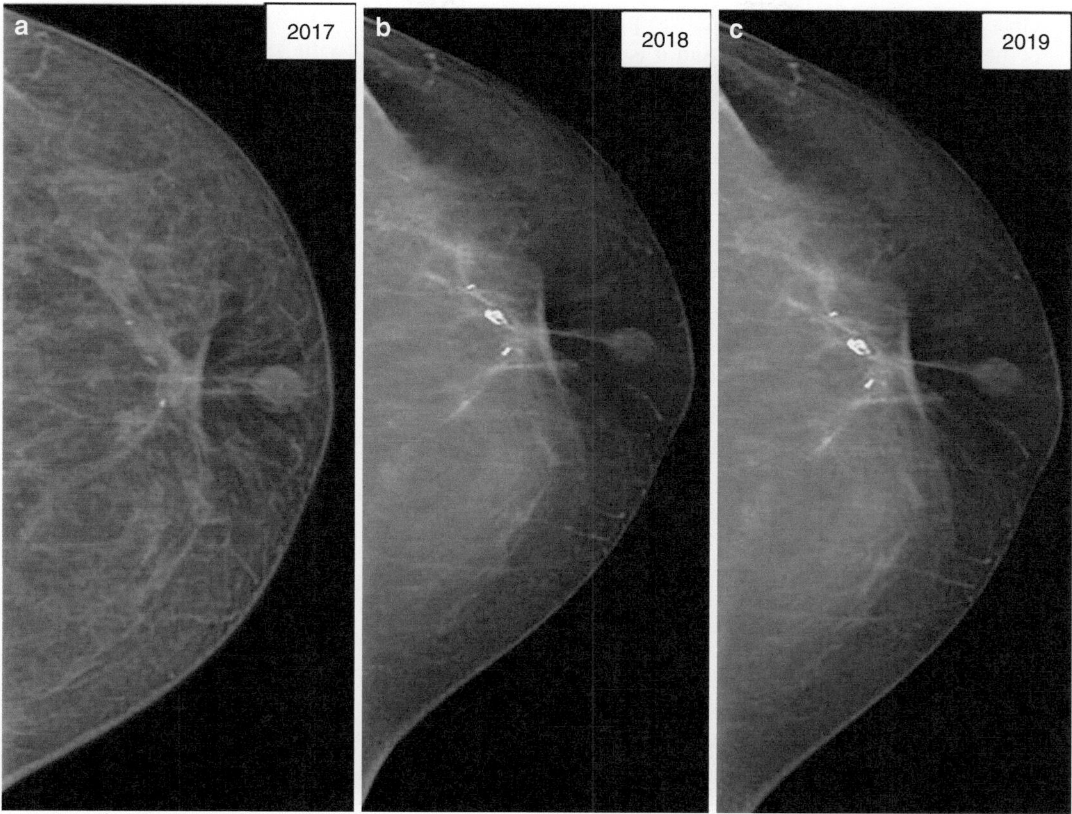

Fig. 27.11 Postoperative scar. (**a**–**c**) Serial CC images of left breast (from year 2017 to 2019)—shows gradual decrease in the density of the scar with no increase in size and appearance of benign calcifications

27.4 Late Postoperative Changes

27.4.1 Lymphedema

It is a late complication after axillary surgical staging of breast cancer. Lymphedema affects 10–20% of women after breast cancer treatment [5]. Lymphedema is a clinical diagnosis.

27.4.2 Recurrence

Recurrent tumors can be invasive or in situ regardless of whether the original tumor was invasive as it is unpredictable. Mammogram and clinical follow-up are complementary in detecting tumor recurrence [7].

On Mammogram, tumor recurrences can appear as follows [6].

- Increasing asymmetry or as an enlarging mass within the operative bed or axilla.
- Increasing edema, overall background trabecular pattern, or skin thickening.
- Pleomorphic, indistinct, coarse heterogeneous, or linear calcifications that have developed within or near the postoperative site.
- Up to 65% of early recurrences occur at or within a few centimeters of the site of original tumor, usually within 6–7 years of treatment.
- At follow up imaging, it is essential to ensure that scar site is visible in two views (CC and MLO or additional views), at least in the first decade after surgery.
- A new lesion or a neodensity which is suspicious may remain stable due to ongoing hormonal treatment; however, the stability

does not indicate benign finding. Morphology is the most important criteria, and it is necessary to achieve a radiological-pathological concordance.

- The most common site of tumor recurrence is the contact line, at the junction of the flap with the native tissue [8].

> Microcalcifications of recurrent disease frequently have the same morphology as those found in the primary cancer. Any neodensity at mammography should be evaluated on ultrasound to determine whether it is solid or cystic, and solid masses should be biopsied [6].

27.4.3 Role of MRI

MRI plays a major role in indeterminate mammography and ultrasound findings. MRI can reliably distinguish posttreatment scar tissue from recurrence when performed at least 12–18 months after completion of breast conservation therapy (Fig. 27.12).

The assessment of dynamic enhancement pattern combined with morphology on contrast-enhanced MRI is crucial.

> The absence of enhancement in the biopsy bed suggests fibrosis, whereas persistent enhancement in the biopsy bed is suspicious for recurrence although fat necrosis can also show enhancement. Hence, it warrants biopsy correlation.

27.4.4 Role of PET CT

The 18-FDG PET CT scan has a major role in detecting local (Fig. 27.13) contralateral breast (Fig. 27.14) recurrence and in distant metastases (Figs. 27.13 and 27.14) in follow-up cases.

BI RADS category: **BI RADS 4C/5**

27.4.5 Management

If calcifications are the only findings. Sterotactic core needle biopsy/vacuum assisted biopsy/

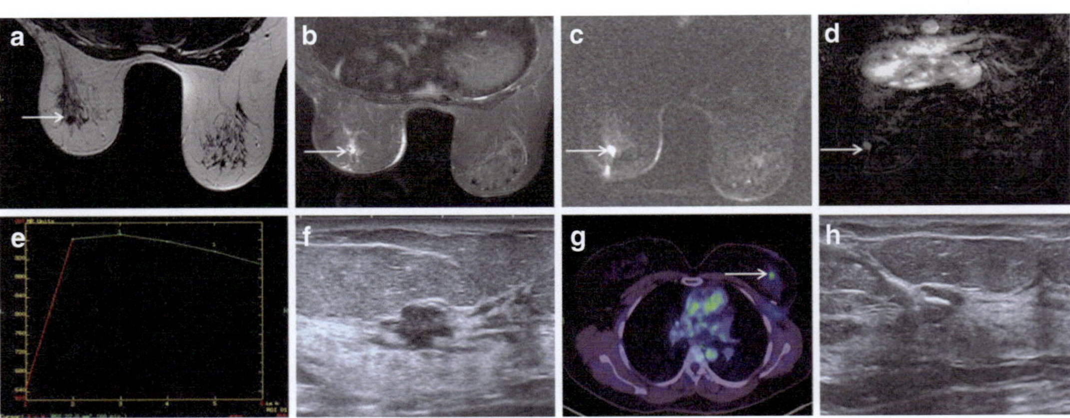

Fig. 27.12 Postoperative recurrence: K/c/o invasive ductal carcinoma of left breast, post-BCS. (**a**) T1w image—left breast is smaller than right (post-BCS status). A circumscribed hypointense mass (arrow) in left breast, appearing hyperintense on STIR (**b**), with diffusion restriction (**c**) and early arterial enhancement (**d**). (**e**) Time kinetics shows type II curve. (**f**) USG reveals an irregular hypoechoic mass showing uptake on PET CT (**g**). (**h**) USG-guided tru cut biopsy revealed invasive ductal carcinoma

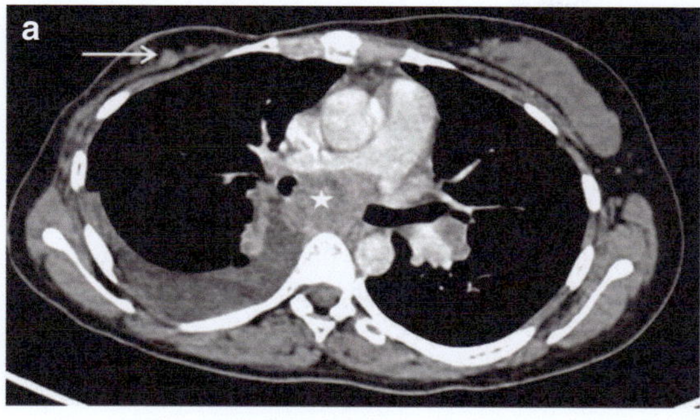

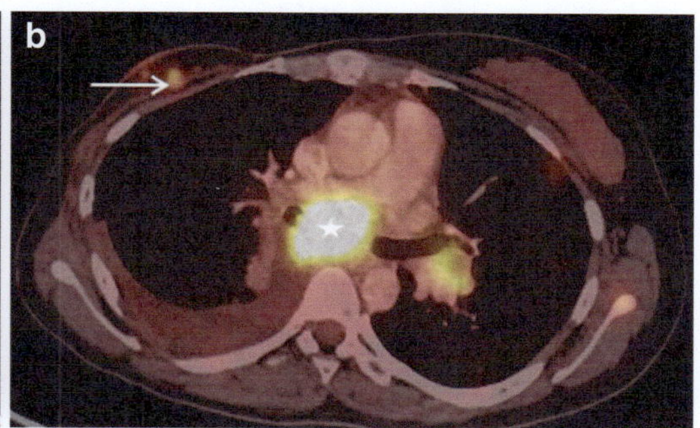

Fig. 27.13 Post-MRM recurrence. (**a**) Focal enhancing mass with uptake on FDG PET CT scan (**b**) noted in right chest wall (arrow), also seen an enlarged subcarinal node (asterix) with left pleural effusion—suggestive of chest wall recurrence with distant metastasis

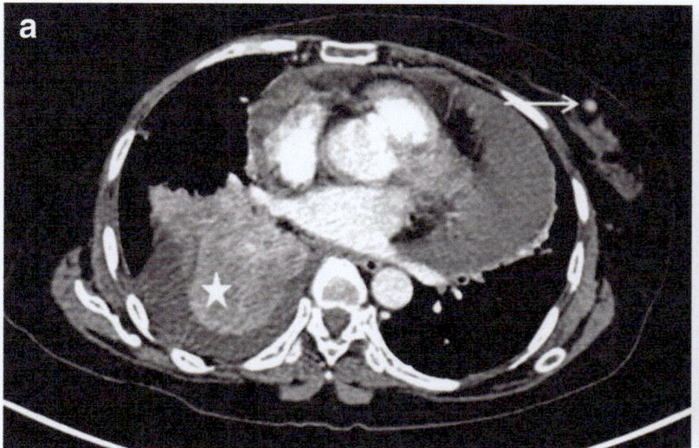

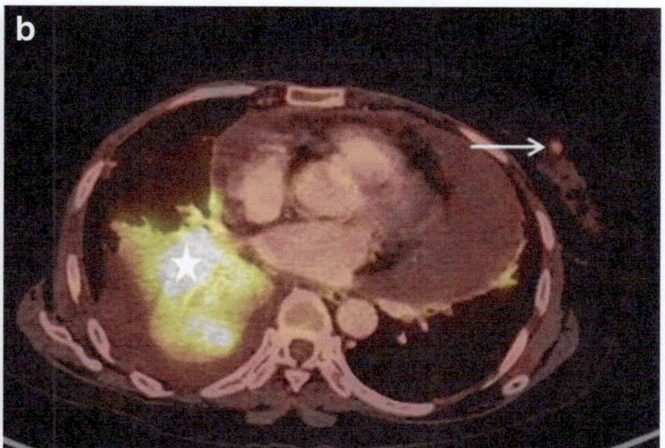

Fig. 27.14 Post-MRM recurrence. (**a**) Focal enhancing lesion in the contralateral breast with increased uptake on FDG PET CT scan (**b**), also seen heterogeneously enhancing mass in the right lung with right pleural effusion—suggestive of recurrence in contralateral breast with distant metastases

wire localization followed by excision can be performed.

If the mass is visualized on ultrasound, ultrasound-guided biopsy or localization is preferred.

If enhancement is seen only on MRI with no obvious ultrasound or mammography correlate, MR-guided biopsy is done.

27.5 Radiation Induced Changes

A chronology of radiation induced changes as explained by Yi A et al. [9] are

1. Early changes (weeks to months post radiation) include skin thickening with breast edema, fat necrosis, dystrophic calcifications, radiation-induced pneumonia, and pleural effusion.
2. Intermediate changes (from months to years) include skin retraction with breast fibrosis, pulmonary fibrosis, and pericardial disease.
3. Late changes (>10 years) include cardiomyopathy and radiation-induced malignancy.

Neoplastic events attributed to radiation of breast cancer are rare. Such occurrences encompass lung cancers, secondary breast cancers, leukemias, and radiation-induced sarcomas including angiosarcomas, osteosarcomas, malignant fibrous histiocytomas, leiomyosarcomas, rhabdomyosarcomas, and fibrosarcomas [7].

Radiation-induced sarcoma is a rare complication, which manifests as *thickening of the skin or prominent trabecular pattern.*

27.6 Conclusion

Imaging plays a major role in postoperative breast diseases to detect early recurrences. A comparison with prior imaging is crucial to avoid unwarranted interventions in benign manifestations. In indeterminate findings, it is always essential to have a clinical and histopathological correlation.

References

1. Margolis NE, Morley C, Lotfi P, Shaylor SD, Palestrant S, Moy L, et al. Update on imaging of the postsurgical breast. RadioGraphics. 2014;34(3):642–60.
2. Swinnen J, Keupers M, Soens J, Lavens M, Postema S, Van Ongeval C. Breast imaging surveillance after curative treatment for primary non-metastasised breast cancer in non-high-risk women: a systematic review. Insights Imaging. 2018;9(6):961–70.
3. Chansakul T, Lai KC, Slanetz PJ. The postconservation breast: part 1, expected imaging findings. Am J Roentgenol. 2012;198(2):321–30.
4. Neal CH, Yilmaz ZN, Noroozian M, Klein KA, Sundaram B, Kazerooni EA, et al. Imaging of breast cancer–related changes after surgical therapy. Am J Roentgenol. 2014;202(2):262–72.
5. Mendelson EB. Evaluation of the postoperative breast. Radiol Clin N Am. 1992;30(1):107–38.
6. Ramani SK, Rastogi A, Mahajan A, Nair N, Shet T, Thakur MH. Imaging of the treated breast post breast conservation surgery/oncoplasty: pictorial review. World J Radiol. 2017;9(8):321–9.
7. Chansakul T, Lai KC, Slanetz PJ. The postconservation breast: part 2, imaging findings of tumor recurrence and other long-term sequelae. Am J Roentgenol. 2012;198(2):331–43.
8. Farras Roca JA, Dao TH, Lantieri L, Lepage C, Bosc R, Meyblum E, et al. Ipsilateral breast cancer recurrence after deep inferior epigastric perforator (DIEP) flap reconstruction: incidence and radiological presentation. Diagn Interv Imaging. 2016;97(2):203–9.
9. Yi A, Kim HH, Shin HJ, Huh MO, Ahn SD, Seo BK. Radiation-induced complications after breast cancer radiation therapy: a pictorial review of multimodality imaging findings. Korean J Radiol. 2009;10(5):496–507.

28 Pathological Assessment of Post-neoadjuvant Therapy Breast Specimen

Ayushi Sahay

Abstract

Neoadjuvant therapy is increasingly being used as a therapeutic option in breast cancer patients, and pathological evaluation of such specimen is the gold standard for documentation of response to treatment. There are multiple response assessment classification systems in use according to local practice. However, pathological assessment of surgical excision specimen after therapy is challenging both macroscopically and microscopically. Thus, a uniform approach, with systematic sampling, in conjunction with clinical and radiological findings is recommended. This chapter outlines the handling of such specimen as per the current guidelines and describes the histopathological features, including the essential elements to be reported according to the most commonly used response assessment classification systems.

Keywords

Neoadjuvant therapy · Response to treatment · Residual disease · Sampling · Cellularity

A. Sahay (✉)
Department of Pathology, Tata Memorial Centre, a CI of Homi Bhabha National Institute (HBNI), Mumbai, India
e-mail: sahayaj@tmc.gov.in

28.1 Pathological Assessment of Post-neoadjuvant Therapy Breast Specimen

Background: Neoadjuvant therapy (NAT), which refers to preoperative treatment of cancer patients with systemic therapy (chemotherapy and/or hormone therapy and/or Her2 receptor monoclonal antibody therapy), is increasingly being offered to locally advanced breast cancer, large operable breast cancer, and even to early stage high-risk breast cancer patients [1–5]. No difference in survival and locoregional control has been noted in patients who receive systemic therapy in adjuvant or neoadjuvant setting [3, 6–8]. However, NAT causes downstaging of tumors to facilitate breast-conserving surgery and makes previously inoperable tumors operable. It also provides an opportunity to assess tumor response to therapy. Good response is a predictor of good outcome. Poor response may indicate need for additional or alternative adjuvant treatment [9–11]. Assessment of response also serves a research tool for studying tumor biology and development of novel therapeutic agents and biomarkers in clinical trials. Pathological complete remission (pCR) (absence of residual invasive tumor in breast and lymph nodes) is recommended as an end point for accelerated approval of new NAT agents by the US Food and Drug Administration [12]. Tumors having a high histological grade, non-lobular histological type,

B. Dev, L. D. Joseph (eds.), *Holistic Approach to Breast Disease*,
https://doi.org/10.1007/978-981-99-0035-0_28

extensive necrosis, dense lymphocytic infiltrates, Her2 positive or triple negative are more likely to show pCR [10, 13–21].

Since clinical and radiological response to NAT does not correlate well with pathologic response, an accurate and reproducible assessment of the post-therapy surgical excision specimen by the pathologist is considered the gold standard. It is needed not only for documenting pCR, but also measuring the degree of response, which correlates with prognosis [22]. Various systems have been devised for the assessment of pathological treatment response, with different criteria; a few of them are shown in Table 28.1 [6, 23–31]. All have their own merits and demerits, and have been validated for correlation with outcome; however, choosing the system depends on institutional or local practice [15, 32, 33]. Most widely prevalent among these are the American Joint Committee on Cancer post-neoadjuvant staging (yAJCC) eighth edition and the Residual Cancer Burden (RCB), as both have shown good correlation with relapse risk and survival independently [14, 28, 30, 34].

It has to be kept in mind, however, that owing to NAT, there is a whole array of changes introduced in the breast and lymph nodes, making pathological assessment following such therapies difficult, both grossly and microscopically [18, 19, 25]. There is also a lot of variation in grossing and reporting protocols followed for post-NAT specimen across the world. To ameliorate this, standardized and universally accepted protocols have been introduced for pathological evaluation of post-NAT specimen recently by the Breast International Group-North American Breast Cancer Group (BIG-NABCG) [13, 35].

Alterations due to NAT: To understand the challenges of post-NAT assessment, the spectrum of possible variations introduced in the tumor and lymph nodes by NAT needs to be recognized [9, 18, 19, 22, 25, 36, 37]. These include:

1. **Changes in the tumor**: Tumor response is highly variable with heterogeneous changes in tumor size and cellularity ranging from complete resolution, concentric contraction, scattered small or large islands of residual disease separated by fibrotic stroma ("buckshot pattern"), to minimal response or even progressive tumor growth. When response is minimal, the tumor may look similar to untreated tumor. Conversely, in dramatic complete response, the tumor bed resembles unremarkable fibrosed breast tissue or may be identifiable only by accompanying calcification, fat necrosis, hemorrhage, or previous biopsy site reaction. There is usually marked softening of the tumor stroma, reduced blood flow, and concomitant with typically reduced cellularity; the tumor becomes ill defined, and difficult to palpate, making locating the tumor and gross T size measurement challenging. Mostly, tumor grade does not change post-NAT, but occasionally, the tumor may appear of higher grade and rarely of lower grade compared to pretherapy biopsy. Similarly, tumor biomarkers (ER, PR, and Her2Neu) usually remain the same before and after treatment, but rare alterations have been recorded, which may be attributed to various factors, including pre-analytical factors, tumor heterogeneity, and type of NAT given. Thus, re-evaluation is usually not recommended unless [38] core biopsy results are negative or equivocal; [9] core biopsy showed only ductal carcinoma in situ (DCIS) or insufficient invasive carcinoma; [13] core biopsy performed at another institute; and [14] no treatment response.
2. **Changes in the nodes**: Lymph node status is the most important prognostic factor in patient receiving NAT. Response in the breast and nodes is usually similar. However, not all nodes respond equally in the same patient; some nodes may show complete response with no evidence of prior involvement or only fibrous tissue, while others show large metastasis. In contrast to patients without NAT, minimetastasis (<1 mm), and micrometastasis (<2 mm) are counted as metastatic nodes in post-NAT patients, as they show similar survival as macrometastasis, and probably represent partial therapy response in macrometastasis. Isolated tumor cells

Table 28.1 Some commonly used systems for evaluating treatment response in breast carcinoma

System	Variables studied	Response evaluation	Comment
Chevallier et al, 1993 [23]	– Presence of in-situ or invasive carcinoma – Treatment effect in breast	Class 1: Disappearance of all tumor, microscopically or macroscopically Class 2: DCIS only, no invasive tumor and negative Lymph nodes Class 3: Presence of invasive carcinoma with stromal alterations Class 4: Few modifications in tumor appearance	Developed for inflammatory carcinoma
Sataloff et al, 1995 [24]	– Treatment effect in invasive carcinoma – Lymph nose status (presence of evidence of response)	Tumor T-A: Total or near total therapeutic effect; <5% tumor surface T-B: >50% therapeutic effect but less than T-A T-C: <50% therapeutic effect T-D: No therapeutic effect Nodes N-A: No metastatic disease with evidence of therapeutic effect N-B: No nodal metastases or therapeutic effect N-C: Metastases present with therapeutic effect N-D: Metastases present without therapeutic effect	Requires comparison with pre-treatment biopsy specimen
Pinder et al, 2007 [25]	– Tumor proportion (%) in remaining breast – Lymph nose status (presence of evidence of response)	Tumor 1. pCR: (a) no residual carcinoma or (b) DCIS only 2. Partial response: (a) <10% tumor cellularity (b) 10–50% tumor cellularity, >50% tumor cellularity compared with pre-treatment biopsy 3. No response to therapy nodes (a) No metastasis and no therapy changes (b) No metastasis but evidence of response (c) Metastasis with evidence of response (d) Metastasis without response	Requires comparison with pre-treatment biopsy specimen
NASBP B-18 [26]	– Treatment effect in invasive carcinoma – Lymph nose status (the number of metastatic lymph node and size of metastatic deposit)	pCR: No invasive tumor cells present pPR: Scattered individual or small clusters of tumor Cells in a desmoplastic/hyalinized stroma pNR: Tumor lacking changes in pCR and pPR	

(continued)

Table 28.1 (continued)

System	Variables studied	Response evaluation	Comment
Miller-Payne system [27]	– Presence of invasive carcinoma – Tumor cellularity	Grade 1: No reduction in overall cellularity Grade 2: Minor loss of tumour cells (<30%) Grade 3: 30–90% reduction in tumor cells Grade 4: >90% loss of tumour cells Grade 5: No invasive cells present, DCIS may be present	Requires comparison with pre-treatment biopsy specimen
Residual Cancer Burden (RCB) [28]	– Size of tumor bed in two dimension – Tumor cellularity – Residual DCIS% – Lymph node status (the number of metastatic lymph node and size of metastatic deposit)	RCB-0: No carcinoma in breast and lymph node RCB-I: Partial response (minimal residual disease) RCB-II: Partial response (moderate residual disease) RCB-III: Chemo-resistant (extensive residual disease)	Based on a mathematical calculator developed by the MD Anderson Cancer Centre. Available freely as a web based online calculator at: http://www.mdanderson.org/breastcancer_RCB
Residual disease in Breast and nodes (RDBN) [29]	– Size of invasive carcinoma – Tumor grade – Lymph nose status (the number of metastatic lymph node)	Residual tumor size (cm) × 0.2 + index of positive lymph nodes (0–3: None, 1–4, 5–7 and > 7) + tumor Grade Level 1: pCR Level 2: 0.1–2.9 Level 3: 3.0–4.3 Level 4: >4.4	Based on modified Nottingham prognostic Index
yAJCC eighth edition [30]	– Size of invasive carcinoma (largest contiguous focus, without intervening fibrosis) – Lymph nose status (the number of metastatic lymph node and size of metastatic deposit)	pCR: No invasive carcinoma in breast and lymph node, No LVI and no ITCs (ypT0 N0, ypTis pN0) pPR: Reduction in T and/or N stage NR: No change or increase in the T or N stage	Anatomical stage groupings based on the TNM staging system

(<0.2 mm) (ypN0i+) are also not regarded as pCR for the same reason.

28.2 Gross Examination of Post-NAT Specimen

Due to these changes, it becomes essential that the pathologist should be aware of detailed clinical and radiological information before grossing. The lab may develop a checklist/surgical requisition form of necessary information needed before grossing. First and foremost, the specimen should be clearly marked as post-NAT. Number, location and presentation of the lesion/s (skin erythema, fixation, etc.), pretherapy clinical and radiological size, pretherapy biopsy histology findings (including tumor type, grade, calcifications, biomarker status), pretherapy nodal status, type of NAT given, and post-therapy clinical and/or radiological response assessment with dimensions of the residual tumor should be known. Any clip placed in situ in the primary tumor or axillary sentinel nodes at the time of biopsy/fine needle aspiration (FNA) to localize the tumor bed should be noted. More

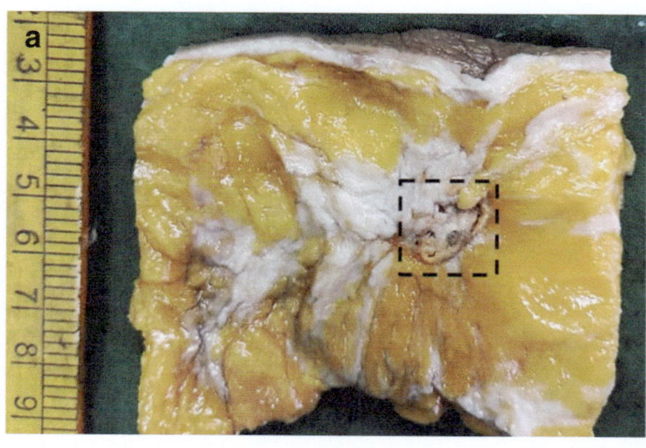

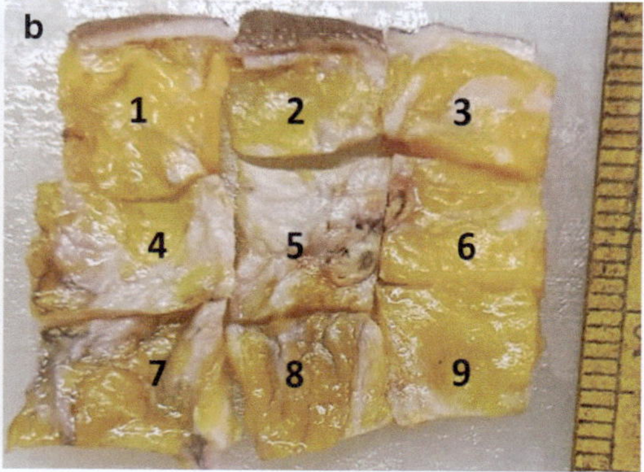

Fig. 28.1 (**a**) Slice of post-NAT simple mastectomy showing largest cross section of tumor bed with a small grossly identifiable residual tumor (broken square) with surrounding fibrotic tumor bed. (**b**) The same slice was processed in grid fashion and numbered serially, and a diagram of the grid made on the accompanying form to enable tumor size estimation and average cellularity. The microscopic sections on slides may be oriented as per the grid diagram and accurate T size calculated. Similar additional grids may be sampled in case of small tumor/ grossly invisible tumor

blocks are generally required than would be usual in an untreated specimen. Careful mapping of the tumor bed slices by photography or with help of tumor grid diagrams (Fig. 28.1) allows reconstruction of the specimen for microscopic tumor measurement, estimation of tumor cellularity, and facilitates correlation of gross and microscopic findings. A systematic mapping and sampling approach is considered more useful rather than exhaustive or blind random sampling [9, 13, 18, 19, 25, 35].

28.3 Grossing Protocol (Post-NAT Lumpectomy and Mastectomy)

1. Specimen should be inked in fresh state, thinly serially sliced at 5 mm intervals and fixed in adequate fixative (10% neutral buffered formalin for 6–72 h) [38, 39].
2. Each slice should be carefully examined to identify residual tumor bed and tumor mass. Note presence of any radiological clip, if any, and prior biopsy site scar.
3. The tumor bed, depending on response, may show almost normal breast or subtle irregular rubbery fibrous tissue/hemorrhage or residual tumor in form of fleshy nodules (Figs. 28.2, 28.3, 28.4, and 28.5). Size of the grossly recognizable tumor bed and any residual tumor should be measured.
4. All margin distances from the tumor bed/ grossly identified tumor mass should be measured. Tumor bed grossly extending to resection margins should be documented, as also distance from the overlying skin and/or nipple areola (if present).
5. The tumor should be sampled to cover the pre-treatment tumor size and just beyond the visible lesion for evaluation of microscopic extent. Small specimens (<5 cm in greatest diameter or < 30 g) can be submitted in their entirety. However, entire tumor bed sampling, though would ensure accuracy, is not practical in larger tumors. As per BIG-NABCG recommendations, if residual tumor is grossly identified, one full-face cross section of the slice with the largest tumor area should be embedded. If no residual tumor is grossly identified, one full-face cross section per centimeter (or for very large tumors, five representative sections per full face for every 1–2 cm) of pre-treatment size is recommended (up to maximum 25 blocks) to determine the full tumor extent [13, 35]. However, as per USFDA, for initial sampling, one to two blocks per centimeter of pre-treatment

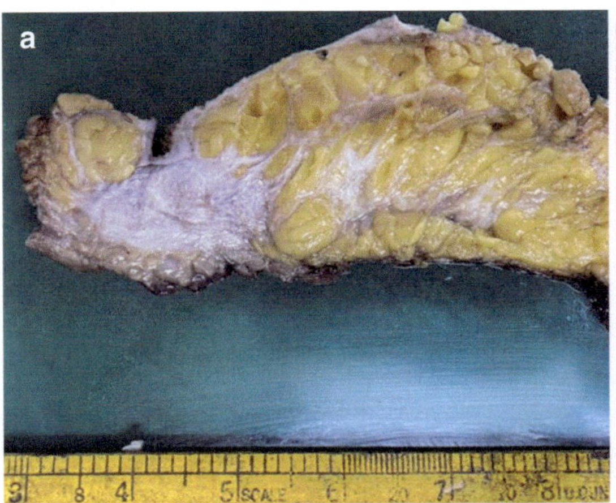

Fig. 28.2 (**a**) Slice of post-NAT simple mastectomy showing a firm fibrotic tumor bed. No residual tumor was grossly identifiable. (**b**) On microscopy, hyalinized loose collagenous stroma without normal glandular breast parenchyma was seen forming the tumor bed. There was complete pathological response (Hematoxylin eosin, ×40)

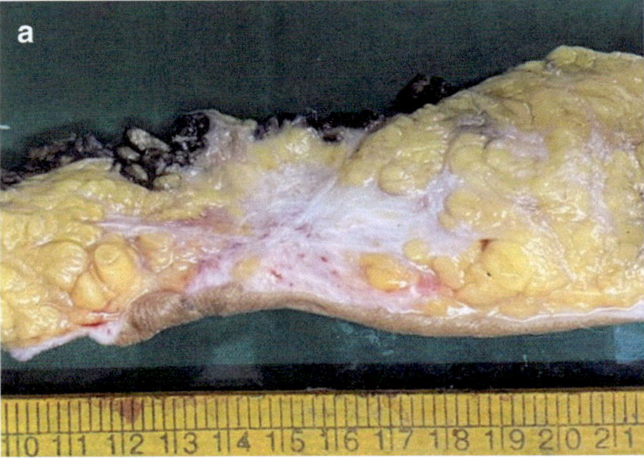

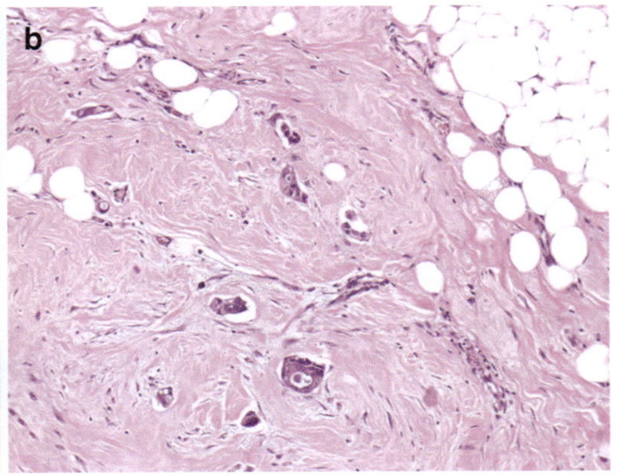

Fig. 28.3 (**a**) Slice of post-NAT simple mastectomy showing fibrotic tumor bed with no grossly identifiable residual tumor. (**b**) Microscopic examination, however, revealed scant scattered foci of residual viable tumor cells amid fibrosis forming approximately 5% cellularity of the entire tumor bed (hematoxylin eosin, ×100)

tumor size, or 10 blocks, whichever is greater, is considered adequate [12]. Grid diagram of the tumor full-face slices should be made to allow microscopic reconstruction (Fig. 28.1). This also allows the pathologist to decide on additional sampling if the microscopic findings do not match the diagram.

6. In case of multifocal disease, each tumor should be handled in the same way, with sampling of the intervening tissue between the tumors. However, for T staging, only the dimension of the largest tumor is considered.
7. In general, lymph nodes are difficult to identify post-NAT, due to atrophy and fibrosis, and the yield may be low [19, 36]. If nodes are difficult to identify grossly, fibrotic areas in axillary fat or around axillary vessels should be entirely sampled to identify microscopic nodes.
8. All identified lymph nodes should be sectioned at 2 mm intervals along the long axis of the lymph node, and if no gross tumor deposit is found, should be entirely submitted.
9. Number and size of all grossly involved nodes should be documented with size of greatest metastatic focus and any grossly evident

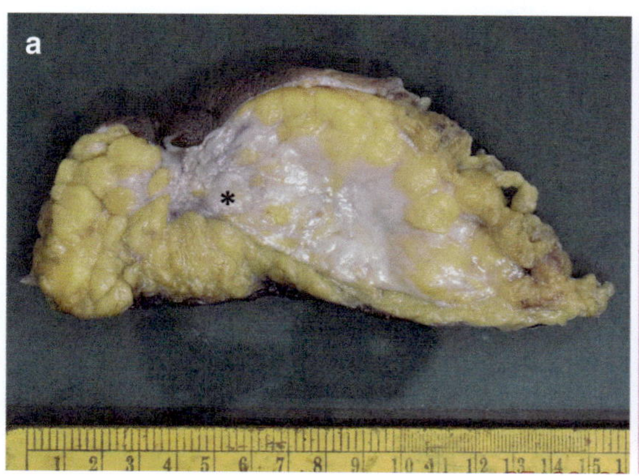

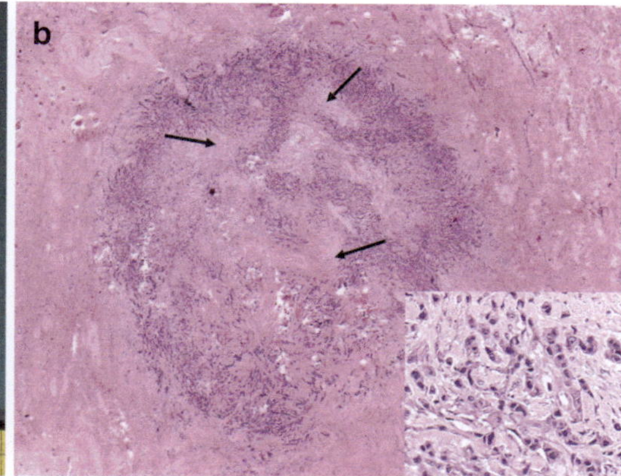

Fig. 28.4 (**a**) Slice of post-NAT simple mastectomy specimen showing a retroareolar solid nodule (black star) with surrounding fibrosis and pale rubbery areas. The nipple appears retracted. The base (posterior margin) is inked. (**b**) Grossly identified nodule on microscopy showed residual viable tumor with surrounding hyalinized stroma. High-power view showed residual viable tumor cells (inset). Therapy-related changes were seen within the nodule (pale areas shown by arrows), reducing the overall cellularity (Hematoxylin eosin, ×10, inset: ×200)

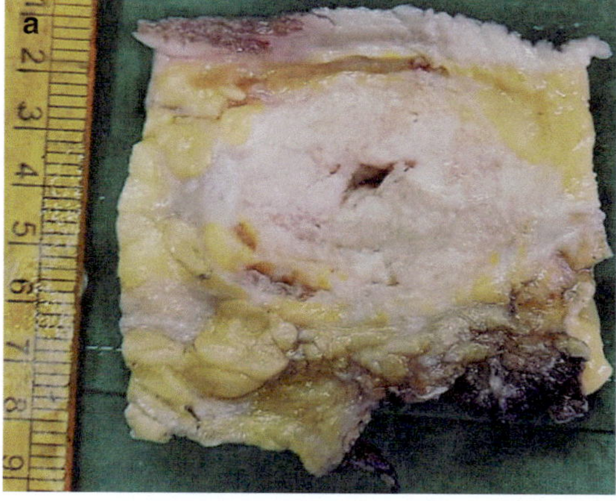

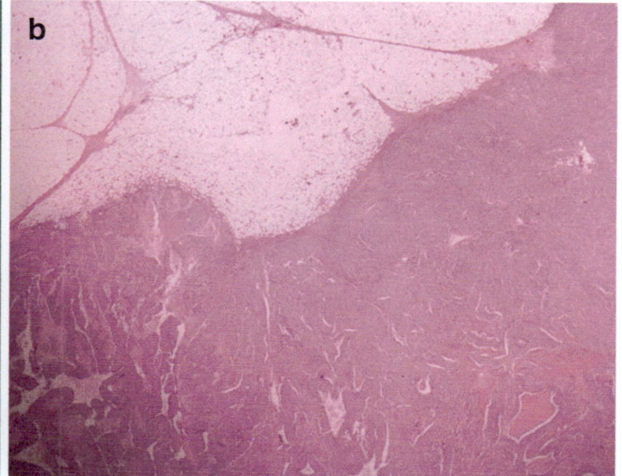

Fig. 28.5 (**a**) Slice of largest cross section of mastectomy with grossly identifiable large residual tumor, appearing similar to an untreated tumor. (**b**) No surrounding therapy-related changes were seen on microscopic examination (Scanner view, Hematoxylin eosin, ×10)

extranodal extension. Representative sections of the grossly involved node with largest focus of metastatic tumor and extranodal extension should be submitted.

Microscopic Examination of Post-NAT Specimen [9, 18, 19, 22, 25, 36, 40, 41]:

Once the tumor bed is adequately sampled, it is essential to confirm presence or absence of residual carcinoma, as even tumors with complete clinical, radiological, and gross response may show microscopic foci of residual tumor (Fig. 28.3). Also, in cases where no residual tumor is identified on microscopy, it is essential to confirm if the tumor bed has been accurately identified and sampled by looking for therapy-related changes, and in their absence, additional gross sampling may be indicated. Additionally, in the presence of residual tumor, percentage response should be assessed microscopically, to provide an estimate of residual tumor cellularity, as per the response assessment system being followed (Table 28.1).

28.3.1 Microscopic Findings Include (Figs. 28.2, 28.3, 28.4, 28.5, and 28.6)

1. **Therapy-related response**: The tumor bed is characterized by loose hyalinized fibrovascular stroma, with edematous, or myxoid changes, mostly with absence of normal breast ducts and lobules. Sheets and infiltrates of foamy histiocytes, cholesterol clefts, hemosiderin laden histiocytes, and chronic inflammation in the form of aggregates of lymphocytes and plasma cells may be noted.

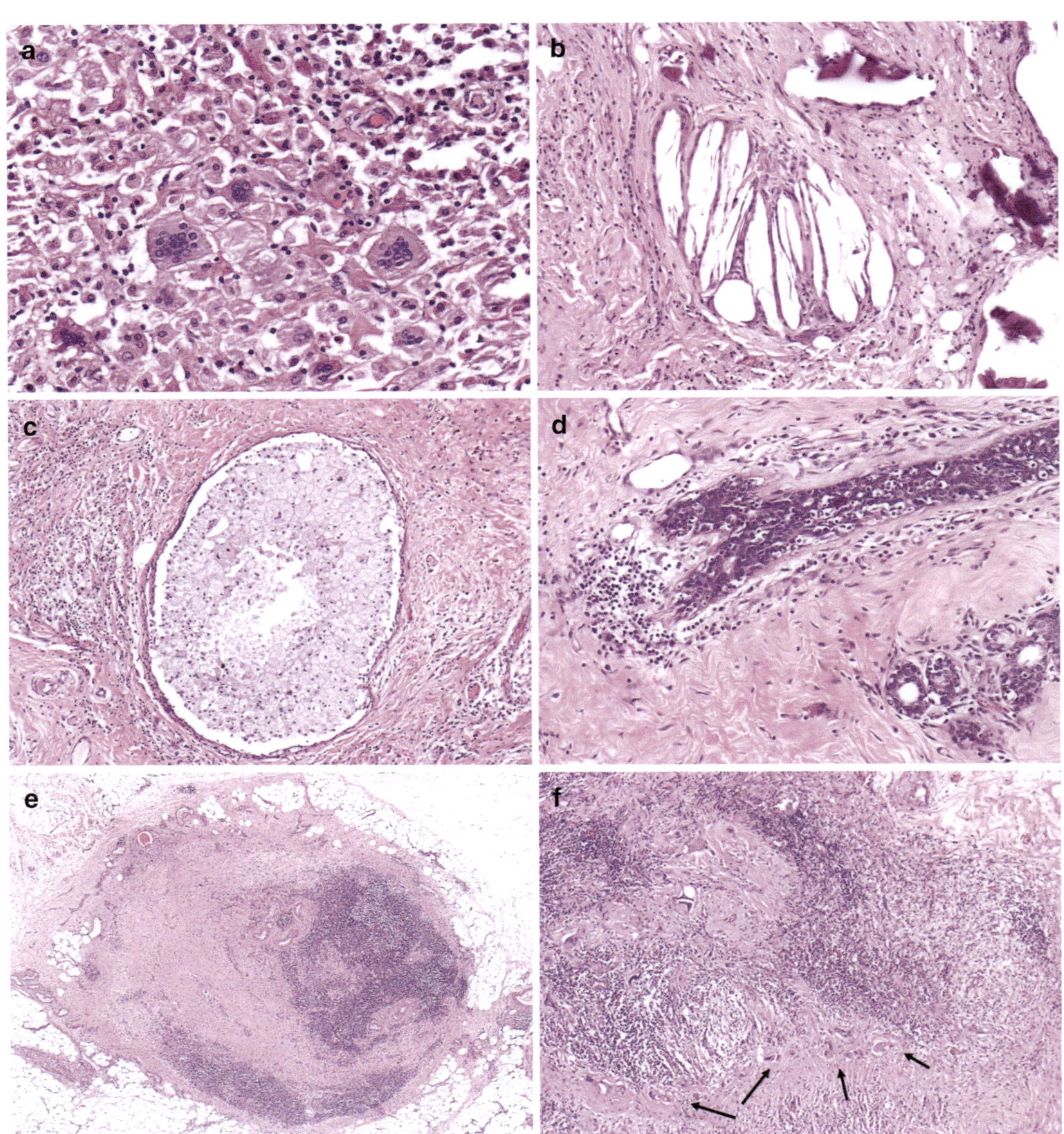

Fig. 28.6 Spectrum of other therapy-related changes identified on microscopy (All hematoxylin eosin): (**a**) Sheets of foamy and hemosiderin laden macrophages with multinucleate histiocytic giant cells (×200); (**b**) cholesterol clefts and calcification (×100); (**c**) complete replacement of in situ carcinoma with sheets of macrophages and surrounding chronic inflammation (×40); (**d**) benign ducts with periductular fibrosis and chronic inflammation (×100); (**e**) lymph node with hyalinzed scar with no viable residual tumor (×10); (**f**) Another lymph node with fibrosis and sheets of macrophages signifying therapy response, along with scattered foci of viable tumor nests (arrows) (×40)

Multinucleate histiocytes, epithelioid granulomas and areas of necrosis may be present.

2. **Residual tumor**: Residual tumor cells, may be identified as infiltrating cords, nests and singly dispersed individual cells resembling lobular carcinoma or histiocytes. Cell distribution varies from uniform to haphazard. Although grade of tumors usually does not change, certain cytological changes may be observed. These include distorted glandular architecture, increased cytoplasm, cytoplasmic vacuolization and eosinophilia, nuclear change in the form of pleomorphic bizarre nuclei, and reduced mitoses. Singly scattered cells may show irregular, hyperchromatic, smudged nuclei, or multinucleation making them difficult to identify. Immunohistochemistry for cytokeratin markers (CK7 or A1/AE3) and histiocytic markers (CD68 or CD163) may help in difficult cases The tumor may have shrunk concentrically, with almost normal cellularity in such regions or in case of "buckshot" response, shows presence of singly scattered or small clusters or islands of tumor cells. Tumor dimension should be reported in the form of largest contiguous focus of invasive carcinoma (for AJCC staging) and size of the largest cross section of residual carcinoma ("span of residual tumor bed") for RCB and other scoring systems. Focality and average cellularity across the largest cross section containing residual carcinoma (including invasive and in situ disease) should be included in the report [13, 28, 30, 31].
   (a) Sometimes, in situ carcinoma or tumor forming lymphovascular invasion (LVI) may be more resistant to treatment than invasive carcinoma and may the only form of residual tumor. LVI is an adverse prognostic factor and needs to be documented in the report but should not be confused with retraction artifacts around the tumor. DCIS may range from minimal alteration to replacement of intraductal cells by macrophages. Description of residual DCIS and quantum (% of tumor) should be included in the report to cover the most common response evaluation systems.
3. **Margin assessment**: The extent of residual tumor bed is difficult to identify clinically, radiologically, and grossly by the operating surgeon and the pathologist. In cases of pCR, the significance of tumor bed changes at the margins is uncertain. However, when there are scattered residual tumor foci, presence of tumor bed changes at the margin should be documented, as it may signify possibility of residual carcinoma in the body.
4. **Adjacent breast parenchyma**: Surrounding non-tumorous breast parenchyma may also show reaction to therapy in the form of periductular, perilobular and/or intralobular fibrosis, lobular atrophy, chronic inflammation, and mild focal cytological atypia, which should not be confused with residual DCIS.
5. **Lymph nodes**: Metastatic deposits in the nodes in case of pCR may show replacement by hyalinized stromal scars, mucin pools, aggregates of histiocytes, necrosis, and cholesterol clefts, similar to response in the breast. The whole node including native lymphoid follicles may be replaced by therapy-related changes. Oftentimes, the metastasis may resolve completely without any evidence of scar. Partial response is seen in the form of isolated tumor cells or small clusters, surrounded by hyaline stromal fibrosis. Total number of nodes, involved nodes, size of the largest contiguous metastatic focus (for AJCC), size of largest focus including intervening fibrosis (for RCB and other systems), and extranodal extension, if any, need to be included in the report. Documentation of treatment response in the nodes should also be included, as it indicates prognosis intermediate between completely node negative and node positive post-NAT patients.

NAT is increasingly being routinely used in clinical practice and though challenging, pathological evaluation of the post-NAT excision specimen remains the gold standard for judging effectiveness of the therapy. Thus, a standardized approach for evaluation of such specimens, with systematic sampling with correlation between clinical, radiological, gross, and microscopic findings is essential. The pathology report should thus provide sufficient information to permit classification by most of the common response evaluation classification systems, specially the AJCC and RCB.

References

1. Early breast cancer trialists' collaborative group (EBCTCG). Long-term outcomes for neoadjuvant versus adjuvant chemotherapy in early breast cancer: meta-analysis of individual patient data from ten randomised trials. Lancet Oncol. 2018;19(1):27–39. https://doi.org/10.1016/S1470-2045(17)30777-5.
2. Kaufmann M, von Minckwitz G, Bear HD, Buzdar A, McGale P, Bonnefoi H, Colleoni M, Denkert C, Eiermann W, Jackesz R, Makris A, Miller W, Pierga JY, Semiglazov V, Schneeweiss A, Souchon R, Stearns V, Untch M, Loibl S. Recommendations from an international expert panel on the use of neoadjuvant (primary) systemic treatment of operable breast cancer: new perspectives 2006. Ann Oncol. 2007;18(12):1927–34. https://doi.org/10.1093/annonc/mdm201.
3. Mauri D, Pavlidis N, Ioannidis JP. Neoadjuvant versus adjuvant systemic treatment in breast cancer: a meta-analysis. J Natl Cancer Inst. 2005;97(3):188–94. https://doi.org/10.1093/jnci/dji021.
4. Schwartz GF, Hortobagyi GN, Masood S, Palazzo J, Holland R, Page D. Consensus conference committee proceedings of the consensus conference on neoadjuvant chemotherapy in carcinoma of the breast, April 26-28, 2003, Philadelphia, PA. Hum Pathol. 2004;35(7):781–4. https://doi.org/10.1016/j.humpath.2004.02.006.
5. Valagussa P, Zambetti M, Bonadonna G, Zucali R, Mezzanotte G, Veronesi U. Prognostic factors in locally advanced noninflammatory breast cancer. Long-term results following primary chemotherapy. Breast Cancer Res Treat. 1990;15(3):137–47. https://doi.org/10.1007/BF01806351.
6. Fisher ER, Wang J, Bryant J, Fisher B, Mamounas E, Wolmark N. Pathobiology of preoperative chemotherapy: findings from the national surgical adjuvant breast and bowel (NSABP) protocol B-18. Cancer. 2002;95(4):681–95. https://doi.org/10.1002/cncr.10741.
7. Mieog JS, van der Hage JA, van de Velde CJ. Preoperative chemotherapy for women with operable breast cancer. Cochrane Database Syst Rev. 2007;2007(2):CD005002. https://doi.org/10.1002/14651858.CD005002.pub2.
8. van der Hage JA, van de Velde CJ, Julien JP, Tubiana-Hulin M, Vandervelden C, Duchateau L. Preoperative chemotherapy in primary operable breast cancer: results from the European organization for research and treatment of cancer trial 10902. J Clin Oncol. 2001;19(22):4224–37. https://doi.org/10.1200/JCO.2001.19.22.4224.
9. Bossuyt V. Processing and reporting of breast specimens in the neoadjuvant setting. Surg Pathol Clin. 2018;11(1):213–30. https://doi.org/10.1016/j.path.2017.09.010.
10. Cortazar P, Zhang L, Untch M, Mehta K, Costantino JP, Wolmark N, Bonnefoi H, Cameron D, Gianni L, Valagussa P, Swain SM, Prowell T, Loibl S, Wickerham DL, Bogaerts J, Baselga J, Perou C, Blumenthal G, Blohmer J, Mamounas EP, Bergh J, Semiglazov V, Justice R, Eidtmann H, Paik S, Piccart M, Sridhara R, Fasching PA, Slaets L, Tang S, Gerber B, Geyer CE Jr, Pazdur R, Ditsch N, Rastogi P, Eiermann W, von Minckwitz G. Pathological complete response and long-term clinical benefit in breast cancer: the CTNeoBC pooled analysis. Lancet. 2014;384(9938):164–72. https://doi.org/10.1016/S0140-6736(13)62422-8.
11. Mamounas EP, Anderson SJ, Dignam JJ, Bear HD, Julian TB, Geyer CE Jr, Taghian A, Wickerham DL, Wolmark N. Predictors of locoregional recurrence after neoadjuvant chemotherapy: results from combined analysis of National Surgical Adjuvant Breast and bowel project B-18 and B-27. J Clin Oncol. 2012;30(32):3960–6. https://doi.org/10.1200/JCO.2011.40.8369.
12. US Food and Drug Administration. Guidance for industry: pathological complete response in neoadjuvant treatment of high-risk early-stage breast cancer: use as an endpoint to support accelerated approval. 2020. http://www.fda.gov/downloads/Drugs/GuidanceComplianceRegulatoryInformation/Guidances/UCM305501.pdf. Accessed 29 July 2020.
13. Bossuyt V, Provenzano E, Symmans WF, Boughey JC, Coles C, Curigliano G, Dixon JM, Esserman LJ, Fastner G, Kuehn T, Peintinger F, von Minckwitz G, White J, Yang W, Badve S, Denkert C, MacGrogan G, Penault-Llorca F, Viale G, Cameron D. Breast international group-north American breast cancer group (BIG-NABCG) collaboration. Recommendations for standardized pathological characterization of residual disease for neoadjuvant clinical trials of breast cancer by the BIG-NABCG collaboration. Ann Oncol. 2015;26(7):1280–91. https://doi.org/10.1093/annonc/mdv161.
14. Campbell JI, Yau C, Krass P, Moore D, Carey LA, Au A, Chhieng D, Giri D, Livasy C, Mies C, Rabban J, Sarode VR, Singh B, Esserman L, Chen YY. Comparison of residual cancer burden, American Joint Committee on Cancer staging and pathologic complete response in breast cancer after neoadjuvant chemotherapy: results from the I-SPY 1 TRIAL (CALGB 150007/150012; ACRIN 6657). Breast Cancer Res Treat. 2017;165(1):181–91. https://doi.org/10.1007/s10549-017-4303-8.

15. Choi M, Park YH, Ahn JS, Im YH, Nam SJ, Cho SY, Cho EY. Assessment of pathologic response and long-term outcome in locally advanced breast cancers after neoadjuvant chemotherapy: comparison of pathologic classification systems. Breast Cancer Res Treat. 2016;160(3):475–89. https://doi.org/10.1007/s10549-016-4008-4.
16. Esserman LJ, Berry DA, DeMichele A, Carey L, Davis SE, Buxton M, Hudis C, Gray JW, Perou C, Yau C, Livasy C, Krontiras H, Montgomery L, Tripathy D, Lehman C, Liu MC, Olopade OI, Rugo HS, Carpenter JT, Dressler L, Chhieng D, Singh B, Mies C, Rabban J, Chen YY, Giri D, van't Veer L, Hylton N. Pathologic complete response predicts recurrence-free survival more effectively by cancer subset: results from the I-SPY 1 TRIAL–CALGB 150007/150012, ACRIN 6657. J Clin Oncol. 2012;30(26):3242–9. https://doi.org/10.1200/JCO.2011.39.2779.
17. Houssami N, Macaskill P, von Minckwitz G, Marinovich ML, Mamounas E. Meta-analysis of the association of breast cancer subtype and pathologic complete response to neoadjuvant chemotherapy. Eur J Cancer. 2012;48(18):3342–54. https://doi.org/10.1016/j.ejca.2012.05.023.
18. Sahoo S, Lester SC. Pathology of breast carcinomas after neoadjuvant chemotherapy: an overview with recommendations on specimen processing and reporting. Arch Pathol Lab Med. 2009;133(4):633–42.
19. Sahoo S, Lester SC. Pathology considerations in patients treated with neoadjuvant chemotherapy. Surg Pathol Clin. 2012;5(3):749–74.
20. von Minckwitz G, Untch M, Nüesch E, Loibl S, Kaufmann M, Kümmel S, Fasching PA, Eiermann W, Blohmer JU, Costa SD, Mehta K, Hilfrich J, Jackisch C, Gerber B, du Bois A, Huober J, Hanusch C, Konecny G, Fett W, Stickeler E, Harbeck N, Müller V, Jüni P. Impact of treatment characteristics on response of different breast cancer phenotypes: pooled analysis of the German neo-adjuvant chemotherapy trials. Breast Cancer Res Treat. 2011;125(1):145–56. https://doi.org/10.1007/s10549-010-1228-x.
21. von Minckwitz G, Untch M, Blohmer JU, Costa SD, Eidtmann H, Fasching PA, Gerber B, Eiermann W, Hilfrich J, Huober J, Jackisch C, Kaufmann M, Konecny GE, Denkert C, Nekljudova V, Mehta K, Loibl S. Definition and impact of pathologic complete response on prognosis after neoadjuvant chemotherapy in various intrinsic breast cancer subtypes. J Clin Oncol. 2012;30(15):1796–804. https://doi.org/10.1200/JCO.2011.38.8595.
22. Mrkonjic M, Berman HK, Done SJ, Youngson B, Mulligan AM. Breast specimen handling and reporting in the post-neoadjuvant setting: challenges and advances. J Clin Pathol. 2019;72(2):120–32. https://doi.org/10.1136/jclinpath-2018-205598.
23. Chevallier B, Roche H, Olivier JP, Chollet P, Hurteloup P. Inflammatory breast cancer. Pilot study of intensive induction chemotherapy (FEC-HD) results in a high histologic response rate. Am J Clin Oncol. 1993;16(3):223–8.
24. Sataloff DM, Mason BA, Prestipino AJ, Seinige UL, Lieber CP, Baloch Z. Pathologic response to induction chemotherapy in locally advanced carcinoma of the breast: a determinant of outcome. J Am Coll Surg. 1995;180(3):297–306.
25. Pinder SE, Provenzano E, Earl H, Ellis IO. Laboratory handling and histology reporting of breast specimens from patients who have received neoadjuvant chemotherapy. Histopathology. 2007;50(4):409–17. https://doi.org/10.1111/j.1365-2559.2006.02419.x.
26. Wolmark N, Wang J, Mamounas E, Bryant J, Fisher B. Preoperative chemotherapy in patients with operable breast cancer: nine-year results from national surgical adjuvant breast and bowel project B-18. J Natl Cancer Inst Monogr. 2001;30:96–102. https://doi.org/10.1093/oxfordjournals.jncimonographs.a003469.
27. Ogston KN, Miller ID, Payne S, Hutcheon AW, Sarkar TK, Smith I, Schofield A, Heys SD. A new histological grading system to assess response of breast cancers to primary chemotherapy: prognostic significance and survival. Breast. 2003;12(5):320–7. https://doi.org/10.1016/s0960-9776(03)00106-1.
28. Symmans WF, Peintinger F, Hatzis C, et al. Measurement of residual breast cancer burden to predict survival after neoadjuvant chemotherapy. J Clin Oncol. 2007;25:4414–22.
29. Chollet P, Abrial C, Durando X, Thivat E, Tacca O, Mouret-Reynier MA, Leheurteur M, Kwiatkowski F, Dauplat J, Penault-Llorca F. A new prognostic classification after primary chemotherapy for breast cancer: residual disease in breast and nodes (RDBN). Cancer J. 2008;14(2):128–32. https://doi.org/10.1097/PPO.0b013e31816bdea2. Erratum in: Cancer J. 2014 Mar-Apr; 20(2): 166.
30. Hortobagyi GN, Connolly JL, D'Orsi CJ, Edge SB, Mittendorf EA, Rugo HS, et al. Breast. In: Amin MB, Edge S, Greene F, Byrd DR, Brookland RK, Washington MK, et al., editors. American Joint Committee on Cancer (AJCC) cancer staging manual. 8th ed. New York: Springer; 2017. p. 589–628.
31. MD Anderson Cancer Center. Residual Cancer Burden calculator and associated documents [guide for measuring cancer cellularity, examples of gross & microscopic evaluation, pathology protocol for macroscopic and microscopic assessment of RCB]. 2018. http://www3.mdanderson.org/app/medcalc/index.cfm?pagename=jsconvert3. Accessed 7 Nov 2018.
32. Corben AD, Abi-Raad R, Popa I, Teo CH, Macklin EA, Koerner FC, Taghian AG, Brachtel EF. Pathologic response and long-term follow-up in breast cancer patients treated with neoadjuvant chemotherapy: a comparison between classifications and their practical application. Arch Pathol Lab Med. 2013;137(8):1074–82. https://doi.org/10.5858/arpa.2012-0290-OA.
33. Lee HJ, Park IA, Song IH, Kim SB, Jung KH, Ahn JH, Ahn SH, Kim HH, Gong G. Comparison of pathologic response evaluation systems after anthracycline with/without taxane-based neoadjuvant chemother-

apy among different subtypes of breast cancers. PLoS ONE. 2015;10(9):e0137885.
34. Peintinger F, Sinn B, Hatzis C, Albarracin C, Downs-Kelly E, Morkowski J, Gould R, Symmans WF. Reproducibility of residual cancer burden for prognostic assessment of breast cancer after neoadjuvant chemotherapy. Mod Pathol. 2015;28(7):913–20. https://doi.org/10.1038/modpathol.2015.53.
35. Provenzano E, Bossuyt V, Viale G, Cameron D, Badve S, Denkert C, MacGrogan G, Penault-Llorca F, Boughey J, Curigliano G, Dixon JM, Esserman L, Fastner G, Kuehn T, Peintinger F, von Minckwitz G, White J, Yang W, Symmans WF. Residual disease characterization working group of the breast international group-north American breast cancer group collaboration. Standardization of pathologic evaluation and reporting of postneoadjuvant specimens in clinical trials of breast cancer: recommendations from an international working group. Mod Pathol. 2015;28(9):1185–201. https://doi.org/10.1038/modpathol.2015.74.
36. Shet T, Agrawal A, Chinoy R, Havaldar R, Parmar V, Badwe R. Changes in the tumor grade and biological markers in locally advanced breast cancer after chemotherapy–implications for a pathologist. Breast J. 2007;13(5):457–64. https://doi.org/10.1111/j.1524-4741.2007.00465.x.
37. Shet T, Pai T, Wadasadawala T, Nair N, Gulia S. Grossing and reporting of breast cancer specimens: an evidence-based approach. Indian J Cancer. 2020;57(2):144–57. https://doi.org/10.4103/ijc.IJC_157_20.
38. Allison KH, Hammond MEH, Dowsett M, McKernin SE, Carey LA, Fitzgibbons PL, Hayes DF, Lakhani SR, Chavez-MacGregor M, Perlmutter J, Perou CM, Regan MM, Rimm DL, Symmans WF, Torlakovic EE, Varella L, Viale G, Weisberg TF, McShane LM, Wolff AC. Estrogen and progesterone receptor testing in breast cancer: ASCO/CAP guideline update. J Clin Oncol. 2020;38(12):1346–66.
39. Wolff AC, Hammond MEH, Allison KH, Harvey BE, Mangu PB, Bartlett JMS, Bilous M, Ellis IO, Fitzgibbons P, Hanna W, Jenkins RB, Press MF, Spears PA, Vance GH, Viale G, McShane LM, Dowsett M. Human epidermal growth factor receptor 2 testing in breast cancer: American Society of Clinical Oncology/College of American Pathologists Clinical Practice guideline focused update. J Clin Oncol. 2018;36(20):2105–22.
40. Fan F. Evaluation and reporting of breast cancer after neoadjuvant chemotherapy. Open Pathol J. 2009;3:58–63.
41. Sharkey FE, Addington SL, Fowler LJ, Page CP, Cruz AB. Effects of preoperative chemotherapy on the morphology of resectable breast carcinoma. Mod Pathol. 1996;9(9):893–900.

Part X

Miscellaneous Topics in the Breast

Diseases of the Nipple

29

Mohana Priya, Mehak Garg, Bhawna Dev, and Sandhya Sundaram

Abstract

Nipple-areolar complex present in the central quadrant of the breast has unique characteristics and can present with a spectrum of diseases such as congenital, inflammatory, benign, and malignant diseases. Approach to diseases of the nipple, especially in cases where the patients present with nipple discharge should be multimodal including clinical, radiological, and pathological evaluation, for an effective management.

Keywords

Nipple · Areola · Discharge · Adenoma · Paget's disease

M. Priya (✉)
Department of Surgery, Sri Ramachandra Institute of Higher Education and Research, Chennai, India
e-mail: mohanapriyadr@sriramachandra.edu.in

M. Garg
Department of Radiology, Sri Ramachandra Institute of Higher Education and Research, Chennai, India

B. Dev · S. Sundaram
Department of Pathology, Sri Ramachandra Institute of Higher Education and Research, Chennai, India
e-mail: bhawnadev@sriramachandra.edu.in

29.1 Embryology and Anatomy

Embryology: During the fetal development stage, there is formation of an epithelial ridge along each side of the body running from the axilla to the inguinal region, known as milk line.

Along this milk line (Fig. 29.1), there are multiple rudiments for future breast development, and in humans, only one rudimentary pair in the pectoral region persists and eventually develops into breast.

Stages of breast and nipple development: At birth, there is elevation of only the nipple. Before puberty, there is elevation of the breast and nipple, called the breast bud stage. At the onset of puberty, the areola enlarges and darkens, and distinct mass of glandular tissue begins to develop beneath the areola. By the onset of menstruation, the breasts are well developed, and there is forward projection of the areola and nipple at the apex of the breast (Fig. 29.2).

Once the breast reaches maturity, only the nipple projects forward, and the areola recedes to the general contour of the breast.

29.1.1 Normal Imaging Appearance of Nipple

The normal position of the nipple is slightly inferior and medial to the center of the breast and lies in the mid-clavicular line. The areola has numerous sweat glands and sebaceous glands, which

B. Dev, L. D. Joseph (eds.), *Holistic Approach to Breast Disease*,
https://doi.org/10.1007/978-981-99-0035-0_29

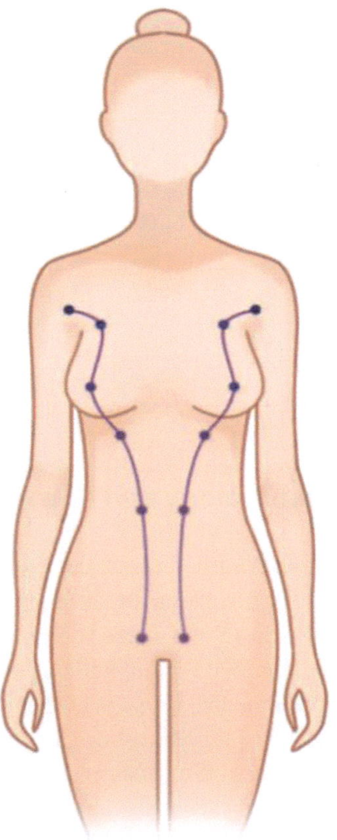

Fig. 29.1 Milk line

enlarge during pregnancy and lubricate the nipple during lactation and are termed as Montgomery's tubercles [1].

X-ray mammogram: Normal nipple is everted and should be depicted in profile (Fig. 29.3a, b) in one of the mammographic views for evaluation of nipple areola complex.

Ultrasound: Nipple appears as a circumscribed semilunar echogenic area in middle of the breast (Fig. 29.4).

Magnetic esonance imaging (MRI) of breasts: In contrast-enhanced MRI, the nipple normally enhances showing mild to intense enhancement patterns, due to presence of tiny vessels within (Fig. 29.5a–c).

MR mammogram plays a major role in differentiating between a tumor confined to retroareolar tissue and the nipple-areolar complex making MR mammogram an essential investigation in patients undergoing nipple-preserving breast-conservation surgery to reduce the rate of local recurrence [2].

Histopathology: The nipple areola complex is lined by pigmented squamous epithelium and contains smooth muscles arranged both concentrically and radially, which makes the nipple an erectile structure.

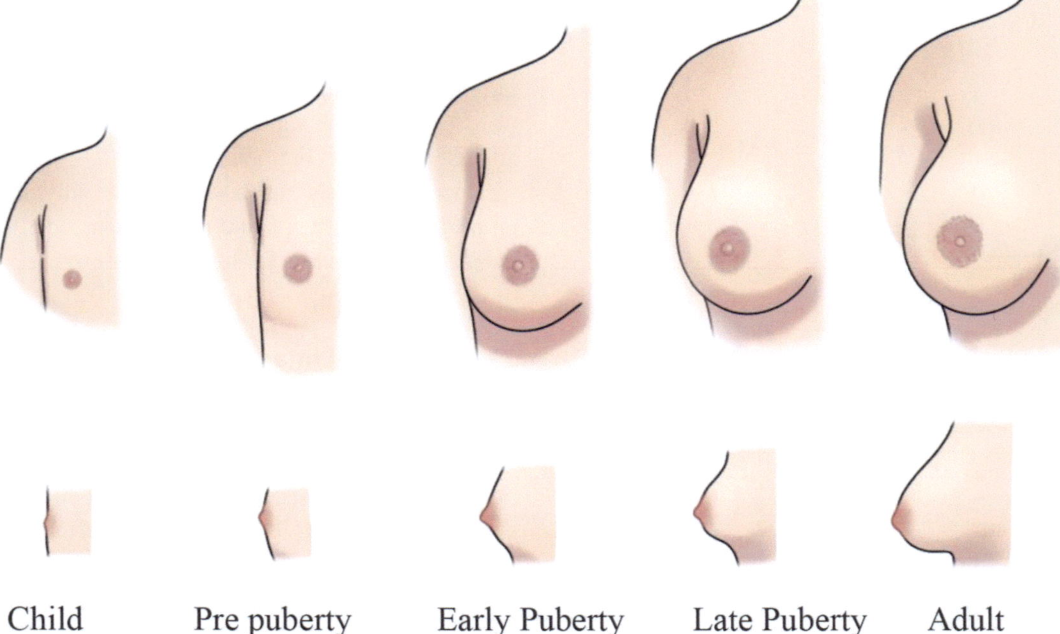

Fig. 29.2 Stages of breast and nipple development

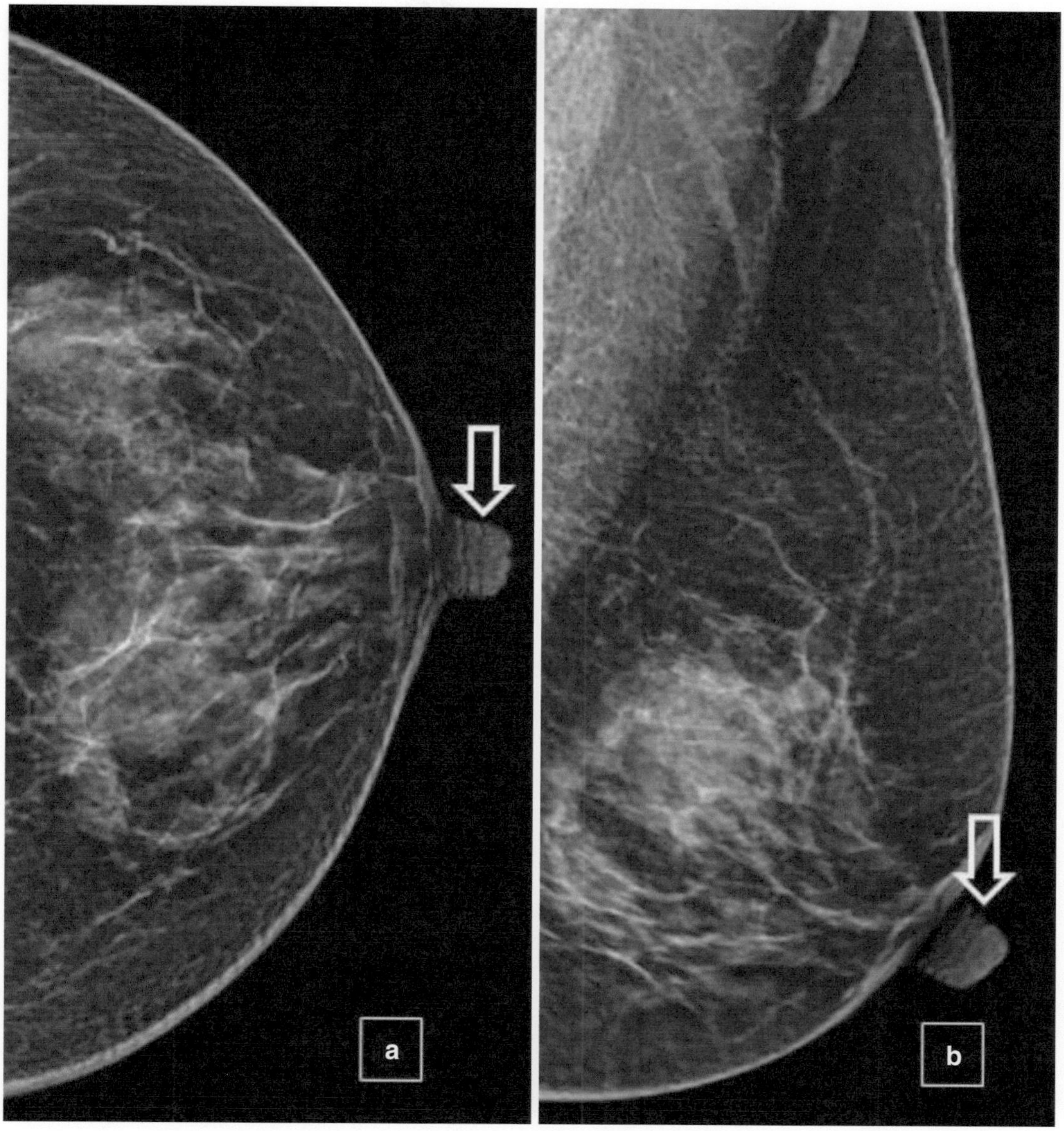

Fig. 29.3 Normal appearance of nipple on mammogram (**a**, **b**) CC and MLO view of the left breast showing nipple in profile (arrow)

Fig. 29.4 Normal appearance of nipple on ultrasound: nipple seen as echogenic semilunar area in center of breast (arrow)

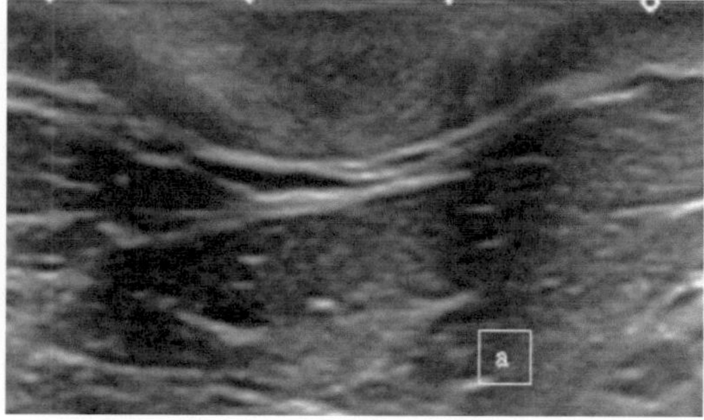

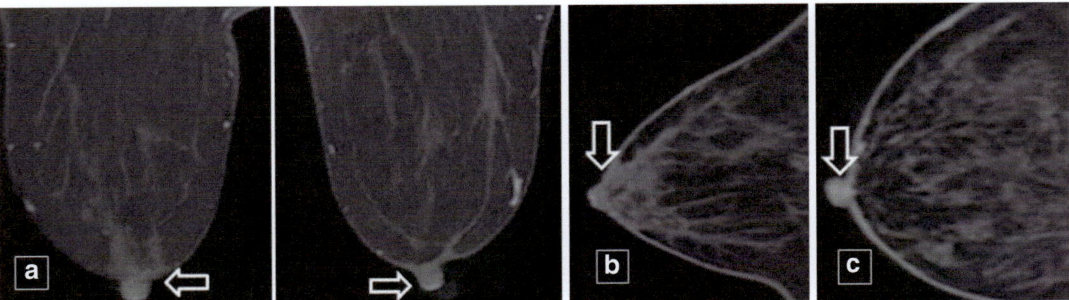

Fig. 29.5 Normal appearance of nipple on MRI breast (**a**) MRI of both breasts—axial view showing symmetric bilateral enhancement of nipple areola complex. (**b**, **c**) sagittal contrast-enhanced T1-weighted fat-suppressed MR images show various degrees of enhancement in a normal nipple, seen as mild enhancement (**b**) and intense enhancement (**c**)

29.2 Congenital Diseases of the Nipple

29.2.1 Athelia

Absence of nipple is a rare condition, which is invariably associated with congenital absence of breast (Amastia).

29.2.1.1 Imaging Features

X-ray mammogram, Ultrasonagram (USG), MR mammogram: No nipple visible in profile.

29.2.1.2 Polythelia/Supernumerary Nipples

Accessory nipple and polythelia is not an uncommon condition with incidence of 0.2–2.5%. It can be seen anywhere along the milk line of Schultz, that extends from the axilla to the groin (Fig. 29.6). This condition occurs due to failure of complete regression of the milk line that happens during gestation. Accessory nipples are a minor congenital anomaly and are mostly a cosmetic problem [2].

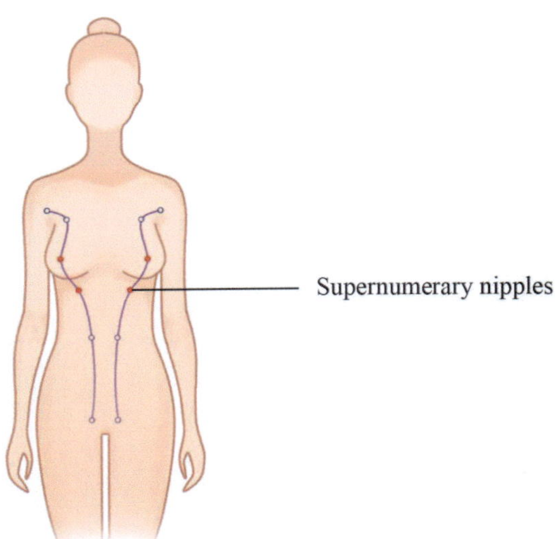

Fig. 29.6 Line diagram showing polythelia

29.2.1.3 Imaging Features

X-ray mammogram: Accessory breast tissue is usually seen below the level of supernumerary nipples.

29.2.2 Inflammatory Diseases of Nipple

29.2.2.1 Cracked Nipple

Cracked nipple mostly occurs during lactation, and if not treated properly, may lead to mastitis or breast abscess. Diagnosis is predominantly by history and clinical examination.

29.2.2.2 Imaging Findings

X-ray mammogram: No specific findings.

USG: Nipple appears dark and large in size with significant increased vascularity.

MR mammogram: Significant increased enhancement is seen in the nipple areola complex, due to increased vascularity.

Treatment is temporary cessation of breastfeeding for 48 hours and expression of milk using breast pump and application of topical lubricants. Later breast feeding may be continued using a nipple guard. Antibiotics can be started if there are signs of inflammation [3].

29.2.2.3 Eczema of the Nipple

Nipple eczema is dermatitis of nipple-areolar complex and is a localized presentation of atopic dermatitis with bilateral presentation. Patient presents with scaling and crusting of the nipple-areolar complex, erythema, serous discharge, and itching (Fig. 29.7).

Clinically, nipple eczema can be confused with Paget's disease with the difference being that eczema is bilateral and involves only the areola with rare nipple involvement, whereas Paget's disease is usually unilateral and involves the nipple first followed by areola.

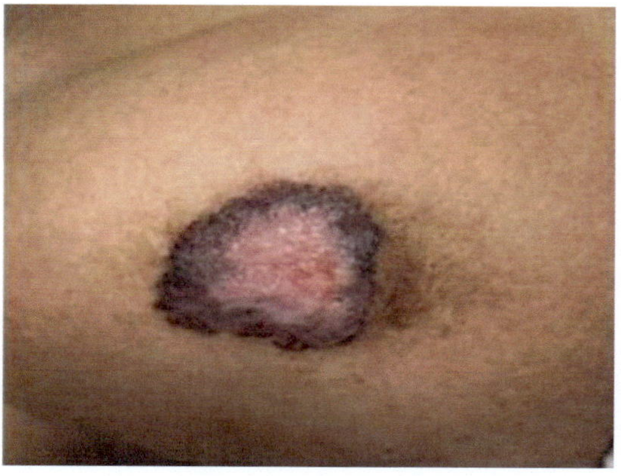

Fig. 29.7 Nipple eczema in a patient showing excoriation, redness, and crusting of nipple

29.2.2.4 Imaging Features

USG: Skin thickening in region of nipple areola with increased vascularity in the subareolar region.

X-ray mammogram, MRI mammogram and skin biopsy is done to rule out Paget's disease in patients with nipple eczema.

Treatment includes topical steroids and antibiotics for preventing secondary infection [4, 5].

29.2.2.5 Nipple Retraction or Inversion

The terms nipple retraction and inversion are used interchangeably and often confused. The term nipple inversion is mainly used when area of nipple appears inverted and is seen slit like (Fig. 29.8). Nipple retraction is used when whole of the nipple is pulled inwards and lies below the surface of breast.

Both retraction and inversion of nipple can be congenital or acquired and can be unilateral or bilateral.

Bilateral and long-standing nipple inversion/retraction is usually benign, whereas the causes of unilateral and acquired nipple retraction

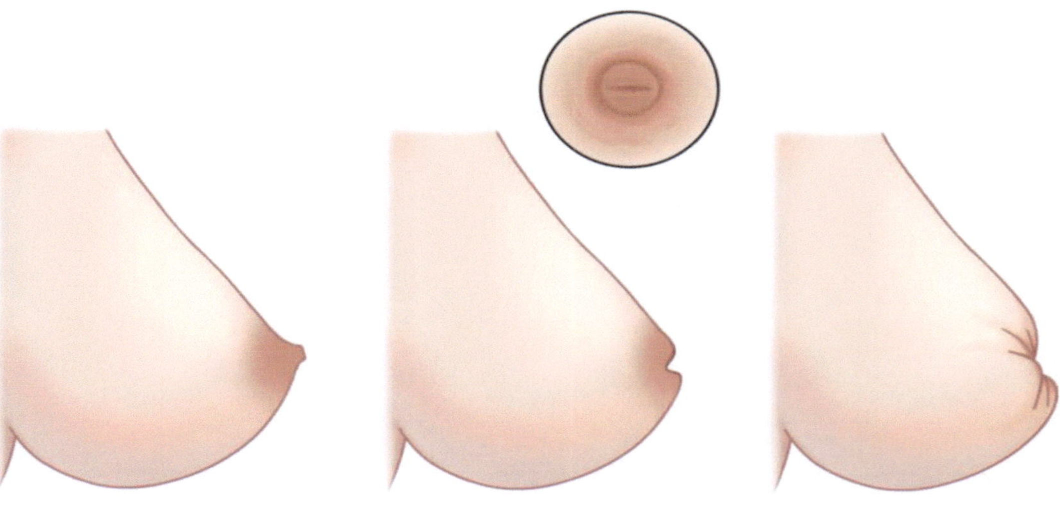

Fig. 29.8 Demonstrates normal nipple, inversion of nipple, and retracted nipple

include duct ectasia, periductal mastitis, or underlying malignancy.

Thus, cases with acquired unilateral nipple retraction should be evaluated with imaging and treated according to the underlying condition.

29.2.2.6 Imaging Features

X-ray mammogram: Inversion of whole nipple with areola distortion and no nipple is seen in profile (Fig. 29.9a, b).

USG breast: Inverted nipple appears as hypoechoic area below the nipple areola complex (Fig. 29.9d).

MR mammogram: Nipple is usually seen pulled inwards with additional detection of underlying cause of nipple inversion (Fig. 29.9c), that is, carcinoma, fat necrosis, postsurgical changes, or duct ectasia.

Management: Benign nipple retraction does not need any intervention; however, if the patient insists on corrective procedure, a total division of the terminal part of the lactiferous ducts with nipple correction may be done. Patient should be warned that breastfeeding will not be possible after the corrective procedure [6].

29.2.2.7 Papilloma of the Nipple (Central Intraductal Papilloma)

It is a benign condition and presents mostly as a pedunculated lesion from the nipple.

Intraductal papillary lesions (papilloma) are breast tumors seen in 2–3% of women and common in the third-sixth decade. These are classified into central and peripheral types.

Central papillomas (aka nipple papilloma) arise in the subareolar space and are usually solitary.

Clinical features: Most common presentation is spontaneous, unilateral, bloody nipple discharge.

29.2.2.8 Imaging Features

X-ray mammogram: Retroareolar linear tubular density lesions are seen, which on galactogram are seen as focal dilatation at level of nipple with filling defects (Fig. 29.10).

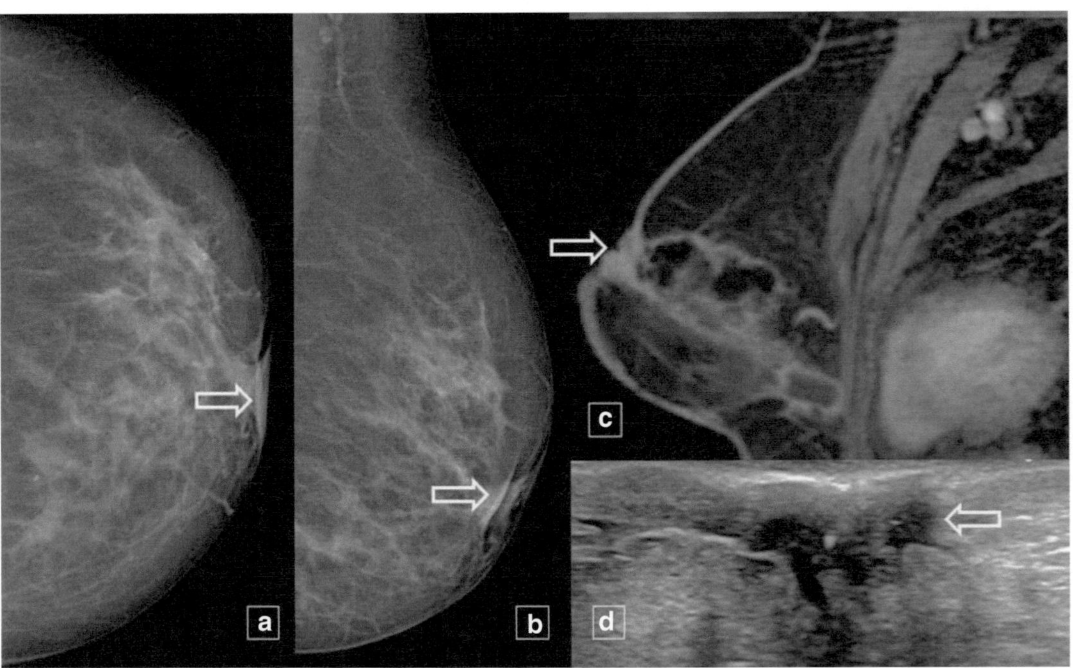

Fig. 29.9 Imaging findings in patients with retracted nipple. (**a**, **b**) Mammogram CC and MLO view of left breast showing inversion of nipple with inward concavity—no nipple seen in profile. (**c**) MRI breast—sagittal T1 + C contrast imaging showing nipple pulled inwards secondary to postsurgical changes. (**d**) USG breast-inverted nipple seen as hypoechoic area in retroareolar region

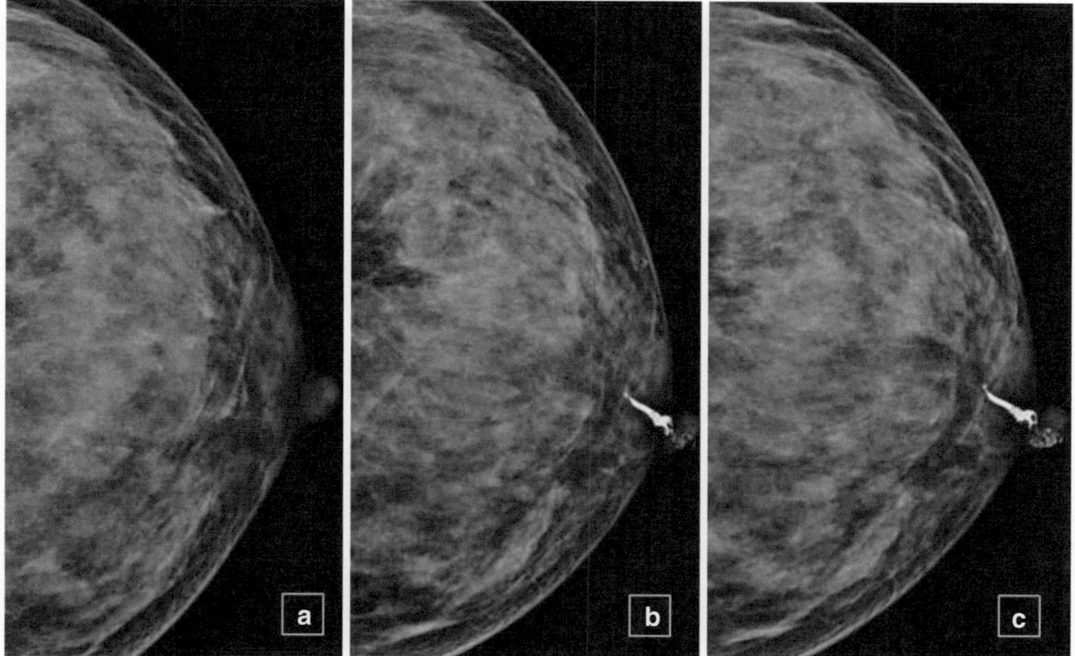

Fig. 29.10 Imaging features of nipple papilloma on mammogram (**a**) CC view of left breast—no obvious lesion noted. (**b**, **c**) galactogram images showing focal dilatation of subareolar duct just at the level of nipple

USG breast: Depicts dilated ducts in subareolar region with internal solid lesion/mass showing varying degrees of internal vascularity.

MR mammogram: Dilated ducts are seen on pre-contrast images in subareolar region, which appear as T2 hyperintense, showing progressive enhancement pattern within the internal solid content on post-contrast images (Fig. 29.11).

Histological features include intraductal proliferation consisting of fibrovascular cores lined by the outer layer of luminal cells and an inner layer of myoepithelial cells.

Management: Papillomas are usually treated by excision [7].

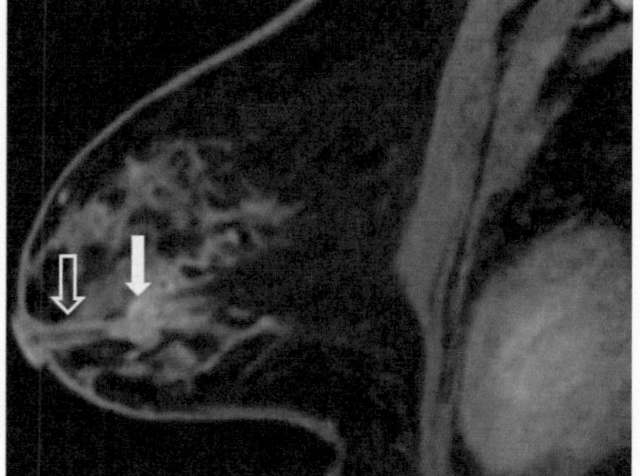

Fig. 29.11 Forty-three year old lady with complaints of bloody nipple discharge MRI breast in same patient,T1 + C sagittal image: Dilated duct (marked with empty arrow) in subareolar region with intensely enhancing internal components (marked with full arrow)—suggestive of central papilloma (nipple papilloma)

29.2.2.9 Nipple Adenoma

Nipple adenoma is also known as florid papillomatosis of the nipple or subareolar sclerosing duct hyperplasia of the nipple. It is a benign proliferative disease of lactiferous ducts and presents in middle-aged women. It can present as a visible or palpable nodule in the nipple or erosion of the nipple with erythema and itching (which is often misdiagnosed as Paget's disease) or as blood-stained or serosanguinous nipple discharge. Rarely, nipple adenoma may be associated with coexisting breast malignancy.

Mammogram: Nipple adenoma on mammogram appears as round/oval equal density nodules in retroareolar region.

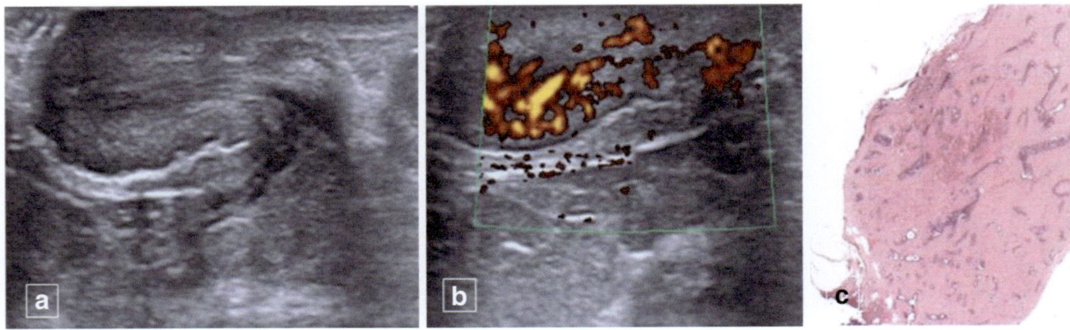

Fig. 29.12 Imaging findings in nipple adenoma (**a**, **b**) USG breast in 45 year old asymptomatic lady—oval hyperechoic circumscribed nodule seen within the nipple showing extensive increased vascularity. (**c**) HPE-Photomicrograph showing ducts with hyperplasia and surrounded by prominent fibrosis (H&E ×100)

USG: Round/oval homogeneous, hypoechoic mass/nodule with circumscribed margins, and intense internal vascularity (Fig. 29.12a, b).

Histopathology: Shows crowded ducts and glands beneath the epidermis with papillomatosis. Fibrosis and keratin cysts may also be seen (Fig. 29.12c).

Deep nipple skin biopsy confirms the diagnosis and helps to rule out Paget's disease.

Management: Complete surgical excision of the nipple-areolar complex [8, 9].

29.2.2.10 Subareolar Abscess (Zuska Disease)

Nonpuerperal subareolar mastitis and abscess, otherwise known as Zuska disease, is a rare condition and affects either young teens or old-aged women. It is not associated with pregnancy or lactation. It is usually seen in females who are cigarette smokers; very rarely, it has been reported in men too.

Causative organism is mostly staphylococcus but recurrent subareolar abscess has multiple organisms as etiology.

The disease has three reported stages. **In the early stage**, blockage and plugging of lactiferous ducts happen followed by the pus and debris formation. Periareolar fistula formation and discharge of pus from the fistula is the third stage.

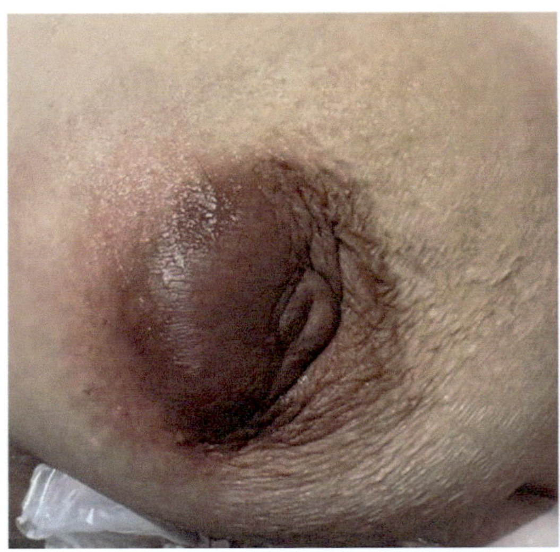

Fig. 29.13 Forty-three year old lady with complaints of painful lump in right nipple areola complex region—on examination, erythematous shiny skin noted over the palpable lump

Symptoms: Patient presents with breast pain and tender swelling in nipple-areolar region (Fig. 29.13).

29.2.2.11 Imaging Findings

X-ray mammogram: Subareolar abscess usually present as retroareolar masses with overlying nipple areola skin thickening (Fig. 29.15a, b). Features are similar to breast neoplasm; thus, clinical history of smoking, fever, and skin erythema is important.

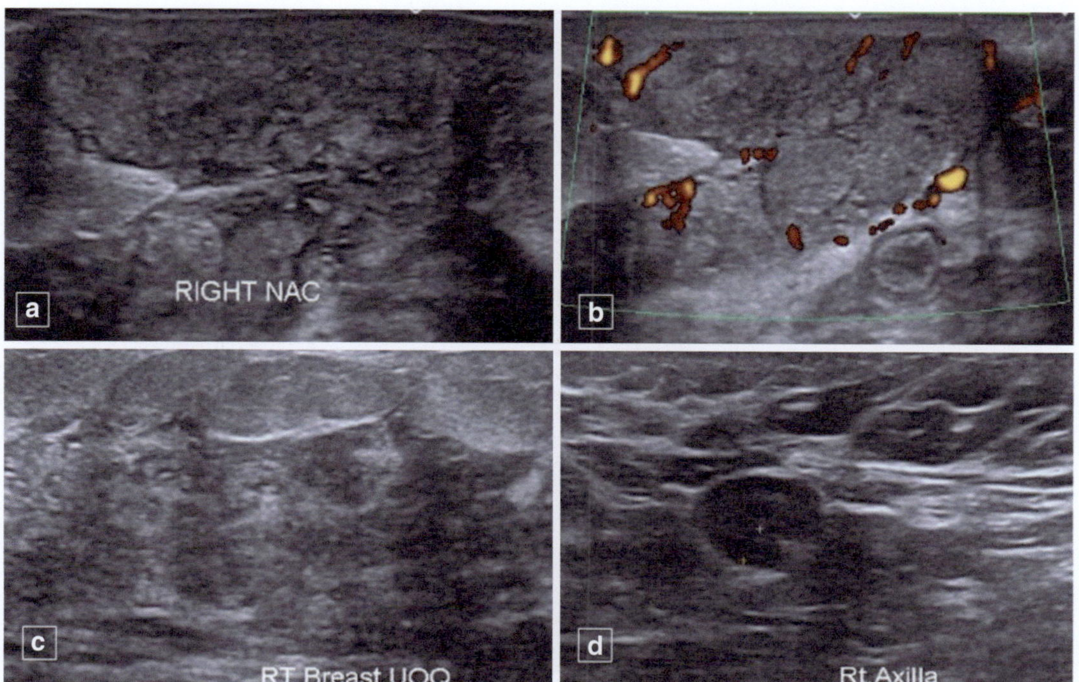

Fig. 29.14 USG in same patient showing (**a**, **b**) ill-defined heteroechoic collection in subareolar region with significant peripheral vascularity, suggestive of subareolar abscess. (**c**) There is surrounding heterogenous parenchyma and inflammatory changes with (**d**) a reactive lymph node in axillary region

Ultrasound: Reveals oval circumscribed collections with internal echoes and surrounding peripheral vascularity (Figs. 29.14a–c and 29.15c). Reactive enlarged lymph nodes may also be present (Fig. 29.14d).

MR mammogram: Shows similar features of abscess—retroareolar circumscribed lesion with peripheral enhancement and diffusion restriction.

Pathology may reveal sheets of neutrophils admixed with foamy macrophages in a proteinaceous background (Fig. 29.15d).

Treatment is ultrasound-guided drainage/surgical drainage and sensitive antibiotics [8]. Unlike lactational abscess, subareolar abscess is known for recurrence and may need repeated drainage procedure.

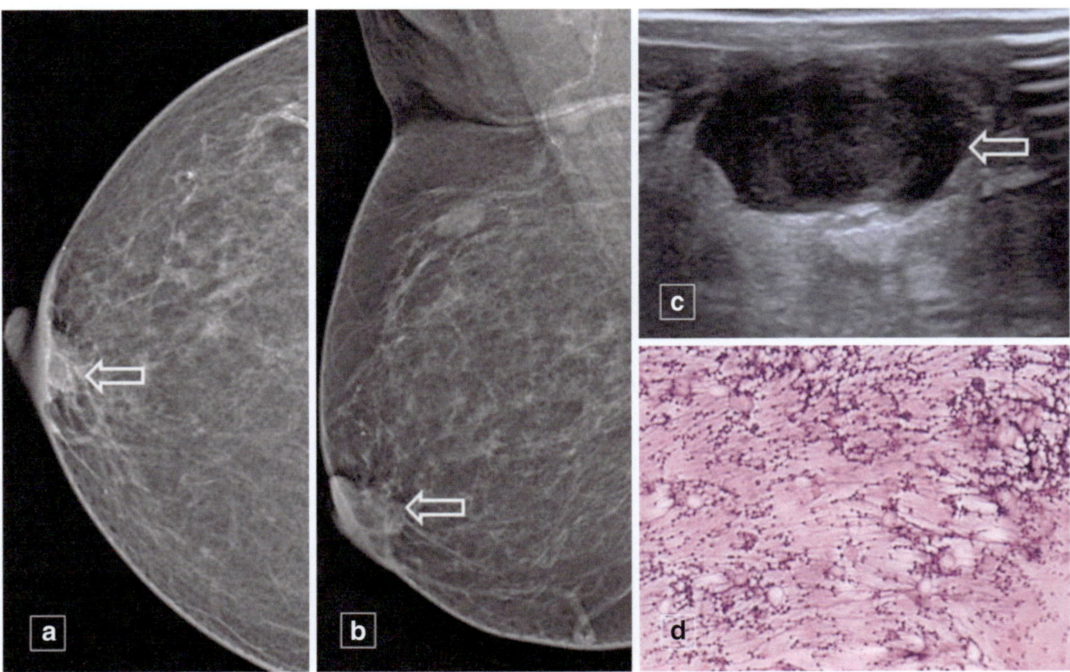

Fig. 29.15 Imaging features of subareolar abscess. (**a**, **b**) Mammogram (CC, MLO views) of right breast showing thickening of the skin over nipple areola complex and a mixed density lesion in the retro areolar region. (**c**) USG breast in same patient showing thick-walled cystic lesion with internal debris in the subareolar region. (**d**) Cytology image showing sheets of neutrophils admixed with foamy macrophages in a proteinaceous background (MGG ×200)

29.3 PAGET'S Disease

Paget's disease accounts for less than 3% of all breast malignancies and is characterized by the presence of malignant cells within the squamous epithelium of the nipple. It may consist of a single self-standing nipple malignancy, but in 95% of cases, it is accompanied by an underlying invasive breast carcinoma or ductal carcinoma in situ (DCIS) both in proximity of or distant from the nipple.

The differential diagnosis of Paget's disease include nipple eczema, Bowen's disease, melanoma, or breast carcinoma involving the nipple by contiguity or invasion.

29.3.1 Clinical Features

It presents as an eczematous lesion centering around nipple initially and later involves the areola and surrounding skin.

The common symptoms are pruritus, pain, or burning sensation in the nipple. Patients may also present with scaling and erythema of the nipple, blood-stained discharge, nipple distortion, or inversion. The presence of underlying small breast lump is an ominous sign of Paget's disease.

29.3.2 Imaging Features

X-ray mammogram—May show malignant calcifications at the level of the nipple or elsewhere in the breast. Other features on X-ray are skin thickening at the nipple-areolar region, nipple retraction, discrete mass behind the nipple (Fig. 29.16a, b) or away from it, and architectural distortion [10].

X-ray mammogram may be normal in approximately 50% of the typical cases of clinically proven Paget's disease [11].

USG findings: Nipple asymmetry/flattening, skin thickening, retroareolar mass, nipple retraction (Fig. 29.16c, d), nipple micro-calcifications (Fig. 29.17a, b), and ductal ectasia.

MRI has a sensitivity of 95% compared with 70% in mammography, in the detection of breast

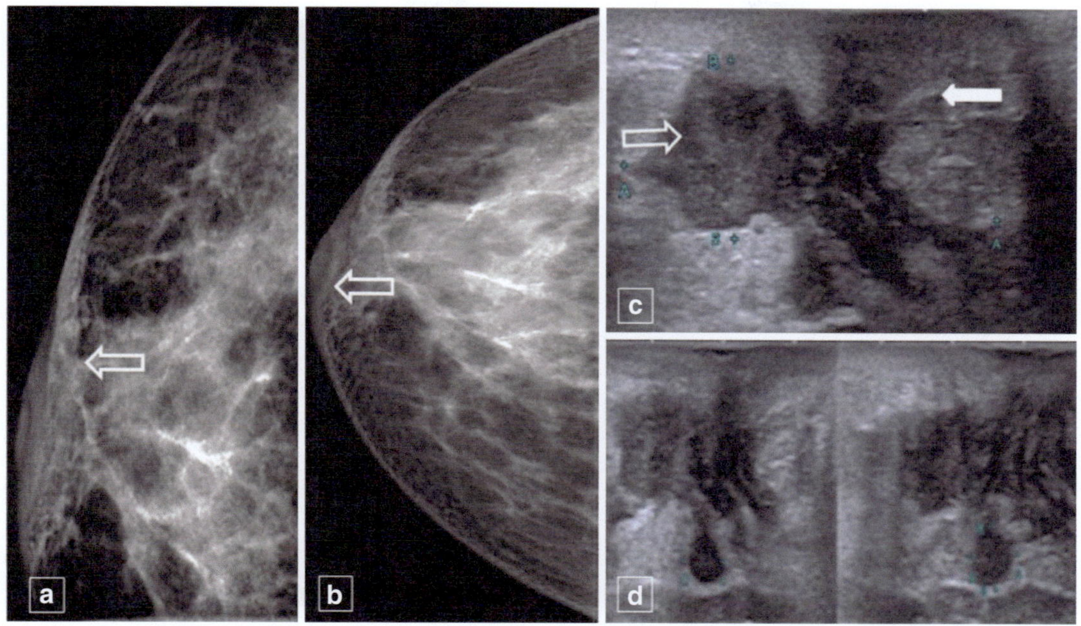

Fig. 29.16 (**a**, **b**) Mammogram—(CC view) of right breast showing skin thickening in nipple areola region (**c**, **d**) USG breast in the same patient showing nipple retraction (marked with white-filled arrow) with irregular retroareolar mass (marked with empty arrow)

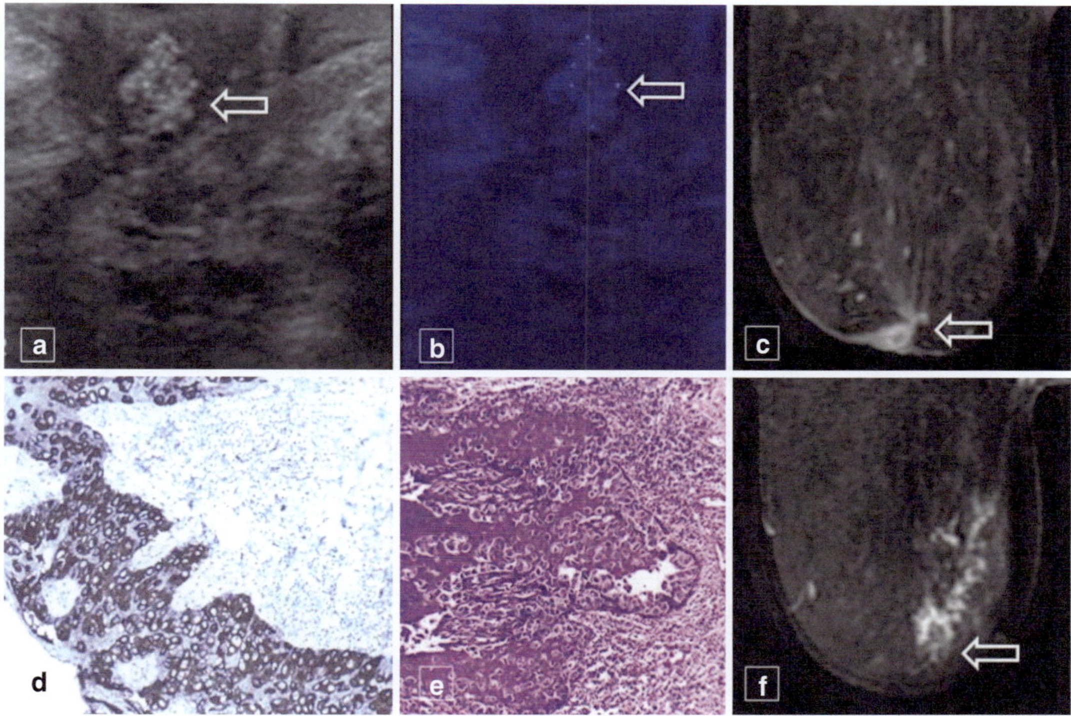

Fig. 29.17 Fifty-two year old lady with complaints of bloody discharge from left nipple (**a**, **b**) USG images showing micro-calcifications within the nipple. (**c**, **f**) MRI of left breast T1 + C Axial: nipple retraction with underlying clumped nonmass enhancement suggestive of Paget's with underlying DCIS. (**d**) HPE-tumor cells in the epithelium of nipple highlighted by EMA (IHC ×200). (**e**) Nipple with single and clusters of atypical cells with clear cytoplasm and nuclear atypia (H&E ×200)

lesions. MRI helps differentiate a normal nipple from abnormal and evaluates the extent of the tumor. Abnormal nipple-areolar skin thickening and asymmetric nipple-areolar enhancement is usually noted (Fig. 29.17c, f). The enhancement may be mild to intense, appear irregular, or irregular discoid. Other findings include enhanced subareolar mass, an associated linear clumped enhancement in cases with associated DCIS [2].

Magnetic resonance imaging can be used as a diagnostic tool to detect clinically occult cancer with nonspecific findings on mammogram and ultrasonogram [12].

Mammary Paget disease can be classified into three categories [12, 13].

1. Paget disease of the nipple without DCIS
2. Paget disease of the nipple with associated DCIS in the underlying lactiferous ducts of the nipple-areolar complex
3. Paget disease of the nipple with associated DCIS in the underlying lactiferous ducts of the nipple-areolar complex and associated DCIS or invasive breast cancer elsewhere in the breast, at least 2 cm from the nipple-areolar complex (Fig. 29.18).

29.3.3 Histopathology

Histopathology is characterized by intraepithelial large atypical cells (Paget cells) arranged as single cells or clusters of cells spread throughout the epidermis. Cells have abundant pale cytoplasm, irregular large nucleus with prominent nucleoli, and underlying dermis with chronic inflammation. Epidermis shows hyperkeratosis, ulceration, or pseudoepitheliomatous hyperplasia (Fig. 29.17d, e). Immunohistochemistry shows positivity for Her2 Neu, CK, CAM5.2 Positivity in over 90% cases.

29.3.4 Treatment

Both clinical and imaging findings are complementary to each other to confirm the diagnosis of mammary Paget's disease. Surgical biopsy is, however, the diagnostic standard, and therefore, nipple skin biopsy is recommended. Image-guided fine needle aspiration cytology (FNAC)/biopsy if there is an underlying breast lump is done. For patients with only nipple involvement, nipple-areolar complex is removed by wide local excision with sentinel lymph node biopsy and

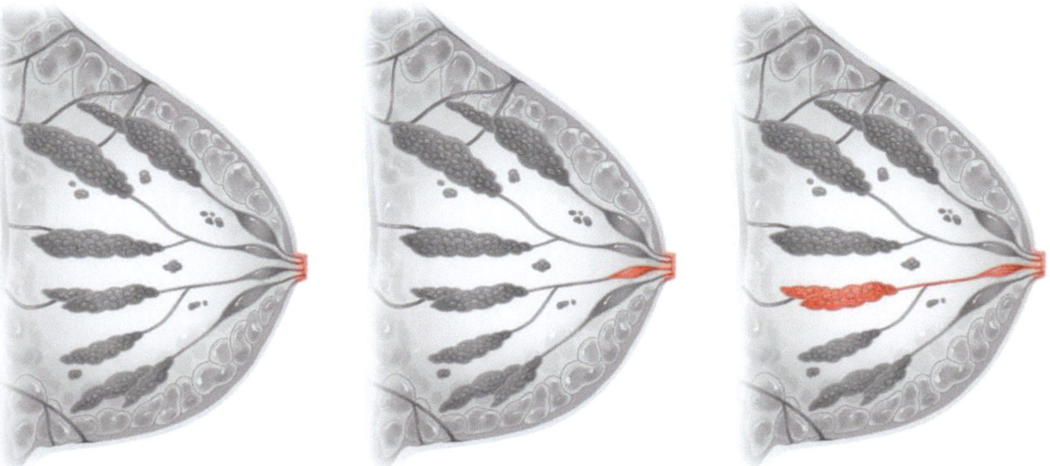

Fig. 29.18 Schematic representation of type 1, 2, and 3 of the mammary Paget's disease

proceeding to axillary dissection if sentinel node is positive. If there is underlying breast lump, primary surgery or neoadjuvant chemotherapy is decided based on the clinicopathological stage of the breast mass, and further adjuvant therapy is also planned accordingly.

29.3.5 Approach to Patient with Nipple Discharge

Nipple discharge constitutes any kind of discharge from the nipple in a nonpregnant, nonbreast-feeding woman. It can be unilateral or bilateral, spontaneous, or only in response to breast manipulation (Fig. 29.19).
Types of nipple discharge

- Serous (yellow)
- Mucinous (clear and watery)
- Milky
- Sanguineous (bloody)
- Purulent
- Multicolored and sticky
- Serosanguinous (pink)

Causes of nipple discharge [14]

- Benign ductal disorders
- Intraductal papilloma
- Mammary duct ectasia
- Fibrocystic changes
- Endocrine disorders
- Breast abscesses or infections

> Intraductal papilloma is the most common cause of a bloody nipple discharge without a breast mass.

Malignant causes (<10% of cases)

- Intraductal carcinoma.
- Invasive ductal carcinoma.

The red flag signs for nipple discharge that warrants further investigations are

- Spontaneous discharge.
- Unilateral

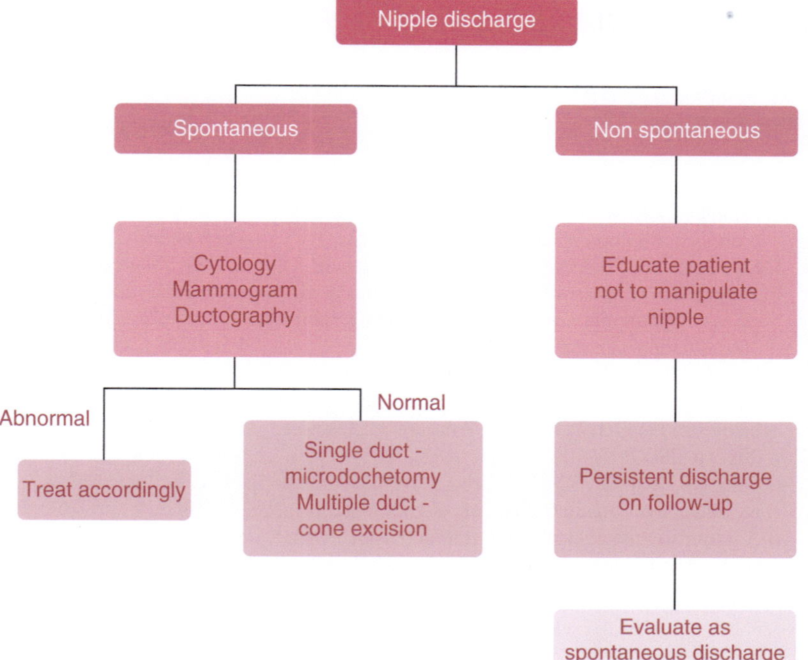

Fig. 29.19 Flowchart showing approach to a patient with nipple discharge

- Age > 40 years
- Palpable mass

29.3.6 Cytology

The nipple discharge is sent for cytology to check for malignant cells. Guaiac test can be done to check for occult blood (in case of malignancy), but these two tests cannot rule out malignancy.

29.3.7 Investigations

- Ductography (Galactography)
- Ultrasound
- Mammogram
- MRI

29.3.8 Treatment

If there is underlying breast disease causing nipple discharge, it is treated accordingly. Otherwise, persistent spontaneous discharge is treated by duct excision/microdochectomy (single-duct discharge) or cone/total duct excision (multiple-duct discharge) [15–18].

References

1. Nicholson BT, Harvey JA, Cohen MA. Nipple-areolar complex: normal anatomy and benign and malignant processes. Radiographics. 2009;29(2):509–23.
2. Da Costa D, Taddese A, Cure ML, Gerson D, Poppiti R, Esserman LE. Common and unusual diseases of the nipple-areolar complex. Radiographics. 2007;27(suppl_1):S65–77.
3. Bland KI, Klimberg VS, Copeland EM, Gradishar WJ. The breast–comprehensive management of benign and malignant diseases. Amsterdam: Elsevier; 2017. p. 38–40, 57–78.
4. Song HS, Jung SE, Kim YC, Lee ES. Nipple eczema, an indicative manifestation of atopic dermatitis? A clinical, histological, and immunohistochemical study. Am J Dermatopathol. 2015;37:284–8. https://doi.org/10.1097/DAD.0000000000000195.
5. Kim SK, Won YH, Kim S. Nipple eczema: a diagnostic challenge of allergic contact dermatitis. Ann Dermatol. 2014;26:413–4. https://doi.org/10.5021/ad.2014.26.3.413.
6. Stone K, Wheeler A. A review of anatomy, physiology, and benign pathology of the nipple. Ann Surg Oncol. 2015;22:3236–40. https://doi.org/10.1245/s10434-015-4760-4.
7. Harris JR, Lipman ME, Morrow M, Osborne CK. Diseases of the breast. 4th ed. Philadelphia: Lippincott; 2002. p. 42–7.
8. Salemis NS. Florid papillomatosis of the nipple: a rare presentation and review of the literature. Breast Dis. 2015;35(2):153–6. https://doi.org/10.3233/BD-150397.
9. Wang C, Wang X, Ma R. Diagnosis and surgical treatment of nipple adenoma. ANZ J Surg. 2015;85:444–7. https://doi.org/10.1111/ans.12744.
10. Sripathi S, Ayachit A, Kadavigere R, Kumar S, Eleti A, Sraj A. Spectrum of imaging findings in Paget's disease of the breast-a pictorial review. Insights Imaging. 2015;6(4):419–29. https://doi.org/10.1007/s13244-015-0415-z.
11. Ikeda DM, Helvie MA, Frank TS, Chapel KL, Anderson IT. Paget disease of the nipple: radiologic-pathologic correlation. Radiology. 1993;189(1):89–94. https://doi.org/10.1148/radiology.189.1.8396786.
12. Babu B, Dev B, Mohanapriya T, Shalini CNS. Bilateral mammary Paget disease in a young adult female. Radiol Case Rep. 2018;13(3):586–91. https://doi.org/10.1016/j.radcr.2018.02.018.
13. Lim HS, Jeong SJ, Lee JS, Park MH, Kim JW, Shin SS. Paget disease of the breast: mammographic, US, and MR imaging findings with pathologic correlation. Radiographics. 2011;31(7):1973–87.
14. Carty NJ, Mudan SS, Ravichandran D, et al. Prospective study of outcome in women presenting with nipple discharge. Ann R Coll Surg Engl. 1994;76:387–9.
15. Simmons R, Adamovich T, Brennan M, et al. Non surgical evaluation of pathogical nipple discharge. Ann Surg Oncol. 2003;10:113.
16. Kasales CJ, Han B, Smith JS, Chetlen AL, Kaneda HJ, Shereef S. Nonpuerperal mastitis and subareolar abscess of the breast. Am J Roentgenol. 2014;202(2):W133–9.
17. Paget J. On disease of the mammary areola preceding cancer of the mammary gland. Cancer J Clin. 1874;10:87–9.
18. Ashikari R, Park K, Huvos AG, Urban JA. Paget's disease of the breast. Cancer. 1970;26(3):680–5. https://doi.org/10.1002/1097-0142(197009)26:3<680::AID-CNCR2820260329>3.0.CO;2-P.

Axillary Lesions

30

Udaya Baskarini Vakamudi, Leena Dennis Joseph, Bhawna Dev, and Mohana Priya

Abstract

Ultrasound is the preferred modality for assessing axillary lymph nodes. Lymph node cortical thickness and uniformity are the most important criteria for distinguishing normal nodes from abnormal ones. In a patient with a known malignancy, normal nodal morphologic features do not necessarily permit the exclusion of metastatic disease from the differential diagnosis, and a sentinel node biopsy may be needed.

Keywords

Axilla · Lymph nodes · Ultrasound · Fatty hilum · Cortical thickening

U. B. Vakamudi (✉) · B. Dev
Department of Radiology, Sri Ramachandra Institute of Higher Education and Research, Chennai, India
e-mail: bhawnadev@sriramachandra.edu.in

L. D. Joseph
Department of Pathology, Sri Ramachandra Institute of Higher Education and Research, Chennai, India

M. Priya
Department of Surgery, Sri Ramachandra Institute of Higher Education and Research, Chennai, India

30.1 Introduction

Axillary adenopathy is a common condition encountered in routine practice during breast imaging and is caused by a broad spectrum of diseases. Knowledge of anatomy, normal and abnormal nodal morphologic features, and patients' appropriate history helps in accurate diagnosis.

The axilla contains both lymph nodes and non-lymphatic tissue such as accessory breast tissue, skin, fat, muscles, nerves, and blood vessels. Hence, there are numerous differential diagnosis pertaining to pathologies in the axilla [1], which have been depicted in Fig. 30.1.

Ultrasound is the first line investigation modality for evaluation of axillary pathologies. While important parameters such as shape, margin, hilar shape, cortical thickness, internal structure, echogenicity, and vascular features can be evaluated on ultrasound, X-ray mammogram, Computed Tomography (CT), and Magnetic Resonance Imaging (MRI) aid in identifying the origin and extent of the axillary mass and evaluating the tissue characteristics and composition [2, 3].

30.1.1 Levels of Axillary Lymph Nodes:

These five groups of axillary lymph nodes, depicted in Fig. 30.2, are divided into three levels with respect to the pectoralis minor muscle.

B. Dev, L. D. Joseph (eds.), *Holistic Approach to Breast Disease*,
https://doi.org/10.1007/978-981-99-0035-0_30

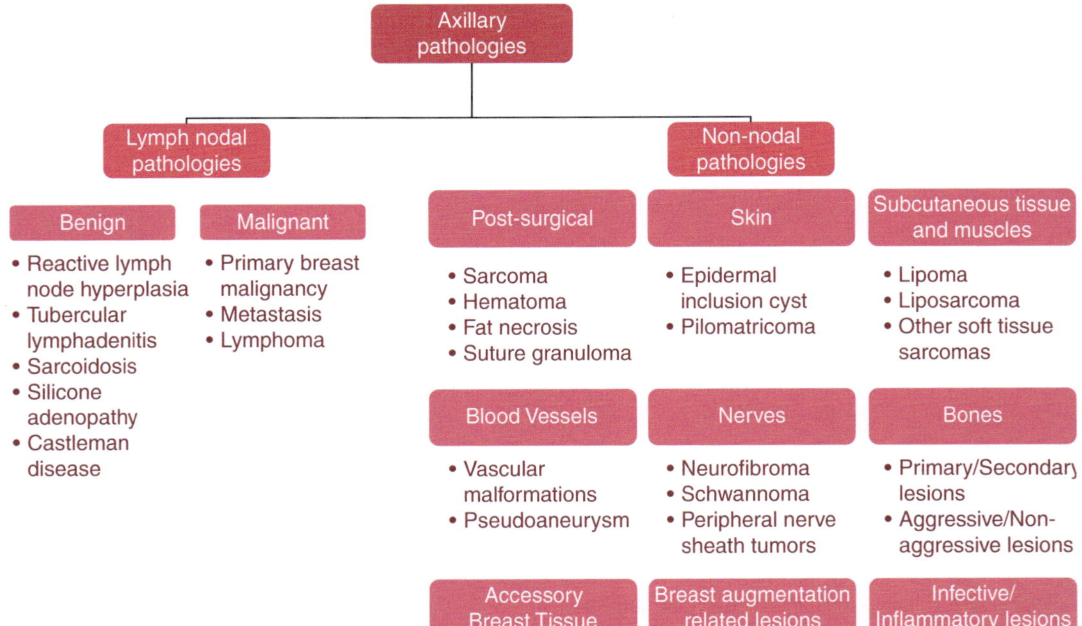

Fig. 30.1 Various lymph nodal and non-lymph nodal pathologies in axilla

Anterior group: Also known as pectoral nodes; located at the inferior border of the pectoralis minor muscle; receive lymph from the major part of the breast.

Posterior group: Also known as subscapular nodes; located at the anterior border of the subscapularis muscle; receive lymph from the axillary tail of the breast and posterior shoulder.

Lateral group: Located behind the axillary vein; this group drains lymph from upper limb.

Central group: Located near the base of the axilla; receive lymph from preceding three groups; most likely the group to be palpable (against the lateral thoracic wall).

Apical group: Located medial to the axillary vein and superior to the pectoralis minor; receive lymph from all other groups and sometimes directly from the breast.

Lymph nodes can also be divided into levels in relationship to pectoralis minor muscle.

Level I: This comprises three groups (lateral, posterolateral, and anteromedial groups) of axillary lymph nodes usually present inferolateral to the pectoralis minor muscle.

Level II: One group of axillary lymph nodes located posterior to the pectoralis minor.

Level III: One group located superomedial to the pectoralis minor muscle.

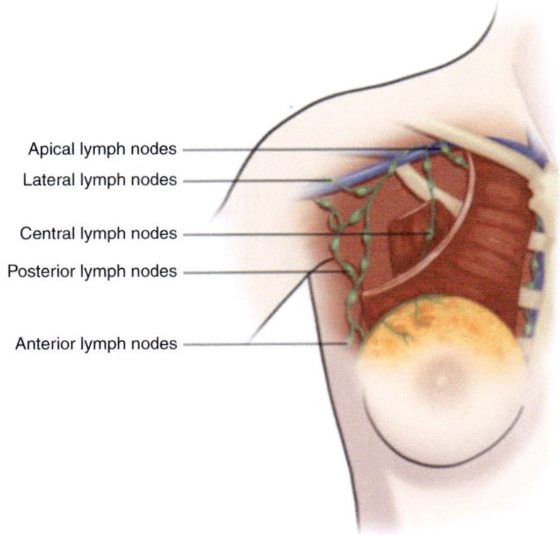

Fig. 30.2 Shown are five groups of axillary lymph nodes

30.1.2 Imaging Appearance of a Non-pathological Lymph Node

Mammogram: In mediolateral oblique view (MLO view), normal lymph node usually appears as well-circumscribed oval density with a central fatty hilum as seen in Fig. 30.3a.

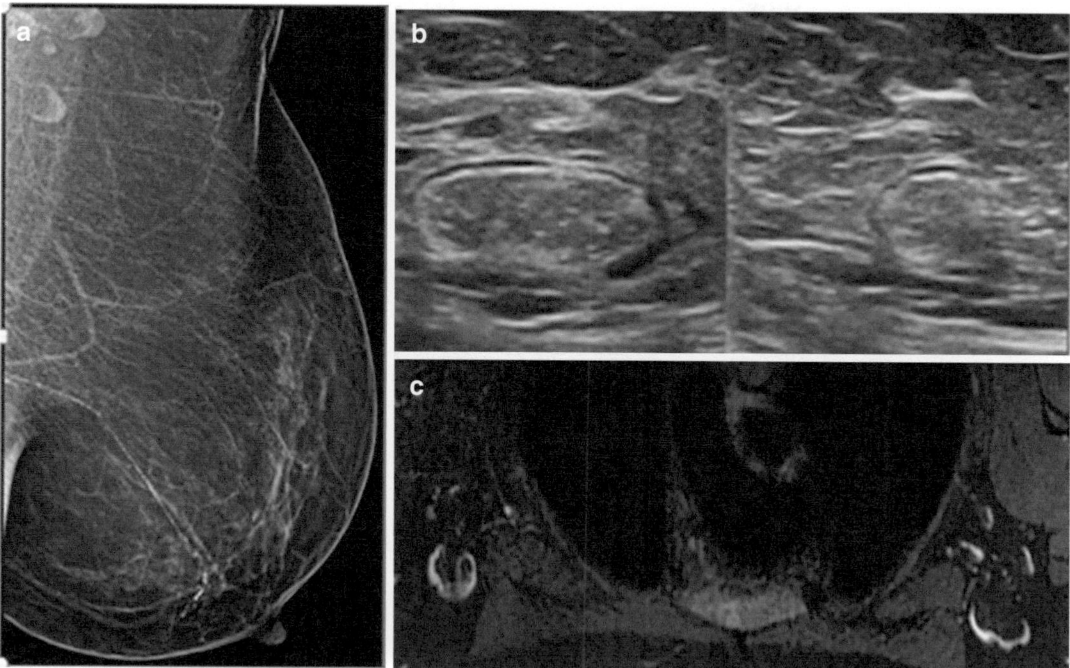

Fig. 30.3 (**a**) MLO view on X-ray mammogram showing few axillary lymph nodes with preserved fatty hilum. (**b**) Ultrasound images showing normal axillary lymph nodes with a pencil thin cortex and fatty hilum. (**c**) Fat-suppressed MRI image showing thin hyperintense cortex with central fatty hilum appearing hypointense

Table 30.1 According to Bedi et al. classification [4]—the cortex of the lymph node is divided into 6 types

Type 1	Without visible cortex	
Type 2	Cortex ≤3 mm	
Type 3	Cortex >3 mm (reactional changes)	
Type 4	Entirely lobulated cortex (probably benign)	
Type 5	with focal lobulation	Suspicious, needs biopsy
Type 6	completely hypoechogenic, without hilum	Suspicious, needs biopsy

Ultrasound: Lymph node shows a reniform shape with smooth margins. The cortex appears uniformly hypoechoic with a maximal thickness of 3 mm. Sometimes cortex may appear as thin and defined as pencil line as shown in Fig. 30.3b. The central echogenic fatty hilum shows vascularity on Doppler.

MRI: The cortex of the lymph nodes appear hypointense on T1 and isohyperintense on T2 weighted images. The hilar fat appears hypointense on fat-saturated sequences as shown in Fig. 30.3c. The nodes show homogenous enhancement post-contrast administration [3].

30.2 Abnormal-Appearing Lymph Node

To label an axillary lymph node abnormal it should have a cortical thickness more than 3 mm (Table 30.1) with eccentric thickening, and irregular margins. The cortical thickening causes hilar displacement with the morphology progressing from uniform thickening to irregular thickening, ultimately leading to absence of the fatty hilum as shown in Fig. 30.4. Change in vascular pattern with either peripheral or mixed vascularity is also observed.

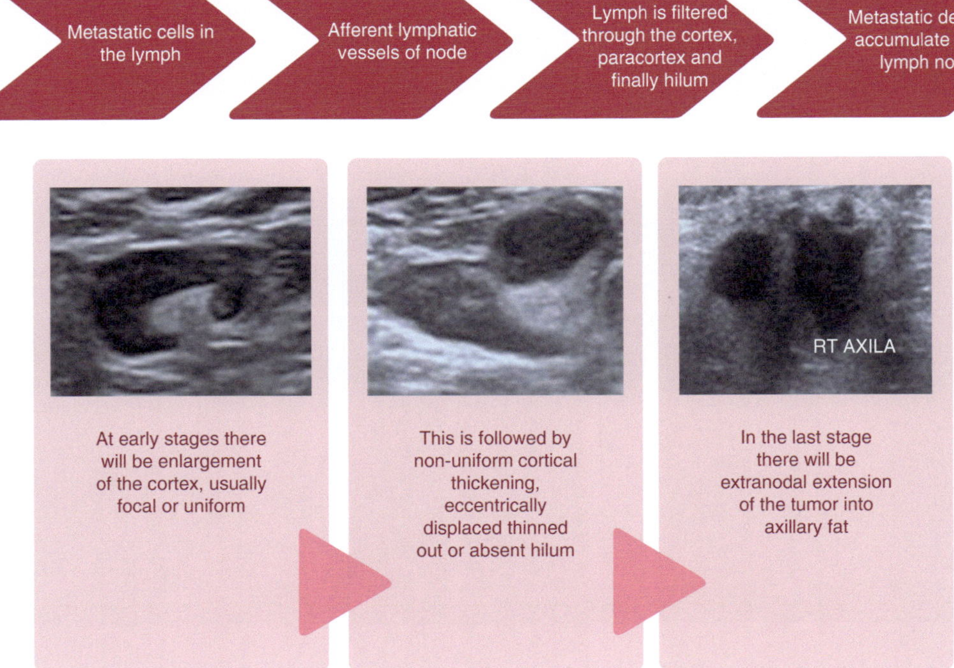

Fig. 30.4 Ultrasound images of the cortex and hilum of the lymph node showing progressive tumor cell infiltration

Absence of the hilum is the most specific finding for metastatic disease, but such finding is present only in cases of advanced disease [5].

30.3 Pathway of Spread of Tumor Cells to Lymph Node

30.4 Lymph Node Characterization and Classification on Ultrasound

Schematic diagrams and corresponding ultrasound images of these five types of lymph nodes are illustrated in Figs. 30.5 and 30.6.

Lymph nodes can also be classified as abnormal with cortex/hilum ratio, instead of an absolute value for the cortex, that is, when the cortical thickness is ≥ the thickness of the fatty hilum (suspicious finding) as shown in Fig. 30.7.

***Sentinel lymph nodes* are the first group of lymph nodes that drain the tumor bed. It is located by injecting blue dye and/or radioactive material at the tumor site and identifying a blue and/or a radioactive lymph node in the axilla.**

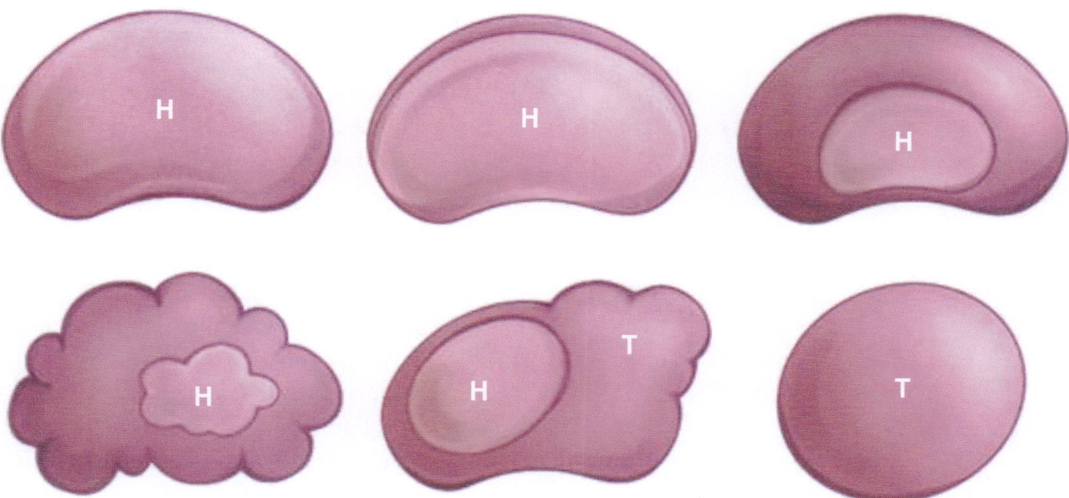

Fig. 30.5 Line diagram of types of lymph nodes—*H* hilum; *T* tumor cell deposit

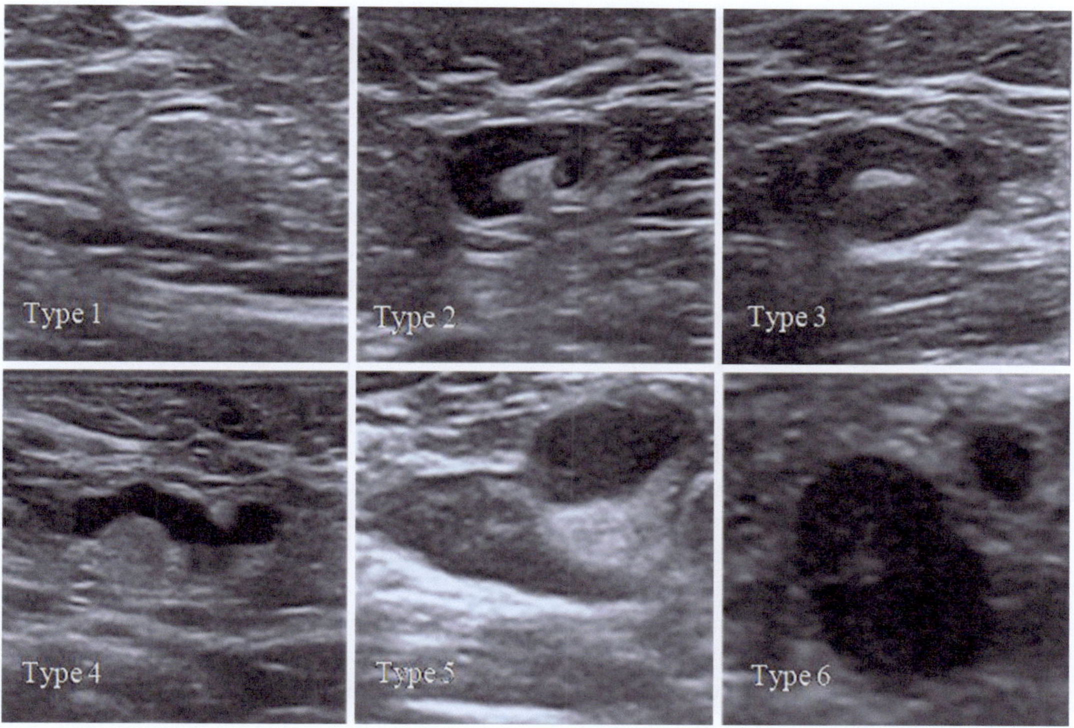

Fig. 30.6 Ultrasound images of types of lymph nodes

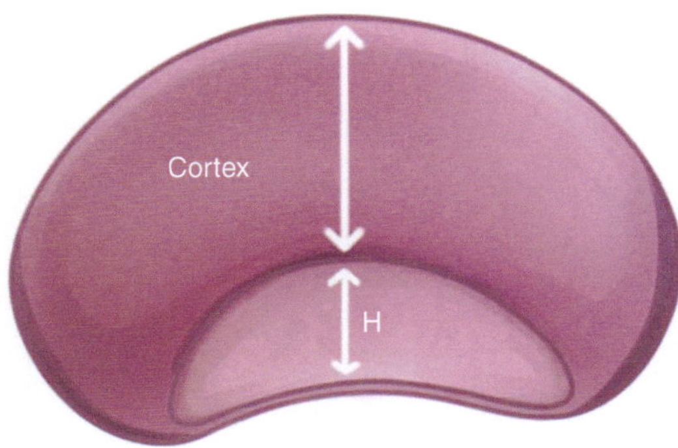

Fig. 30.7 Showing cortical thickness > fatty hilum thickness

30.5 Differential Diagnosis to Be Considered During Imaging

Pathologies occuring in axilla can be broadly classified into nodal and non-nodal pathology.

30.5.1 Benign Lesions

30.5.1.1 Congenital: Accessory Breast Tissue

It is a common congenital variant in which there is accessory breast tissue in the axilla that occurs due to failure of regression of primitive mammary tissue along the embryonic milk line. Normal breast tissue is also present. This can be seen in any location along the milk line extending from axilla to inguinal region. A palpable mass develops during menarche, pregnancy, or lactation due to hormonal stimulation.

Mammogram and ultrasound show an area of normal-appearing fibroglandular breast tissue similar to normal breast tissue in unilateral/bilateral axillae (Fig. 30.8a–d) or anywhere along the milk line. Any disease that arises in breast parenchyma can occur in the accessory breast tissue, including benign, malignant, infective, and inflammatory disease [2].

Management: Accessory breast tissue does not need any specific treatment. Surgical Excision can be done for cosmetic reasons.

30.5.1.2 Benign Reactive Lymph Node Hyperplasia

Benign axillary lymph node hyperplasia is the most frequently encountered axillary pathology [2].

Causes of benign unilateral axillary lymphadenopathy commonly include infection such as mastitis [5] and postvaccination reactions [6, 7]; bilateral axillary lymphadenopathy can be due to systemic etiologies such as wide-spread infection, rheumatoid arthritis, collagen vascular disease, lymphoma, leukemia, and metastatic breast and non-breast lesions [6].

Calcifications in abnormal axillary lymph nodes may represent calcified metastasis from breast, thyroid or ovarian cancer, collagen vascular disease, or granulomatous infections [8].

Reactive lymph node hyperplasia can be caused by local skin infections, inorganic dusts (silica, coal), and systemic infections (tuberculosis, HIV, etc.). It could be unilateral or bilateral.

Mammogram: It may appear as a enlarged lymph node with increased density as seen in Fig. 30.10a.

Ultrasound: Usually seen as oval or elongated lymph node (long/short axis ratio (LSR) >2) with low to moderate echogenicity, sharp or blurred margins, preserved central echogenic hilum, and concentric cortical thickening (Table 30.1) as seen in Fig. 30.10b. Color doppler may show prominent hilar vascularity due to increased blood flow. Nodal vascularity on Doppler ultrasound (US) generally follows two patterns: central or peripheral [5, 6] as shown in Fig. 30.9.

CT: Node appears as oval shaped or elongated with preserved central hypodense fatty hilum,

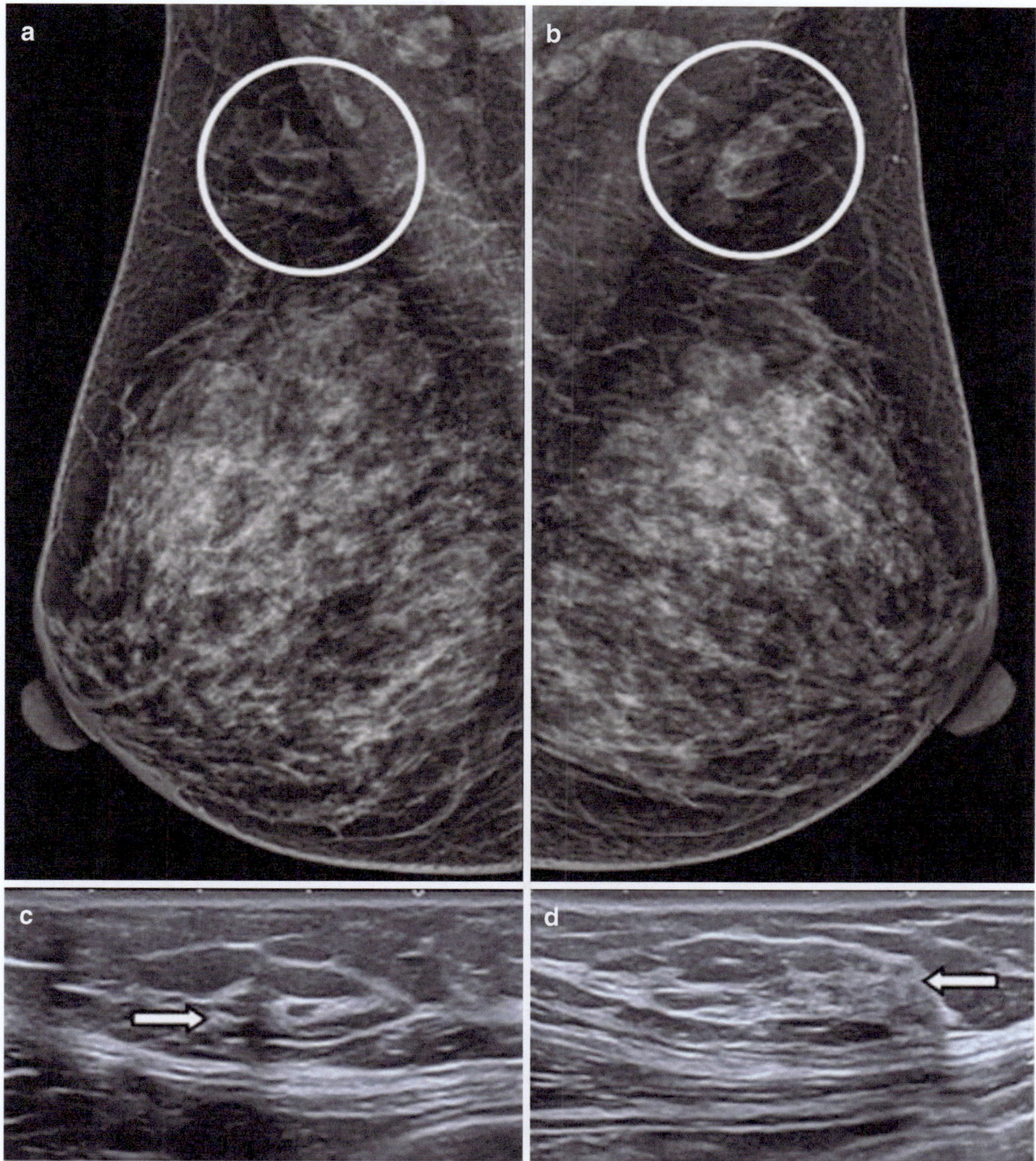

Fig. 30.8 (**a**, **b**) X-ray mammogram showing an area of accessory fibroglandular breast tissue in both axillae (white circles), more pronounced in the left axilla. (**c**, **d**) ultrasound of accessory breast parenchyma bilaterally

smooth margins, homogenous density, and concentric cortical thickening.

MRI: The cortex shows low signal intensity in T1weighted images, intermediate-high signal intensity on T2 weighted images, and enhances avidly and homogenously on post contrast sequences. The fatty hilum demonstrates increased intensity in nonfat saturation sequences [2].

Pathology: Reactive lymphadenitis manifests as lymph node enlargement, due to hyperplasia of cellular components, secondary to antigenic stimulation. The histopathological appearance may be that of reactive follicular

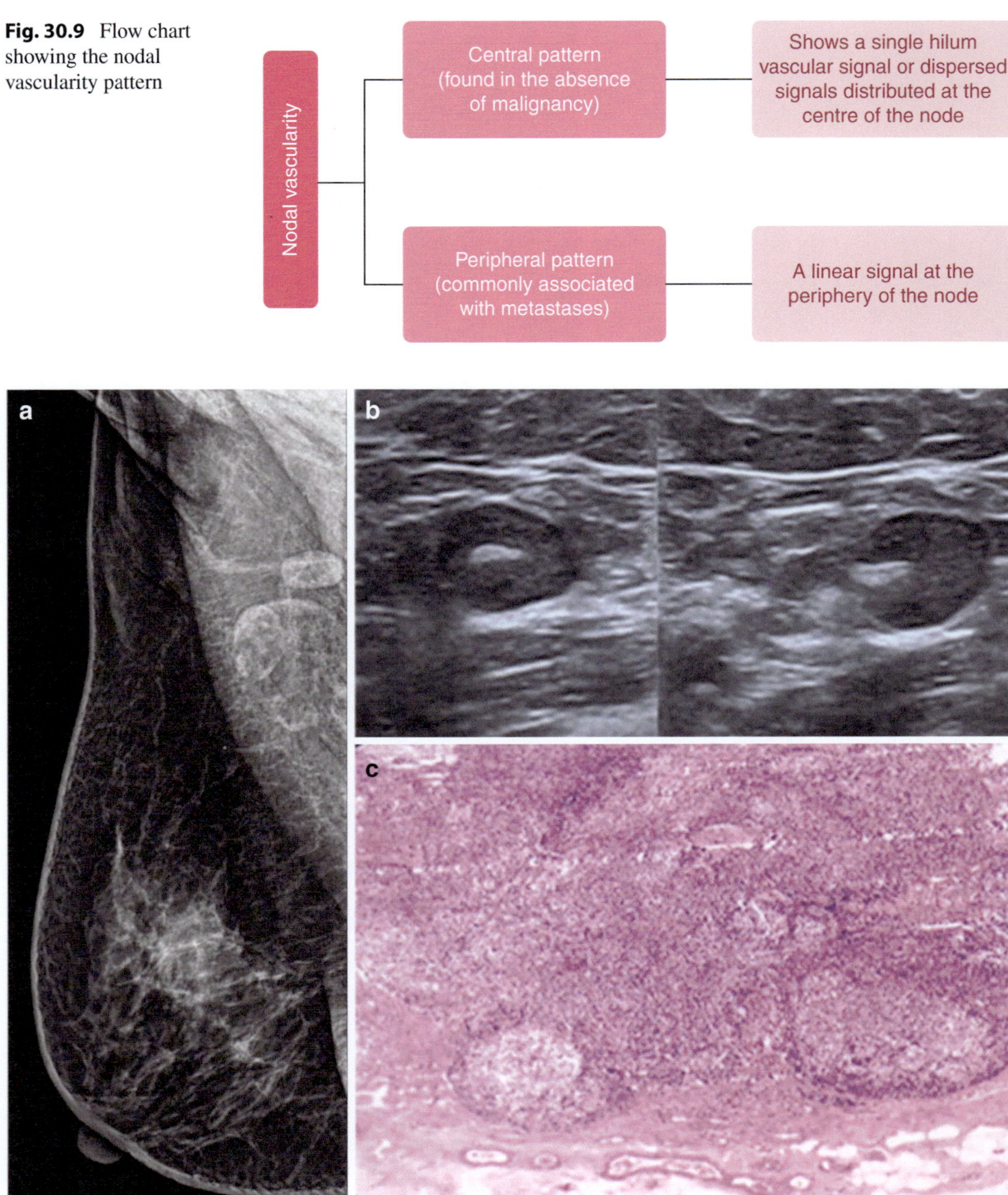

Fig. 30.9 Flow chart showing the nodal vascularity pattern

Fig. 30.10 (**a**) X-ray mammogram showing rounded lymph nodes with preserved fatty hilum. (**b**) Ultrasound shows an axillary lymph node with uniform cortical thickening with preserved fatty hilum. (**c**) Reactive lymph node—enlarged lymphoid follicles of varying sizes in the cortex (H&E ×200)

hyperplasia, diffuse paracortical hyperplasia, sinus histiocytosis pattern, or a mixed pattern. Reactive follicular hyperplasia shows enlarged follicles of varying size and shape with prominent germinal centers and mantle zones as seen in Fig. 30.10c. This pattern is due to B cell response. Germinal centers show mixed population of centrocytes and centroblasts. The diffuse paracortical hyperplasia is mainly a T cell response, where there is expansion of paracortical or interfollicular zones with numerous small lymphocytes admixed with immunoblasts.

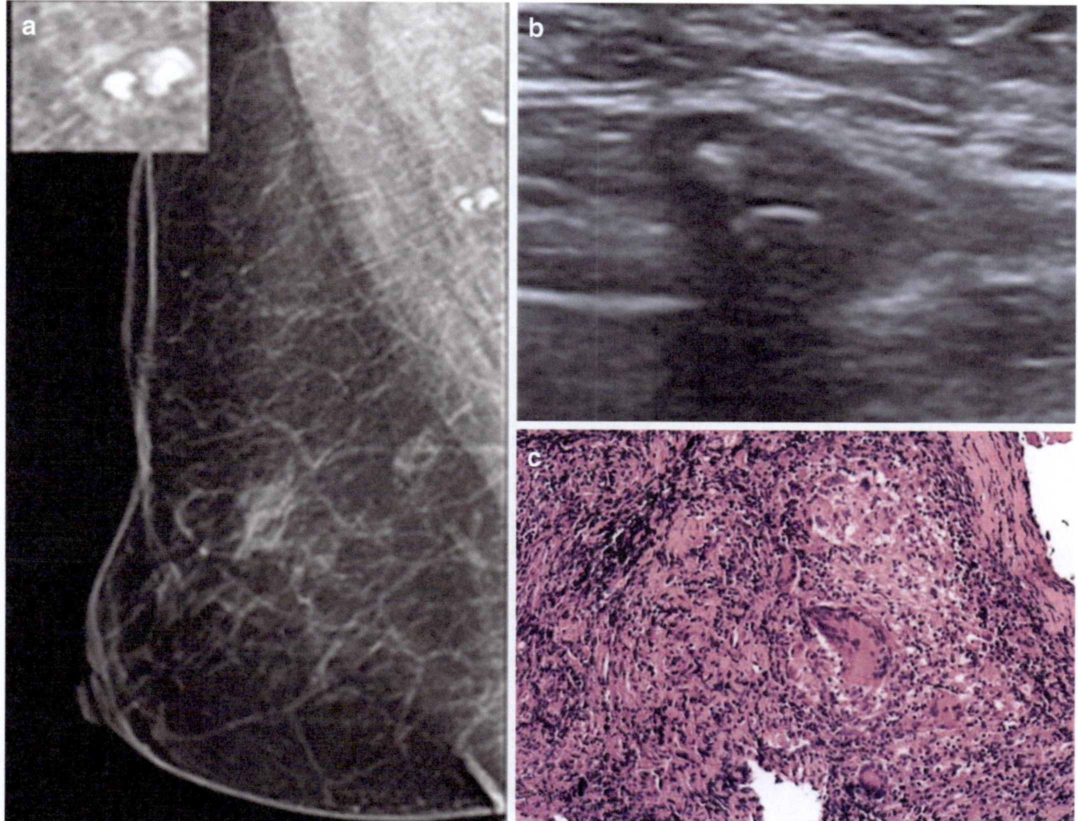

Fig. 30.11 (**a**) X-ray mammogram showing axillary lymph nodes with coarse calcifications, which have been depicted clearly in zoomed image inset. (**b**) Corresponding ultrasound shows axillary lymph with coarse internal calcifications with posterior acoustic shadowing. (**c**) TB lymph node—epithelioid granulomas with giant cells and focal necrosis (H&E ×400)

Sinus histiocytosis shows prominent sinuses, which are lined by hyperplastic sinus histiocytes.

Management: Benign lymph node hyperplasia does not need any specific management. Major concern is to rule out malignancy/tuberculosis.

Few unique features involving the axillary lymph nodes may be present in specific pathological conditions as demonstrated below:

30.5.1.3 Tuberculous Lymphadenitis

Tuberculosis is a common cause of benign peripheral lymphadenopathy. Cervical group involvement is most common. Imaging appearances vary depending on the stage of the disease, from subtle inflammatory change to abscess formation with rupture and fistula, followed by fibrosis and calcifications.

Mammogram: Enlarged, dense nodes sometimes with coarse calcifications as shown in Fig. 30.11a.

Ultrasound: Enlarged, hypoechoic axillary nodes with coarse internal calcifications as seen in Fig. 30.11b. Tuberculous lymphadenitis usually has indistinct borders due to periadenitis and surrounding soft tissue edema, unlike malignant lymphadenopathy, which has circumscribed borders. Matting of lymph nodes is a common feature of tuberculosis. The conglomerate of lymph nodes with necrosis can lead to rupture, resulting in severe inflammatory change [2].

Pathology: Histopathology of the lymph node shows multiple epithelioid granulomas with presence of multinucleated giant cells, characteristically called langhan giant cells as shown in Fig. 30.11c. Caseous necrosis maybe seen admixed with the epithelioid granulomas. The necrotic focus maybe surrounded by granulomas. In most of the cases, there is a lymphocytic cuffing around the granulomas. The necrotic foci may also show dystrophic calcification. Occasionally, acid fast bacilli can be detected by Zeihl Nelson stain in the necrotic foci, where the bacilli are seen as pink rods.

Management: Fine Needle Aspiration Cytology (FNAC) of the axillary node confirms the diagnosis. Once the diagnosis of tuberculosis is confirmed, patient is started on antituberculous drugs based on newer revised national tuberculosis control programme guidelines. For patients representing with cold abscess, nondependent aspiration/drainage of abscess is done.

30.5.1.4 Silicone Adenopathy

Migrated silicone from an augmented breast can mimic calcifications in lymph nodes and can usually be differentiated by a relevant clinical history. Migrated gold particles in rheumatoid arthritis are seen in patients receiving gold therapy, which can also mimic as calcifications in lymph nodes [6].

In silicone implant rupture or silicone gel bleed, silicone droplets migrate into the axilla or are taken up by axillary lymph nodes.

Mammogram: Silicone adenopathy is extremely dense, which distinguishes it from adenopathy due to other benign causes [9].

Ultrasound: Silicone droplet is a hypoechoic mass indistinguishable from a cyst. Silicone granuloma is seen as a highly echogenic area of scattered and reverberating echoes, giving a "snowstorm" appearance (free silicone droplets mixed with breast tissue giving a characteristic heterogeneous echogenic appearance—considered as a reliable sign of extracapsular breast implant rupture), or a highly echogenic area with posterior shadowing. Similar appearances are seen in breast tissue and axillary adenopathy [2].

Pathology: The lymph nodes show a pattern of diffuse follicular hyperplasia, with many vacuolated histiocytes in the sinusoids. The histiocytes may elicit a foreign body granulomatous response with presence of giant cells. The giant cells may demonstrate refractile and nonrefractile particles.

Management: Silicone adenopathy is a rare entity. Major concern is to rule out malignancy. It is more of a diagnosis of exclusion. Diagnosis is by mammogram followed by core needle biopsy/lymph node biopsy. If patient presents with pain and/or palpable lump, then excision can be done.

30.5.1.5 Castleman Disease

Castleman disease is a rare inflammatory lymphoproliferative disorder of unknown cause. It commonly occurs in the mediastinum and rarely in the axilla. It is classified into two clinical types, localized and disseminated. Most cases are disseminated type with a worse prognosis.

Ultrasound: Shows multiple well-defined homogeneous hypoechoic masses with associated hypervascularity.

CT (Post-contrast): Shows intense homogeneous enhancement.

MRI: Homogeneous architecture with hypointensity on T1-weighted images, hyperintensity on T2-weighted images, and early rapid enhancement and washout on dynamic scan [2].

Pathology: Castleman disease is an unusual nonmalignant lymphoproliferative disorder, due to polyclonal proliferation of B lymphocytes. It may be unicentric or multicentric. Histologically, there are three subtypes, hyaline vascular type, plasma cell type, and mixed hyaline vascular plasma cell type. Hyaline vascular type is characterized by prominent vascular proliferation and hyalinization of the vessel walls as seen in Fig. 30.12. Atretic germinal centers traversed by penetrating vessels are common. Mantle zones are thickened with lymphocytes arranged in layers.

Sheets of mature plasma cells are seen in the interfollicular areas, which is the characteristic feature of plasma cell type; follicles also show hyperplastic germinal centers.

Management: Diagnosis is by lymph node biopsy. Radiotherapy is treatment of choice for localized (unicentric) disease. Immunotherapy/

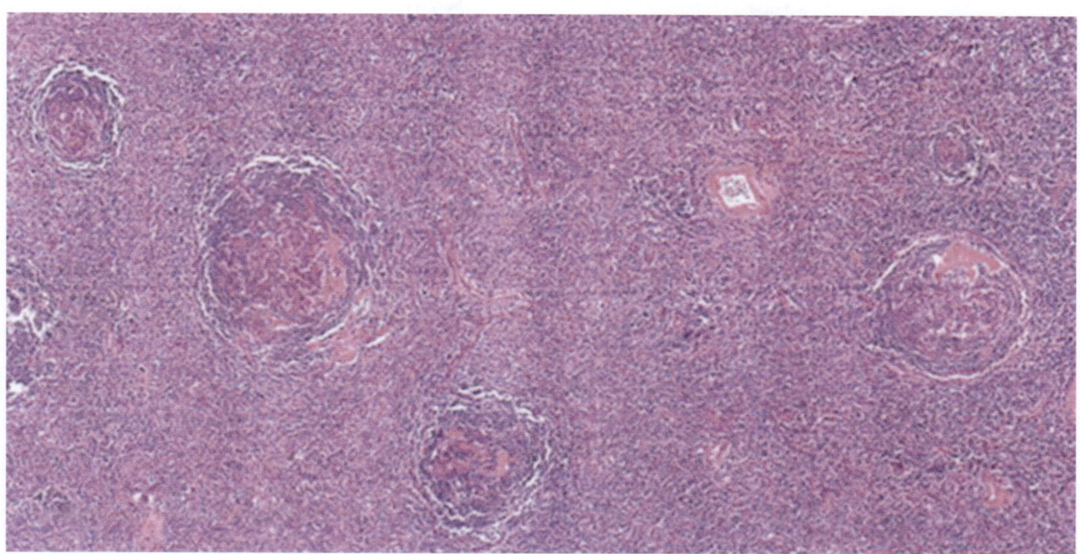

Fig. 30.12 Castleman disease—hyaline vascular type with prominent vascular proliferation and hyalinization of the vessel walls (H&E ×200)

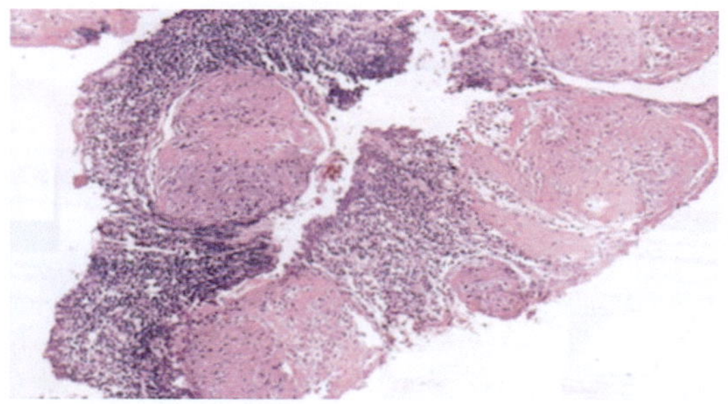

Fig. 30.13 Sarcoidosis—non-necrotising granulomas (H&E ×200)

Steroids are the treatment option for disseminated/multicentric disease.

30.5.1.6 Sarcoidosis

Sarcoidosis is a noncaseating granulomatous multisystem disease that can cause lymphadenopathy. Imaging findings for nodes involved with sarcoidosis are nonspecific, and differentiation from metastatic carcinoma or lymphoma may be difficult.

Pathology: Histologically, sarcoidosis is characterized by the presence of noncaseating granulomas as seen in Fig. 30.13. The architecture of the lymph node is effaced by these granulomas, which are tight and discrete and arranged back to back.

Management: Sarcoidosis of axillary nodes can be diagnosed only after excluding other diseases causing granulomatous inflammation like fungal, tuberculosis, and foreign body; if needed, image guided biopsy is done to confirm the diagnosis. Treatment is similar to pulmonary sarcoidosis.

30.5.2 Malignant Lesions

30.5.2.1 Metastatic Lymphadenopathy

Metastasis to axillary lymph nodes can occur from mammary and extra mammary tumors and are nonspecific at imaging, especially when the metastasis is early and small.

Mammogram: Enlarged, circumscribed borders, ill-defined (Figs. 30.14a and 30.16a) or spiculated borders as shown may be seen with extranodal spread. Rarely, tumoral calcifications are seen within metastatic lymph nodes from invasive ductal carcinoma or serous papillary carcinoma of the ovary.

Ultrasound: Lymph node usually show spherical or round shape, eccentric, or nonuniform cortical thickening with or without loss of fatty hilum (Table 30.1) as seen in Fig. 30.14b

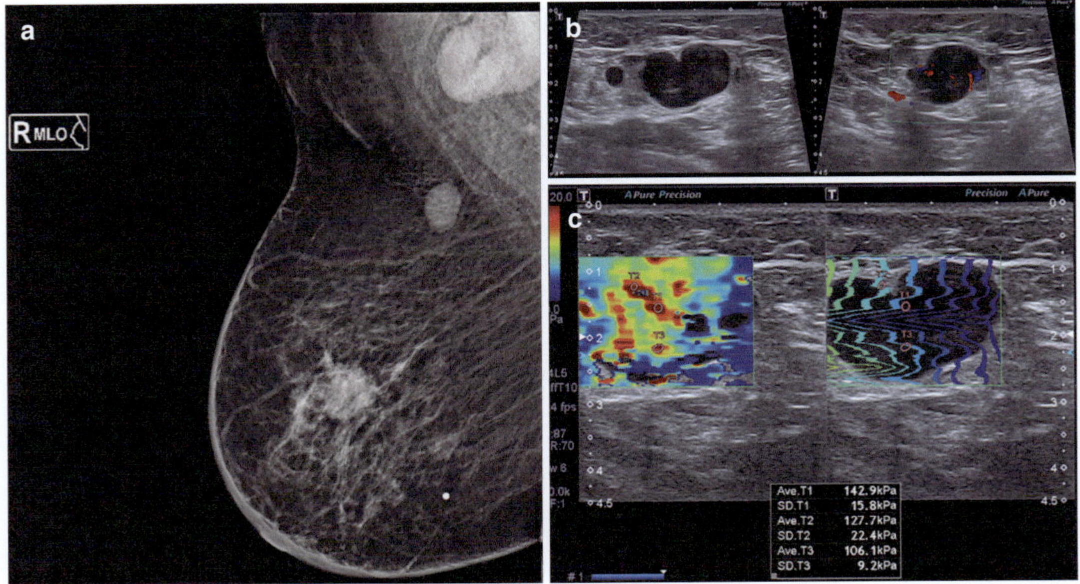

Fig. 30.14 (**a**) X-ray mammogram shows a high-density mass with spiculated margins in the central quadrant of the breast and enlarged axillary lymphnodes with thickened cortex tiny eccentrically displaced fatty hilum, (**b**) corresponding ultrasound shows enlarged axillary lymph nodes with thickened cortex and pinched up hilum (**c**) Elastography shows the nodes to be hard (104–142 kPa) consistent with malignancy

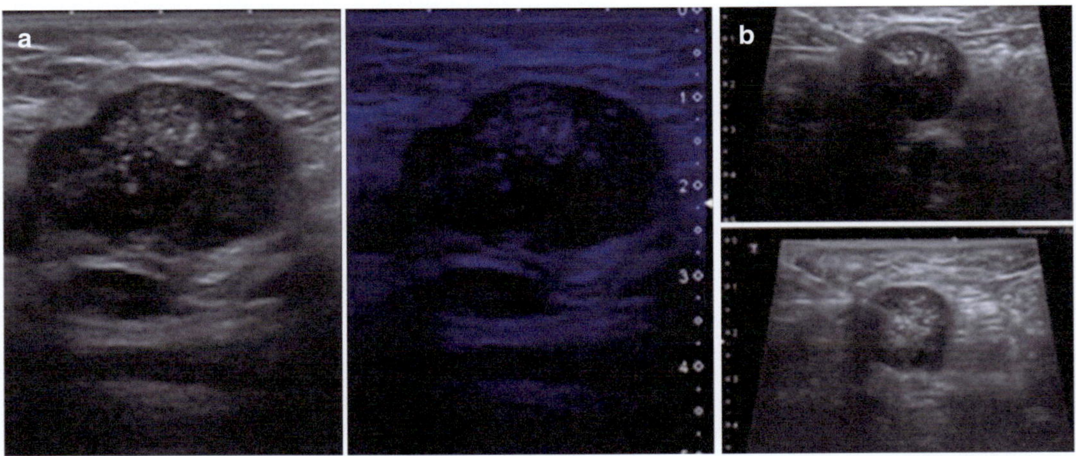

Fig. 30.15 (**a**) Ultrasound performed in a patient with carcinoma breast shows enlarged axillary lymph nodes with microcalcifications, which is depicted as starry sky appearance on micropure application (**b**) Core biopsy performed confirmed the diagnosis of nodal metastasis

and sometimes necrotic center. The metastatic lymph nodes are hard on elastography as shown in Fig. 30.14c. Intranodal microcalcifications can be present in a few cases which can be visualized better by micropure technique as depicted in the image (Fig. 30.15a). Cystic changes can occur in few types of tumors, including squamous cell carcinoma, thyroid papillary carcinoma, serous papillary carcinoma of the ovary or endometrium, and malig-

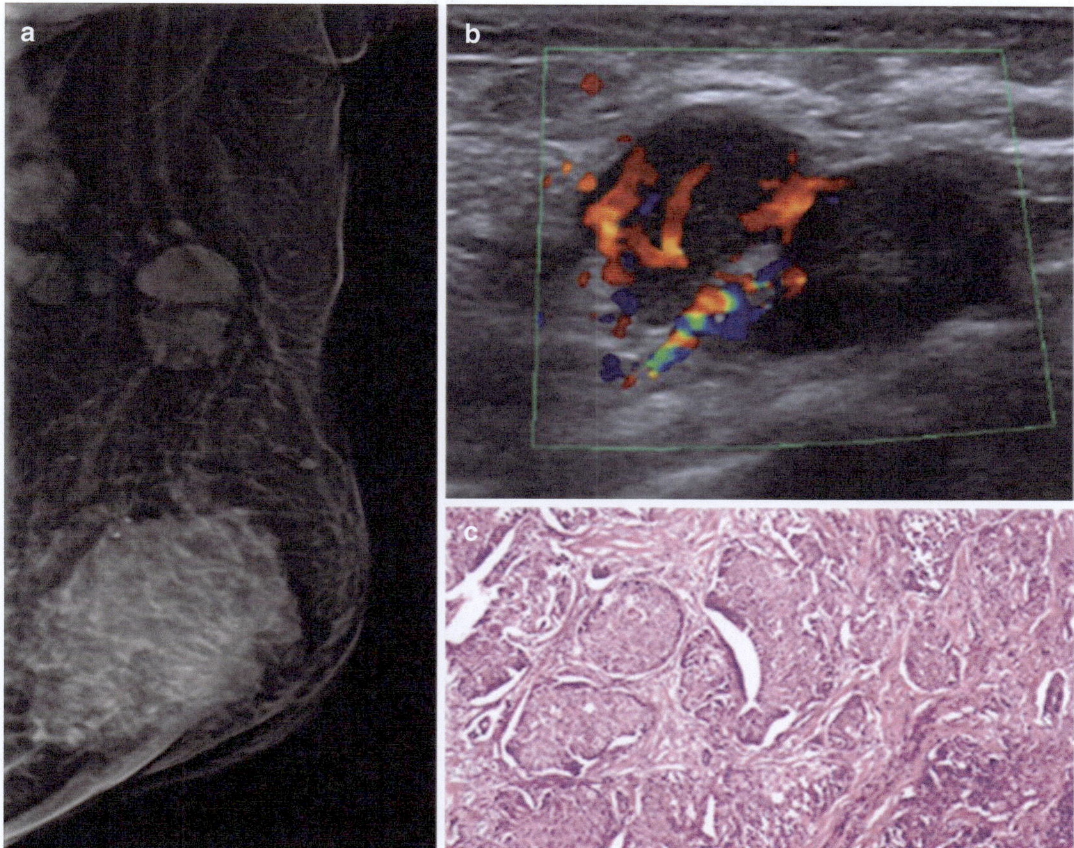

Fig. 30.16 (**a**) X-ray mammogram showing a large high-density lesion with microcalcifications and multiple enlarged axillary lymph nodes with thickened cortex, (**b**) corresponding ultrasound shows an enlarged axillary lymph node with significantly thickened cortex and peripherally pushed pinched hilum and increased increased hilar and peripheral vascularity (**c**) Metastasis in node-tumor deposits in the lymph node (H&E ×400)

nant melanoma. Metastatic nodes tend to have peripheral or mixed (both peripheral and hilar) vascularity on doppler as shown in Fig. 30.16b. Transcapsular feeding vessels are highly specific for metastasis [2].

MRI: Typically demonstrate heterogeneous enhancement. Dynamic contrast-enhanced MRI shows rapid enhancement in comparison with benign lymph node. Diffuse enhancement may occur with total replacement of the lymph node (LN) by tumor.

Pathology: The microscopic examination of the lymphnode usually shows clusters of tumor cells in the cortex and medulla as shown in Fig. 30.16c. At times, few tumor cell clusters are seen in the subcapsular space. The morphology of the metastatic deposit may or may not resemble the tumor at the primary site.

Extranodal extension of tumor: It denotes extracapsular growth of tumor cells and spread into the extranodal axillary fat.

Mammogram: Shows an irregular axillary lymph node with loss of fatty hilum as shown in Fig. 30.17a.

Ultrasound: Shows an irregular axillary lymph node with extranodal extension of the tumor into the adjacent axillary fat as shown in Fig. 30.17b. Perinodal oedema is a specific sign of extranodal extension and appears as

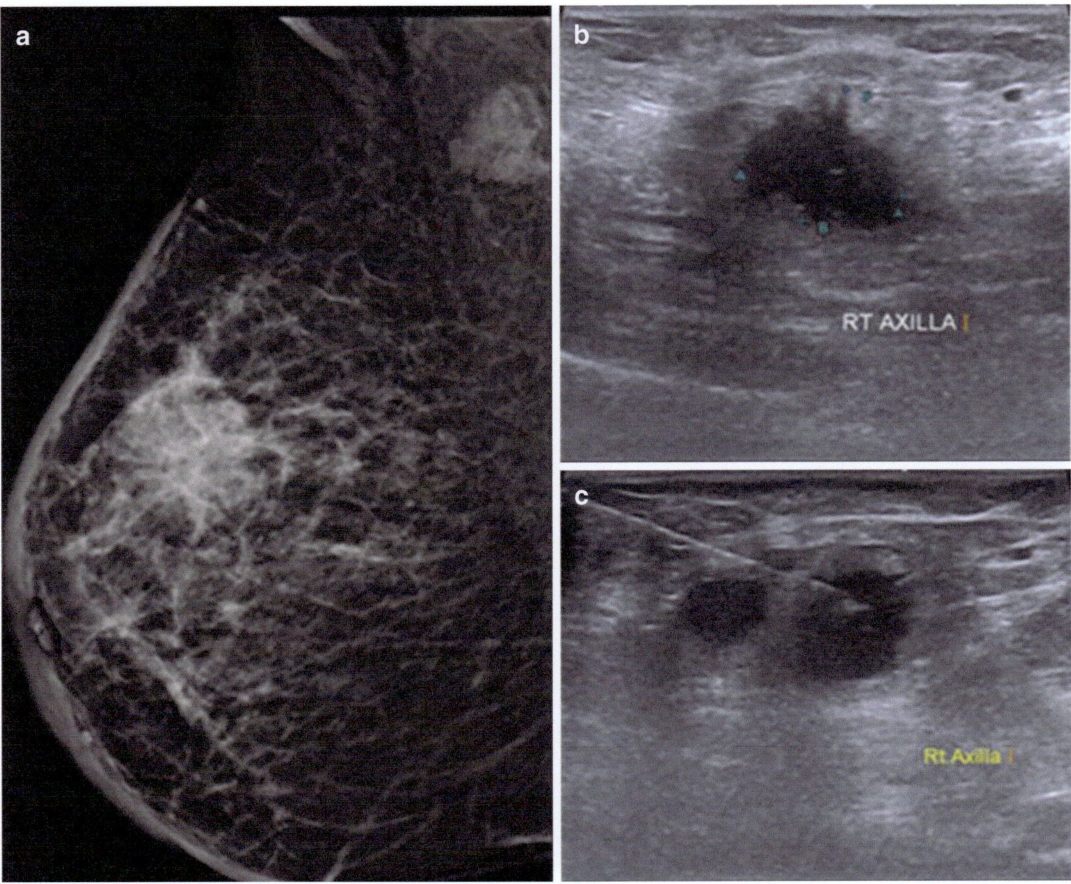

Fig. 30.17 (**a**) x-ray mammogram showing an irregular axillary lymph node with loss of fatty hilum and a high density lesion with spiculated margins in the upper quadrant of the breast with diffuse skin thickening. (**b**) corresponding ultrasound performed in the patient showed an irregular axillary lymph node with extranodal extension of the tumor into the adjacent axillary fat. (**c**) Lymph node biopsy performed, confirmed the same

a hyperechoic halo around the node on ultrasound.

Cross-sectional imaging: CT and MRI shows irregularity of the cortical margin or a spiculated appearance. Blurring of the margins on CT and areas of T2 hyperintensity in the perinodal fat on MR. A fused appearance could denote perinodal spread and should be considered as a poor prognostic factor and warrants adjuvant radiotherapy. [2]

Management: Diagnosis is by FNAC or image guided core needle biopsy of the lymph node as shown in Figs. 30.15b and 30.17c. Treatment depends on the stage of primary malignancy.

- Size of lymph node cannot be used to accurately predict the benign versus malignant status of an axillary LN; even a normal sized node may contain microscopic metastasis.
- Perinodal edema is a feature of tuberculous adenitis and extranodal extension of tumor and is not a common feature in metastases when the tumor cells are contained within the lymph node.

30.5.2.2 Lymphoma

Lymphomas are tumors arising from reticuloendothelial and lymphatic systems. It can be localized or disseminated, with frequent involvement of the axilla. Non-Hodgkin's lymphoma commonly affects the axilla.

Mammogram: Enlarged, well-defined, homogenously high-density mass.

Ultrasound: well-defined, rounded, and hypoechoic node, usually with a preserved echogenic hilum. Lymphomatous nodes show mixed hilar and peripheral vascularity.

Perinodal oedema and intranodal calcification are uncommon. Calcification before therapy in mediastinal node denotes more aggressive disease [2].

Management: Diagnosis is by node biopsy. Treatment is chemotherapy according to the stage of the disease.

30.5.3 Non-nodal Pathologies

30.5.3.1 Postsurgical Lesions

Postsurgical lesions in the axilla include seromas or hematomas, fat necrosis, and suture granulomas.

Seromas appear as loculated fluid collections, with or without fluid debris as seen in Fig. 30.18a, b.

Hematomas show variable internal architecture depending on the evolution of the blood products [2]. Postsurgical seromas and hematomas do not warrant any intervention if small as they resolve spontaneously. Persistent lesions can be subjected to image guided aspiration or surgical evacuation.

Fat necrosis is a benign inflammatory process resulting from vascular insult to fat cells, and its imaging findings are reported to correspond to the stage of development and maturation. Imaging findings correlates with the stage of development, from an oil cyst to a spiculated mass [10].

Suture granuloma characterized by hyperechoic double or single line (representing surgical sutures) within a hypoechoic lesion on ultrasound. Sometimes these postsurgical lesions may be difficult to differentiate from malignancy, and biopsy is required [2]. Treatment is surgical exploration and removal of the suture material.

30.5.4 Breast Augmentation–Related Lesions

They are mainly related to migration of ruptured implants or injected materials. Examples include

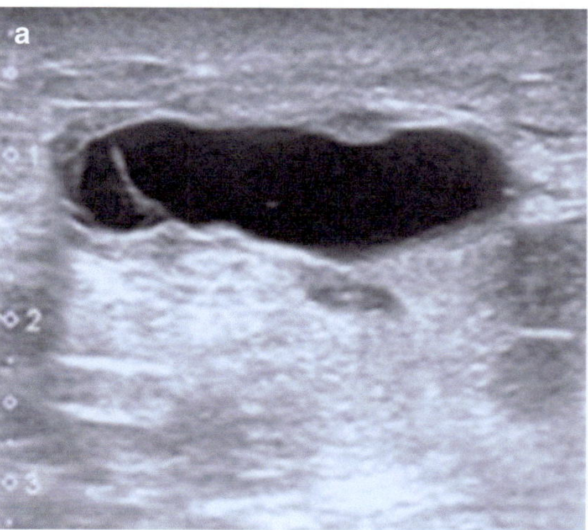

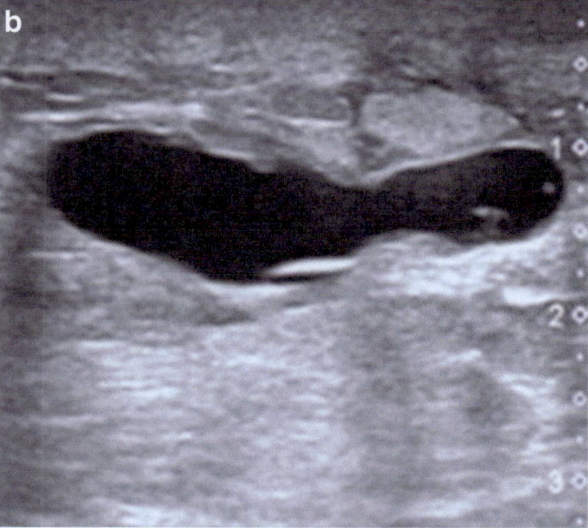

Fig. 30.18 (**a**, **b**) Ultrasound images showing an anechoic collection (seroma) with thin internal septations in a patient post-modified radical mastectomy

silicone deposits in axillary lymph nodes as described previously and polyacrylamide gel migration into the axilla as a consequence of breast augmentation. Migrated polyacrylamide gel appears as either small loculations with MRI signal intensity being similar to that of water in the axilla [10].

30.5.5 Infective or Inflammatory Lesions

This entity includes abscesses. Local injury, sweat or sebaceous gland obstruction, and hair follicle infection can result in abscess formation. Abscesses can also occur within the lymph nodes as a result of bacterial or tuberculosis lymphadenitis [11].

Ultrasound: They can appear as a hypoechoic fluid collection with internal debris or loculations and a hypervascular echogenic wall (Fig. 30.19a, b).

On contrast-enhanced cross-sectional imaging, they usually show peripheral rim enhancement.

30.5.6 Axillary Tail Lesions

Axillary tail is a continuous extension of the upper outer quadrant breast tissue. Therefore, benign lesions such as cyst can develop in the axillary tail as in the rest of the breast. Breast carcinoma in the axillary tail is extremely rare [12].

30.5.7 Skin

Ultrasound is the optimal imaging modality to differentiate lesions in the dermis and epidermis (e.g. sebaceous cyst, epidermal inclusion cyst) from lesions in that are located within the subcutaneous fat of the breast. US features that suggest a lesion of dermal origin include an acute angle between the lesion and the dermal line, and a "claw"[12] (a schematic ofwhich has been depicted in Fig. 30.20).

Epidermal inclusion cyst is a benign dermal lesion containing keratin and is lined by epidermis. Its appearance on ultrasound varies with its content, ranging from cystic to hypoechoic (as shown in Fig. 30.21) or heterogeneous. The presence of a tract to the skin, which represents the hair follicle extending from the dermis up through the epidermis, is diagnostic [13].

Pilomatricom: is more common in children but occasionally encountered in adults. It arises from the lower dermis and extends into the subcutaneous fat as it grows, with thinning of the overlying dermis. On US, it appears as a well-defined hypoechoic mass with echogenic calcific foci, or a completely calcified mass showing strong posterior acoustic shadow [14].

Management: All skin lesions in the axilla require surgical excision.

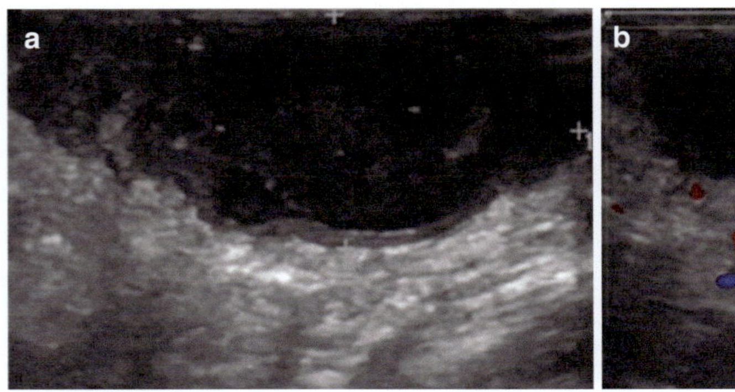

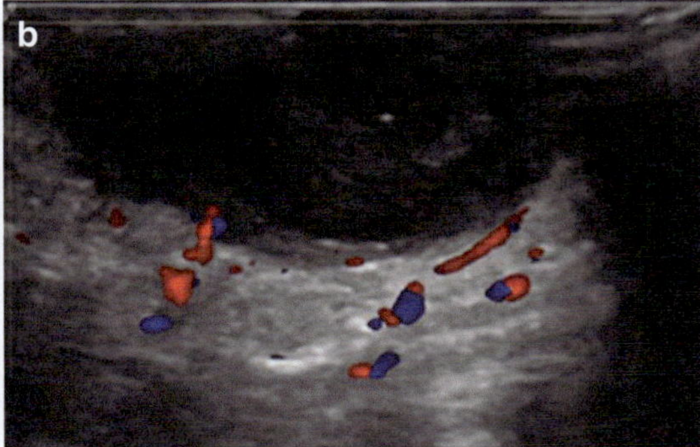

Fig. 30.19 (**a**, **b**) Ultrasound images showing an anechoic thick-walled abscess with increased peripheral vascularity seen in the axilla

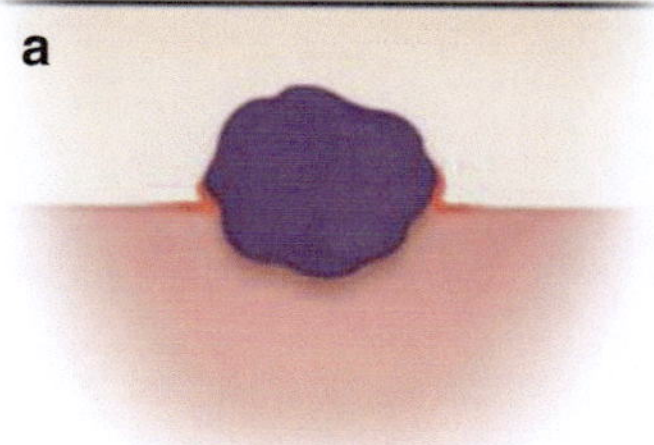

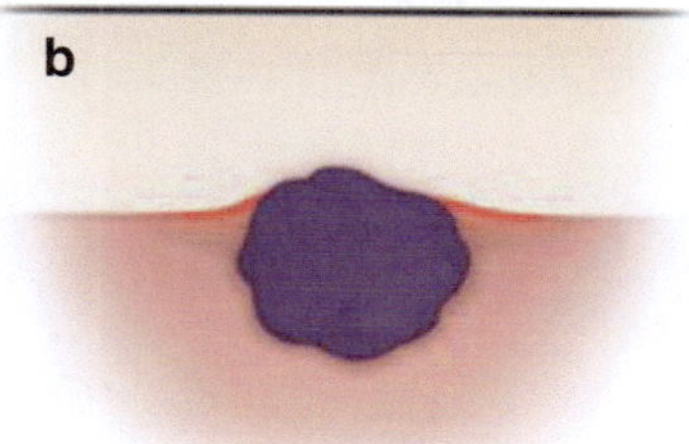

Fig. 30.20 Illustrated diagrams showing a dermal lesion-within the skin like dermatofibrosis, a lesion arising from the dermal/subcutaneous junction depicted by acute angle (claw sign) it forms with the skin (**a**) and a subcutaneous lesion, which forms an obtuse angle with the skin like apocrine breast cancer (**b**)

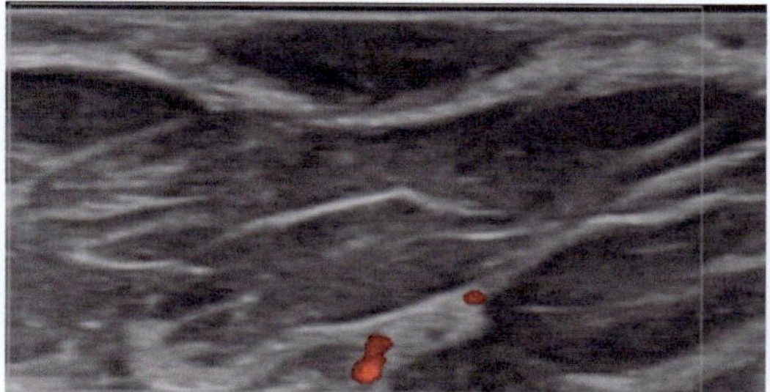

Fig. 30.21 An epidermal inclusion cyst seen as a circumscribed hypoechoic lesion is seen in the right axilla

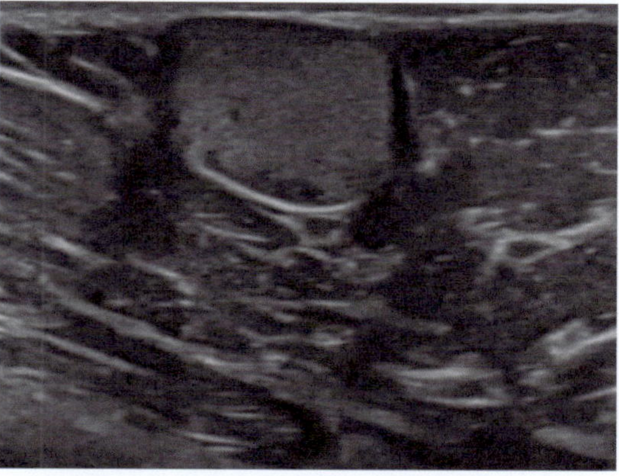

Fig. 30.22 An oval circumscribed hyperechoic lesion with few cystic spaces within is seen in the axilla, suggestive of a subcutaneous lipoma

30.5.8 Subcutaneous Tissues and Muscles

Lipomas: They are usually subcutaneous in origin but can also arise intramuscularly, including from the pectoralis muscle in the axilla.

Ultrasound: Lipomas often have a homogeneous circumscribed appearance as shown in Fig. 30.22, some of which may have septations or may show variable appearance and may be encapsulated.

Mammography and CT: manifest as a low density area and show fat density.

MRI: They typically demonstrate fat signal with minimal contrast enhancement [11].

Management: Surgical excision can be done for cosmetic reasons.

30.5.9 Liposarcoma

When a lipomatous mass shows atypical features including heterogeneity and contrast enhancement on cross-sectioned imaging, a liposarcoma should be considered [11]. On ultrasound, a well-differentiated liposarcoma appears heterogeneous, multilobulated (as seen in Fig. 30.23a, b), and typical well-defined sonographic identification of hyperechoic fat may be difficult and variable. On CT and MRI scans, it usually presents as a predominantly lipomatous mass with non-lipomatous components, most often as thickened septa with or without nodularity [15].

Other Soft Tissue Masses include other soft tissue sarcomas, nodular fasciitis, desmoid fibromatosis, and benign muscular neoplasms such as intramuscular myxoma [5, 12].

Pathology: Histopathology shows a diffuse infiltrate of spindle cells with nuclear atypia and

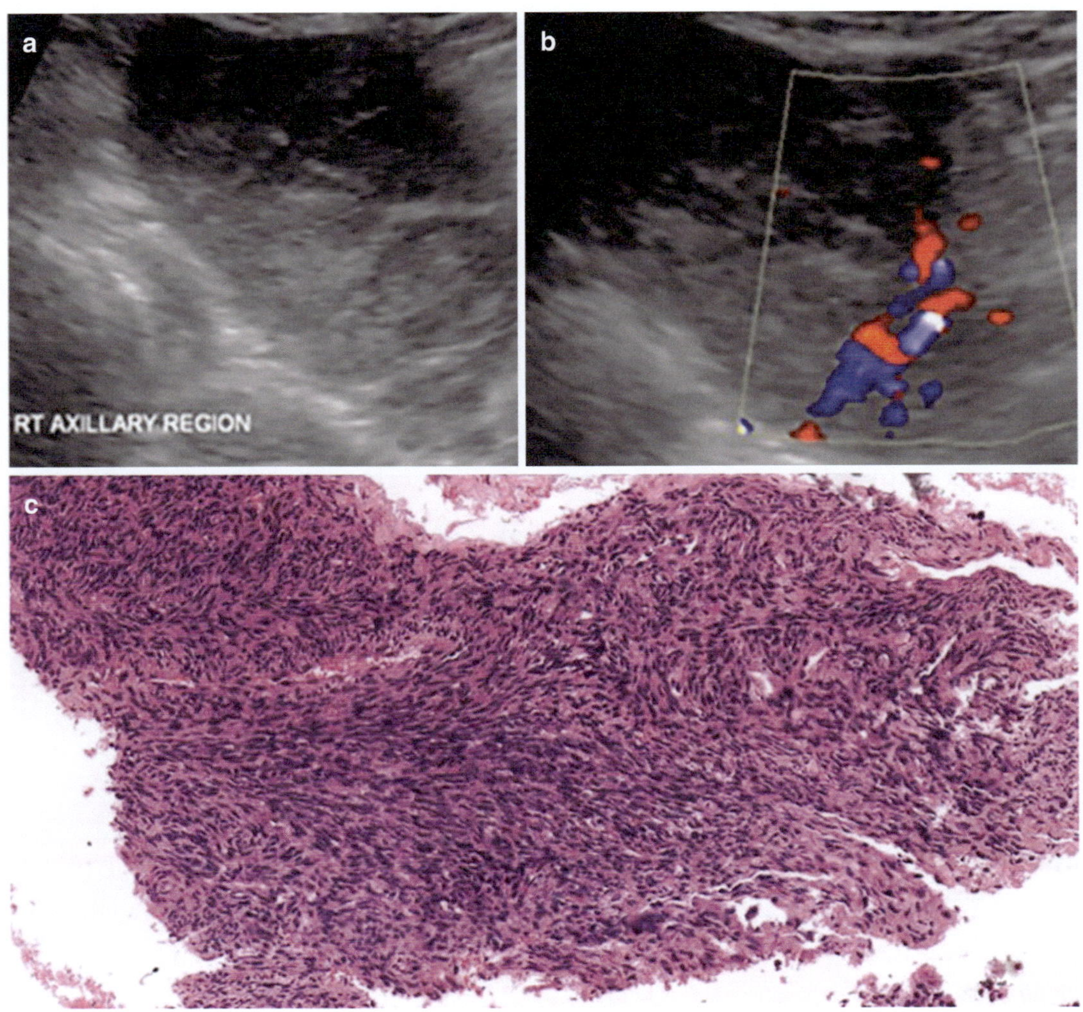

Fig. 30.23 (**a**, **b**) ultrasound images of a heteroechoic mass with marked internal vascularity in the right axilla; (**c**) HPE shows a diffuse infiltrate of spindle cells with nuclear atypia and arranged in a vague fascicular pattern

arranged in a vague fascicular pattern shown in Fig. 30.23c.

Management: Diagnosis is by image-guided core needle biopsy, and treatment is wide local excision with appropriate skin cover.

30.5.10 Blood Vessels

Vascular lesions: Vascular malformation and pseudoaneurysms, axillary vein thrombosis (shown in Fig. 30.24a, b) are encountered. Pseudoaneurysms can be spontaneous or trauma related. On colour flow typical findings include the "yin-yang" sign and a "to-and-fro" waveform is seen on Doppler, both of which are turbulent blood flow in the lesion.

Different types of angiography (conventional or CT) may also help, especially in identifying the donor artery. Pseudoaneurysm can appear as a low-density lesion on CT with enhancement similar to the donor artery while a non-enhanced region within the lesion may signify thrombosis [16].

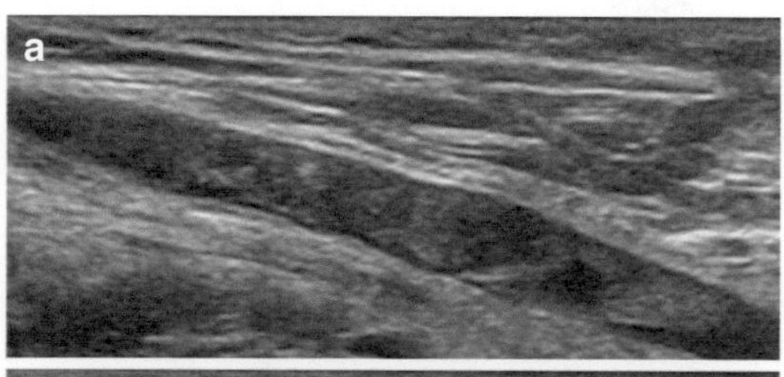

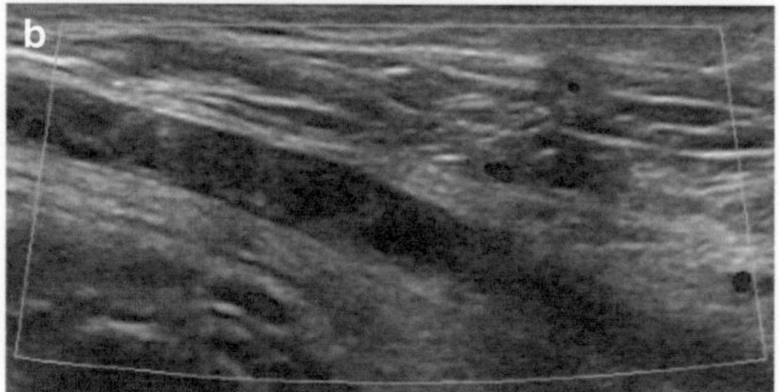

Fig. 30.24 (**a**) B-mode ultrasound shows echogenic thrombus; (**b**) doppler ultrasound image showing echogenic thrombus with absent flow seen within the right axillary vein

30.5.11 Nerves

Peripheral nerve sheath tumors are divided into two benign entities, neurofibroma and schwannoma, and a malignant form, malignant peripheral nerve sheath tumor. MRI plays an important role in the identification and characterization of these tumors. They commonly appear as fusiform masses and demonstrate low to intermediate signal intensity on T1-weighted sequence and high signal intensity on T2-weighted sequence. Some other suggestive imaging features include the "entering or exiting nerve sign," the "split-fat" sign, the "target sign," the "fascicular sign," and atrophy of the muscles supplied by the involved nerve [17].

30.5.12 Bones

Tumors arising from bones such as the proximal humerus, scapula or ribs, primary or secondary, aggressive or nonaggressive, can present as focal swelling or mass in the axilla due to indentation or local invasion. Examples include benign osteochondroma and primary bone malignancy such as osteogenic sarcoma. Metastasis should be considered especially in patients with a known history of primary malignancy elsewhere.

References

1. Lai TKB, Wong T, Chau CM, Fung WY, Chan RLS, Yung AWT, Ma JKF. Differential diagnoses of axillary lesions: a pictorial essay. Hong Kong J Radiol. 2021;24:219–28. https://doi.org/10.12809/hkjr2117394.
2. Park YM, Park J-S, Yoon HK, Yang WT. Imaging-pathologic correlation of diseases in the axilla. AJR Am J Roentgenol. 2013;200:W130–42. https://doi.org/10.2214/AJR.12.9259.
3. Net JM, Mirpuri TM, Plaza MJ, et al. Resident and fellow education feature: US evaluation of axillary lymph nodes. Radiographics. 2014;34:1817. https://doi.org/10.1148/rg.347140081.
4. Bedi DG, Krishnamurthy R, Krishnamurthy S, et al. Cortical morphologic features of axillary lymph nodes as a predictor of metastasis in breast cancer: in vitro sonographic study. AJR Am J Roentgenol. 2008;191:646–52.
5. Pinheiro DJ, Elias S, Nazário AC. Axillary lymph nodes in breast cancer patients: sonographic evaluation. Radiol Bras. 2014;47:240–4.
6. Ikeda DM, Miyake KK. Breast imaging: the requisites. 3rd ed. Amsterdam: Elsevier; 2017. p. 422–5.
7. Mehta N, Sales RM, Babagbemi K, Levy AD, McGrath AL, Drotman M, et al. Unilateral axillary adenopathy in the setting of COVID-19 vaccine. Clin Imaging. 2021;75:12–5.
8. Dialani V, James DF, Slanetz PJ. A practical approach to imaging the axilla. Insights Imaging. 2015;6:217–29.
9. Leibman AJ, Wong R. Findings on mammography in the axilla. AJR. 1997;169:1385–90.
10. Wong T, Lo LW, Fung PY, Lai HY, She HL, Ng WK, et al. Magnetic resonance imaging of breast augmentation: a pictorial review. Insights Imaging. 2016;7:399–410.
11. Gupta A, Metcalf C, Taylor D. Review of axillary lesions, emphasising some distinctive imaging and pathology findings. J Med Imaging Radiat Oncol. 2017;61:571–81.
12. Oliff MC, Birdwell RL, Raza S, Giess CS. The breast imager's approach to nonmammary masses at breast and axillary US: imaging technique, clues to origin, and management. Radiographics. 2016;36:7–18.
13. Giess CS, Raza S, Birdwell RL. Distinguishing breast skin lesions from superficial breast parenchymal lesions: diagnostic criteria, imaging characteristics, and pitfalls. Radiographics. 2011;31:1959–72.

14. Hwang JY, Lee SW, Lee SM. The common ultrasonographic features of pilomatricoma. J Ultrasound Med. 2005;24:1397–402.
15. Murphey MD, Arcara LK, Fanburg-Smith J. From the archives of the AFIP: imaging of musculoskeletal liposarcoma with radiologicpathologic correlation. Radiographics. 2005;25:1371–95.
16. Saad NE, Saad WE, Davies MG, Waldman DL, Fultz PJ, Rubens DJ. Pseudoaneurysms and the role of minimally invasive techniques in their management. Radiographics. 2005;25Suppl 1:S173–89.
17. Chee DW, Peh WC, Shek TW. Pictorial essay: imaging of peripheral nerve sheath tumours. Can Assoc Radiol J. 2011;62:176–82.

Breast Implants

31

Priya K. Palanisamy, Bhawna Dev, and Anupama Chandrasekharan

Abstract

With the number of women having breast implants increasing, it is only essential for the radiologists to be aware of the normal and abnormal imaging findings of breast implants. Implant rupture is the most common complication and cause for implant removal. Although mammography and ultrasound are still the basic steps in diagnostic evaluation, magnetic resonant imaging (MRI) is recognized to be the accurate modality in assessing the implant integrity due to its ability to suppress and enhance the signals from the silicone. It also aids in detecting other implant-associated abnormalities like anaplastic large-cell lymphoma (ALCL) and breast cancers unrelated to implants.

Keywords

Breast implants · Implant rupture · Magnetic resonant imaging · ALCL · Siliconoma

31.1 Introduction

In 1895, the first breast augmentation was attempted by transplanting lumbar lipoma from a patient to enhance her breast after the removal of a fibroadenoma [1]. Since then, a wide variety of breast implants have evolved, with saline and silicone being the prototype mostly commonly used. There is a recent increase in the number of patients having breast implants for various reasons, namely, reconstruction after mastectomy (most common), cosmetic augmentation of the breast and correction of congenital malformations. Breast reconstruction may involve insertion of various types of implants or modelling of autologous myocutaneous flaps.

31.2 Types of Breast Implants [1]

The most used implants consist of silicone envelops (rubber bags), which contain either silicone gel or saline within. The various types of implants are illustrated in Table 31.1.

P. K. Palanisamy (✉)
Department of Radiology, Maidstone and Tunbridge Wells NHS Trust, Kent, UK
e-mail: p.palanisamy@nhs.net

B. Dev · A. Chandrasekharan
Department of Radiology, Sri Ramachandra Institute of Higher Education and Research, Chennai, India
e-mail: bhawnadev@sriramachandra.edu.in

B. Dev, L. D. Joseph (eds.), *Holistic Approach to Breast Disease*,
https://doi.org/10.1007/978-981-99-0035-0_31

Table 31.1 Types of breast implants

S. no	Implant type	Material used
1.	Single lumen	Silicone/saline gel filled (Fig. 31.1)
2	Single lumen-adjustable	Silicone. Saline gel filled, to which variable amount of saline can be added at the time of placement (Figs. 31.1 and 31.2)
3	Standard double lumen	Silicone gel inner lumen, saline outer lumen (Fig. 31.3)
4	Reverse double lumen	Saline inner lumen, silicone outer lumen
5	Reverse-adjustable, PVP filled	Silicone gel inner and outer lumens, variable amount of saline added to inner lumen at time of placement
6	Gel-gel double lumen	Silicone gel in inner and outer lumen
7	Triple lumen	Silicone gel in inner and middle lumen with saline in the outer lumen
8	Saline-filled, dextran-filled	Dextran-filled (some early implants), PVP-filled (Bioplasty), and the rest saline-filled

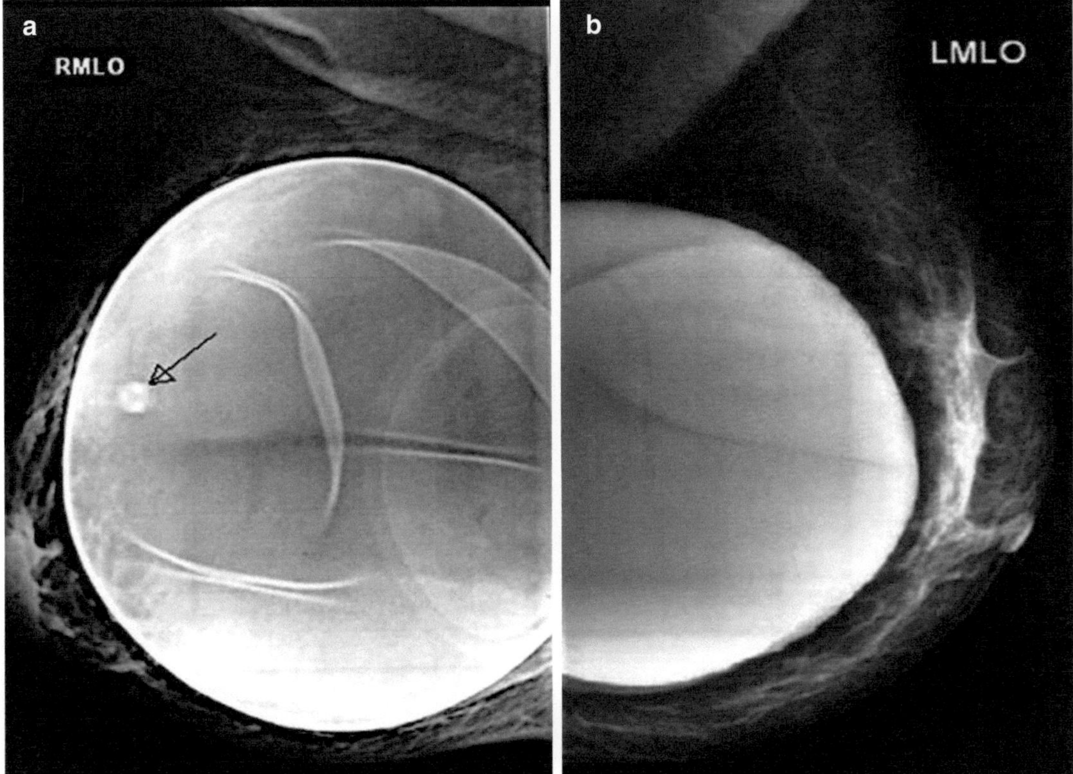

Fig. 31.1 Difference between single lumen saline and silicone implant. (**a**) shows a relatively less dense single lumen saline implant with valve within (black arrow). (**b**) shows a dense single lumen silicone implant

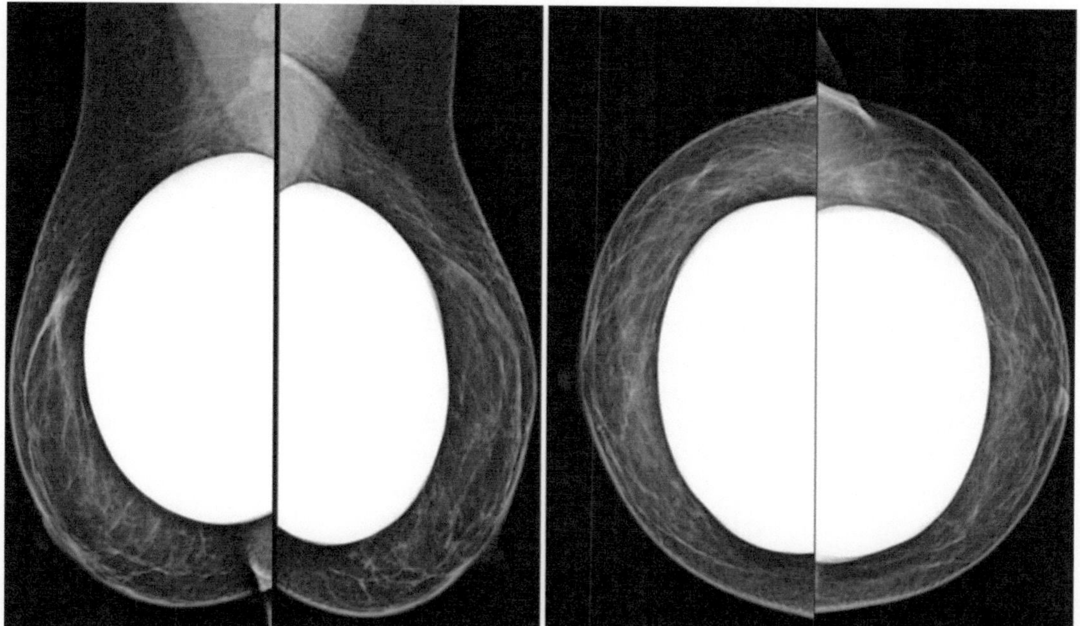

Fig. 31.2 A 35-year-old women with bilateral breast augmentation—silicone implants. Standard MLO and CC view mammograms of both breasts show homogenously hyperdense oval mass-like silicone implants obscuring most of the underlying normal breast parenchyma

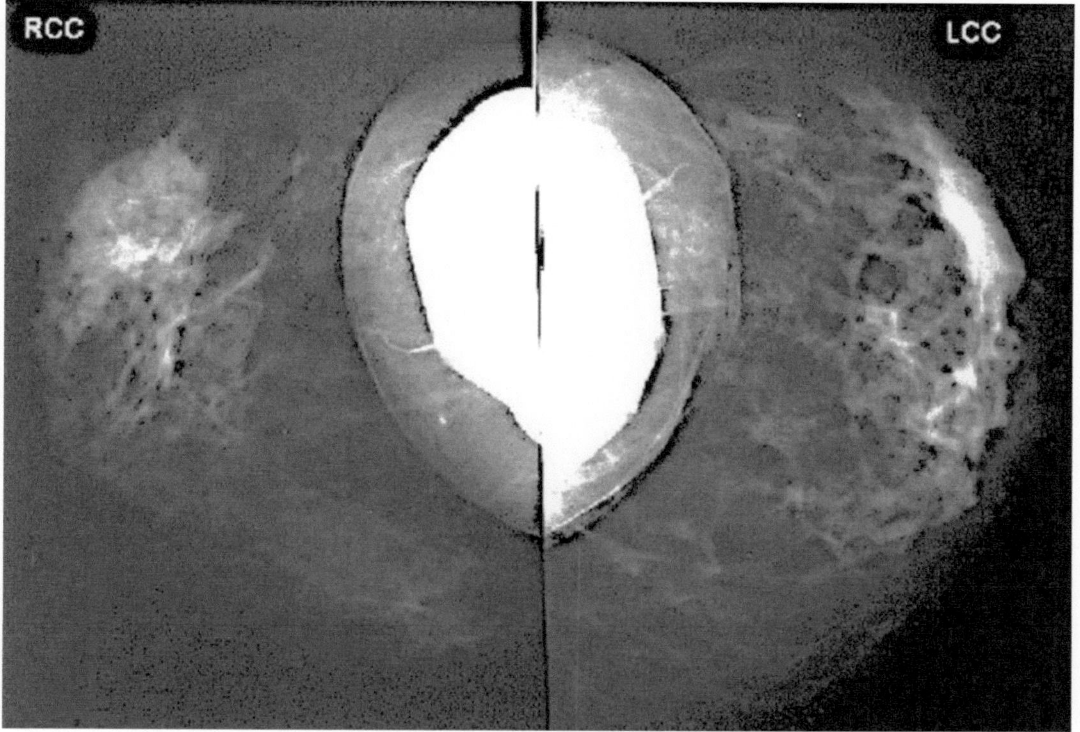

Fig. 31.3 CC view mammograms of both breasts showing retroglandular double lumen implants with inner denser silicone lumen and outer less-dense saline lumen

31.3 Tissue Expanders

Tissue expanders are inserted into the mastectomy site post-oncoplastic breast surgery in a small to moderate-sized breast with or without ptosis. These expanders are inserted between the skin and muscle before the implant augmentation as a preparation step in order to stretch the remaining skin. These expanders are like inflatable balloons and inserted in collapsed form, and fluid is injected slowly later; hence, it is important to note that the multiple folds seen in these expanders on imaging do not represent rupture.

Fibrous encapsulation of the implants: The silicone breast implants are not biologically inert. A thin fibrous capsule forms around the implant after placement (encapsulation) as physiological response to the foreign body.

31.4 Location of Implants

The surgical approach to placing implant varies. Implants are positioned either through following **incision types**—inframammary incisions, through periareolar incision or through axilla. There are two major locations of implant placement.

1. **Subglandular (retroglandular)**—implant placed behind the glandular tissue but anterior to the pectoralis major muscle (Fig. 31.4a, b).

   Advantage—most commonly used location due to easy surgical accessibility.

   Disadvantage—occurrence of capsular contracture.
2. **Subpectoral**—posterior to the pectoralis major muscle as shown in Fig. 31.4c, d.

   Advantage—less incidence of capsular contracture as the motion of the muscle over the muscle prevents the capsule formation. Another advantage of the location is

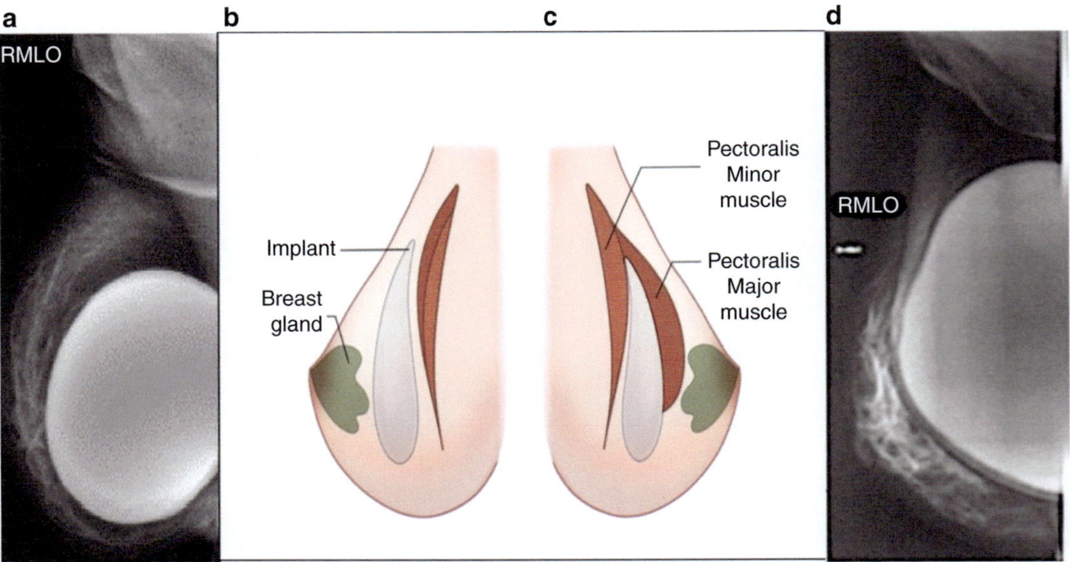

Fig. 31.4 **Location** of breast implants in a schematic diagram (**b**, **c**) and mammograms (**a**, **d**). (**Left**) subglandular implant located anterior to the pectoralis muscle (**a**, **b**). (**Right**) submuscular implant located behind the pectoralis major muscle (**c**, **d**)

that it facilitates the implant displacement imaging in mammography and permits better compression of the breast tissue for cancer detection.

31.5 Implant Imaging

31.5.1 Mammography

Mammography is of little value in evaluating the implant integrity; however, it is useful in assessing the surrounding breast tissue. The screening mammogram in an augmented breast should include the following views.

(a) Implant displaced—**Eklund technique**
(b) Craniocaudal (CC)
(c) Mediolateral oblique (MLO) views

Eklund technique (Fig. 31.5): also known as **implant displacement view**. In 1988, Eklund et al. introduced the displacement technique to facilitate mammography in augmented women, especially in subglandular location of the implant [2]. Displacing the implant allows more breast tissue to be visualized than the standard compression views (Fig. 31.6). A woman with breast implants attending the breast unit for mammograms should be offered a standard MLO and CC views of both breasts along with Eklund Technique. The standard views help in assessing the position (subglandular/retro pectoral) of the implants, which helps the mammographer to position for Eklund View as subglandular implants need more posterior displacement than the retropectoral. Even though there is no evidence to support, the patient must be informed of the small possibility of implant rupture/migration secondary to compression and positioning for Eklund views, and consent needs to be obtained for the same from the patient.

Saline implants in the mammogram are seen as oval mass, which is relatively less radio dense through which breast tissue can be visualized, and sometimes, a dense round structure which is the valve can be seen, that is used to fill the saline (Fig. 31.1a). Silicone implants are relatively dense when compared to the saline implants (Fig. 31.1b).

Advantage: Can easily detect extracapsular implant rupture, since free silicone is radio dense within the breast parenchyma.

Disadvantage:
1. Uses ionizing radiation
2. Probability of implant rupture during compression mammogram, especially in women who had intracapsular rupture prior to the mammogram

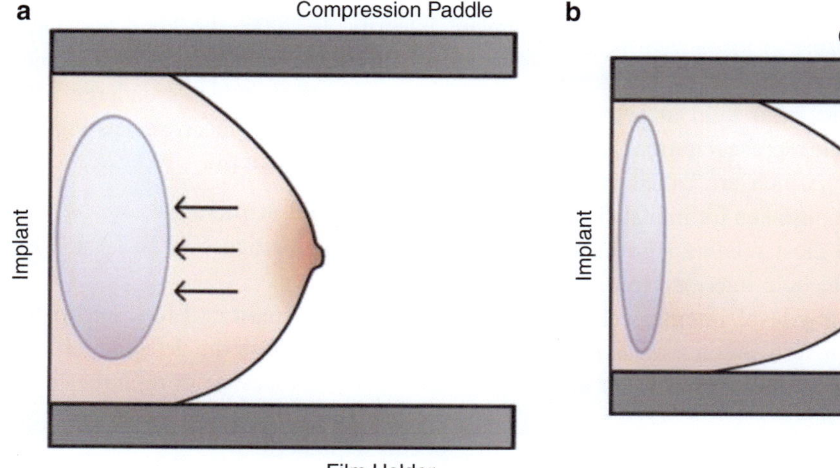

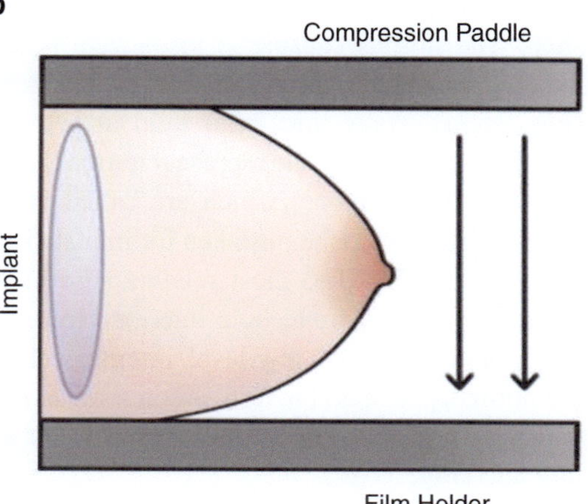

Fig. 31.5 Eklund Displacement view allows better visualization of the breast tissue (**a**) than the standard compression mammography (**b**)

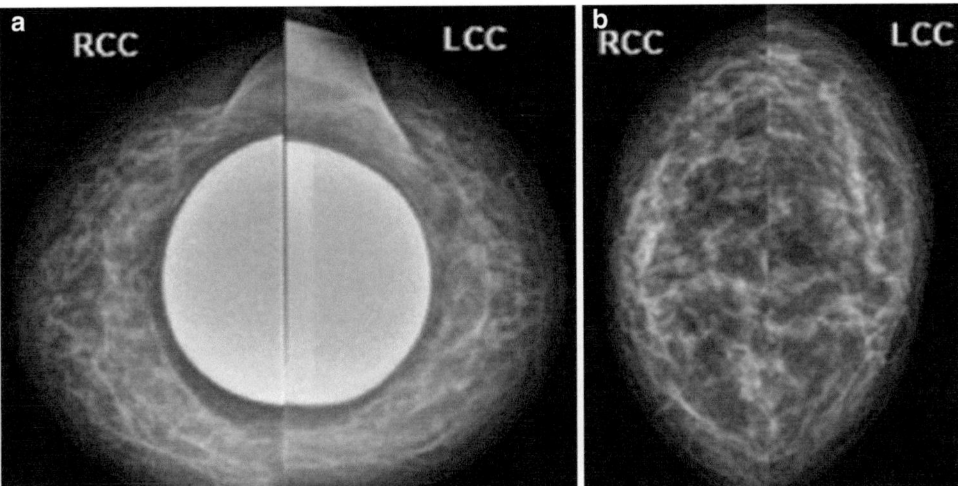

Fig. 31.6 A 45-year-old patient with bilateral breast implants. (**a**) CC view of both breasts shows sub glandular position of silicone implants. (**b**) shows the Eklund mammogram, which has facilitated the visualization of more breast tissue due to posterior displacement of the implant, which is not included in the mammogram field

31.5.2 Ultrasound

> **NOTE**: Reverberation artifacts seen anteriorly, and echoes produced behind the implant should not be confused with loss of implant integrity.

On ultrasonography (USG), saline and silicone implants have a similar appearance and are seen as anechoic structures surrounded by a linear echogenic envelope, which is the implant shell. The fibrous capsule is visualized as two parallel echogenic lines anterior to the shell (Fig. 31.7a). Wavy lines with fluid in between along the implant capsule represent normal undulation of the envelope, which are called radial folds and should not be mistaken for implant rupture (Fig. 31.7b). The most reliable sign of an intact implant is an anechoic interior. However, more often, minimal low-level internal echoes are normally seen and reverberation artefact secondary to highly reflective internal surface of the implants (Fig. 31.7c).

Advantage: Does not use ionizing radiation.

Disadvantage:

1. The posterior wall of the implant and the breast tissue behind the implant could not be evaluated due to the attenuation of the ultrasound beam by the silicone.
2. Another disadvantage of ultrasound evaluation of implant is operator dependency.

31.5.3 Magnetic Resonance Imaging (MRI)

The ability of MRI to suppress or emphasize the signal from water, fat, or silicone makes it the most ideal modality for evaluating breast implants. It is the most accurate technique in diagnosing the implant integrity. In 2006, the Food and Drug Administration (FDA) recommended that women with silicone gel breast implants undergo MRI screening 3 years after they receive a new implant and every 2 years after that [3].

Requirements and Sequences:

1. High field strength magnets of at least 1.5 T are preferred.
2. A dedicated MRI breast coil for high spatial resolution—those aid in the detection of subtle signs of implant leakage or rupture.
3. **Sequences**—T1 TSE, T2 TSE, DWI

   Special sequences:

   STIR silicone excited (Silicone-hyperintense, water-suppressed)

   STIR silicone suppressed (Silicone—suppressed, water-hyperintense)

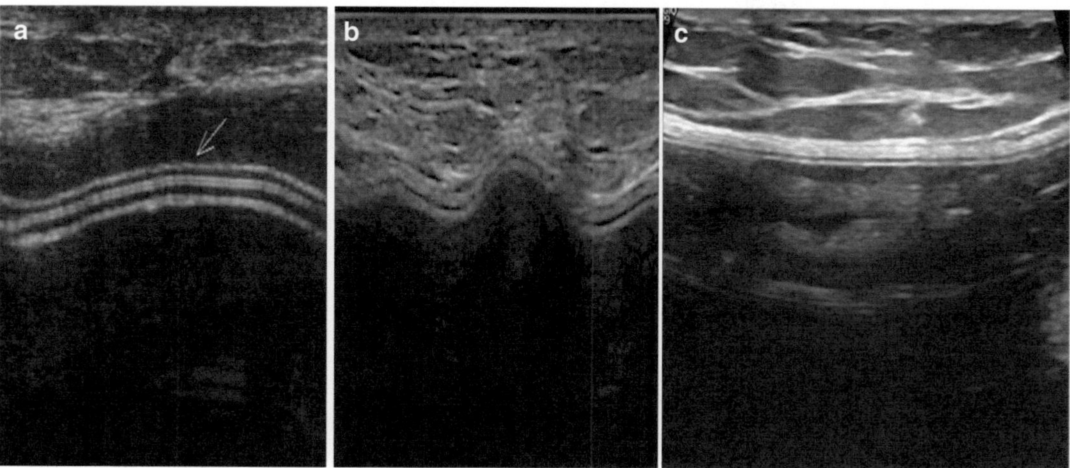

Fig. 31.7 High-resolution ultrasound image of a women with intact breast impact, (**a**) demonstrates the triple line of the envelope—inner single line is the shell and outer double line is the fibrous capsule. (**b**) demonstrates the normal undulation (without intervening fluid) in an intact breast implant. (**c**) shows the reverberation artefact posterior to the implant capsule

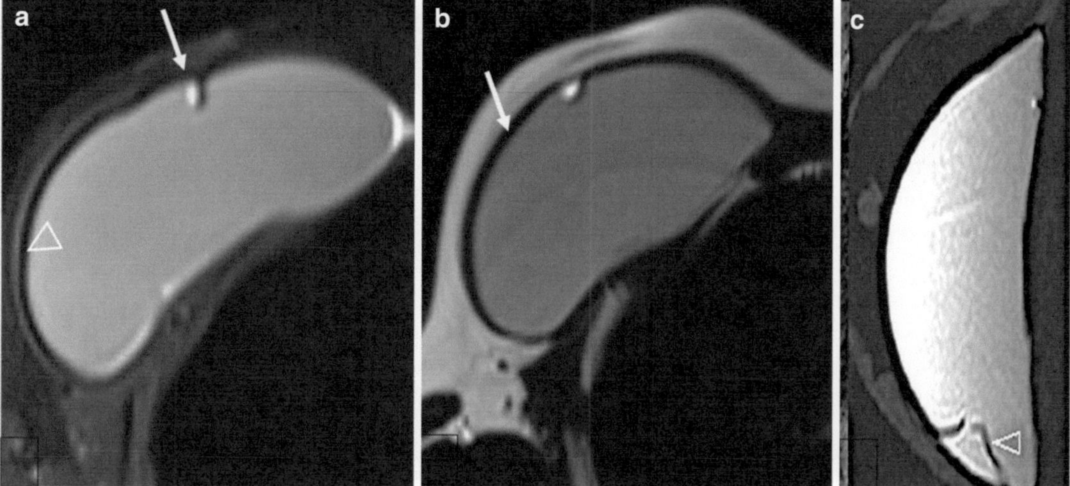

Fig. 31.8 MRI images of breast implant—Axial T1 TRIM image (**a**) shows hyperintense silicone implant with a small pocket of peri-implant-free fluid (arrow) and capsule seen as low signal intensity along the margins (arrowhead). Axial Silicon suppressed T2 image (**b**) shows the implant capsule again seen as low signal intensity along the periphery (arrow). Sagittal T2 weighted image (**c**) shows two dark signal radial folds along the inferior aspect of the implant (arrowhead)

Silicone appears hypointense on T1-weighted image and hyperintense on T2-weighted image. The envelope and capsule have low signal on all sequences (Fig. 31.8). MRI often shows low signal intensity radial folds extending to the periphery of the implant. Radial folds and periprosthetic fluid are considered normal findings and should not be mistaken for rupture.

Note: The use of contrast-enhanced MRI for assessing implant integrity is generally not recommended unless the priority of the imaging is to detect any residual/recurrent tumor, and BI-RADS category cannot be assigned for breast implants.

Advantage:

1. High spatial and soft tissue resolution
2. Lack of ionizing radiation
3. High-sensitivity and specificity in detecting implant rupture

Disadvantage:

1. Contraindicated—in patients with cardiac pacemakers, aneurysm clips, metallic foreign body and claustrophobia
2. Expensive
3. Not used for diagnosing saline implant ruptures, which are primarily a clinical diagnosis

31.5.4 Computed Tomography (CT)

On CT, an intact silicone implant is characterized by an oval shape and homogeneous gray density within a surrounding high-density ring, which represents the capsule (Fig. 31.9).

Advantage: Easy availability

Disadvantage:

1. Radiation exposure
2. Low sensitivity and specificity in detecting extracapsular implant rupture, as both silicone and soft tissue are both radio dense

A summary of the various imaging appearances of the saline and silicone implants are described in brief in Table 31.2.

31.5.4.1 Variant Imaging Appearances of Normal Breast Implant

There are variant appearances of an intact breast implant in the imaging modalities; the presence of which should not be mistaken for implant rupture and have been briefly presented below.

(a) Intact breast implant shell with a **fibrous capsule** surrounding.
(b) Mild to moderate **Periprosthetic fluid**—probably due to inflammatory response and does not indicate rupture.
(c) **Radial folds** (simple or complex)—Lines extending from the surface of the implant

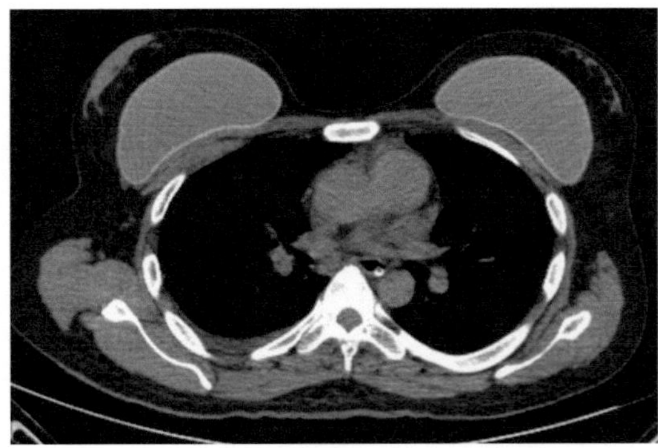

Fig. 31.9 Axial noncontrast CT chest section of a 45-year-old transgender woman with bilateral breast augmentation with sub glandular implants

Table 31.2 Summary of imaging appearance of breast implants [4]

	Implant type	
Imaging modality	Saline implant	Silicone implant
Mammography	Less dense center through which breast tissue is visible, denser outer envelope. Valve seen	Dense center, envelope not visible separately
Ultrasound	Anechoic with surrounding echogenic envelope	Anechoic surrounded by echogenic envelope
Magnetic resonant imaging	T1 hypointense, T2 hyperintense. The envelope and fibrous capsule hypointense on all pulse sequences and valve seen as mural nodule	Similar to saline implants on T1 and T2 weighted images. **On special sequences like silicone suppressed imaging, the implant looks homogenously hypointense**
Computed tomography	Hypodense mass with dense outer envelope and valve	Homogenous gray mass with dense outer envelope

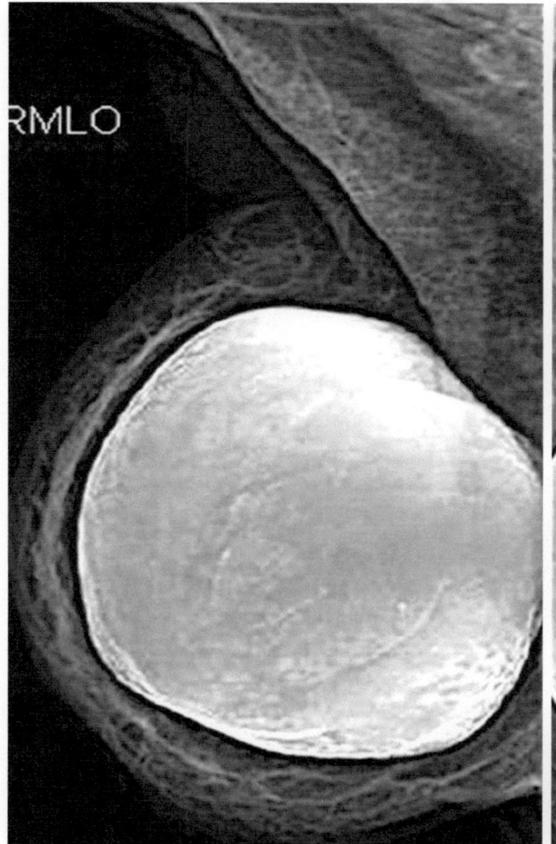

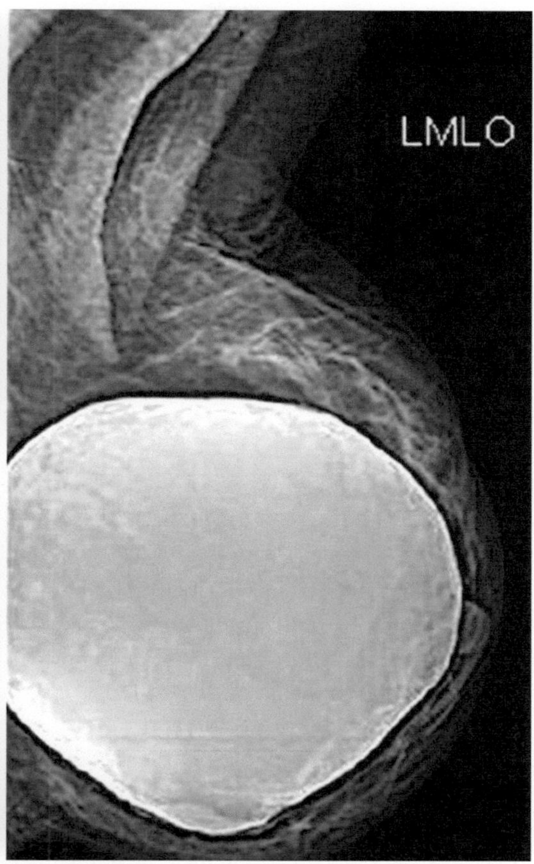

Fig. 31.10 Standard MLO view mammograms of both breasts show subglandular silicone implant. We can notice the rim of calcification seen along the fibrous implant capsule. This is a benign finding and can be seen in patients with longstanding breast implants and can also be seen secondary to implant contractures in which case positioning Eklund view can get difficult

inwards in a perpendicular manner. Frequently occurs in capsular contracture. These are one of the major causes of false positive cases of implant rupture in MRI.

(d) **Calcification and thickening of fibrous capsule** (Fig. 31.10).

31.6 Complications

Early complications: Occurs immediately in the postsurgical period and includes

1. Peri-implant collections/infection
2. Hematoma

Delayed complications:

1. Capsule formation and contracturec
2. Implant rupture
3. Gel bleed

Peri-implant collections/infection: Breast implant infections usually present in a bimodal fashion, during the acute postoperative period (6 days to 6 weeks after surgery) or with subacute or late onset (more than 6 weeks to months after surgery). About 2.9% of people develop surgical site infection after aesthetic breast surgeries with average onset time of 10–12 days postsurgery [5].

Risk factors for breast implant infections include the patient's underlying clinical comorbidities as well as intraoperative and postoperative factors. Women undergoing reconstructive surgery following mastectomy, axillary dissection, chemotherapy, or radiation therapy are at significantly increased risk of infection, up to 10 times higher than women undergoing nonreconstructive augmentation for cosmetic purposes [6]. The increased risk of infection is likely due to preexisting tissue scarring, ischemia, and delayed wound healing. Infection is less likely to occur with delayed placement of the implant in postmastectomy patients, as part of a two-stage procedure.

Clinical presentation: Patient presents with swelling, pain, and erythema.

Imaging features: On ultrasound, there may be thick-walled fluid collection/abscess with internal debris within. On MRI, there may be skin thickening, edema, and capsular enhancement.

Management: Ultrasound has an important role in the management of these infection by USG-guided drainage. Target therapy after identifying the organism from the aspirant via culture and antibiogram are of prime importance. Sometimes implants removal becomes inevitable in case of patients with systemic infections and poor general conditions.

Hematoma: It can occur in immediate postsurgical period, or it could be post traumatic.

Clinical presentation: Patient presents with swelling, pain, and erythema.

Imaging features: On mammography, well-defined hyperdense or heterogeneous density masses may be seen. USG, computed tomography (CT), and MRI can be used to demonstrate the hematoma.

Management: Acute hematoma seen in immediate postsurgical period requires drainage. Small hematoma can be treated conservatively for spontaneous resolution. Late hematomas, which are relatively rare, may require surgical removal.

Capsular contraction: It is the most common delayed complication of silicone breast implants. It is due to the abnormal constriction of the fibrous capsule surrounding the breast implant resulting in hardening and deformity of the implant.

Clinical presentation: Predominantly, a clinical diagnosis often presents with deformed, tense, and painful breast.

Imaging features: On imaging (mammogram, USG, and MRI)—presents as spherical in shape rather than oval with an increased anteroposterior diameter than the transverse diameter (Figs. 31.11 and 31.12). There may be unusual areas of irregularity, bulging, and tenting seen on the surface of the implant shell. Thickening of fibrous capsule with calcification and increase in the number of radial folds may also be seen.

Management: The management of capsular contraction depends upon the location of the implant (subglandular/subpectoral). Capsulectomy, site change, and implant exchange have been referred to as the gold standard treatment of clinically significant contractures [7]. The routine management of the capsular contraction is capsulectomy or capsulotomy, but recent studies state that anterior and posterior capsulectomy can be attempted in selective cases [7].

Implant rupture: It is the most common complication of breast implants. About 10–15 years of implant placement the incidence of implant rupture increases as the placement, and by 9–12 years, the estimated cumulative incidence was 15.1% [8].

Clinical presentation: Decrease in the size of the implant due to the extrusion of the fluid is the main clinical feature. Silicone implant ruptures can be difficult to identify as size change might not be as significant as in saline implant. The patient may or may not have pain due to rupture, and absence of pain does not exclude implant rupture. Ruptures are most often silent; using the physical examination as a screening method results in missed silent ruptures and leads to an underestimation of the true rupture rate.

Risk factors for rupture include excessive force to the chest, for example, during closed capsulotomy (strongly advised against), seat belt contusion injury, blunt trauma, compression during mammographic imaging, or severe capsular contracture. Case reports of implant damage as a consequence of mammography were associated primarily with thinner shell, earlier second generation device [9].

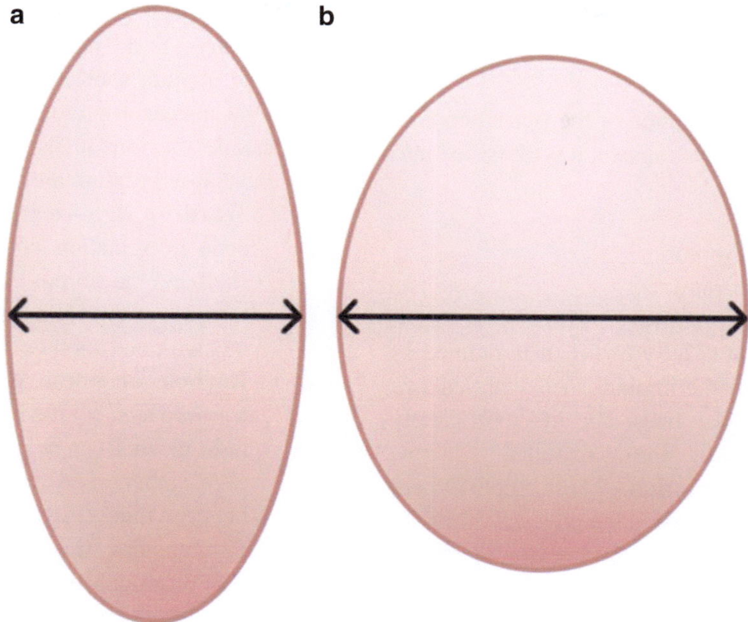

Fig. 31.11 Schematic representation of implant contracture. (**a**) Normal implant: oval with normal anteroposterior diameter (shown as arrow) and (**b**) contracted implant, which is spherical in shape with increased anteroposterior diameter

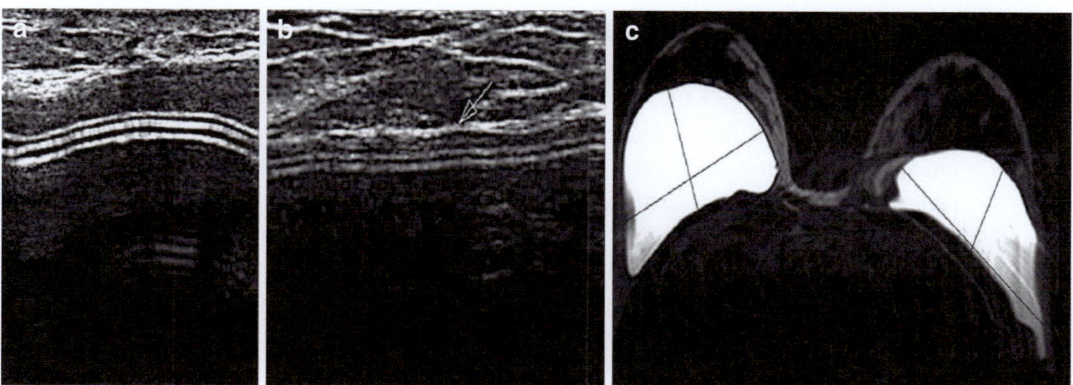

Fig. 31.12 Implant contracture imaging features in USG and MRI. In ultrasound, implant contracture is evident by thickened appearance of the implant capsule (**arrow in b**) compared to the normal appearance of the capsule in (**a**) MRI breast STIR sequence image (**c**) shows contracted right implant with increased anteroposterior diameter when compared to the normal left implant

31.7 Types of Silicone Implant Rupture

Depending on the location of the free silicone in relation to the fibrous capsule, it is classified into two categories:

1. Intracapsular rupture
2. Extracapsular rupture

1. **Intracapsular rupture**: This is the most common type (77–89%) [4]. It is defined as the rupture of the implant shell with leakage of silicone that does not macroscopically extend beyond the fibrous capsule.

   Clinical presentation: These ruptures are most often silent; using the physical examination as a screening method results in missed silent ruptures, leading to an underestimate of the true rupture rate.

   Imaging features:

   (a) **Magnetic resonance imaging (MRI)**: Various signs seen in MRI indicate intracapsular rupture, and it depends if the implant is collapse or not due to the rupture. The ruptures are as follows:

   Collapsed intracapsular silicon rupture:

   - **Linguine sign—**Most reliable sign of intracapsular rupture in MRI. Presence of multiple curvilinear low-signal intensity lines within the T2 bright silicone gel. These lines represent the collapsed implant membrane (Fig. 31.13a) floating within the implant gel and is a feature of collapsed implant rupture.

   Uncollapsed intracapsular silicone rupture—is defined as a tear of the silicone implant shell and is considered an intracapsular rupture with silicone gel outside the implant shell. The signs of uncollapsed rupture are

   - **Teardrop sign—**represents focal silicone invagination between the inner shell and the fibrous capsule, with the margins of the collapsing shell in contact with one another (Fig. 31.13b).
   - **Keyhole or noose sign—**Similar to teardrop sign but the margin of the collapsing shell is not in contact with each other, and there is silicone between them (Fig. 31.13c).
   - **Subcapsular line—**Subcapsular line sign represents a thin layer of silicone between the shell and the fibrous capsule (Fig. 31.13d).

   (a) **Mammography**: Mammography does not confidently detect intracapsular rupture. A contour bulge may indicate intracapsular rupture; however, the differential diagnosis includes implant herniation.

   (b) **Ultrasound (USG)**: Horizontally stacked echogenic lines traversing through the implant interior at various levels, termed the "**stepladder sign**" (Fig. 31.14). Isoechoic silicone may be found between the fibrous capsule, and the implant surface and low-level internal echoes may be indicative of minimal prosthetic collapse; however, these findings should be confirmed with MRI.

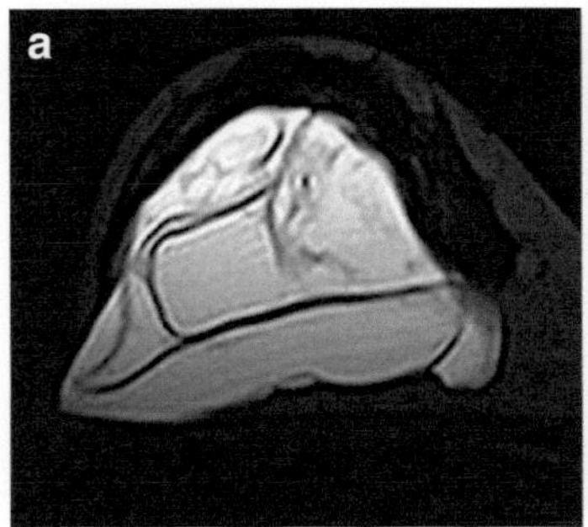

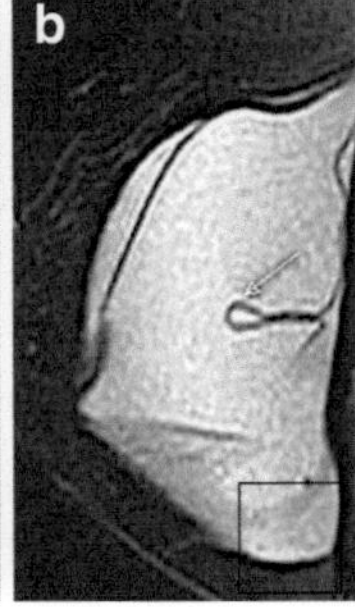

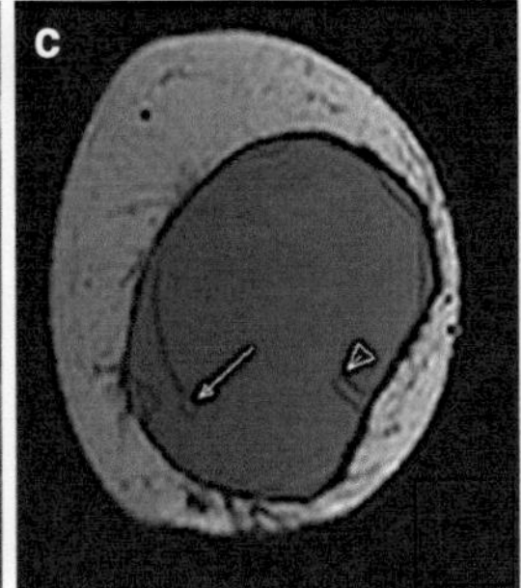

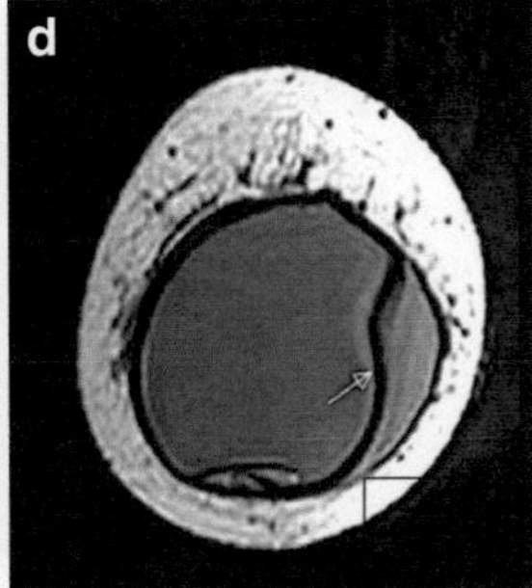

Fig. 31.13 MRI signs of the intracapsular implant rupture—axial T2 TRIM image shows linguine sign (**a**), sagittal T2 fat-saturated image shows teardrop sign (**b**), coronal T2 images shows noose sign (arrow) and teardrop sign (arrowhead) (**c**). Coronal T2 image with subcapsular sign (**d**)

Management: Treatment of intracapsular rupture consists of removal of the ruptured device, complete evacuation of any free silicone, capsulectomy, and, if desired by the patient, insertion of a new implant. In patients with capsular contracture, insertion of the new implant into a virgin pocket is advisable to reduce the risk of recurrent contracture.

2. **Extracapsular rupture**: This occurs secondary to the rupture of both implant shell and fibrous capsule, with macroscopic silicone leakage that extends beyond the fibrous capsule into surrounding parenchymal tissues.

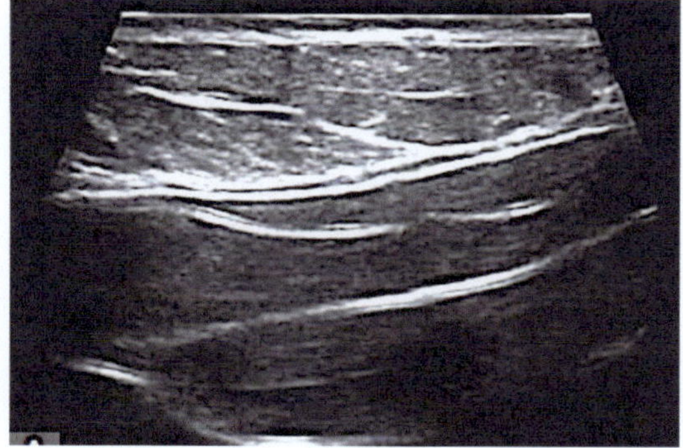

Fig. 31.14 High-resolution transverse ultrasound image of the patient with intracapsular implant rupture showing multiple echogenic lines in **stepladder pattern**

This leads to silicone granuloma formation within the breast parenchyma and axillary lymph nodes, which may be mistaken for carcinoma.

Clinical presentation: Patients are usually symptomatic. There may be a change in breast shape, palpable lumps, axillary adenopathy, or inflammatory changes of the overlying skin caused by silicone infiltration into the dermis.

Imaging Features:

(a) **Mammography**: Extravasated silicone can be seen as dense material extending into the breast parenchyma or within the axillary lymph nodes.
(b) **Ultrasound**: Free silicone can be seen as an echogenic nodule with posterior dirty acoustic shadowing, termed as "**snowstorm sign**" (Fig. 31.15a).
(c) **MRI**: Extracapsular free silicone is visualized as discrete foci of isointense to low signal intensity on T1 fat-suppressed images and of high signal intensity on water-suppressed T2-weighted images (Fig. 31.15b).

Management: Extracapsular leakage often leads to granuloma formation and silicone mastitis secondary to inflammation. If the sili-

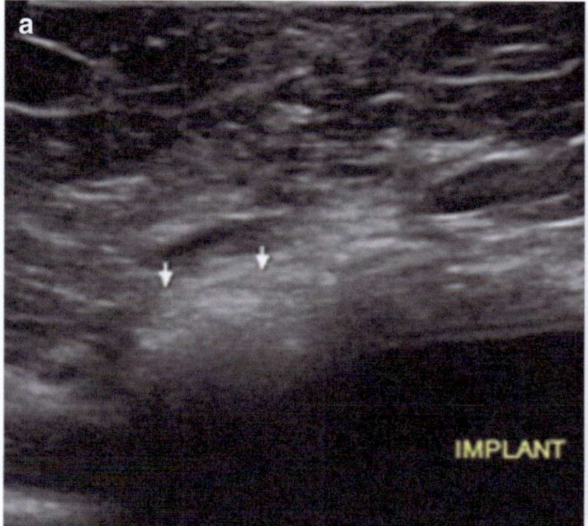

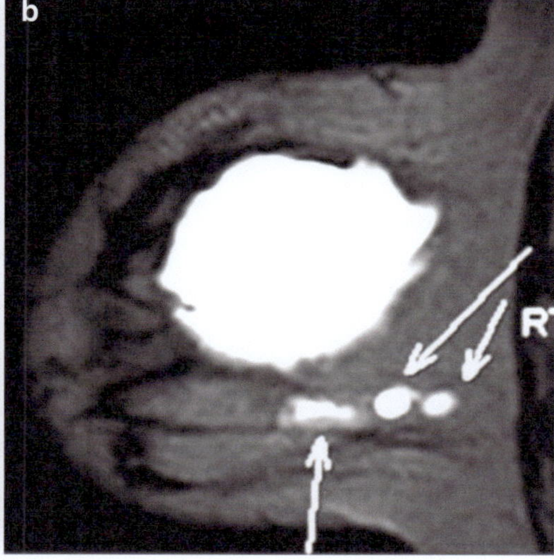

Fig. 31.15 Imaging features of extracapsular implant rupture: (**a**) high-resolution transverse USG image shows extravasated silicone outside the implant capsule with posterior dirty shadowing (arrows). (**b**) Sagittal T2 silicone sequence showing hyperintense extravasated silicone within the breast parenchyma (arrow)

conoma formation/inflammation is small, then it can be resected without causing major changes to the breast appearance. However, if there is a large area of inflammatory changes/ granuloma then it is advised to do subtotal resection with removal of the rupture implant and placement of new implant in a virgin pocket to isolate it from the field of gel contamination [10].

3. **Gel bleed**: defined as microscopic transudation of silicone through an **intact breast prosthesis** membrane into the surrounding tissues and lymphatics. Silicone can migrate, even reaching the upper limbs, the liver, the inguinal lymph nodes, the synovium, the skin, and the pleura fluid. For this reason, the silicone found in axillary nodes always does not imply extracapsular rupture.

   Imaging Features: Gel bleed is difficult to identify on USG and MRI unless it is extensive. Only when a gel bleed is extensive can silicone gel be detected. In MRI, gel bleed can produce subtle high signal intensity on both sides of the implant shell on silicone selective sequences.

A summary of the breast associated complications has been listed in Table 31.3 with their MRI features.

31.8 Other Conditions Associated with Breast Implants

The remaining breast tissue can develop both benign and malignant conditions. Benign cysts and fibroadenoma are the commonest. The risk of breast cancer is **not increased** in augmented women [11]. There is no difference in survival rates in women with breast cancer and implants compared to those without implants. The sensitivity of mammography and ultrasound (US) for cancer detection may be reduced in augmented woman [1]. However, the presence of the implant does not seem to decrease the sensitivity of breast MRI. A correlation between physical examination and mammography findings should be first done. Any palpable abnormality can then be subjected to a USG or contrast-enhanced MRI. Suspicious findings should be further evaluated with biopsy with maximum caution to avoid damage to the implant.

Breast implant associated anaplastic large cell lymphoma (BIA-ALCL) is a newly included category in the World health Organization (WHO) category of lymphoid neoplasm in 2016 with its rising incidence in association with the increase in the use of textured breast implants for aesthetic and reconstructive purposes. [12] They occur as late-onset swelling of the breast with a

Table 31.3 Summary of findings of implant complication in MRI

S. no	Implant complication		MRI findings
1	Infection		Peri implant heterogenous fluid collection, skin thickening and edema, capsular enhancement **(Note: Contrast MRI can be performed if clinically suspicious of infection)**
2	Hematoma		Variable signal intensity in T1/T2 sequences depending on the age of the bleed
3	Capsular contracture		Increasing anteroposterior diameter in imaging. Thickening of fibrous capsule, peri-implant calcification and increase in the number of radial folds
4	Implant rupture	(a) Intracapsular	Linguine sign—in case of **collapsed implant** Keyhole/noose sign Tear drop sign **Uncollapsed** Subcapsular line
		(b) Extracapsular	Water suppressed sequence—high T2 signal intensity outside the implant capsule, within the breast tissue, axillary nodes, intramammary and internal mammary nodes
5	Gel bleed		No specific imaging features

median period of 1–10 years post-implant reconstruction with either peri-implant effusion along the medial aspect to begin within or mass forming type. On imaging, mammograms are usually not sensitive/specific in diagnosing BIA-ALCL. Ultrasound is most preferred and is a simpler modality to diagnose ALCL. On USS, there is homogenous anechoic peri-implant free fluid (effusion), requires USS-guided aspiration fine needle aspiration of this fluid for cytological confirmation. However, peri-implant fluid of <10 mL volume is usually considered physiological. There can be associated thickening of the fibrous capsule and inflammatory changes in the surrounding breast tissue. In mass forming type there can be either solid/complex solid cystic masses and requires biopsy. A detailed discussion about BIA-ALCL is given in the hematolymphoid neoplasm (Chap. 24).

31.9 MRI-Based Preoperative Breast Volumetry

The principle aesthetic objective of breast augmentation is to restore and achieve volumetric symmetry. MRI-based breast volumetry is a simple and convenient solution to assessing breast volume and composition of breast tissue for initial operative planning, postsurgical follow-up, and calculating the implant size [13]. Breast MRI has been shown to have the highest correlation with the actual breast volume. The entire augmented breast with the elliptical implant in situ is traced onto axial slices. The breasts with the implant inside are traced on a bilateral axial slice and the borders of the implant are outlined. After marking all slices, a software program is used to determine the implant volume and the volume of the entire breast.

Acknowledgement We would like to extend our sincere and heartfelt thanks and gratitude to Dr. Bijal Jankharia of Dr. Jankharia's imaging center for contributing images (Fig. 31.1, 31.3, 31.4a, d, 31.6, 31.7a, b, 31.10, 31.12, 31.13, 31.14, and 31.15) to this chapter.

Conflict of Interest There is no conflict of interests.

References

1. Middleton MS, McNamara MP. Breast implant classification with MR imaging correlation. RadioGraphics. 2000;20(3):e1.
2. Juanpere S, Perez E, Huc O, Motos N, Pont J, Pedraza S. Imaging of breast implants—a pictorial review. Insights Imaging. 2011;2(6):653–70.
3. Chung KC, Malay S, Shauver MJ, Kim HM. Economic analysis of screening strategies for rupture of silicone gel breast implants. Plast Reconstr Surg. 2012;130(1):225–37.
4. Shah AT, Jankharia BB. Imaging of common breast implants and implant-related complications: a pictorial essay. Indian J Radiol Imaging. 2016;26(2):216–25.
5. Rubino C, Brongo S, Pagliara D, Cuomo R, Abbinante G, Campitiello N, et al. Infections in breast implants: a review with a focus on developing countries. J Infect Dev Ctries. 2014;8(9):1089–95.
6. Lalani T. Breast implant infections: an update. Infect Dis Clin N Am. 2018;32(4):877–84.
7. Wan D, Rohrich RJ. Revisiting the management of capsular contracture in breast augmentation: a systematic review. Plast Reconstr Surg. 2016;137(3):826–41.
8. Berg WA, Caskey CI, Hamper UM, Anderson ND, Chang BW, Sheth S, et al. Diagnosing breast implant rupture with MR imaging, US, and mammography. RadioGraphics. 1993;13(6):1323–36.
9. Brown S, Todd J, Luu HM. Breast implant adverse events during mammography: reports to the food and drug administration. J Women's Health. 2002;13:371–8. discussion 379.
10. Handel N, Garcia ME, Wixtrom R. Breast implant rupture: causes, incidence, clinical impact, and management. Plast Reconstr Surg. 2013;132(5):1128–37.
11. Bryant H, Brasher P. Breast implants and breast cancer—reanalysis of a linkage study. N Engl J Med. 1995;332(23):1535–9.
12. Sharma B, Jurgensen-Rauch A, Pace E, Attygalle AD, Sharma R, Bommier C, Wotherspoon AC, Sharma S, Iyengar S, El-Sharkawi D. Breast implant–associated anaplastic large cell lymphoma: review and multiparametric imaging paradigms. RadioGraphics. 2020;40(3):609–28.
13. Yoo A, Minn KW, Jin US. Magnetic resonance imaging-based volumetric analysis and its relationship to actual breast weight. Arch Plast Surg. 2013;40(3):203–8.

32 Male Breast Abnormalities

M. C. Sheela, Bhawna Dev, Archana,
and Ramya Ramakrishnan

Abstract

The morphology and histology of a male breast is different as compared to female breast due to hormonal influences. Similarly, the pathology in male breast is limited to ductal and stromal proliferation. Although there are few pathological conditions common to both the genders, the lesions pertinent to male breast like gynecomastia are discussed in detail.

Keywords

Gynecomastia · Dendritic gynecomastia · Nodular gynecomastia · Pseudogynecomastia · Male breast cancer

M. C. Sheela (✉) · B. Dev
Department of Radiology, Sri Ramachandra Institute of Higher Education and Research, Chennai, India
e-mail: sheelamc@sriramachandra.edu.in; bhawnadev@sriramachandra.edu.in

Archana
Department of Pathology, Sri Ramachandra Institute of Higher Education and Research, Chennai, India

R. Ramakrishnan
Department of Surgery, Sri Ramachandra Institute of Higher Education and Research, Chennai, India

32.1 Introduction

The breast composition of normal adult male breasts is skin, subcutaneous fat, atrophic ducts, and stromal elements. Cooper ligaments and lobules are absent in male breasts. Therefore, conditions secondary to lobular proliferation, such as fibroadenoma, phylloides tumor, invasive lobular carcinoma, and lobular carcinoma in situ, are extremely rare in men. Conditions related to ductal and stromal proliferation, such as gynecomastia, invasive ductal carcinoma, ductal carcinoma in situ, and papillary neoplasm, may occur [1].

The most common clinical presentation is the lump with or without pain in the breast.

The other causes are as similar to female breast diseases spectrum like

1. Infectious and inflammatory conditions
   Mastitis, abscess
2. Benign lesion
   Cysts, lipoma, hamartoma, and fibroadenoma (extremely rare)
3. Vascular conditions like Mondor's disease and venous malformations.
4. Miscellaneous:
   Diabetic mastopathy, post-traumatic hematoma, and fat necrosis
5. Malignant lesions:
   Ductal carcinoma in situ (DCIS), invasive ductal carcinoma, invasive lobular carcinoma, lymphoma, and metastases

B. Dev, L. D. Joseph (eds.), *Holistic Approach to Breast Disease*,
https://doi.org/10.1007/978-981-99-0035-0_32

Lesions pertinent to the male breast include gynecomastia, pseudogynecomastia, and malignant lesions, which are discussed in detail as follows.

32.2 Gynecomastia

32.2.1 Introduction

It is the enlargement of the male breast. It is the most common abnormality in a male breast and is extremely common in newborns due to the exposure of maternal estrogens.

32.2.2 Etiopathogenesis [2]

It can be physiologic or nonphysiological, caused due to disruption of estrogen to testosterone ratio further leading to breast glandular proliferation.

The common nonphysiological causes are

- Systemic conditions like hyperthyroidism, hypogonadism, cirrhosis, chronic renal failure, and chronic pulmonary disease
- Hormone use such as exogenous estrogen, androgens
- Drug use such as digitalis, finasteride, cimetidine, spironolactone, tricyclic antidepressants, and marijuana.
- Neoplasms like testicular germ cell tumors, lung carcinoma

32.2.3 Clinical Presentation

It has a bimodal presentation with a peak incidence in peripubertal and after 50 years, probably due to hormonal instability.

It can be unilateral (commonly left breast) or bilateral [3].

They may present as a discrete, nodular subareolar mass (rarely peripheral) or as a diffuse enlargement with or without pain or tenderness.

32.2.4 Imaging Protocol

The most recent ACR Appropriateness Criteria for the evaluation of the symptomatic male breast published in 2015 [4] proposed imaging protocol in male breast as follows:

- Men with typical symptoms of gynecomastia or pseudogynecomastia do not usually need imaging.
- For men with an indeterminate palpable mass, begin with ultrasound if the patient is <25 years of age, because breast cancer is highly unlikely. Mammogram should be performed if ultrasound shows a suspicious finding.
- For men ≥25 years of age, or men with a highly concerning physical examination, begin with mammogram. Ultrasound is useful if mammogram is inconclusive or suspicious [4, 5].

32.2.5 Mammogram

The conventional Craniocaudal (CC) and Mediolateral Oblique (MLO) views are obtained.

32.2.5.1 Findings [6]

Three patterns of gynecomastia are identified:

1. Nodular
2. Dendritic
3. Diffuse glandular

32.2.5.2 Nodular Pattern

It is the early, florid phase of ductal and stromal proliferation usually seen within 1 year of onset of gynecomastia.

It appears as a fan-shaped subareolar density that blends into the surrounding subcutaneous fat, resulting in indistinct borders. This phase is *reversible* if the causative factor is eliminated.

32.2.5.3 Dendritic Pattern

It represents the quiescent, fibrotic phase.

It classically manifests as a "flame-shaped" subareolar density radiating from the nipple with linear projections interdigitating into the deeper adipose tissues (Fig. 32.2). The dendritic pattern may extend into the upper outer quadrant. Due to fibrosis, it is **irreversible** finding both on clinical palpation and mammography.

32.2.5.4 Diffuse Glandular Pattern

It is typically seen in patients receiving high-dose estrogen therapy.

It is characterized by heterogeneously dense breast consisting of both nodular and dendritic components that closely resemble female breasts. It can be unilateral (Figs. 32.1 and 32.2) or bilateral (Fig. 32.3).

32.2.6 Ultrasound [7]

32.2.6.1 Nodular Pattern

A subareolar, hypoechoic mass, which may have typical nodular features and a long axis that is parallel to the skin (Fig. 32.4).

32.2.6.2 Dendritic Pattern

It is seen as a subareolar hypoechoic lesion with an anechoic star-shaped posterior border, which can be described as finger-like projections or "spider legs" insinuating into the surrounding echogenic fibrous breast tissue (Fig. 32.5).

32.2.6.3 Diffuse Gynecomastia

It resembles a female breast with both nodular and dendritic components (Fig. 32.6).

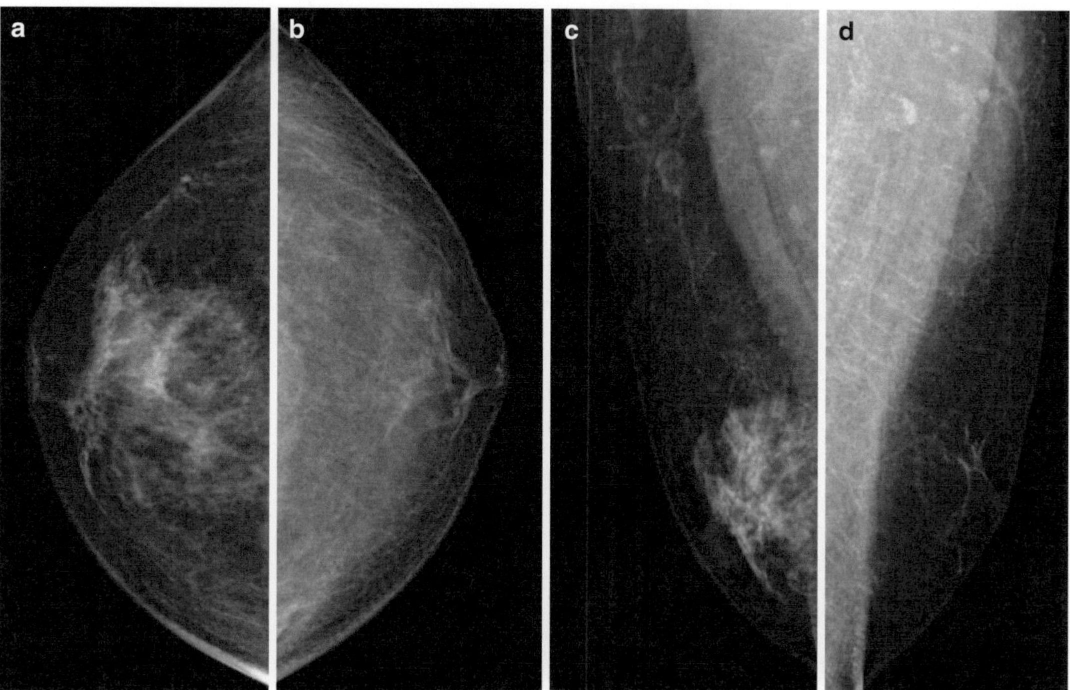

Fig. 32.1 Diffuse glandular pattern. CC (**a**, **c**) and MLO (**b**, **d**) views of both breasts. An asymmetric glandular tissue is noted in the right breast (**a**, **c**) in contralateral to normal fatty left breast (**b**, **d**)

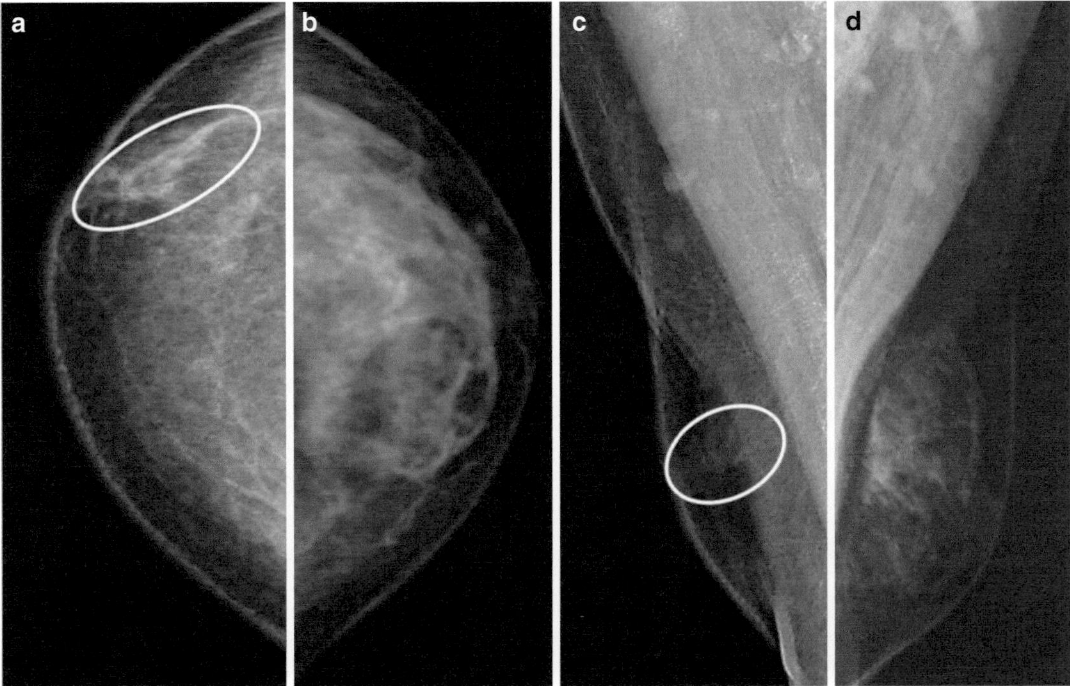

Fig. 32.2 Dendritic pattern: CC (**a**, **c**) and MLO (**b**, **d**) views of both breasts. A flame-shaped glandular tissue is noted in the right breast subareolar region—**dendritic pattern** (circled in **a** and **c**). Diffuse glandular tissue in left breast—**diffuse glandular pattern**

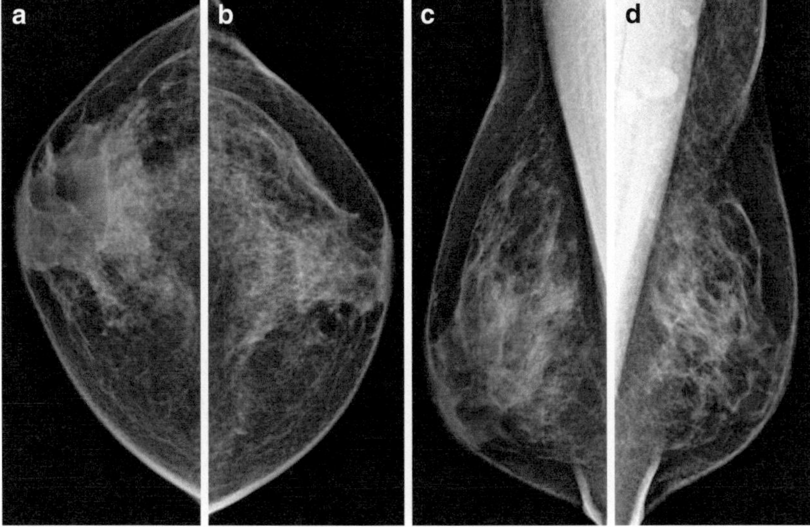

Fig. 32.3 Diffuse glandular pattern. CC (**a**, **c**) and MLO (**b**, **d**) views of both breasts. Diffuse glandular proliferation of both the breasts resembling female breast

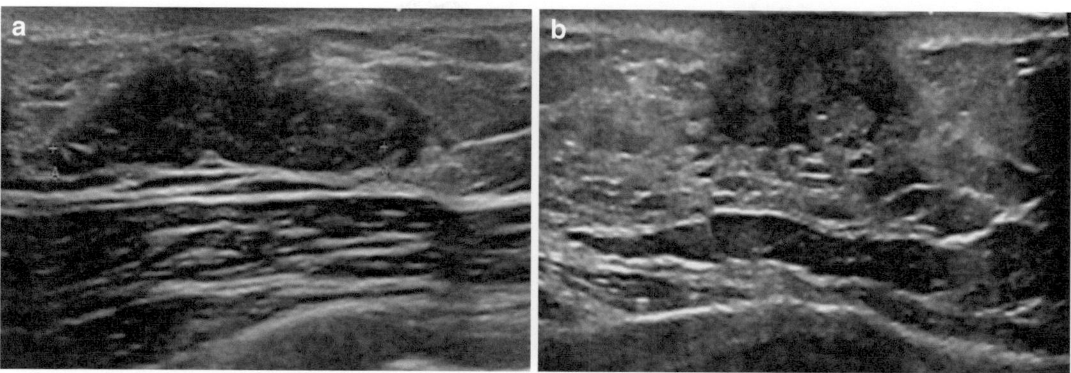

Fig. 32.4 Nodular type of gynecomastia. (**a**, **b**) USG reveals a well-circumscribed oval hypoechoic lesion in the subareolar region

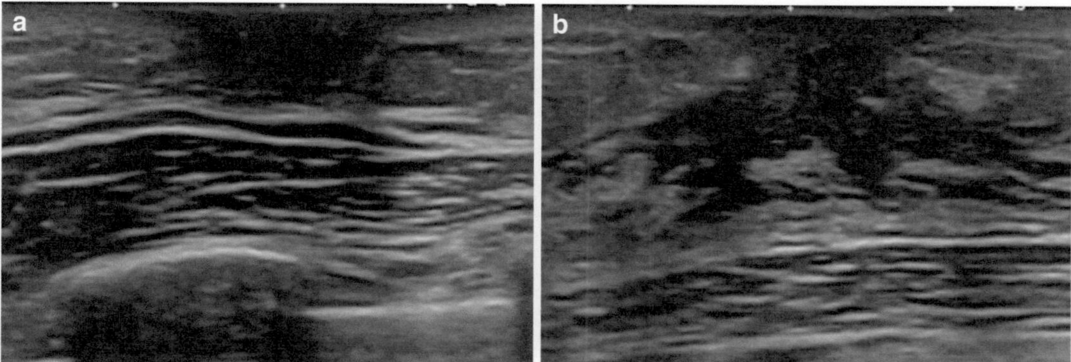

Fig. 32.5 Dendritic type of gynecomastia. USG reveals a subareolar hypoechoic lesion with star-shaped posterior borders—s/o dendritic gynecomastia (**b**) in contrast to normal subareolar region is some other patient (**a**)

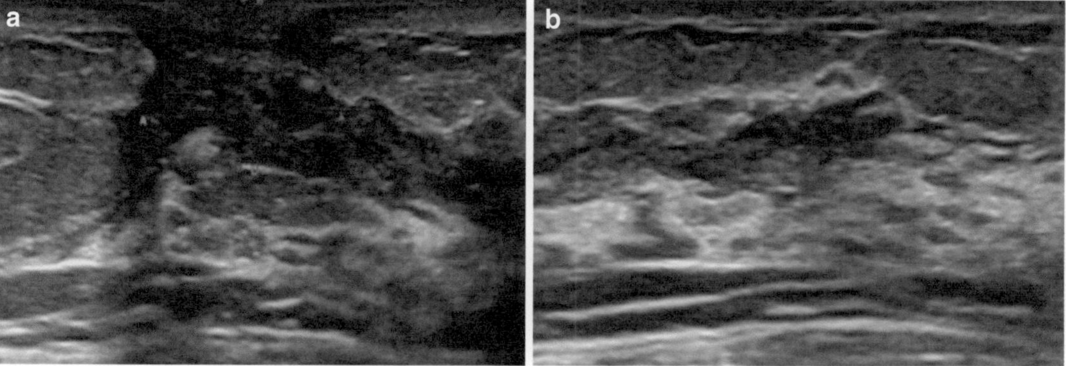

Fig. 32.6 Diffuse gynecomastia. USG reveals a subareolar hypoechoic area with finger-like projections (**a**) with glandular component extending into the adjacent breast parenchyma (**b**)

If unilateral, occasionally, it can mimic malignancy [6].

32.2.7 Computed Tomography (CT) and Magnetic Resonance Imaging (MRI)

Not indicated for evaluation of gynecomastia.

32.2.8 BI-RADS Category: BI-RADS 2

32.2.8.1 Pathology

Gross Examination

Soft, rubbery, or firm gray white that forms a discrete mass or an ill-defined induration on cut surface. Rarely, fat is seen dispersed in the tissue.

Histopathology [8]

Three phases of proliferative changes are described by microscopy:

- Florid gynecomastia characterized by ductal epithelial hyperplasia (Fig. 32.7a), periductal stromal cellularity, vascularity with myxoid, and edematous stroma. It occurs within 1 year of onset.
- Intermediate gynecomastia characterized by a florid component and increased fibrosis tends to last up to 6 months. It represents a transitional phase in the maturation of the lesion.
- Fibrous phase characterized by more collagenous stroma and lesser epithelial proliferation with less edema and less vascularity (Fig. 32.7b). It occurs after the lesion has been present for 1 year or more.

Other findings include PASH (pseudoangiomatous stromal hyperplasia), lobule formation, pseudolactational hyperplasia, apocrine, and squamous metaplasia.

Cytologic atypia (atypical ductal hyperplasia) with mitosis may be present and related to finasteride therapy for prostate cancer and alopecia [9].

Fine needle aspiration cytology (FNAC) usually yields a sparsely cellular aspirate and may not be of much value. Biopsy is preferred.

32.2.8.2 Immunohistochemistry

Gynecomastia will show positivity for estrogen receptor (ER), progesterone receptor (PR), androgen receptor (AR) in the epithelial cells and P63, CK5, CK14 in the myoepithelial cells. Prostate specific antigen (PSA) will be positive in the ductal epithelium, and prostatic acid phosphatase (PAP) will be negative in the epithelium [10].

32.2.8.3 Microscopic Differential Diagnosis

Difficulty in differentiating atypical hyperplasia from carcinoma is noted on FNAC.

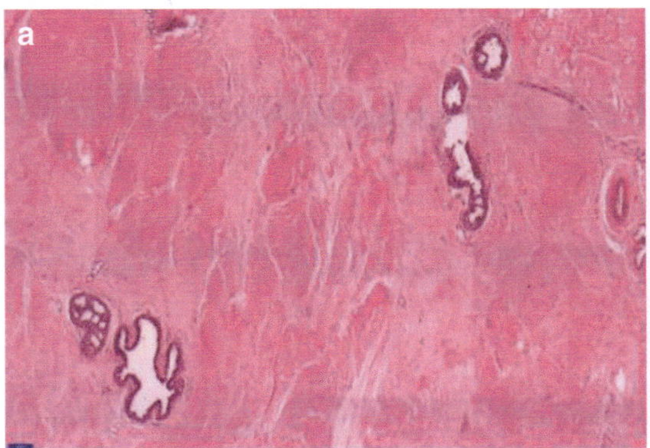

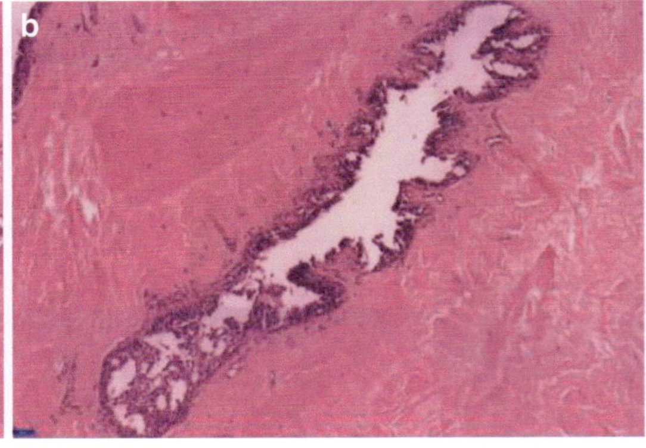

Fig. 32.7 (**a**) H&E image of gynecomastia showing scattered ducts in a dense hyalinized hypocellular stroma (20×). (**b**) H&E image of gynecomastia demonstrating an irregular branching duct with epithelial hyperplasia surrounded by a fibrous stroma (40×)

32.2.8.4 Management and Treatment

The aim is to rule out reversible cause of gynecomastia.

Image guided/excisional biopsy is performed to rule out carcinoma. For idiopathic gynecomastia, for cosmetic reasons on patient's request, Webster Procedure (subcutaneous mastectomy) or liposuction can be done.

32.2.8.5 Follow Up and Prognosis

Regression has been noted in hyperthyroidism and alcoholic liver disease when the underlying conditions were treated. Evidence of increased risk of carcinoma arising from gynecomastia remains debated.

32.3 Pseudogynecomastia

32.3.1 Introduction

Pseudogynecomastia is more commonly seen in overweight or obese individuals.

32.3.2 Etiopathogenesis

It is caused by benign diffuse proliferation of normal fatty tissue without stimulation of ductal and stromal elements.

32.3.3 Clinical Presentation

Bilateral enlarged breast with no definite palpable mass/nipple retraction is presented. It is usually seen in an obese individual, sometimes seen in normal built males also.

32.3.4 Imaging Findings

32.3.4.1 Mammogram

Mammogram can be performed if physical examination findings are inconclusive and will demonstrate increased lucent subareolar fat or diffuse fatty proliferation (Fig. 32.8).

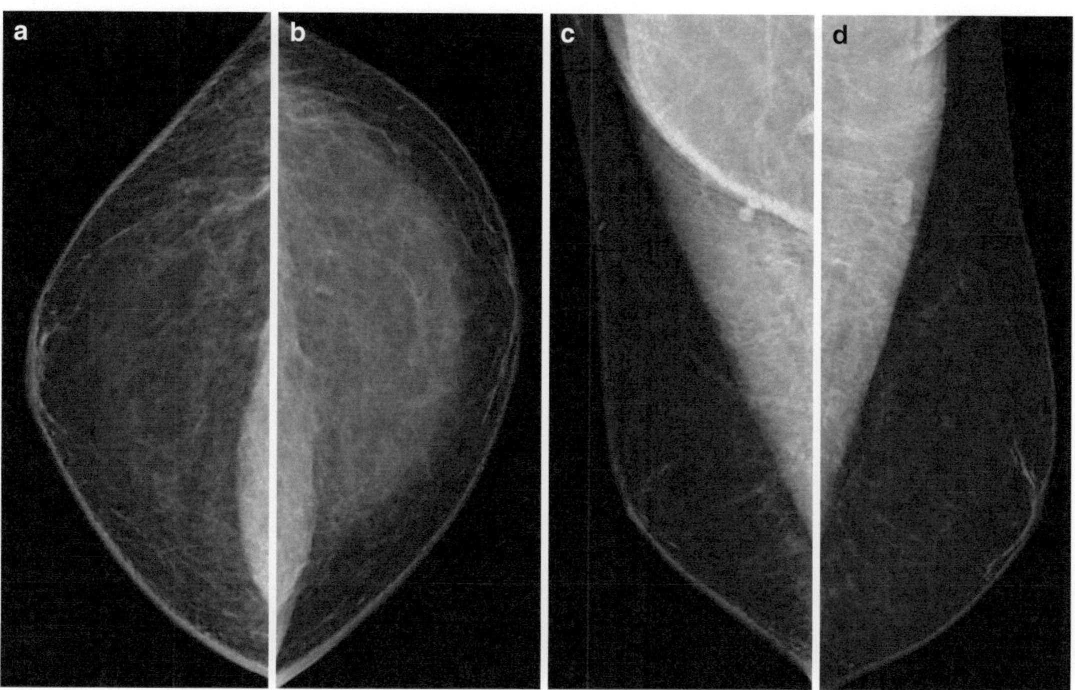

Fig. 32.8 Pseudogynecomastia. CC (**a**, **c**) and MLO (**b**, **d**) views of both breasts. Diffuse enlargement of both the breasts showing fatty proliferation

32.3.4.2 Ultrasound

Ultrasound is typically not necessary, but if performed due to clinical concern, will demonstrate normal-appearing subcutaneous adipose tissue.

32.3.5 BI-RADS Category: BI-RADS 1

32.3.5.1 Clinical Management

Reassurance. No active intervention needed.

32.4 Cysts

In men, cysts are actually dilated ducts rather than the actual cysts as seen in females.

32.4.1 Clinical Presentation

Usually an incidental finding if small. It may be associated with gynecomastia. They are generally solitary.

32.4.2 Imaging

Breast cysts can be simple, complicated, or complex.

On ultrasound, simple cysts are characterized by well-defined margins, anechoic contents, with posterior acoustic enhancement.

Cysts are of greater alarm if clinically they have a firm consistency that are relatively fixed to underlying structures. It is crucial to rule out subtle papillary projections in the walls as it can be a papillary neoplasm.

32.4.3 BI-RADS Category: BI-RADS 2

32.4.3.1 Histology

The cells composing the ductal epithelium often have abundant, eosinophilic, granular cytoplasm, and roundish hyperchromic nuclei. The epithelium resembles that of the apocrine sweat glands. The secretions may be calcified.

32.4.3.2 Clinical Management

Isolated simple cysts with no ominous features are managed conservatively.

If large and painful, aspiration can be performed for symptomatic relief.

If associated with gynecomastia, primary treatment is directed toward gynecomastia.

32.5 Fibroadenoma

Fibroadenomas are rare in the male breast owing to the absence of glandular lobules.

32.5.1 Etiopathogenesis

It has been proposed that many of these have developed during estrogen stimulation [11–13].

32.5.2 Clinical Presentation

Usually presents as a painless palpable lump.

32.5.3 Imaging

32.5.3.1 Mammogram

A well-circumscribed equal density lesion with no omnious features.

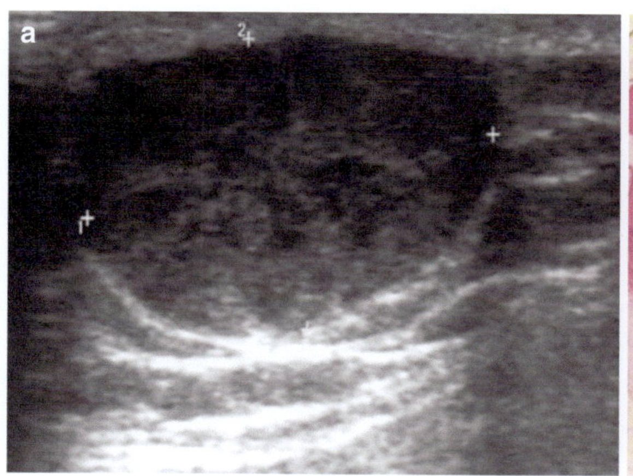

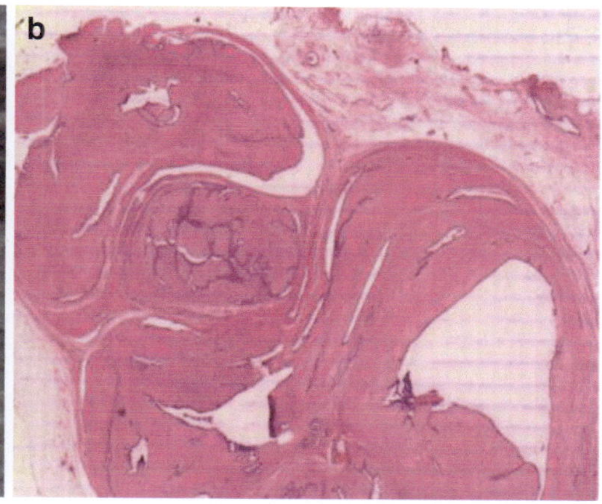

Fig. 32.9 Fibroadenoma. (**a**) USG reveals a circumscribed heteroechoeic lesion with posterior enhancement. (**b**) H&E-Fibroadenoma showing a circumscribed lesion composed of glandular epithelium with a few dilated ducts in a fibrous stroma (2.5×)

32.5.3.2 Ultrasound

Imaging findings are similar to those of fibroadenomas in the female breast (Fig. 32.9).

It appears as an oval, hypoechoic mass that is circumscribed, with well-defined margins, and some cases may show few soft lobulations.

32.5.4 BI-RADS Category: BI-RADS 3

32.5.5 Clinical Management

In case of positive family history/discordant clinical findings, image-guided biopsy/excision biopsy is indicated.

32.6 Intraductal Papilloma

32.6.1 Introduction

Benign intraductal papillomas, although rare, can occur in the male breast.

32.6.2 Clinical Presentation

As in women, breast papillomas in men usually manifest as nipple discharge or a palpable subareolar mass. Most intraductal papillomas are solitary and are located in the central breast.

32.6.3 Imaging

32.6.3.1 Mammogram

It can be visualized as well-circumscribed round or oval, equal density lesion, usually in the subareolar region (Fig. 32.10).

32.6.3.2 Ultrasound

It is more sensitive than mammography or galactography for the detection of papillomas, which typically manifest as an intraluminal mass within a dilated duct or as an solid cystic lesion (Fig. 32.11).

32.6.3.3 Color Doppler

A "stalk" of internal vascularity can be seen.

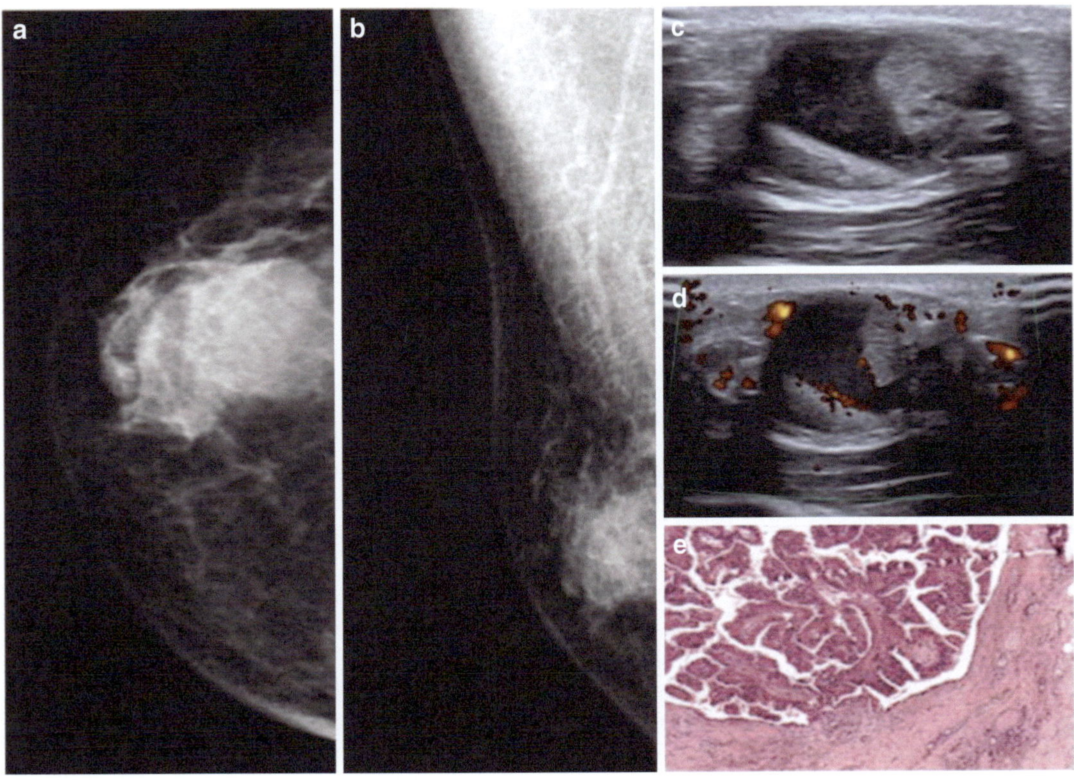

Fig. 32.10 Benign intraductal papilloma. (**a**, **b**) CC and MLO view of the right breast shows a partly obscured high-density lesion in the upper outer quadrant. (**c**) USG shows a solid cystic lesion with vascularity within the solid component (**d**). (**e**) H&E stained photomicrograph of a benign papillary neoplasm composed of benign epithelial and myoepithelial cells enclosing a prominent fibrovascular core within a large, dilated duct (20×)

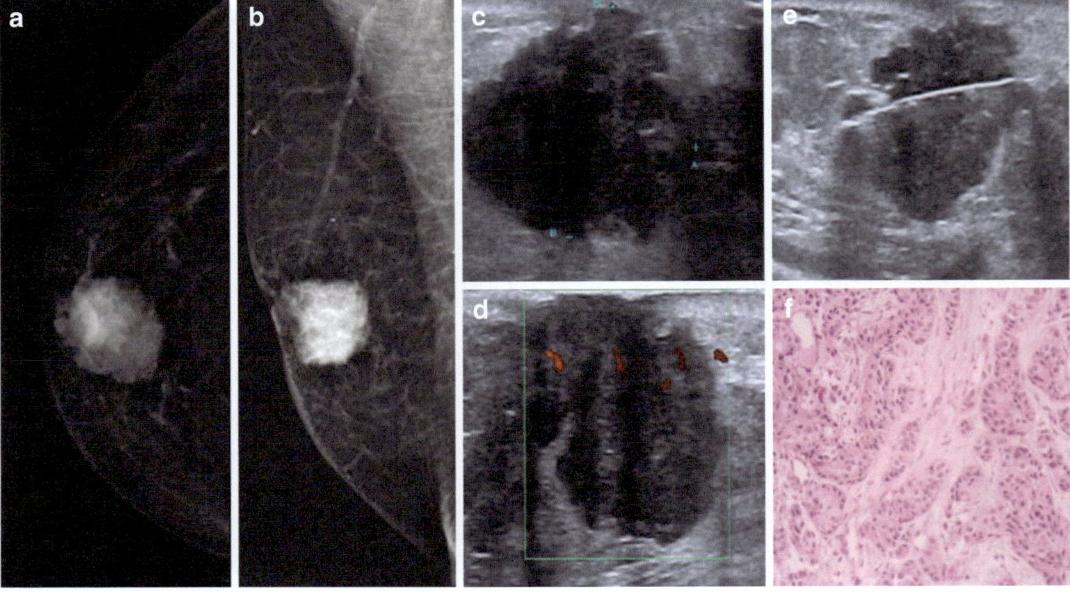

Fig. 32.11 Invasive ductal carcinoma. (**a**, **b**) CC and MLO view of the right breast reveals an irregular high-density mass in the subareolar region with mild nipple retraction. (**c**) Ultrasound reveals irregular hypoechoic lesion with increased vascularity (**d**). (**e**) USG guided tru cut biopsy. (**f**) H&E stained photomicrograph of invasive carcinoma of the breast, no special type (NST) composed of nests of pleomorphic cells infiltrating the stroma (20×)

An ultrasound with no identifiable lesion in patient with nipple discharge does not allow exclusion of intraductal papilloma, since at times it is difficult to visualize when the duct is not distended with fluid at the time of examination.

32.6.4 BI-RADS Category: BI-RADS 4A

32.6.4.1 Histology

Benign papillary lesions are composed of two layers of cells, one ductal epithelial cell layer and an underling myoepithelial cell layer supported by a vascular core.

32.6.4.2 Clinical Management

Excision biopsy to rule out occult invasive component.

32.7 Carcinoma of the Male Breast

32.7.1 Introduction

Male breast cancer is uncommon accounting for <1% of all male cancers and less than 0.1% of male cancer deaths [14].

The common malignant lesions are ductal carcinoma in situ, invasive ductal carcinoma (most common ~85% cases), and papillary neoplasm (~2.6% are papillary carcinomas) and rarely lobular carcinoma (~1.5%) [15].

32.7.2 Etiopathogenesis

1. Increased levels of estradiol and estrogenic hormones [16].
2. Undescended testis, testicular atrophy post-orchitis, late puberty, and infertility.
3. Prostate cancer [17].
4. Trauma, radiationexposure, pituitarydysfunction, Klienfelter's syndrome [18, 19].
5. Gynecomastia and its risk for developing breast cancer is unclear.
6. Familial history: Cutuli et al. found a positive family history of breast cancer in 5.6% of 397 men with breast carcinoma. Another study by Casagrande et al. reported a two-fold increased risk of breast carcinoma among first degree relatives of male breast cancer patients.
7. Genes such as BRCA1/2, loss of heterozygosity on chromosome 11q13, RAD51B, CHEK2, PTEN, and CYP17 have been implicated in the etiology of male breast cancer [20–23].

32.7.3 Clinical Presentation

The usual presentation is a palpable, firm, painless, immobile mass, bloody nipple discharge (25% of cases), and palpable ipsilateral axillary lymphadenopathy. Sometimes lesions are identified due to nipple ulceration and retraction. The average age at diagnosis is between 60 and 67 years; however, it can be seen in all ages [24].

Coexisting gynecomastia has been reported in up to 40% of cases, although it as a risk factor is debatable [15].

In men, breast cancer is diagnosed at age approximately 5–10 years older than the age at which it is diagnosed in women. Due to delay in diagnosis, men usually present at a more advanced stage of cancer than women.

Most of the lesions are in the retroareolar region. Lesions in the upper outer quadrant have also been described. Rarely bilateral lesions have been found.

32.7.4 Imaging Features

Overall, there is no significant difference in the imaging findings as compared to female breast malignancy changes.

32.7.5 Invasive Ductal Carcinoma

32.7.5.1 Mammogram

An irregular high-density spiculated/round/oval mass, or irregular subareolar mass with circumscribed, indistinct, spiculated, or microlobulated margins (Fig. 32.11).

The other secondary features such as skin thickening, nipple retraction, and axillary lymphadenopathy may be associated.

Microcalcifications are uncommon in male breast cancers and are seen in only 13–30% of cases [15].

32.7.5.2 Ultrasound

An ill-defined poorly circumscribed hypoechoic mass with spiculated/angular margins. It may or may not be associated with posterior features (Fig. 32.11).

However, up to 20% of male breast carcinomas are circumscribed [25].

Malignant mass in men is usually seen in the subareolar region that is eccentric to the nipple, a feature distinguishing it from gynecomastia.

On color Doppler, it may show internal or peripheral vascularity.

32.7.5.3 MRI

Generally not indicated. It can be reserved for cases with inconclusive imaging findings/discordant clinical findings.

MRI helps to distinguish gynecomastia from malignancy based on the contrast enhancement pattern, that is, the early enhancement and washout characteristics on dynamic contrast scan. It follows the type I kinetic curve.

32.7.6 Papillary Carcinoma of Breast

It accounts for approximately 2.6% of male breast cancer.

The majority of male papillary carcinomas are intracystic type and noninvasive.

32.7.7 Clinical presentation

The most common presentation is bleeding per nipple/nipple discharge/palpable mass.

32.7.7.1 Imaging

Mammogram

Typically present as a subareolar mass that may have circumscribed, irregular, or spiculated margins (Fig. 32.12).

Ultrasound

Usually seen as a complex cyst or as a mixed solid cystic mass. The solid component typically presents as a mural nodule or papillary projection arising from the cyst wall (Fig. 32.12).

Color Doppler

The solid component shows internal vascularity.

32.7.8 Lobular Carcinoma of Breast

Invasive lobular carcinoma is a rare histologic subtype in men, accounting for only 1.5% of cases. Associations with Klinefelter syndrome and increased estrogen exposure have been reported.

32.7.8.1 Clinical Presentation

It usually presents a palpable mass in the breast.

32.7.8.2 Imaging

Mammogram

The typical presentation at mammography is a spiculated mass or area of architectural distortion.

Ultrasound

Ultrasound typically shows an irregular, hypoechoic, or mixed echogenicity mass.

Invasive lobular carcinoma can be found in conjunction with invasive ductal carcinoma.

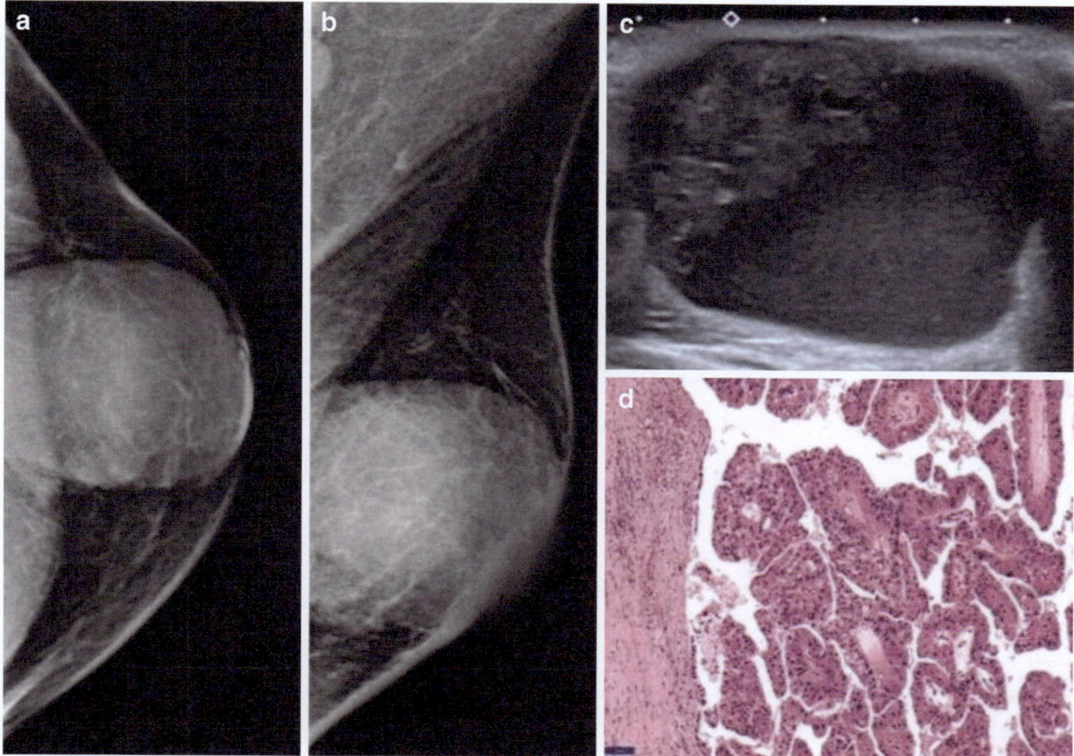

Fig. 32.12 Encapsulated papillary carcinoma. (**a**, **b**) CC and MLO view of the left breast reveals a high density lesion in the subareolar region. (**c**) Correlative ultrasound reveals solid cystic lesion. (**d**) H&E stained photomicrograph, demonstrating a complex branching papillary growth pattern lined by columnar cells enclosing a fibrovascular core suggestive of an encapsulated papillary carcinoma (40×)

32.7.8.3 BI-RADS Category: BI-RADS 4C/5

Pathology of Male Breast Cancers

FNAC

Fine needle aspiration usually shows dispersed cells with atypia and mitosis. Caution to be excised as findings may overlap with gynecomastia. Background myoepithelial cells and cohesive sheets give a clue to the diagnosis of gynecomastia.

Gross Examination

Identical to female breast cancers. Cystic papillary carcinomas may present with striking features grossly.

Histopathology

Majority (85%) are of invasive ductal carcinoma (IDC), no special type. Two percent can be lobular type, and 13% are papillary, mixed, other morphologies. Papillary carcinomas are usually intracystic (encapsulated papillary carcinoma), and they are more commonly seen in men than in women [26]. DCIS may be found in 35–50% male breast carcinomas. Rare isolated lobular carcinomas have been described. Other carcinomas like micropapillary, medullary, adenoidcystic, mucinous, secretory and carcinoma with osteoclastic giant cells have been reported [27].

Immunohistochemistry

Eighty to ninety percent cases are estrogen and progesterone receptor positive [28]. Her 2 neu positivity have also been found to a different degree in various studies [29]. Positivity for EGFR (epithelial growth factor receptor) and TP53 have been observed in various studies. AR, cyclin D1, and Bcl2 expressions have also been documented.

32.7.8.4 Clinical Management

Total mastectomy and axillary dissection is recommended. This may be followed by radiation in patients with large tumors with risk of recurrence.

Hormonal therapy with tamoxifen is considered effective. Chemotherapy with methotrexate is also used routinely.

32.7.8.5 Follow Up and Prognosis

Prognosis is related to the stage at diagnosis, tumor size, and nodal status. Tumor size larger than 2 cm and poor histologic differentiation are considered unfavorable prognostic factors.

References

1. Kopans DB. Breast imaging. Philadelphia: Lippincott; 1998. p. 497–509.
2. Johnson RE, Kermott CA, Murad MH. Gynecomastia–evaluation and current treatment options. Ther Clin Risk Manag. 2011;7:145–8.
3. Dickson G. Gynecomastia. Am Fam Physician. 2012;85(7):716–22.
4. Mainiero MB, Lourenco AP, Barke LD, Argus AD, Bailey L, Carkaci S, et al. ACR appropriateness criteria evaluation of the symptomatic male breast. J Am Coll Radiol. 2015;12(7):678–82.
5. Chesebro AL, Rives AF, Shaffer K. Male breast disease: what the radiologist needs to know. Curr Probl Diagn Radiol. 2019;48(5):482–93.
6. Nguyen C, Kettler MD, Swirsky ME, Miller VI, Scott C, Krause R, et al. Male breast disease: pictorial review with radiologic-pathologic correlation. Radiographics. 2013;33(3):763–79. https://doi.org/10.1148/rg.333125137.
7. Draghi F, Tarantino CC, Madonia L, Ferrozzi G. Ultrasonography of the male breast. J Ultrasound. 2011;14(3):122–9.
8. Cuhaci N, Polat SB, Evranos B, Ersoy R, Cakir B. Gynecomastia: clinical evaluation and management. Indian J Endocrinol Metab. 2014;18(2):150.
9. Zimmerman RL, Fogt F, Cronin D, Lynch R. Cytologic atypia in a 53-year-old man with finasteride-induced gynecomastia. Arch Pathol Lab Med. 2000;124(4):625–7.
10. Gatalica Z, Norris BA, Kovatich AJ. Immunohistochemical localization of prostate-specific antigen in ductal epithelium of male breast. Potential diagnostic pitfall in patients with gynecomastia. Appl Immunohistochem Mol Morphol. 2000;8(2):158–61.
11. Lemmo G, Garcea N, Corsello S, Tarquini E, Palladino T, Ardito G, et al. Breast fibroadenoma in a male-to-female transsexual patient after hormonal treatment. Eur J Surg Suppl. 2003;588:69–71.
12. Kanhai RC, Hage JJ, Bloemena E, van Diest PJ, Karim RB. Mammary fibroadenoma in a male-to-female transsexual. Histopathology. 1999;35(2):183–5.
13. Ansah-Boateng Y, Tavassoli FA. Fibroadenoma and cystosarcoma phyllodes of the male breast. Mod Pathol. 1992;5(2):114–6.
14. Sharma D, Singh G. Male breast cancer: an overview. J Radiat Cancer Res. 2017;8(2):98–102.
15. Chau A, Jafarian N, Rosa M. Male breast: clinical and imaging evaluations of benign and malignant entities with histologic correlation. Am J Med. 2016;129(8):776–91.
16. Nirmul D, Pegoraro RJ, Jialal I, Naidoo C, Joubert SM. The sex hormone profile of male patients with breast cancer. Br J Cancer. 1983;48(3):423–7.
17. Sobin LH, Sherif M. Relation between male breast cancer and prostate cancer. Br J Cancer. 1980;42(5):787–90.
18. Eldar S, Nash E, Abrahamson J. Radiation carcinogenesis in the male breast. Eur J Surg Oncol. 1989;15(3):274–8.
19. Dodge OG, Jackson AW, Muldal S. Breast cancer and interstitial-cell tumor in a patient with Klinefelter's syndrome. Cancer. 1969;24(5):1027–32.
20. Ford D, Easton DF, Stratton M, Narod S, Goldgar D, Devilee P, et al. Genetic heterogeneity and penetrance analysis of the BRCA1 and BRCA2 genes in breast cancer families. The breast cancer linkage consortium. Am J Hum Genet. 1998;62(3):676–89.
21. Sanz-Ortega J, Chuaqui R, Zhuang Z, Sobel ME, Sanz-Esponera J, Liotta LA, et al. Loss of heterozygosity on chromosome 11q13 in microdissected human male breast carcinomas. J Natl Cancer Inst. 1995;87(18):1408–10.
22. Wasielewski M, den Bakker MA, van den Ouweland A, Meijer-van Gelder ME, Portengen H, Klijn JGM, et al. CHEK2 1100delC and male breast cancer in the Netherlands. Breast Cancer Res Treat. 2009;116(2):397–400.
23. Young IE, Kurian KM, Annink C, Kunkler IH, Anderson VA, Cohen BB, et al. A polymorphism in the CYP17 gene is associated with male breast cancer. Br J Cancer. 1999;81(1):141–3.
24. Hill T, Khamis H, Tyczynski J, Berkel H. Comparison of male and female breast cancer incidence trends, tumor characteristics, and survival. Ann Epidemiol. 2005;15:773–80.

25. Yitta S, Singer CI, Toth HB, Mercado CL. Image presentation. Sonographic appearances of benign and malignant male breast disease with mammographic and pathologic correlation. J Ultrasound Med. 2010;29(6):931–47.
26. Norris HJ, Taylor HB. Carcinoma of the male breast. Cancer. 1969;23(6):1428–35.
27. Burga AM, Fadare O, Lininger RA, Tavassoli FA. Invasive carcinomas of the male breast: a morphologic study of the distribution of histologic subtypes and metastatic patterns in 778 cases. Virchows Arch. 2006;449(5):507–12.
28. Jaggessarsingh D, Catalano J, Akram M, Brogi E, Murray M. Male breast carcinoma: clinicopathologic and molecular analysis of 89 cases. In: Laboratory investigation. vol. 93. New York: Springer Nature; 2013. p. 47a–48a.
29. Rayson D, Erlichman C, Suman VJ, Roche PC, Wold LE, Ingle JN, Donohue JH. Molecular markers in male breast carcinoma. Cancer. 1998;83(9):1947–55.

Familial Breast Cancer

33

Suma Chakrabarthi

Abstract

Breast cancer is the commonest cancer amongst women in the world today, and about 5–10% of breast cancers have a strong inherited component. The aim of this chapter is to give an overall idea to specialists of all disciplines including general practitioners about familial breast cancers. We look at the genes that increase the risk of breast cancer, learn about methods of risk assessment and delve into the concepts of absolute and relative risks of breast cancer. The clinical features, imaging findings and pathology characteristics of these cancers that differ from sporadic breast cancers have been discussed. Genetic testing and risk reduction options have also been discussed. An attempt has also been made to understand how the knowledge of high-risk breast cancer can be exploited positively for targeted treatment of breast cancer.

Keywords

Familial breast cancer · Hereditary breast cancer · High risk of breast cancer · High penetrance genes of breast cancer · Risk assessment for breast cancer · Genetic testing for breast cancer · BRCA1 and BRCA2 mutation carriers · Risk reduction options for familial breast cancer

33.1 Introduction

Breast cancer is the commonest cancer amongst women in the world today and is in most cases associated with somatic mutation in breast cells that are acquired in one's lifetime. Hence, the mutations are not inherited, and the cases are not clustered in families. However, germline mutations can lead to hereditary or familial breast cancer with the specific genetic factors involved determining the inherited cancer risk [1, 2]. The first known reference to familial breast cancer was made in 1866 by the French doctor Pierre P. Broca in his treatise Traité des tumours [3–5].

Of all the known risk factors for breast cancer, family history is the strongest, and studies estimate that about 5–10% of breast cancers have a strong inherited component. About 4–5% breast cancers are due to high penetrance genes transmitted in an autosomal dominant (AD) fashion [6]. Lower risk genes have been identified from association studies, and it is likely that hereditary factors play a role in a proportion of the remaining breast cancers, but it is hard to quantify this perfectly [7, 8]. Twin studies estimate that up to 27% of breast cancers are due to hereditary factors [9].

S. Chakrabarthi (✉)
Department of Radiology and Imaging, Peerless Hospital, Kolkata, India

B. Dev, L. D. Joseph (eds.), *Holistic Approach to Breast Disease*,
https://doi.org/10.1007/978-981-99-0035-0_33

33.2 Genes That Increase Risk of Breast Cancer

A specific predisposing gene is identified in less than 30% of cases with a suggestive personal and/or family history. The breast cancer susceptibility genes and alleles identified so far can be classified into high, moderate and low penetrant categories based on the risk they confer [10]. Some of the genes also increase the risk of other malignancies such as ovarian, prostate, pancreas and melanoma.

Mutations in one of the rare highly penetrant genes such as BRCA1, BRCA2, PTEN, TP53, CDH1 and STK11 confer about 40–85% lifetime risk of breast cancer. Of these, the BRCA1 and BRCA2 germline mutations are the commonest and attribute to about 15–20% of the familial breast cancer risk [10]. Hereditary breast and ovarian cancer, a genetic tumour syndrome of breast and ovarian malignant tumours, is most commonly caused by BRCA1 and BRCA2 mutations [11]. BRCA1 plays a role in DNA repair including homologous recombination and nucleotide excision repair and regulation of cell-cycle progression in particular checkpoint control [12]. BRCA2 is a mediator of the core mechanism of homologous recombination [12]. A mutation in these genes hampers their normal protective function leading to formation of tumours. Germline mutations in *PTEN, TP53, STK11* and *CDH1* are very rare and account for <1% of the familial breast cancers [8, 10] (Table 33.1).

Mutation in moderate penetrance genes such as CHEK2, BRIP, ATM and PALB account for an additional 2–3% cases, with a lifetime risk of about 20–40% [6, 13]. Low-risk genes such as single nucleotide polymorphisms (SNP) have been identified by genome-wide association studies, but an individual SNP is likely to contribute to a risk quite small [6, 13, 14].

Men with BRCA1 and BRCA2 mutation have a lifetime risk of 1.2% and 6.8% (by age 70 years), respectively, compared to a risk of 0.1% in the general population [15, 16]. Among men diagnosed with breast cancer, approximately 10% and 40% carry BRCA1 and BRCA2 mutation, respectively [16]. The risk of developing breast cancer in men is highest in their 30 s and 40 s and decreases with age. This is more pronounced in BRCA2 mutation carriers whose relative risk at 30 years is 22.3 times that at the age of 70 years [15].

Table 33.1 High penetrance genes [2, 6, 13, 14, 17–20]

Gene	Chromosome (cr) location	Lifetime risk of breast cancer in women	Proportion of familial breast cancer risk	Inheritance pattern	Other associated tumours
BRCA1	cr17	60–85%	5–10%	AD	Ovary, pancreas
BRCA2	Cr 13	40–85%	5–10%	AD	Ovary, prostate, gastric, cholangiocarcinoma, melanoma, pancreas
TP53 (Li Fraumeni syndrome)	Cr 17	80–90%	0.1%	AD	Sarcoma, glioma, adrenal, leukemia
PTEN (Cowden syndrome)	Cr 10	25–50%	0.02%	AD	Thyroid, colorectal, endometrium, kidney, multiple hamartomas
E-cadherin (CDH1)	cr16	40–60%	0.1%	AD	Gastric, colon
STK11 (Peutz-Jeghers syndrome)	Cr 19	50%	0.04%	AD	Colorectal, small bowel, pancreas, gastric, oesophagus, sex-cord stromal tumours, gastrointestinal hamartomatous polyps

33.3 Risk Assessment

An accurate family history with data of three generation pedigree including both maternal and paternal history is the most important information. In families where breast cancer shows an AD inheritance, risk assessment is easier and depends on the prior probability of inheriting mutation and the penetrance of the gene. Risk estimation has to be based on large epidemiological studies in the absence of dominant family history [6].

There are a number of risk assessment/prediction models available, which can be used to estimate the risk of carrying the BRCA genes and the overall breast cancer risk for the individual. These include Claus, Ford, BRCAPRO, Tyrer-Cuzic, Breast and ovarian analysis of disease incidence and carrier estimation algorithm (BOADICEA) models and Manchester Scoring System [21–29]. The assessment is best carried out in dedicated high-risk clinics.

33.4 Absolute Versus Relative Risk

Risk is a quantitative measure of the probability of developing or dying from a particular disease such as cancer. Absolute risk is a measure of the probability of developing cancer over a specified time interval [30]. Lifetime risk is an absolute risk. An overall lifetime risk for developing invasive breast cancer is approximately one in eight for women in the United States, which means a lifetime risk of 12.9% [31]. Lifetime risk varies across the world. For example, only 1 in 29 Indian women will develop breast cancer during their lifetime (0–74 years) [32].

Relative risk of breast cancer is a ratio of the probability of developing breast cancer in the exposed group versus the probability of breast cancer occurring in the non-exposed group. The exposure can be to any risk factor [33]. BRCA1 and BRCA2 carriers have a relative risk of 10. Family history of breast cancer in first degree relative aged ≤50 years increases risk for an individual, with a relative risk of ≥2. This means the risk of developing breast cancer almost doubles for this individual. The risk triples if two first degree relatives have breast cancer [14]. The risk is also higher if the cancer was diagnosed in the relatives at a younger age [6]. For example, women have three to four times population risk if they have one first degree relative diagnosed under the age of 40 years or two first or second degree relatives diagnosed under the age of 60 years [14]. Bilateral breast cancer, multiple cases on one side of the family, association with other cancers such as ovarian cancer, early onset sarcoma or male relative with early onset prostate cancer also increase the risk [6]. To make sense of the relative risk one needs to know the absolute risk [34].

33.5 Clinical Features

Usually there are no phenotypic changes or external markers to help us identify a faulty gene. In a small proportion of cases when the genetic abnormality is associated with clinical features of a syndrome, phenotypic changes can be detected. Mucocutaneous manifestations and macrocephaly in Cowden's Disease (CD) predate breast neoplasms [14, 35]. Bannayan-Riley—Ruvalcaba Syndrome (BRRS) is characterised by macrocephaly, pigmented maculae on the glans penis, developmental delay and mental retardation [36]. Both CD and BRRS are characterised by hamartomas and are part of the PTEN hamartoma tumour syndrome [37]. Mucocutaneous pigmentation may be detectable in Peutz-Jegher's syndrome [38].

Familial breast cancers are more likely to present earlier in life, more so in Asian countries where it is known that women develop breast cancer in general at a younger age when compared to the Caucasian population [39–41]. Bilateral breast cancer, second ipsilateral primary breast cancer and association with other cancers such as ovarian, colon, prostate, pancreatic, endometrial, and male breast cancers and sarcomas are recognised features [41–43]. *BRCA1/2* mutation carriers diagnosed with breast cancer have a long-term risk of developing a contralateral tumour as high as 60% to 70% as opposed to only 11% of patients with breast cancer in the general population [16, 41].

33.6 Radiological Features

The sensitivity of mammography is lower in BRCA carriers due to multiple factors such as dense breasts in younger women and mammographic appearance overlapping with benign lesions [16]. These can present as interval cancers in a screening programme due to the above reasons and because they have a higher growth rate and hence a short lead time [44]. The more easily identifiable suspicious features of spiculated mass, architectural distortion and malignant calcifications are less frequent in BRCA mutation carriers [16]. A common mammographic feature of BRCA-associated breast cancers is a well-defined mass described by some as fibroadenoma-like masses without calcifications, but with internal enhancement or enhancement kinetics not fibroadenoma-like at breast MR imaging [45] (Fig. 33.1). The shape can be round or oval. BRCA1 carriers are more likely to demonstrate such masses when compared to BRCA2 carriers. Suspicious microcalcifications are more common in BRCA2 carriers, who may present as pure ductal carcinoma in situ (DCIS) disease

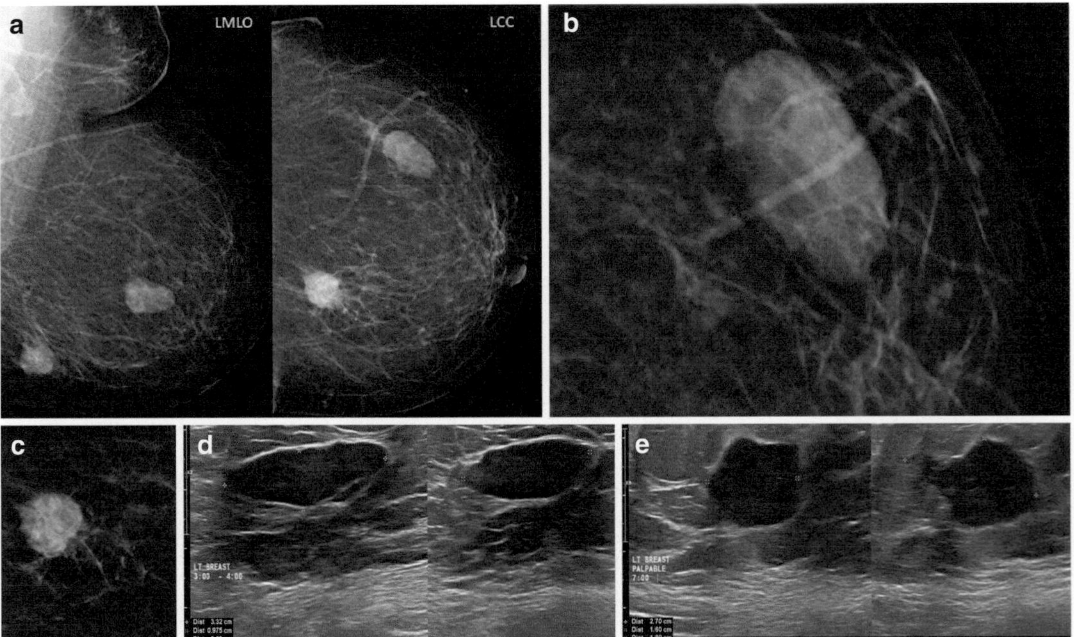

Fig. 33.1 (**a**) Left mediolateral oblique (MLO) and craniocaudal (CC) mammography images of a 43 year-old high-risk lady. There is a mass in the left lower inner breast, which corresponds to the palpable mass with which the lady presented. Another mass is seen in the outer central breast. (**b**) CC spot compression view of the left outer central breast mass demonstrates an oval, low density mass with circumscribed margin, in keeping with a fibroadenoma. (**c**) CC spot compression view of the left lower inner breast mass demonstrates that its margin is partly circumscribed and partly indistinct, its density is high and its shape is irregular rather than oval. Overall, it has a fibroadenoma-like appearance, although upon careful observation the sinister features are obvious. (**d**) Ultrasound image demonstrates a 3.3 × 1 × 2.6 cm oval parallel circumscribed hypoechoic mass in the left lower outer (3–4 o'clock position) breast. This was confirmed to be a fibroadenoma on core biopsy. (**e**) Ultrasound image demonstrates a 2.7 × 1.6 × 1.8 cm mass in the left lower inner (7 o'clock position) breast. It has a margin that is mostly circumscribed but is indistinct at places, an irregular shape and parallel orientation. This fibroadenoma-like mass shows sinister features upon careful assessment. Core biopsy demonstrated a triple negative grade 3 invasive ductal carcinoma

[46]. Prevalence of malignant calcifications in BRCA2 carriers is similar to the 30–50% seen in sporadic invasive cancers [16]. Women at high risk should have ultrasound and biopsy of all mammography masses even if they are well defined [47]. At ultrasound, BRCA1-associated cancers are often round, well circumscribed, homogeneously hypoechoic and demonstrate posterior accentuation [16, 48].

MRI is more sensitive for detecting breast cancers than mammography or ultrasound alone in BRCA1 and BRCA2 mutation carriers [16, 49]. On post-contrast sequences, they are more likely to demonstrate rim enhancement in keeping with their aggressive nature [50]. They may demonstrate homogeneous enhancement or non-mass like enhancement also, and they often demonstrate malignant type kinetic properties on dynamic imaging [16, 45]. DCIS is best detected by a combination of mammography and MRI [51]. BRCA-related cancers in men are more likely to be of higher grade, and biopsy of breast masses in men is advised even if the mass looks well defined as approximately a fifth of these cancers have been reported to be well defined [16]. BRCA1 carriers are known to develop fewer bone metastases but more lung and distant lymphnode metastases, whereas BRCA2 carriers and non-carriers develop bone metastases more often [52, 53].

33.7 Histopathology

BRCA1 mutation carriers are more likely to be diagnosed with triple negative breast cancer, p53 positivity, a basal-like immunophenotype and a higher histologic grade when compared to women with no BRCA1 mutation. High mitotic count, continuous pushing margins and lymphocytic infiltrate are noted in BRCA1 mutations [54]. Medullary carcinoma and invasive ductal carcinoma with medullary features are associated with BRCA1 mutation, with 7.8–19% medullary carcinomas and 35–60% showing some medullary features, in contrast to only 2% in sporadic and BRCA2 mutation-associated breast tumours [55, 56] (Fig. 33.2). The most frequently mutated

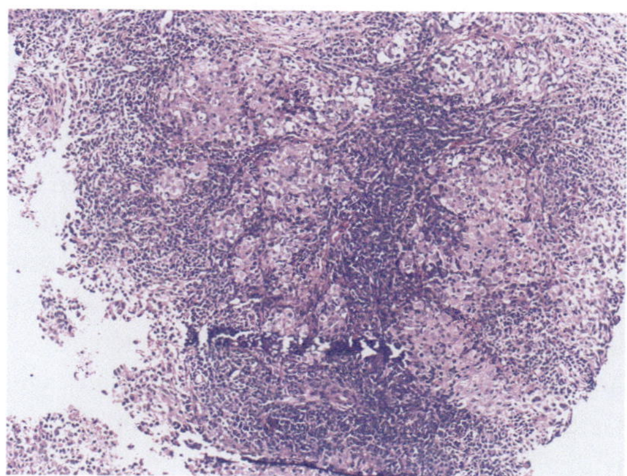

Fig. 33.2 Histology of a palpable mass of a high-risk 41 year-old lady demonstrates grade 3 triple negative medullary carcinoma with pushing borders, syncytial growth pattern, high-grade nuclei and prominent lymphoid infiltrate. (Image contributed by Dr. Sugat Sanyal, Department of Pathology, Peerless Hospital, Kolkata)

gene in invasive breast cancer is TP53 (p53) and is seen in 30–35% of all cases of breast cancer, although p53 is mutated in approximately 80% of triple-negative tumours [57, 58]. DCIS is almost never identified in BRCA1-associated breast cancer [16]. BRCA2 mutation carriers have clinicopathologic features that are more similar to sporadic breast carcinomas [59–62]. However, they tend to have a higher grade when compared to cancers in age-matched control patients with sporadic cancers [16]. They tend to be luminal-type tumours, positive for oestrogen receptor (ER) and progesterone receptor (PR) and lack expression of HER2 [11]. They also have a high rate of male breast cancer and lower incidence of ovarian cancer [54].

33.8 Genetic Testing

Molecular genetic testing options include BRCA1 and BRCA2 gene panel and multigene panel [63]. The best test candidate in a family is a person who has a BRCA1 or BRCA2-associated cancer such as a breast cancer diagnosed very early in life [63]. Guidelines are available for genetic/familial high-risk assessment and genetic counselling [39]. Testing criteria for high penetrance genes includes known mutation in a blood relative, personal history of breast cancer at <45 years of age, triple negative breast cancer diagnosed at <60 years of age and male breast cancer at any age. Genetic testing is advisable for women diagnosed with breast cancer between the ages of 46 and 50 years who have unknown/limited family history available, diagnosis of a second breast cancer at any age, more than one close blood relative with breast, ovarian, pancreatic or high-grade/intraductal prostate cancer at any age. Genetic testing is also appropriate for women with a personal history of epithelial ovarian cancer, including fallopian tube and peritoneal cancer at any age [64]. These guidelines are likely to vary from place to place, and following the national/regional/local guidelines is advisable. The individual must be appropriately counselled prior to genetic testing. Psychological assessment and support must be provided, and pros and cons of genetic testing must be discussed before obtaining informed consent for testing [65]. All male patients with breast cancer should undergo genetic counselling [39].

33.9 Risk Reduction

Screening and surveillance programmes for early detection reduce risk by reducing mortality. Mammography and/or MRI Breast are used for screening women at high risk [66, 67].

The extreme step of undergoing bilateral prophylactic mastectomy reduces the risk of breast cancer by approximately 90% in women with BRCA1/2 mutations [68]. BRCA-positive women with stage I or II breast cancer are less likely to die from breast cancer if they undergo bilateral mastectomy when compared to women who are treated with unilateral mastectomy [69, 70]. Surgery does not give a 100% protection from breast cancer as it is not possible to remove all breast tissue. Counselling about possible surgical complications, long-term psychosocial and sexual consequences is necessary, and the decision should be patient led rather than clinician led [71].

Chemoprevention with selective oestrogen receptor modulators (SERMs) is seen to reduce incidence of invasive oestrogen receptor-positive breast cancer, and they work by binding to the oestrogen receptor and inhibiting the stimulus for cell division [72]. Tamoxifen treatment of the first cancer is shown to reduce the risk of developing a subsequent contralateral cancer [73]. SERMs tamoxifen and raloxifene and aromatase inhibitors anastrazole and exemestane have been advised in guidelines for women at high risk, although a meticulous check for contraindications must be made, which includes bilateral mastectomy. Of these, anastrozole, exemestane and raloxifene are not to be used in premenopausal women [71, 74].

Most guidelines recommend risk-reducing salpingo-oophorectomy to be performed between the ages of 35 and 40 years in women with BRCA1/2 mutation for prevention of ovarian cancer [75–82]. However, the effect of oophorectomy on breast cancer for premenopausal women with no personal history of breast cancer has been debated and may be considered after careful counselling and should be managed by a multidisciplinary team [71, 79–81]. In premenopausal women diagnosed with breast cancer, oophorectomy is used as adjuvant treatment for ER-positive cancers. This also allows the use of adjuvant aromatase inhibitors, which are effective only in postmenopausal women and are superior to tamoxifen [83, 84].

33.10 Impact on Treatment

At present, treatment recommendations for BRCA-associated breast cancer include mainly surgery, radiotherapy and chemotherapy, similar to sporadic breast cancers [41]. Knowledge specific to BRCA-associated tumours can be used to make an impact on treatment of breast cancer in these patients. Studies suggest that platinum-containing chemotherapy may benefit women with BRCA1 mutation with a high rate of pathologic complete response noted after neoadjuvant chemotherapy with Cisplatin [85–88]. Polyadenosine diphosphate-ribose polymerase (PARP) proteins like BRCA proteins help repair DNA damage in cells. PARP inhibitors acting on cancer cells may lead to further DNA damage and cell death in a cell that already has a defect in DNA repair due to BRCA mutation. Olaparib, a PARB inhibitor, given after completion of local treatment and adjuvant or neoadjuvant chemotherapy has shown significant improvement in survival free of invasive or distant disease [89, 90].

33.11 Conclusion

It is hard to objectively quantify the physical and psychological trauma that familial breast cancers cause. The information that is available to us is largely based on the BRCA gene mutations, and we are aware that there is a large gap in our knowledge of familial breast cancers. Further studies on identification, assessment, treatment and prophylaxis are required to treat this condition effectively. Counselling prior to risk assessment and genetic testing as well as after a positive result is of paramount importance in coping with this inherited condition.

References

1. Sung H, Ferlay J, Siegel RL, Laversanne M, Soerjomataram I, Jemal A, et al. Global cancer statistics 2020: GLOBOCAN estimates of incidence and mortality worldwide for 36 cancers in 185 countries. CA Cancer J Clin. 2021;71(3):209–49.
2. Godet I, Gilkes DM. BRCA1 and BRCA2 mutations and treatment strategies for breast cancer. Integr Cancer Sci Ther. 2017; 4(1). https://doi.org/10.15761/ICST.1000228.
3. Van der Groep P, van der Wall E, van Diest PJ. Pathology of hereditary breast cancer. Cell Oncol (Dordr). 2011;34(2):71–88.
4. Broca P. Traité des tumeurs. Paris: P. Asselin; 1869.
5. Krush AJ. Contributions of Pierre Paul Broca to cancer genetics. In: Transactions of the Nebraska Academy of Sciences. Lincoln: Nebraska Academy of Sciences; 1979.
6. Lalloo F, Evans DG. Familial breast cancer. Clin Genet. 2012;82:105–14.
7. Seal S, Thompson D, Renwick A, Elliott A, Kelly P, Barfoot R, et al. Truncating mutations in the Fanconi anemia J gene BRIP1 are low-penetrance breast cancer susceptibility alleles. Nat Genet. 2006;38(11):1239–41.
8. Stratton MR, Rahman N. The emerging landscape of breast cancer susceptibility. Nat Genet. 2008;40(1):17–22.
9. Peto J, Mack TM. High constant incidence in twins and other relatives of women with breast cancer. Nat Genet. 2000;26(4):411–4.
10. Rivandi M, Martens JWM, Hollestelle A. Elucidating the underlying functional mechanisms of breast cancer susceptibility through post-GWAS analyses. Front Genet. 2018;9:280.
11. Hodgson A, Turashvili G. Pathology of hereditary breast and ovarian cancer. Front Oncol. 2020;10:531790. https://www.frontiersin.org/article/10.3389/fonc.2020.531790.
12. Roy R, Chun J, Powell SN. BRCA1 and BRCA2: different roles in a common pathway of genome protection. Nat Rev Cancer. 2012;12(1):68–78.
13. Shiovitz S, Korde LA. Genetics of breast cancer: a topic in evolution. Ann Oncol. 2015;26(7):1291–9.
14. Dixon JM. ABC of breast diseases. 4th ed. New York: Wiley; 2009. PDF Free Download. https://www.allthingsmedicine.com/abc-of-breast-diseases-4th-edition-pdf/.
15. Tai YC, Domchek S, Parmigiani G, Chen S. Breast cancer risk among male BRCA1 and BRCA2 mutation carriers. J Natl Cancer Inst. 2007;99(23):1811–4.
16. Lee MV, Katabathina VS, Bowerson ML, Mityul MI, Shetty AS, Elsayes KM, et al. BRCA-associated cancers: role of imaging in screening, diagnosis, and management. Radiographics. 2017;37(4):1005–23.
17. Carbognin L, Miglietta F, Paris I, Dieci MV. Prognostic and predictive implications of PTEN in breast cancer: unfulfilled promises but intriguing perspectives. Cancers (Basel). 2019;11(9):1401.
18. Rivlin N, Brosh R, Oren M, Rotter V. Mutations in the p53 tumor suppressor gene. Genes Cancer. 2011;2(4):466–74.
19. Amos CI, Bali D, Thiel TJ, Anderson JP, Gourley I, Frazier ML, et al. Fine mapping of a genetic locus for Peutz-Jeghers syndrome on chromosome 19p. Cancer Res. 1997;57(17):3653–6.
20. Shenoy S. CDH1 (E-cadherin) mutation and gastric cancer: genetics, molecular mechanisms and guidelines for management. Cancer Manag Res. 2019;11:10477–86.
21. Claus EB, Risch N, Thompson WD. Autosomal dominant inheritance of early-onset breast cancer. Implications for risk prediction. Cancer. 1994;73(3):643–51.
22. Engel C, Fischer C. Breast cancer risks and risk prediction models. Breast Care (Basel). 2015;10(1):7–12.
23. Amir E, Evans D, Shenton A, Lalloo F, Moran A, Boggis C, et al. Evaluation of breast cancer risk assessment packages in the family history evaluation and screening programme. J Med Genet. 2003;40(11):807–14.
24. Mazzola E, Chipman J, Cheng S-C, Parmigiani G. Recent BRCAPRO upgrades significantly improve calibration. Cancer Epidemiol Biomark Prev. 2014;23(8):1689–95.
25. Himes DO, Root AE, Gammon A, Luthy KE. Breast cancer risk assessment: calculating lifetime risk using the Tyrer-Cuzick model. J Nurse Pract. 2016;12(9):581–92.

26. Kurian AW, Hughes E, Simmons T, Bernhisel R, Probst B, Meek S, et al. Performance of the IBIS/Tyrer-Cuzick model of breast cancer risk by race and ethnicity in the Women's health initiative. Cancer. 2021;127(20):3742–50.
27. Lee AJ, Cunningham AP, Kuchenbaecker KB, Mavaddat N, Easton DF, Antoniou AC. BOADICEA breast cancer risk prediction model: updates to cancer incidences, tumour pathology and web interface. Br J Cancer. 2014;110(2):535–45.
28. NICE. Familial breast cancer: classification, care and managing breast cancer and related risks in people with a family history of breast cancer. 2022. https://www.nice.org.uk/guidance/cg164/chapter/recommendations#genetic-testing.
29. Kast K, Schmutzler RK, Rhiem K, Kiechle M, Fischer C, Niederacher D, et al. Validation of the Manchester scoring system for predicting BRCA1/2 mutations in 9,390 families suspected of having hereditary breast and ovarian cancer. Int J Cancer. 2014;135(10):2352–61.
30. Joy JE, Penhoet EE, Petitti DB, Institute of Medicine (US) and National Research Council (US) Committee on New Approaches to Early Detection and Diagnosis of Breast Cancer. Saving women's lives: strategies for improving breast cancer detection and diagnosis. Washington (DC): National Academies Press (US); 2005.
31. Feuer EJ, Wun LM, Boring CC, Flanders WD, Timmel MJ, Tong T. The lifetime risk of developing breast cancer. J Natl Cancer Inst. 1993;85(11):892–7.
32. Mathur P, Sathishkumar K, Chaturvedi M, Das P, Sudarshan KL, Santhappan S, et al. Cancer statistics, 2020: report from National Cancer Registry Programme, India. JCO Glob Oncologia. 2020;6:1063–75.
33. Tenny S, Hoffman MR. Relative risk. In: StatPearls. Treasure Island, FL: Stat Pearls Publishing; 2022. http://www.ncbi.nlm.nih.gov/books/NBK430824/.
34. Noordzij M, van Diepen M, Caskey FC, Jager KJ. Relative risk versus absolute risk: one cannot be interpreted without the other. Nephrol Dial Transplant. 2017;32(suppl_2):ii13–8.
35. Miguelote S, Silva R, Fougo JL, Barbosa LE, Araújo Teixeira JP. Cowden syndrome is a risk factor for multiple neoplasm: a case report. World J Surg Oncol. 2020;18(1):211.
36. Hendriks YMC, Verhallen JTCM, van der Smagt JJ, Kant SG, Hilhorst Y, Hoefsloot L, et al. Bannayan-Riley-Ruvalcaba syndrome: further delineation of the phenotype and management of PTEN mutation-positive cases. Familial Cancer. 2003;2(2):79–85.
37. Yehia L, Eng C. PTEN hamartoma tumor syndrome. In: Adam MP, editor. GeneReviews. Seattle: University of Washington; 2021. https://www.ncbi.nlm.nih.gov/books/NBK1488/.
38. McGarrity TJ, Amos CI, Baker MJ. Peutz-Jeghers syndrome. In: Adam MP, editor. GeneReviews. Seattle: University of Washington; 2021. https://www.ncbi.nlm.nih.gov/books/NBK1266/.
39. Daly MB, Pal T, Berry MP, Buys SS, Dickson P, Domchek SM, et al. Genetic/familial high-risk assessment: breast, ovarian, and pancreatic, version 2.2021, NCCN clinical practice guidelines in oncology. J Natl Compr Cancer Netw. 2021;19(1):77–102.
40. Brandt A, Bermejo JL, Sundquist J, Hemminki K. Age of onset in familial breast cancer as background data for medical surveillance. Br J Cancer. 2010;102(1):42–7.
41. Kim E-K, Park SY, Kim S-W. Clinicopathological characteristics of BRCA-associated breast cancer in Asian patients. J Pathol Transl Med. 2020;54(4):265–75.
42. Breast Cancer Linkage Consortium. Cancer risks in BRCA2 mutation carriers. J Natl Cancer Inst. 1999;91(15):1310–6.
43. Thompson D, Easton DF. Breast cancer linkage consortium. Cancer incidence in BRCA1 mutation carriers. J Natl Cancer Inst. 2002;94(18):1358–65.
44. Komenaka IK, Ditkoff B-A, Joseph K-A, Russo D, Gorroochurn P, Ward M, et al. The development of interval breast malignancies in patients with BRCA mutations. Cancer. 2004;100(10):2079–83.
45. Schrading S, Kuhl CK. Mammographic, US, and MR imaging phenotypes of familial breast cancer. Radiology. 2008;246(1):58–70.
46. Hamilton LJ, Evans AJ, Wilson ARM, Scott N, Cornford EJ, Pinder SE, et al. Breast imaging findings in women with BRCA1- and BRCA2-associated breast carcinoma. Clin Radiol. 2004;59(10):895–902.
47. Kaas R, Kroger R, Hendriks JHCL, Besnard APE, Koops W, Pameijer FA, et al. The significance of circumscribed malignant mammographic masses in the surveillance of BRCA 1/2 gene mutation carriers. Eur Radiol. 2004;14(9):1647–53.
48. Rhiem K, Flucke U, Schmutzler RK. BRCA1-associated breast carcinomas frequently present with benign sonographic features. Am J Roentgenol. 2006;186(5):E11–2.
49. Warner E, Plewes DB, Hill KA, Causer PA, Zubovits JT, Jong RA, et al. Surveillance of BRCA1 and BRCA2 mutation carriers with magnetic resonance imaging, ultrasound, mammography, and clinical breast examination. JAMA. 2004;292(11):1317–25.
50. Veltman J, Mann R, Kok T, Obdeijn IM, Hoogerbrugge N, Blickman JG, et al. Breast tumor characteristics of BRCA1 and BRCA2 gene mutation carriers on MRI. Eur Radiol. 2008;18(5):931–8.
51. Kuhl CK, Schrading S, Bieling HB, Wardelmann E, Leutner CC, Koenig R, et al. MRI for diagnosis of pure ductal carcinoma in situ: a prospective observational study. Lancet. 2007;370(9586):485–92.
52. Albiges L, André F, Balleyguier C, Gomez-Abuin G, Chompret A, Delaloge S. Spectrum of breast cancer metastasis in BRCA1 mutation carriers: highly increased incidence of brain metastases. Ann Oncol. 2005;16(11):1846–7.
53. Song Y, Barry WT, Seah DS, Tung NM, Garber JE, Lin NU. Patterns of recurrence and metastasis in

BRCA1/BRCA2-associated breast cancers. Cancer. 2020;126(2):271–80.
54. Lakhani SR. The pathology of familial breast cancer: morphological aspects. Breast Cancer Res. 1999;1(1):31–5.
55. Stratton MR. Pathology of familial breast cancer: differences between breast cancers in carriers of BRCA1 or BRCA2 mutations and sporadic cases. Lancet. 1997;349(9064):1505–10.
56. Limaiem F, Mlika M. Medullary breast carcinoma. In: Stat Pearls. Treasure Island, FL: Stat Pearls Publishing; 2021. https://www.ncbi.nlm.nih.gov/books/NBK542292/.
57. Duffy MJ, Synnott NC, Crown J. Mutant p53 in breast cancer: potential as a therapeutic target and biomarker. Breast Cancer Res Treat. 2018;170(2):213–9.
58. Peng L, Xu T, Long T, Zuo H. Association between BRCA status and P53 status in breast cancer: a meta-analysis. Med Sci Monit. 2016;22:1939–45.
59. Li WF, Hu Z, Rao NY, Song CG, Zhang B, Cao MZ, et al. The prevalence of BRCA1 and BRCA2 germline mutations in high-risk breast cancer patients of Chinese Han nationality: two recurrent mutations were identified. Breast Cancer Res Treat. 2008;110(1):99–109.
60. Musolino A, Bella MA, Bortesi B, Michiara M, Naldi N, Zanelli P, et al. BRCA mutations, molecular markers, and clinical variables in early-onset breast cancer: a population-based study. Breast. 2007;16(3):280–92.
61. Noguchi S, Kasugai T, Miki Y, Fukutomi T, Emi M, Nomizu T. Clinicopathologic analysis of BRCA1- or BRCA2-associated hereditary breast carcinoma in Japanese women. Cancer. 1999;85(10):2200–5.
62. Atchley DP, Albarracin CT, Lopez A, Valero V, Amos CI, Gonzalez-Angulo AM, et al. Clinical and pathologic characteristics of patients with BRCA-positive and BRCA-negative breast cancer. J Clin Oncol. 2008;26(26):4282–8.
63. Petrucelli N, Daly MB, Pal T. BRCA1- and BRCA2-Associated Hereditary Breast and Ovarian Cancer. In: Adam MP, editor. GeneReviews. Seattle: University of Washington; 1993. https://www.ncbi.nlm.nih.gov/books/NBK1247/.
64. Daly MB, Pilarski R, Yurgelun MB, Berry MP, Buys SS, Dickson P, et al. NCCN guidelines insights: genetic/familial high-risk assessment: breast, ovarian, and pancreatic, version 1.2020: featured updates to the NCCN guidelines. J Natl Compr Cancer Netw. 2020;18(4):380–91.
65. Genetic/Familial high-risk assessment: breast and ovarian. NCCN clinical practice guidelines in oncology, version 3.2019. 2022. https://www2.tri-kobe.org/nccn/guideline/gynecological/english/genetic_familial.pdf.
66. Monticciolo DL, Newell MS, Moy L, Niell B, Monsees B, Sickles EA. Breast cancer screening in women at higher-than-average risk: recommendations from the ACR. J Am Coll Radiol. 2018;15(3):408–14.
67. American College of Radiology. ACR Appropriateness Criteria ® Breast Cancer Screening. J Am Coll Radiol. 2017;14(11S):S383–90. https://acsearch.acr.org/docs/70910/narrative/. Accessed 28 Mar 2022.
68. Rebbeck TR, Friebel T, Lynch HT, Neuhausen SL, van't Veer L, Garber JE, et al. Bilateral prophylactic mastectomy reduces breast cancer risk in BRCA1 and BRCA2 mutation carriers: the PROSE study group. J Clin Oncol. 2004;22(6):1055–62.
69. Metcalfe K, Gershman S, Ghadirian P, Lynch HT, Snyder C, Tung N, et al. Contralateral mastectomy and survival after breast cancer in carriers of BRCA1 and BRCA2 mutations: retrospective analysis. BMJ. 2014;348:g226.
70. Teoh V, Tasoulis M-K, Gui G. Contralateral prophylactic mastectomy in women with unilateral breast cancer who are genetic carriers, have a strong family history or are just young at presentation. Cancer. 2020;12(1):140.
71. National Collaborating Centre for Cancer (UK). Familial breast cancer: classification and care of people at risk of familial breast cancer and management of breast cancer and related risks in people with a family history of breast cancer, vol. 2013. Cardiff: National Collaborating Centre for Cancer (UK); 2013. p. 253.
72. Cuzick J, Sestak I, Bonanni B, Costantino JP, Cummings S, DeCensi A, et al. Selective oestrogen receptor modulators in prevention of breast cancer: an updated meta-analysis of individual participant data. Lancet. 2013;381(9880):1827–34.
73. Gronwald J, Robidoux A, Kim-Sing C, Tung N, Lynch HT, Foulkes WD, et al. Duration of tamoxifen use and the risk of contralateral breast cancer in BRCA1 and BRCA2 mutation carriers. Breast Cancer Res Treat. 2014;146(2):421–7.
74. Visvanathan K, Fabian CJ, Bantug E, Brewster AM, Davidson NE, DeCensi A, et al. Use of endocrine therapy for breast cancer risk reduction: ASCO clinical practice guideline update. J Clin Oncol. 2019;37(33):3152–65.
75. Kauff ND, Satagopan JM, Robson ME, Scheuer L, Hensley M, Hudis CA, et al. Risk-reducing salpingo-oophorectomy in women with a BRCA1 or BRCA2 mutation. N Engl J Med. 2002;346(21):1609–15.
76. Rebbeck TR, Lynch HT, Neuhausen SL, Narod SA, van't Veer L, Garber JE, et al. Prophylactic oophorectomy in carriers of BRCA1 or BRCA2 mutations. N Engl J Med. 2002;346(21):1616–22.
77. Rebbeck TR, Kauff ND, Domchek SM. Meta-analysis of risk reduction estimates associated with risk-reducing Salpingo-oophorectomy in BRCA1 or BRCA2 mutation carriers. J Natl Cancer Inst. 2009;101(2):80–7.
78. Kauff ND, Domchek SM, Friebel TM, Robson ME, Lee J, Garber JE, et al. Risk-reducing salpingo-oophorectomy for the prevention of BRCA1- and BRCA2-associated breast and gynecologic cancer: a multicenter prospective study. J Clin Oncol. 2008;26(8):1331–7.
79. Eleje GU, Eke AC, Ezebialu IU, Ikechebelu JI, Ugwu EO, Okonkwo OO. Risk-reducing bilateral salpingo-oophorectomy in women with BRCA1 or

BRCA2 mutations. Cochrane Database Syst Rev. 2018;2018(8):CD012464.
80. Mai PL, Miller A, Gail MH, Skates S, Lu K, Sherman ME, et al. Risk-reducing salpingo-oophorectomy and breast cancer risk reduction in the gynecologic oncology group Protocol-0199 (GOG-0199). JNCI Cancer Spectr. 2019;4(1):pkz075.
81. Mavaddat N, Antoniou AC, Mooij TM, Hooning MJ, Heemskerk-Gerritsen BA, Noguès C, et al. Risk-reducing salpingo-oophorectomy, natural menopause, and breast cancer risk: an international prospective cohort of BRCA1 and BRCA2 mutation carriers. Breast Cancer Res. 2020;22:8.
82. Walker JL, Powell CB, Chen LM, Carter J, Bae Jump VL, Parker LP, Borowsky ME, Gibb RK. Society of Gynecologic Oncology recommendations for the prevention of ovarian cancer. Cancer. 2015;121(13):2108–20. https://doi.org/10.1002/cncr.29321.
83. Meiser B, Tucker K, Friedlander M, Barlow-Stewart K, Lobb E, Saunders C, et al. Genetic counselling and testing for inherited gene mutations in newly diagnosed patients with breast cancer: a review of the existing literature and a proposed research agenda. Breast Cancer Res. 2008;10(6):216.
84. Howell A, Cuzick J, Baum M, Buzdar A, Dowsett M, Forbes JF, et al. Results of the ATAC (Arimidex, tamoxifen, alone or in combination) trial after completion of 5 years' adjuvant treatment for breast cancer. Lancet. 2005;365(9453):60–2.
85. Gronwald J, Byrski T, Lubinski J, Narod SA. Cisplatin in breast cancer treatment in BRCA1 carriers. Hered Cancer Clin Pract. 2012;10(Suppl 4):A17.
86. Turner NC, Tutt AN. Platinum chemotherapy for BRCA1-related breast cancer: do we need more evidence? Breast Cancer Res. 2012;14(6):115.
87. Torrisi R, Zuradelli M, Agostinetto E, Masci G, Losurdo A, de Sanctis R, et al. Platinum salts in the treatment of BRCA-associated breast cancer: a true targeted chemotherapy? Crit Rev Oncol Hematol. 2019;135:66–75.
88. Byrski T, Gronwald J, Huzarski T, Grzybowska E, Budryk M, Stawicka M, et al. Response to neoadjuvant chemotherapy in women with BRCA1-positive breast cancers. Breast Cancer Res Treat. 2008;108(2):289–96.
89. Tutt ANJ, Garber JE, Kaufman B, Viale G, Fumagalli D, Rastogi P, et al. Adjuvant Olaparib for patients with BRCA1- or BRCA2-mutated breast cancer. N Engl J Med. 2021;384(25):2394–405.
90. Tung NM, Garber JE. BRCA1/2 testing: therapeutic implications for breast cancer management. Br J Cancer. 2018;119(2):141–52.

34 Visual Morbidity and Ocular Disease in Metastatic Breast Carcinoma

Radha Annamalai and Bhawna Dev

Abstract

All over the world, breast carcinoma is the most common tumour to affect women. Ocular metastatic foci in breast carcinoma leading to visual morbidity can occur both as a complication of active cancer and as an adverse effect of treatment. Metastases may cause both intra- and extraocular sequelae. Uveal tissue is the predominant site of metastatic disease due to its high vascularity, increased blood flow and architecture of blood vessels. Choroidal metastases are usually detected 3 years after diagnosis of primary breast carcinoma and are rarely the initial manifestation. Metastatic lesions appear as yellow, plateau-shaped, ill-defined masses of 3 mm thickness with subretinal fluid.

Complaints are usually painless blurred vision or may be asymptomatic. The various ophthalmic treatment options for choroidal metastases are external beam radiotherapy, plaque radiotherapy systemic chemotherapy, adjuvant hormone therapy, enucleation and observation. Ocular tumour regression is comparable in those who receive radiotherapy or systemic treatment. In those with ocular metastases, the mean survival time is about 21 months. The ophthalmologist has an important role in the detection of metastatic disease and during follow-up. Prompt management with local and systemic therapy will improve visual prognosis.

Keywords

Uveitis · Choroidal infiltrates · Masquerade syndrome · Optic neuropathy · Breast carcinoma

34.1 Introduction

Metastatic breast cancer is the most common secondary tumour that spreads to the eye and orbit followed by lung, kidney, bone, liver, prostrate and skin. The frequency of involvement of the eye and visual pathways is reported to be as high as 30% in patients with known metastatic disease [1].

Any ocular structure can be involved as a site of metastases, but the most frequent part to be affected is the choroid in nearly 80% with a diagnosis of the primary tumour [2]. A diverse presentation of ocular features can occur with all

R. Annamalai (✉)
Department of Ophthalmology, Sri Ramachandra Institute of Higher Education and Research, Chennai, India
e-mail: radhaannamalai@sriramachandra.edu.in

B. Dev
Department of Radiology, Sri Ramachandra Institute of Higher Education and Research, Chennai, India
e-mail: bhawnadev@sriramachandra.edu.in

B. Dev, L. D. Joseph (eds.), *Holistic Approach to Breast Disease*,
https://doi.org/10.1007/978-981-99-0035-0_34

types of breast carcinoma. Ophthalmic involvement usually occurs during the advanced stages. Uveal metastases are the first indication of breast cancer in only 3%, and asymptomatic patients are more common [3] (Fig. 34.1).

An improvement in diagnostic facilities and therapy for breast carcinoma has increased the incidence and detection of ocular involvement. This in turn has enhanced prognosis and survival of these patients. More commonly, ocular features follow systemic involvement, but rarely, the eye can present as the initial manifestation of a primary breast carcinoma. The time between breast cancer diagnosis and ophthalmic spread is 20–40 months, and usually non-ocular metastatic lesions precede ocular involvement [4].

Signs of ocular involvement: Ocular metastases should be suspected when the patient develops morphological or functional changes such as blurred vision, floaters or photophobia, but asymptomatic involvement has been reported in 7% [5]. In the asymptomatic, metastatic foci are detected during routine examination as part of systemic evaluation. In those with ocular metastases, the mean survival time is about 21 months. Both the ophthalmologist and oncologist should be aware of the spectrum of ophthalmic disorders that occur both directly and indirectly.

Types of ocular involvement: Ophthalmic invasion can be intraocular, extraocular, neuroophthalmic or paraneoplastic based on the anatomical and functional involvement (Table 34.1). The uvea is the first site of systemic metastasis in about 14% of patients with a diagnosis of carcinoma breast [6]. Uveal tissue is involved in 8–10% of metastatic disease. Among all types of uveal metastases, the incidence has been reported to be highest in the choroid accounting for 81%, iris in 9% and the ciliary body in less than 2% [7].

34.1.1 Intraocular Involvement

Choroidal metastasis: The most common primary site for choroidal metastases is breast carcinoma, which is found in 40–53% [8]. They are usually unilateral, multinodular and multifocal. The most common symptom is defective vision with or without metamorphopsia. Choroidal infiltrates appear elevated, yellow and ill-defined with subretinal fluid and an intact overlying retinal pigment epithelium. The most common sites of involvement are in the superior and temporal quadrants of the post-equatorial choroid. An abundant blood supply of the posterior choroid by the posterior ciliary artery is the cause of post-equatorial location of choroidal metastasis (CM). Pain indicates the development of uveitis or glaucoma.

Based on clinical suspicion, various modalities available for the diagnosis of choroidal

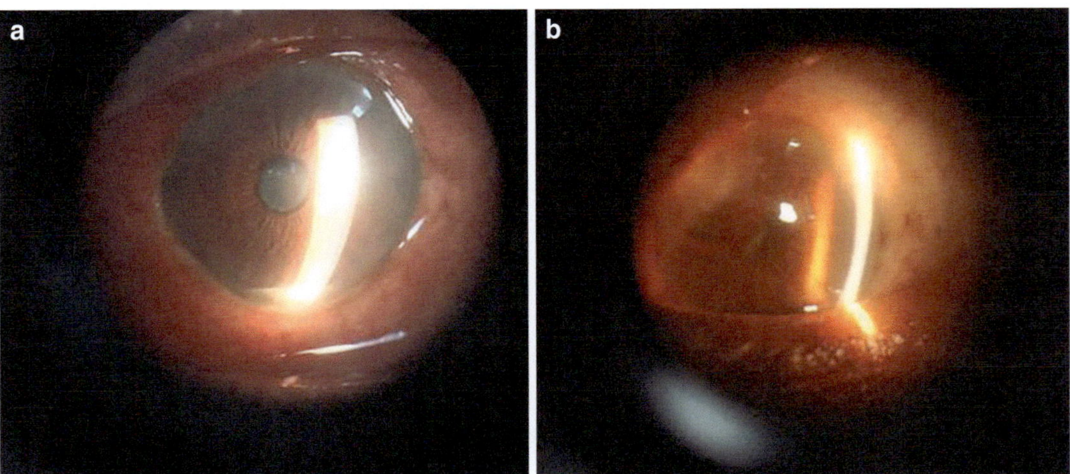

Fig. 34.1 Slit lamp photograph of the left eye. (**a**) At initial presentation showing anterior chamber reaction with hypopyon and chemosis of conjunctiva. (**b**) Pthisis bulbi after one year despite treatment

Table 34.1 Ocular involvement in carcinoma of breast

Site	Percentage	Symptoms	Signs
Iris	9%	Aymptomatic Symptomatic with defective vision or pain	Uveitis Glaucoma Pseudo-hypopyon Iris mass(superior)
Ciliary body	2%	Aymptomatic Symptomatic with defective vision or pain	Mass (dome shaped or sessile) Uveitis Sectorial cataract Shallow anterior chamber causing angle closure glaucoma Subluxation of lens
Choroid	81%	Aymptomatic Blurred vision Metamorphopsia Rare-pain, diplopia	Placoid lesion(superior and temporal) Serous retinal detachment Choroidal detachment RPE abnormalities
Vitreous	Rare	Floaters	Vitritis
Orbit	2–3%	Pain Diplopia Blurred vision	Proptosis Palpable mass Restriction of EOM
Eye lids	Less than 1%	Painless or painful swelling	Nodular or diffuse mass
Cerebral	Rare	Visual field defects Colour vision defects Diplopia defective vision	Strabismus Hemianopias

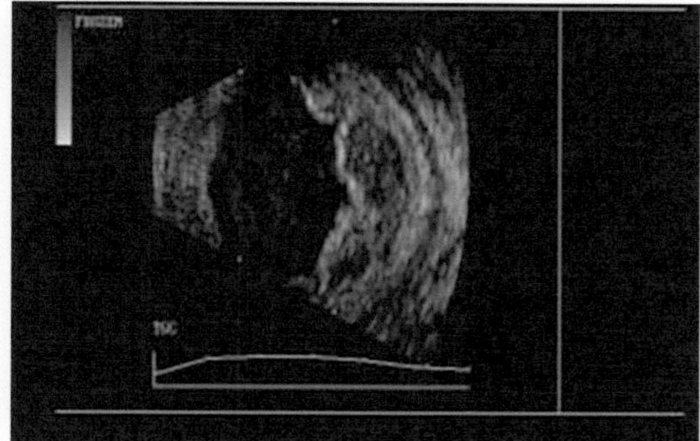

Fig. 34.2 Ultrasound of the left eye B-scan mode showing irregular, lobulated retinochoroidal elevation with retinal detachment, marked choroidal thickening in the peri-papillary area, exudative retinal detachment and T sign in a patient with breast carcinoma

metastasis are ultrasonography (Fig. 34.2), fundus fluorescein angiography, indocyanine angiography (ICG) and optical coherence tomography (OCT). Choroidal tumour biopsy is performed in diagnostic dilemmas to confirm the histopathology of tumour. Biopsy of a small choroidal lesion is difficult with a chance of inadequate sample and risk of intraocular injury. Hence, ancillary investigations help with characterisation of the lesions. Intraocular biopsy using vitreous cutter or a transcleral incisional biopsy with forceps can penetrate directly into the tumour and is more effective in obtaining a tissue sample. Ophthalmic ultrasound shows a flat or dome-shaped mass with medium to high non-homogenous reflectivity. ICGA is very useful and is seen as hypocyanescence on an isocyanescent background. It shows a larger area of choroidal involvement than with other investigations [9]. OCT helps in the identification of anatomical features. OCT angiography guides follow-up of tumour size regression and development of retinal complications. Enhanced depth OCT can identify very small lesions, which show lumpy anterior surface, and this helps differentiate choroidal metastases from other choroidal tumours such as melanoma and hemangioma [10]. Treatment for patients with choroidal metastases includes chemotherapy, external beam irradiation, plaque radiotherapy, proton beam, hormone therapy or enucleation in very advanced patients.

Ciliary body metastases have an incidence of 1% [11]. The ciliary body may be affected directly or through extension from a choroidal tumour with focal deposits commonly involving the antero-inferior parts. They appear as dome-shaped or sessile masses but are not easily visible due to their anterior location. The presence of a conjunctival sentinel vessel indicates an anterior extension of the choroidal metastases and confirms the presence of a tumour in the same quadrant. Pain or decreased vision due to uveitis or glaucoma occur when there has been invasion of the iris root or the trabecular meshwork. Other presentations are subluxation of the lens with sectoral cataract and a shallow anterior chamber due to the mass effect, which may resemble acute angle closure glaucoma.

Iris metastases occur in about 3% [12]. Symptoms are usually very mild and noticed by chance. Pain is associated with the development of uveitis or secondary glaucoma. A vascular iris mass localised to the mid-periphery and inferior quadrant causing pupillary distortion is noted on slit lamp examination. Development of a pseudo-hypopyon where the tumour cells settle in the inferior angle can occur if the lesion is friable and can resemble a granulomatous uveitis. Other complications are secondary glaucoma, rubeosisirides and hyphema. Iris metastasis may be mistaken for a primary iris melanoma. A differentiation is made based on its potential for rapid growth, peripheral location and poor response to treatment.

Systemic investigations performed by the radiologist can identify the extent and type of carcinoma breast (Fig. 34.3).

34.1.2 Neuro-ophthalmic Involvement

Optic nerve metastases is relatively rare and results from emboli in the microcirculation, as an extension from an adjacent choroidal tumour or hematogenous through the posterior ciliary arteries, which supply the optic nerve head [13].

Infiltration on the optic disc can be a diffuse or nodular mass with secondary optic disc oedema and splinter haemorrhages. Most masses are yellow or white and are located adjacent to or on the optic disc (Fig. 34.4). Retinal deposits and infiltrates with exudates and haemorrhages can cause vitreous involvement because of the poorly cohesive nature of tumour cells. Unilateral loss of visual acuity is the most common feature. Sixteen percent of optic disc metastases present as a nodule on the optic disc and few have diffuse thickening [14].

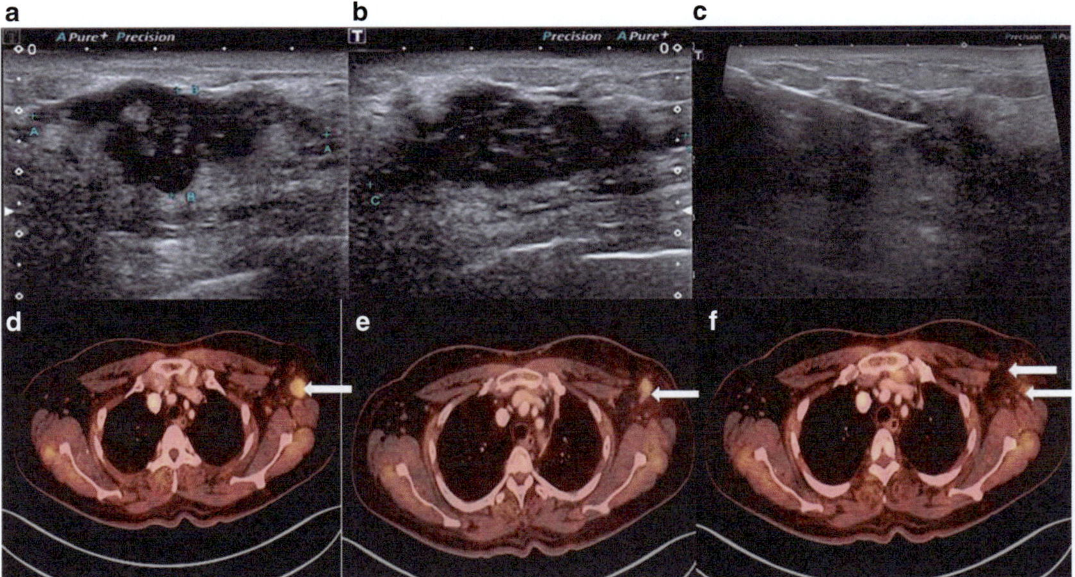

Fig. 34.3 (**a**, **b**) Left breast ultrasound showing irregular illdefined-BI-RADS 5 mass. (**c**) Ultrasound guided core needle biopsy of the mass. (**d–f**) PET-CT showing multiple lesions in the left breast (arrows)

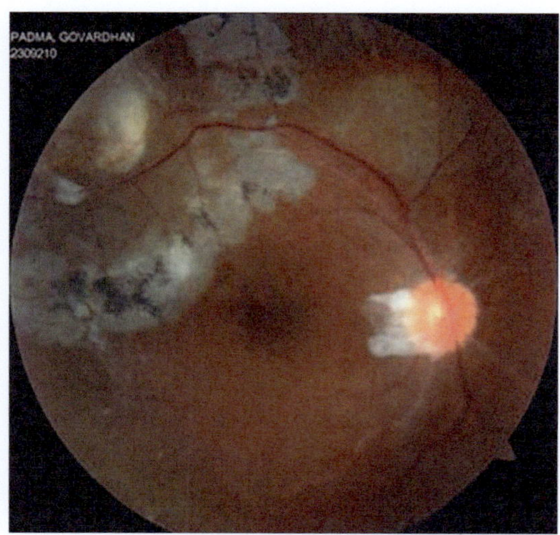

Fig. 34.4 Choroidal infiltrates with involvement of optic disc secondary to carcinoma breast

Extension to the subarachnoid space can cause leptomeningeal carcinomatosis (LPC) [15]. LPC occurs in 5% of patients with carcinoma of breast, and visual loss in these patients is due to neoplastic infiltration, optic nerve sheath cuffing or vascular compromise. Optic disc metastases can be a diagnostic dilemma, and prompt recognition can facilitate early treatment.

Differential diagnosis:

- Retinal astrocytic hamartoma, is a raised, multilobulated, mulberry appearance and hyper-autofluorescence is typical of hamartoma.
- Calcific drusen.
- Involvement of both optic nerves and invasion of the lamina cribrosa can resemble a meningioma or papilloedema.

Compression at the orbital apex can result in palsy of cranial nerves 3, 4, 5, 6 [16].

Deposits that compress sympathetic neurons between the sympathetic chain and the superior cervical ganglion can resemble Pancoast's tumour and cause preganglionic Horner's syndrome.

Cerebral metastases: The most common site for metastases in carcinoma of breast is the brain and cerebral involvement has the potential to lead to visual loss. Homonymous hemianopia and dyschromatopsia occurs when the visual pathway is affected, and involvement of the cerebellum or brainstem causes nystagmus, saccades and oscillatory eye movements [17]. Pituitary metastases can cause bitemporal hemianopia, headache and decreased visual acuity.

34.1.3 Extraocular Involvement

Orbital metastases have been reported in 2–3% of patients [18]. Pain, proptosis and diplopia, exophthalmos and a palpable mass indicate spread to the orbit and adnexa. Enophthalmos is an infrequent feature but occurs in scirrhous adenocarcinoma of the breast as the tumour infiltrates the surrounding nerve and muscles causing the eye to become immobilised and pulled posteriorly. Motility defects in breast cancer can be due to infiltration of the extraocular muscles and surrounding fat but is rare probably because the constant contractile activity makes it a less favourable site for tumour seeding [19]. The prognosis of orbital metastases is poor. After establishing the diagnosis, palliative treatment can provide relief to an extent.

Eyelid metastases indicates advanced stages of the tumour and extensive systemic spread. Systemic combined therapy of cyclophosphamide, 5 fluorouracil (FU) and adriamycin as intravenous injections and good response noted with eye lid metastases. 47% of eyelid metastases are solitary nodules [20], and the lesion can resemble more common inflammatory nodules such as chalazion or primary eyelid tumours. A high index of suspicion is required for any painless eyelid lesion in a patient with a history of breast tumour. Biopsy and histopathological examination should be done as the average survival after diagnosis of metastases is about 1.5 years [21].

34.1.4 Paraneoplastic Reactions

Tumour cells can incite an immune response and cause rare but significant effects against antigens produced in normal cells resulting in bilateral visual loss, scotoma, nyctalopia and photopsia. Cancer-associated retinopathy is a retinal degeneration in which electroretinogram and pattern reversal visual evoked responses are reduced in amplitude [22].

34.2 Ocular Effects of Treatment in Breast Carcinoma

Treatment may be administered in the form of oral medications, cytotoxic chemotherapy or targeted therapy. The most frequent ocular adverse effects of treatment are keratoconjunctivitis sicca (KCS), retinopathy and cataracts. Toxic effects occur with tamoxifen, 5-fluorouracil and aromatase inhibitors. A temporary chemical conjunctivitis occurs when there has been drug leakage into the conjunctiva.

- **Tamoxifen** is a non-steroidal antagonist of oestrogen and causes crystalline retinopathy, maculopathy, cataracts and KCS. It is a selective oestrogen receptor modulator and acts by blocking breast cancer cells by occupying estrogen receptors. Oestrogen receptors are present in the eye and can affect visual processing, lacrimal and meibomian gland functioning. Hence tamoxifen use is typically associated with dry eye. The risk of posterior subcapsular cataract is increased when the drug has been used for longer than 6 years. KCS or dry eye that develops in these patients can be treated with lubricant eye drops. A temporary chemical conjunctivitis occurs when there has been drug leakage into the conjunctiva.
  Retinopathy develops in patients on tamoxifen at doses more than 180 mg daily for longer than 12 months [23]. White to yellow refractile deposits around the macula in the inner retinal layers have been reported in 0–6% and can cause symptoms such as floaters, pigmentary retinopathy, macular oedema or rarely permanent loss of vision [24]. Doses used now are lower in the range of 20 mg/day and toxicity is rare and reversible with this.
- Corneal deposits are seen in the form of a whorl like pattern called cornea verticillata [25]. This is believed to occur due to a hydrophobic mechanism and positive charge of side chains in the chemical structure of tamoxifen resulting in intracellular and intralysosomal-lipidosis. Oxidative stress has also been implicated as a cause of axonal degeneration and retinal damage.

Tamoxifen induced optic neuritis can occur but is reversible. Raloxifene is an alternative to tamoxifen used off label in breast carcinoma and has fewer side effects.

Cytotoxic chemotherapy is sometimes used as an adjuvant treatment especially in those who are refractory to endocrine treatment. Chemotherapy can be toxic to cells causing harm to cell division and renewal is delayed. Agents used include cyclophosphamide, methotrexate 5-fluorouracil and cyclophospamide as either part of combination therapy or single agent chemotherapy.

Patients may complain of blurred vision, dry eyes or excessive lacrimation and mild conjunctivitis, loss of eyelashes and eyebrows as part of the general alopecia associated with many cytotoxic regimens. These symptoms usually start within 7–14 days of chemotherapy and will resolve after treatment has finished. Certain toxic effects of specific drugs listed in Table 34.2.

Table 34.2 Ocular side-effects of cytotoxic drugs used in breast cancer

Drug	Adverse effects
Alkylating agents	Keratoconjunctivitissicca Blepharoconjunctivitis Miosis Cataract and blurred vision Stevens–Johnson syndrome
5 fluorouracil	Epiphora, conjunctivitis, keratitis, cicatricialentropion, canalicular stenosis, optic neuropathy, nystagmus
Methotrexate	Blepharitis, ocular surface disease, lacrimation
Anthracyclines	Lacrimation and conjunctivitis
Paclitaxel and docetaxel	Scintillating scotomas Epiphora (stenosis of tear drainage and irregularities in the lacrimal apparatus

Aromatase inhibitors are popular in the treatment of carcinoma breast and ocular toxicity rarely occurs with this. Aromatase inhibitors are prescribed to postmenopausal breast cancer patients after few years of treatment with tamoxifen. They work by inhibiting estrogen synthesis and estrogen suppression can cause accelerated aging in women and an exaggerated menopause. Short term effects are mild but long term adverse effects such as posterior vitreous detachment and small retinal haemorrhages have been reported [26]. Excessive traction on the retina caused by estrogen depletion can cause dry eye and photopsia.

Progestins when used in metastatic breast carcinoma are associated with adverse effects of corticosteroid treatment. Ocular side effects are posterior subcapsular cataract, secondary glaucoma or ocular hypertension, reactivation of herpetic keratitis.

Chemotherapy can cause can cause ocular toxicity but adverse effects are rare with hormonal therapy [27].

Local treatment of ocular metastases: The objective of local treatment is to preserve vision and prevent further deterioration. Drugs are delivered to the eye by topical, intraocular and systemic routes. The various modalities of local treatment include laser, radiotherapy, intravitrealantivascular endothelial growth factors, photodynamic therapy and enucleation if all other modalities of treatment fail.

Principle of treatment in ocular metastases: Local treatment is considered for isolated CM, if the general prognosis is good. In such patients, brachytherapy, proton therapy or stereotactic body radiation is an option. In case of multifocal metastatic disease which is life threatening combined systemic and local treatment is required. Local ocular treatment is done only after systemic metastatic disease is controlled.

Radiotherapy is the primary management of orbital and ocular metastatic lesions and 80% of patients show improvement [28]. Modalities of radiotherapy include external beam radiotherapy (EBRT), charged particle radiotherapy, plaque radiotherapy (PRT), stereotactic radiosurgery and proton beam therapy. Retinal vasculature is destroyed by ionizing radiation. Radiation is associated with side effects, and the extent depends on the host and type of radiation delivery. Complications can occur months or years after irradiation and the regimen is 30 Gyrons in 10 fractions.

Most common complications of irradiation include skin erythema, conjunctivitis, cataract, iris neovascularisation, neovascular glaucoma, radiation retinopathy, exposure keratitis,, radiation retinopathy and papillopathy.. Cataract is more common in patients with metastases in the anterior segment. Radiation retinopathy has been reported at 3–8%. The severity of retinopathy does not correlate with the dose of radiation and has been reported to occur with doses as low as 50cG. Radiation-induced retinopathy shows features resembling diabetic retinopathy, such as microaneurysma, haemorrhages, telengiectasia, exudation and neovascularisation of the retina and optic disc. It is more severe in those affected by other microvascular abnormalities such as in diabetic retinopathy. Simultaneous use of chemotherapy may potentiate the injury due to interference with DNA synthesis and vascular endothelial cell division and repair. In radiation optic neuropathy, patient has an oedematous hyperaemic optic disc. Visual loss in these patients occurs because of optic atrophy.

External beam radiotherapy is used extensively in ocular metastases. It is reported to cause tumour regression in about 63–83% of patients with metastatic uveal tumours [29]. External beam irradiation is very effective in blurred vision secondary to foveal involvement

Proton beam radiotherapy is useful in unifocal-tumours and peripheral tumours which are radio resistant and has the advantage of localised intraocular delivery of radiation, less destruction of surrounding tissues and decreased ocular toxicity. Solitary lesions are treated with episcleral plaques, and tumour regression is reported in about 84% [30]. PRT has been proven effective in solitary, solid uveal metastases and in those who did not respond to EBRT. Tumour regression starts as early as 2–3 days after PRT.

Plaque brachytherapy: a radioactive isotope sutured to the sclera above the tumour delivers radiation to the target tissue. The plaque is left in place till the entire therapeutic dose is delivered.

Transpupillary thermotherapy using diode laser and laser photocoagulation causes tumour necrosis by vascular occlusion and is used in small foci [31].

Intravitreal injections of antivascular endothelial growth factors using bevacizumab may be effective in choroidal metastases who did not respond to other forms of treatment.

Photodynamic therapy with vertiporfin causes tumour regression in 78% by producing highly reactive oxygen particles which activate immune responses against tumour cells [32]. Oxygen particles bind to vascular endothelial cells and induce thrombosis. It is a non-invasive technique in which a light sensitive compound such as vertiporfin is administered. It gets activated after light exposure. Photochemical effects are produced in the tissue due to accumulation of photosensitive molecules in the target tissue.

Chemotherapy and hormonal therapy are other options that are reported to cause tumour regression.

Laser photocoagulation is used to treat macular oedema and neovascularisation.

Enucleation is considered only for intractable ocular pain, secondary glaucoma or very rapid tumour growth.

Newer Modalities of Treatment

- Navigation-assisted surgical biopsy is used to diagnose orbital metastasis.
- Novel targeted systemic treatment and systemic treatment with biphosphonate are increasingly used in choroidal metastases.
- A favourable response has been noted with complete regression of choroidal metastasis after treatment with anastrazole and combined chemotherapy. Stabilisation of vision occurs in 50% and improvement in 36% of patients [33].

Follow-up: All patients need a baseline ophthalmic evaluation at diagnosis, within the first year of treatment and every 4–6 months thereafter. Those with symptoms should be seen earlier with monitoring of colour vision and visual fields during each review. The risk of ocular side effects is cumulative and usually effects of toxicity are seen after 1 year of therapy. The detection of asymptomatic refractile bodies alone does not warrant discontinuation but the onset of colour vision or central vision, retinal haemorrhages and cystoid macular oedema while on tamoxifen requires consideration to stop the drug. Almost all ocular side effects with tamoxifen are reversible after the drug is discontinued. The only serious adverse effect is progressive visual loss in which case the drug needs to be stopped immediately.

Conclusion: The survival time of breast cancer has increased due to more awareness, extensive screening programmes, early detection of cancer and effective treatment. This, however, has increased the incidence and detection of ocular metastases. Also, visual loss may occur not only due to the tumour but as an adverse effect of treatment (Table 34.3). Adjuvant therapy of ocular and orbital metastases is aimed at providing an improvement in the quality of patient's life, in restoring visual function, to eradicate metasatases, to prevent further development of metastatic foci or as a palliative measure. Routine ophthalmic evaluation is controversial but altered vision requires immediate examination. A multidisciplinaryy approach is required in the management of these patients.

Table 34.3 Common Causes of visual loss in carcinoma breast

Due to disease	Due to treatment
Choroidal metastasis with macular involvement Exudative retinal detachment	Radiation retinopathy
Proptosis/orbital mass	Posterior subcapsular cataract
Secondary glaucoma	Neovascular glaucoma
Uveitis	Blepharitis
Cortical blindness	Meibomian gland disease
Diplopia/strabismus	Conjunctivitis
Cancer associated retinopathy	Lid scarring/ ectropion

References

1. Jemal A, Siegel R, Ward E, et al. Cancer statistics. CA Cancer J Clin. 2009;59:225–49.
2. Demirci H, Shields CL, Chao A, Shields JA. Uveal metastasis from breast cancer in 264 patients. Am J Ophthalmol. 2003;136:264–71.
3. Shields CL, Shields JA, Gross NE, Schwartz GP, Lally SE. Survey of 520 eyes with uveal metastases. Ophthalmology. 1997;104:1265–76.
4. Mejia-Novelo A, Varado-Miranda A, Morales-Vazquez F, et al. Ocular metastases from breast carcinoma. Med Oncol. 2004;21:217–21.
5. Fenton S, Kemp EG, Harnett AN. Screening for ophthalmic involvement in asymptomatic patients with metastatic breast carcinoma. Eye (Lond). 2004;18(1):38–40.
6. d'Abbadie I, Arriagada R, Spielmann M, Le MG. Choroid metastases: clinical features and treatments in 123 patients. Cancer. 2003;98:1232–8.
7. Mathis T, Jardel P, Loria O, Delaunay B, Nguyen AM, Lanza F, Mosci C, Coujolle JP, Kodjikian L, Thariat J. New concepts in the diagnosis and management of choroidal metastases. Prog Retin Eye Res. 2019;68:144–17.
8. Arepalli S, Kaliki S, Shields CL. Choroidal metastases: origin, features and therapy. Indian J Ophthalmol. 2015;63(2):122–7.
9. Merrill CF, Kaufman DI, Dimitrov NV. Breast cancer metastatic to the eye is a common entity. Cancer. 1991;68:623–7.
10. Vishnevskia-Dai V, Zur D, Yaacobi S, Moroz I, Newman H, Neudorfer M. Optical coherence tomography: an adjunctive tool for differentiating between choroidal melanoma and metastasis. J Ophthalmol. 2016;2016:9803547.
11. Swampillai AJ, Boothe AP, Cohen VM. Ciliary body and iris metastases with anterior chamber angle infiltration L a rare complication from invasive ductal breast cancer. J Glaucoma. 2020;29(3):e12–5.
12. Suhr KS, Sperber LT, Marr P, Kahn JB. Unusual case of iris metastases from breast carcinoma. JCRS Online Case Reports. 2015;3(1):8–11.
13. Kim CU, Pearce WA. Metastatic breast carcinoma involving the optic disc. Am J Ophthalmol Case Rep. 2020;18:100698.
14. Fox B, Pacheco P, De Monte F. Carcinoma of the breast metastatic to the optic nerve mimicking an optic nerve sheath meningioma: case report and review of the literature. Skull Base. 2005;15(4):281–7.
15. Scott BJ, Kesari S. Leptomeningeal metastases in breast cancer. Am J Cancer Res. 2013;3(2):117–26.
16. Madgula IM, Hemmerdinger CM, Clark P. Metastatic breast cancer presenting as sequential cranial nerve-palsy: a case report. J Med Case Rep. 2014;8:430.
17. Massot-Punyer R, Almajano J, Camacho JM. Cerebral metastasis. Rev Neurol. 2000;31:1242–7.
18. Ahmad SM, Esmaeli B. Metastatic tumours of the orbit and ocular adnexa. Curr Opin Ophthalmol. 2007;18(5):405–13.
19. Framarino-Dei-Malatesta M, Chiarito A, Bianciardi F, Fiorelli M, Ligato A, Pecorella I. Metastases to extraocular muscles from breast cancer: case report and up-to-date review of the literature. BMC Cancer. 2019;19(1):36.
20. Fonseca NL, Lucci LMD, Cha SB, Rosetti C, Rehder JRCL. Metastatic eyelid disease associated with primary breast carcinoma: case report. Arq Bras Oftalmol. 2009;72(3):390–3.
21. Martin J, Fung MA, Lin LK. Breast cancer metastasis masquerading as the great masquerader: sebaceous cell carcinoma. Case Rep Oncol. 2017;10(2):485–8.
22. Hojlo MM, Ejma M, Gorczyca WA, Szymaniec S, Witkowsk D, Fortuna W, Miedzybrodzki R, Rogozinska-Szczepka J, Bartnik W. Cancer-associated retinopathy in patients with breast carcinoma. Arch Immunol Ther Exp. 2007;55(4):261–5.
23. Alwitry A, Gardner I. Tamoxifenmaculopathy. Arch Ophthalmol. 2002;120:140.
24. Ugurlu S, Karagoz A, Ekin MA. Ocular findings in breast cancer patients using tamoxifen. Cutan Ocul Toxicol. 2015;34(1):16–20.
25. Zinchuk O, Watanabe M, Hayashi N, et al. A case of tamoxifenkeratopathy. Arch Ophthalmol. 2006;124:1046–8.
26. Manquez ME, Brown MM, Shields CL, Shields JA. Management of choroidal metastases from breast carcinomas using aromatase inhibitors. Curr Opin Ophthalmol. 2006;17(3):251–6.
27. Gianni L, Panzini I, Li S, Gelber RD, Collins J, Holmberg SB, Crivellari D, Castiglione-Gertsch M, Goldhirsch A, Coates AS, Ravaiolo A, International Breast Cancer Study Group (IBCSG). Ocular toxicity during adjuvant chemoendocrine therapy for early breast cancer: results from International Breast Cancer Study Group trials. Cancer. 2006;106(3):505–13.
28. Shaik R, Tariq K, Sharma S, Tang S-C. Metastatic breast cancer presenting as orbital mass: a case report with literature review. J Glob Oncol. 2018;4:1–4.
29. Amer R, et al. Treatment options in the management of choroidal metastases. Ophthalmologica. 2004;218(6):372–7.
30. Lim JI, Petrovich Z. Radioactive plaque therapy for metastatic choroidal carcinoma. Ophthalmology. 2000;107:1927–31.
31. Lin CJ, Tsai YY. The effect of intravitreal bevacizumab and transpupillary thermotherapy on choroidal metastases and literature review. Indian J Ophthalmol. 2015;63(1):37–41.
32. Kaliki S, Shields CL, Dahmash SA, Mashayekhi A, Shields JA. Photodynamic therapy for choroidal metastasis in 8 cases. Ophthalmology. 2012;119(6):1218–22.
33. Chen CJ, McCoy AN, Brahmer J, Handa JT. Emerging treatments for choroidal metastases. Surv Ophthalmol. 2011;56(6):511–21.

Part XI
Recent Advances

35 Advances in Breast Imaging and Intervention

Soujanya Gadde

Abstract

Over the past couple of decades, screen-film mammography has been replaced by full-field digital mammography (FFDM) improving the mammographic quality. However, sensitivity of mammography is often limited by breast density. Majority of recent advances like the digital breast tomosynthesis (DBT), contrast-enhanced spectral mammography (CESM), abbreviated breast magnetic resonance imaging (MRI), and automated breast ultrasound (US) have been developed to either to overcome the limitations in standard mammography or to offer alternative imaging methods to improve detection of early breast cancer. In addition, other advances such as elastography offer better specificity and prehistological characterization of lesions especially when initial imaging findings are equivocal. Advances in image-guided intervention such as vacuum-assisted biopsy (VAB) helps in better sampling ability or option for lesion excision (VAE), thereby reducing the need for open surgical biopsies. Newer localization methods like radioactive/magnetic seeds and radiofrequency tags have offered flexibility for the breast surgeons, radiologists, and the patient in terms of time frame between the surgery and the localization.

Keywords

DBT · Tomosynthesis · CEDM · CESM · ABUS · Elastography · Nonwire localization · VAB · VAE · Abbreviated breast MRI

The incidence of breast cancer has increased by more than 20% since 2008, and with 2.3 million newly detected cases worldwide in 2020, breast cancer has surpassed lung cancer as the most common malignancy [1]. Several studies have demonstrated that early detection of breast cancer by screening asymptomatic women does reduce mortality and morbidity [2]. This led to a wider adaptation of breast screening with mammography as the primary screening tool.

Over the past couple of decades, screen-film mammography has been replaced by full-field digital mammography (FFDM) improving the mammographic quality. However, sensitivity of mammography is often limited by breast density. Due to the masking effect caused by tissue superimposition, lesion detection is significantly lower in women with heterogeneously dense or extremely dense breasts [3]. Majority of recent advances like the digital breast tomosynthesis (DBT), contrast-enhanced spectral mammography (CESM), abbreviated breast MRI, and auto-

S. Gadde (✉)
Nightingale breast centre, Manchester University Hospital NHS Trust, Manchester, UK
e-mail: soujanya.gadde@mft.nhs.uk

B. Dev, L. D. Joseph (eds.), *Holistic Approach to Breast Disease*,
https://doi.org/10.1007/978-981-99-0035-0_35

mated breast US outlined in this chapter have been developed to either to overcome the limitations in standard mammography or offer alternative imaging methods to improve detection of early breast cancer. In addition, other advances such as elastography offer better specificity and prehistological characterization of lesions especially when initial imaging findings are equivocal. Advances in image-guided intervention such as vacuum-assisted biopsy (VAB) helps in better sampling ability or option for lesion excision (VAE) thereby reducing the need for open surgical biopsies. Especially in cases of indeterminate B3 lesions like papilloma without atypia, LCIS and ADH, the newer techniques like vacuum-assisted excision (VAE) with 9 g needles make it possible to obtain larger tissue samples, which in turn aids in the histological upgrade and detection of underlying malignancies without open surgical excision.

Newer localization methods like radioactive/magnetic seeds and radiofrequency tags have offered flexibility for the breast surgeons, radiologists, and the patient in terms of time frame between the surgery and the localization. Especially in times of pandemic like this, flexibility in time frame reduces the load on the patients turning up in the hospital before the surgery.

35.1 Digital Breast Tomosynthesis (DBT)

DBT is a promising new technology, which has shown to improve accuracy in screening and diagnostic breast imaging in the recent past. This imaging technique, facilitated by digital detectors, employs a limited-angle tomographic evaluation of breast tissue and was developed specifically to overcome the issue of tissue superimposition [4]. Unlike the full-field digital mammography (FFDM), which offers single image acquisition in the MLO and CC planes each, DBT acquires multi-projection images in both planes. This facilitates a three-dimensional visualization of breast tissue and helps to evaluate it in a greater detail thereby improving the diagnostic accuracy (Figs. 35.1 and 35.2). Occasionally, standard mammography can lead to misinterpretation of complex yet normal of breast tissue as suspicious. These "pseudo positive lesions" can also be better evaluated on DBT as it offers an option to scroll through a stack of reconstructed sections of confounding superimposed breast tissue for better evaluation. This in turn has shown to increase specificity and reduce false-positive recall rate for breast cancer. DBT in practice also offers better lesion characterization and triangulation. Further targeted evaluation with US at this stage can lead to successful work up of the suspicious features initially detected in the mammogram with biopsy for early diagnosis. In cases where a suspicious abnormality can only be seen on DBT images, DBT technique also offers the ability to biopsy and localize lesions for excision, which is widely termed as stereotactic biopsies/excisions.

Technique: Most DBT systems employ an X-ray tube, which moves in a smooth arc of approximately 60 degrees overhead, executing several exposures, each from a different angle, resulting in a series of low-dose images. Images are then reconstructed into stacks in standard MLO and CC projections. Objects seen in a specific plane are in focus, while objects in planes on either side are blurred out.

Practical Applications of DBT

- Screening in high-risk patients or dense breasts
- Further assessment of standard mammographic abnormalities
- Accurate estimation of the lesion size/extent
- Detection of multifocal disease (Fig. 35.3)
- Aids in biopsy of lesion/subtle architectural distortion, which are only visible in the tomosynthesis

35.1.1 Limitations of DBT

Despite the advantages that DBT can offer, there are certain limitations. There is an increased risk of radiation to the breast tissue with DBT compared to a standard full-field digital mammogra-

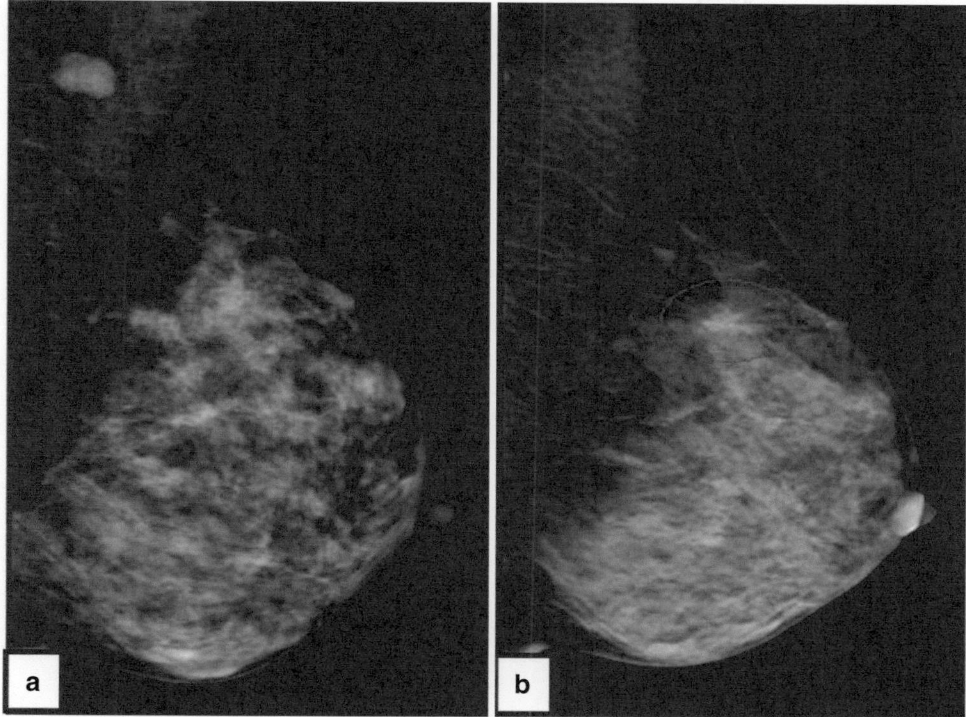

Fig. 35.1 (**a**) The 2D screening mammogram MLO view of the left breast shows suspicious architectural distortion in the upper quadrant with a malignant appearing axillary lymph nodes. (**b**) Tomosynthesis MLO view of the same left breast confirms a spiculate malignant mass in the left upper breast; it was not every obvious in the background of dense glandular breast tissue on standard 2D mammogram

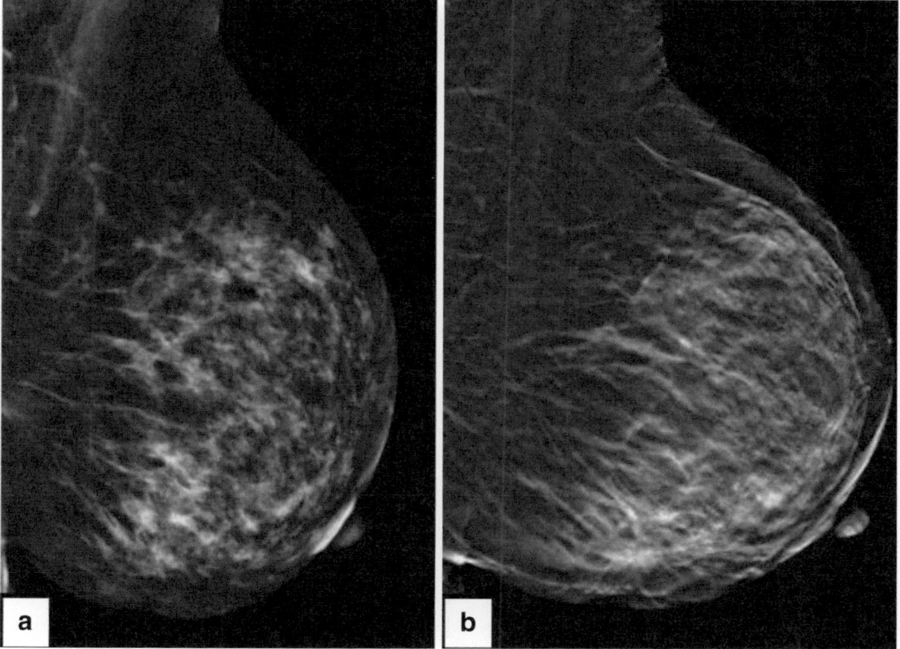

Fig. 35.2 (**a**) FFDM mammogram MLO view of the left breast—essentially appears normal. (**b**) Due to the presence of a clinically palpable lump, DBT was performed, which demonstrated a mammographically occult malignant mass in the lower left breast and its extent which aids in surgical planning

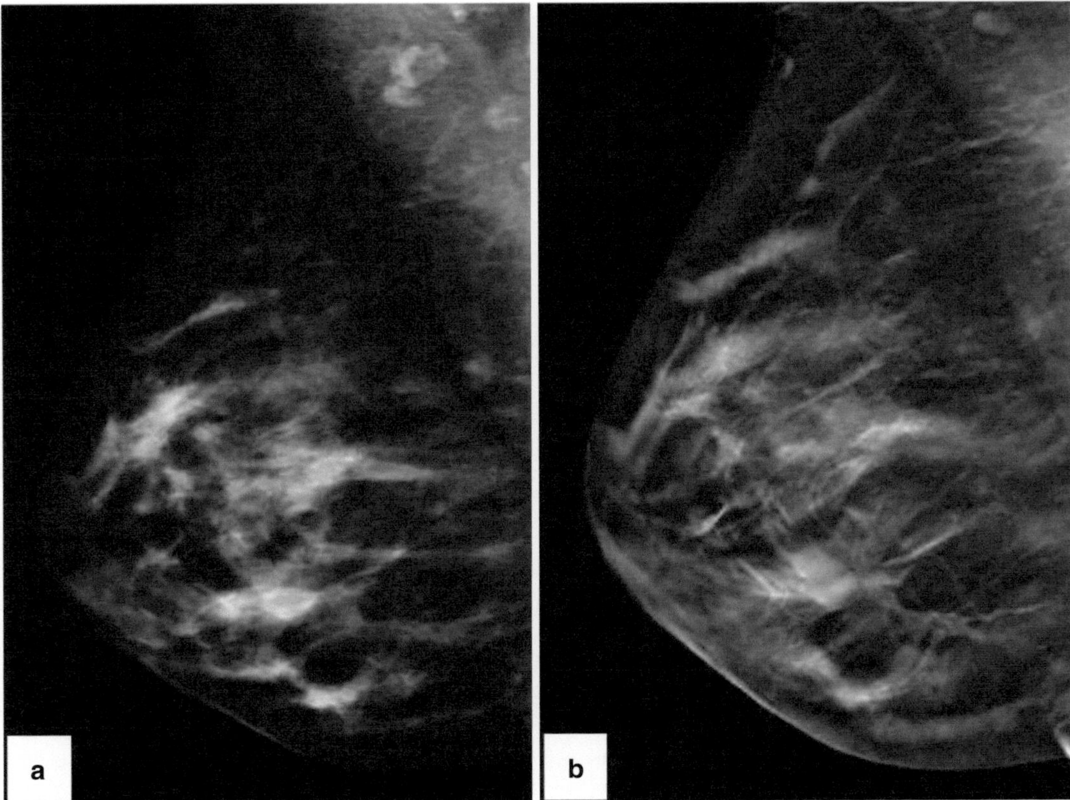

Fig. 35.3 (**a**) Full-field digital mammogram MLO view of the right breast—essentially appears normal. (**b**) DBT demonstrates extensive multifocal architectural distortion in the upper and in the lower quadrant thereby playing a major role in the surgical planning

phy (FFDM). The radiation risk, measured as the mean glandular dose, is variable depending on factors such as the size and density of a breast and/or the compressed breast thickness [5]. A combo mode of FFDM with supplemental DBT, is shown to double the radiation dose of FFDM. Synthesis of a digital mammogram from DBT has shown to reduce the radiation dose compared to the combo mode.

Because of reduced overlap of breast tissue, benign lesions such as cysts and lymph nodes that would have been previously concealed are more readily detected at DBT and may lead to an increase in unnecessary further assessment.

Although masses and architectural distortion are often better detected and better characterized with DBT, if a malignancy does not demonstrate these imaging characteristics, it may not be detectable with DBT [6]. DBT has shown a risk of false-negative assessment especially when evaluating mammographic asymmetries where in a true abnormality can be incorrectly interpreted as normal background glandular breast tissue.

Like any new imaging technology, there is a substantial learning curve in interpreting DBT. Several studies have shown that the average interpretation time for DBT reconstructions were substantially higher than for FFDM [7]. While DBT may offer a reduction in recall rate thereby reducing the time and resources for diagnostic evaluation, the increased interpretation time should be considered for resource and workflow management purposes. DBT also requires a more compliant patient as the acquisition times are longer compared to FFDM.

35.2 Breast MRI

Breast MRI has shown to be the most sensitive modality for the detection of breast cancer (Fig. 35.4). MR imaging allows detection of more breast cancers, both invasive and in situ, than the other available techniques. Although developed before the turn of the century, breast MRI has grown to become a great diagnostic tool more recently with far wider application in breast evaluation. It has now become a part of standard evaluation of lobular and suspected multifocal breast cancer. Breast MRI has been also shown to be a highly sensitive screening tool in patients with increased risk of developing breast cancer especially with those who are young with dense breasts.

Technique: A minimum field strength of 1.5 T and utilization of a dedicated breast coil are required to achieve high spatial resolution imaging of diagnostic quality. Women lie in the prone position with the breasts hanging free in the recesses of the coil.

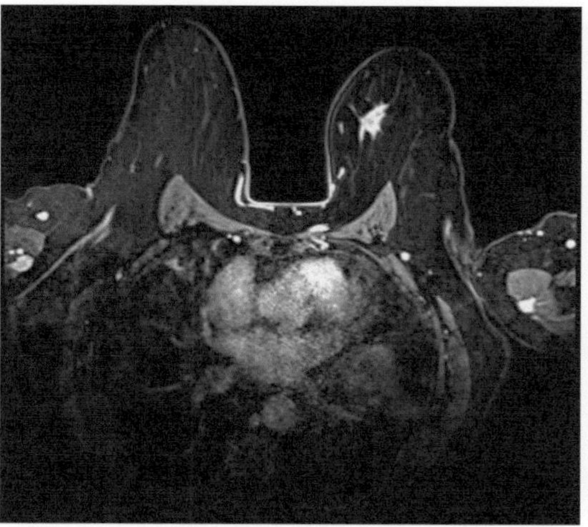

Fig. 35.4 MRI of both breasts T1 post-contrast subtracted image shows an ill-defined enhancing mass in the lower inner quadrant of the left breast, which is highly suspicious for malignancy. Other than detection, MRI also helps in accurate sizing, extent, multifocality, presence of satellite lesion, involvement of the nipple areolar complex and chest wall, and evaluation of contralateral breast and axillary lymph nodes. Presence of internal mammary, subpectoral lymph nodes, which otherwise cannot be evaluated with mammogram and/or ultrasound, also can be detected by MRI breast, thus playing an important role in staging and treatment planning

Breast MRI can be undertaken either a contrast-enhanced examination or a non-contrast scan depending on the indication. Contrast-enhanced breast MRI helps in assessing both lesion morphology and rate of contrast uptake (kinetics) by obtaining precontrast T1, T2, and fat saturation sequences through the desired breast plane followed byT1-weighted contrast-enhanced dynamic scanning. Image subtraction technique helps in increasing lesion conspicuity and highlight the enhancement characteristics while diffusion-weighted imaging can be used to improve lesion characterization. The resultant multiparametric imaging can be evaluated for morphologic features and enhancement pattern using time-intensity curves. Dynamic analysis investigates the permeability of the vessels that supply a lesion, which is reflected in the shape of the time–signal intensity curves. The underlying principle of a time-intensity curve is that neovascularization of aggressive breast tumors leads to formation of leaky vessels allowing for faster contrast agents extravasation resulting in rapid local enhancement. This in turn helps in differentiating benign and malignant breast lesions. The morphologic features and kinetic enhancement are described using the BI-RADS lexicon.

Non-contrast MRI is generally used in assessment of breast implant integrity. This can be achieved by utilizing MR parameters specific for highlighting water and silicone signal.

Indications for Contrast-Enhanced Breast MRI

- Preoperative extent of disease evaluation (especially lobular carcinoma)
- Screening high-risk patients
- Assessment of neoadjuvant chemotherapy response
- Problem solving in dense breasts
- Further evaluation in occult breast primary or carcinoma of unknown origin
- MRI-guided biopsy or lesion localization for surgery
- Evaluation breast implants—rupture (intra/extracapsular), Anaplastic Large B cell Lymphoma (ALBL)

35.2.1 Limitations of Breast MRI

Apart from requiring a high level of patient cooperation, general MRI compatibility issues, and contrast-related problems, false-positive findings seem to be a specific disadvantage to breast MRI. Also, in a screening setting, breast MRI is not cost or time efficient when compared to other screening modalities.

35.3 Abbreviated MRI

This more recently developed MRI protocol helps in addressing some of the issues faced with standard dynamic breast MRI. With shorter image acquisition and interpretation times, abbreviated MRI has shown to improved utilization of scanner time more effectively and reduce the costs. Kuhl et al. introduced the concept of an abbreviated protocol that consisted of one pre- and one post-contrast T1-weighted acquisition and found equivalent diagnostic accuracy for the abbreviated and full protocols [8]. Dynamic information obtained by scanning at repeated intervals during post-contrast phase on a standard breast MRI is not obtained in abbreviated MRI. This thereby reduces the MRI acquisition and interpretation time to make it more effective especially in high-risk breast screening programs. Supplemental ultrafast sequences can be used in conjunction to obtain dynamic information without lengthening the protocol and maintaining a high diagnostic accuracy.

35.4 Contrast-Enhanced Spectral Mammography (CESM)

Contrast-enhanced spectral mammography (CESM) is a more recent development, which is being increasingly adapted into clinical practice. MRI, which allowed better disease evaluation than standard mammography and US, is not always readily available, can be time consuming, and is contraindicated in certain patients [9]. CESM technique which simply adds contrast-enhanced information to standard mammograms based on the presence or absence of neoangiogenesis in a breast lesion can be an efficient alternative (Fig. 35.5). A CESM examination is typically shorter than that of MRI, and both modalities have similar rates of sensitivity to

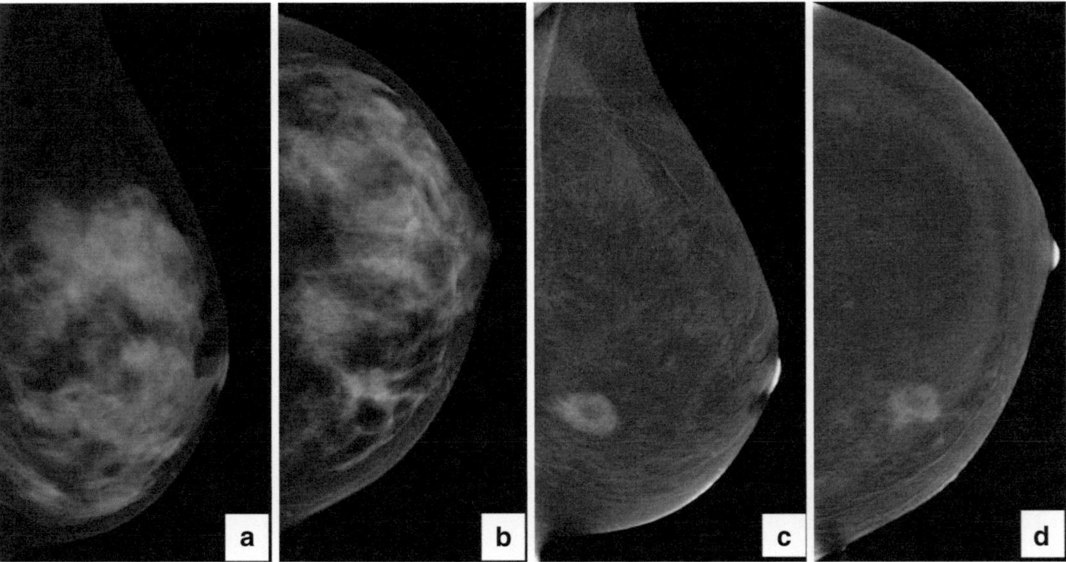

Fig. 35.5 (**a**, **b**) Digital mammography of the left breast shows no abnormality; (**c**, **d**) CESM helps to identify the mammographically occult grade 3 invasive ductal cancer in a dense breast lesion and to confirm unifocal nature. Image courtesy Dr. Penny Moyle, Cambridge Breast Unit, UK

detect lesions with CESM being more cost-effective.

Combining the diagnostic elements of mammography and MRI, CESM can evaluate breast lesion for its density, morphological characteristics, and neovascularity simultaneously. This provides a superior sensitivity and specificity compared to mammography or MRI on its own.

35.4.1 Technique

CESM is performed by using standard mammography equipment, which can be upgraded to include copper filtration and additional software to make it capable of performing dual-energy imaging.

Prior to imaging, nonionic low-osmolar iodinated contrast material is administered intravenously to the patient. Following this, standard CC and MLO images were performed using a dual-energy technique in order to obtain low-energy and high-energy images. Low-energy imaging is undertaken below the k-edge of iodine (33.2 keV). This results in no iodinated contrast material to be depicted. High-energy imaging is undertaken above the k-edge of iodine to reveal contrast material uptake. Low- and high-energy images are then superimposed; the resulting recombined image highlights areas of contrast enhancement while suppressing the normal background breast tissue.

Currently no CESM-specific BI-RADS lexicon is available for lesion classification; hence, BI-RADS mammography lexicon is used for low-energy images, and the BI-RADS MRI lexicon is used for recombined image evaluation. CESM is associated with a level of radiation exposure like that of digital mammography.

35.4.2 Application in Clinical Practice

At present, the main application for CESM appears to be as an adjunct to diagnostic imaging in further evaluation of a breast abnormality. This is often used in conjunction with US, which is required for guided biopsy. The main role of CESM when evaluating mass lesions is to identify any additional abnormalities in the ipsilateral or contralateral breast especially if the initial lesion is suspicious for malignancy. Studies have also demonstrated that CEM has a high sensitivity and negative predictive value (NPV) in patients with architectural distortion (AD) [10] The data suggest that the absence of enhancement associated with AD in patients with minimal background enhancement is a strong indication of benignity. With microcalcifications CESM demonstrates their morphology on low-energy images and associated enhancement on recombined images.

35.4.3 Limitations

The most significant challenge of CESM relates to the administration of iodinated contrast material, which is more frequently associated with risk of allergic reactions and extravasation. Also, the additional upgrade needed for a normal mammography machine in terms of copper filtration and software for dual energy imaging is not available in all mammogram vendors.

CESM-guided biopsy is not yet available. When lesions are found on recombined CESM images, it becomes imperative to find a correlate on alternative imaging modality, such as mammography, US, or MRI for biopsy or localization purposes.

As with other imaging modalities, false-positive and false-negative results also occur with CESM where benign entities such as fibroadenoma, pseudoangiomatous stromal hyperplasia (PASH), abscesses, and papilloma can show enhancement, resulting in unnecessary biopsies while low-grade carcinomas may be missed due to lack of enhancement or being obscured by significant surrounding background enhancement.

35.5 Automated Breast Ultrasound (ABUS)

Handheld ultrasound used either for screening or diagnostic purposes is largely operator dependant. This also has limited value in evaluation certain early breast cancer and in situ malignancies features such as distortions, asymmetries, and microcalcifications.

ABUS has been introduced as a supplementary screening modality mainly in women with dense breasts [11] where tissue overlap limits mammographic sensitivity. This technique is particularly useful in detection of early invasive cancers.

Benefits of ABUS over handheld US include structured acquisition and evaluation of whole breast. With additional advantage of being non-operator dependent, it allows for true comparison. Its three-dimensional volumetric acquisition helps overcome the issue of glandular overlap while the ability to undertake multiplanar reformatting, allows for true comparison with other cross-sectional imaging (Fig. 35.6). One of the most unique features of ABUS is the retraction phenomenon on coronal reformatted images. Retraction tends to appear as a stellate pattern, caused by desmoplastic reaction in the normal tissue surrounding even small cancers. This phenomenon is rarely seen with benign findings but accompanies almost all breast cancers making it the one of the most distinguishing and useful features to identify on ABUS.

Technique: Most ABUS systems acquire either two or three overlapping B-mode US volumes per breast with a high-frequency linear-array transducer. The transducer is automatically driven by a mechanical arm. By acquiring overlapping volumes, the entire breast area between the midsternal line and the midaxillary line can be imaged. Images are then reconstructed in axial and coronal reformats prior to interpretation.

Image interpretation is performed using the BI-RADS standard US lexicon, which has been accepted as being sufficient for screening and diagnostic purposes.

The main advantages of ABUS are that it is relatively inexpensive, could be used as a standalone or supplemental screening test in women

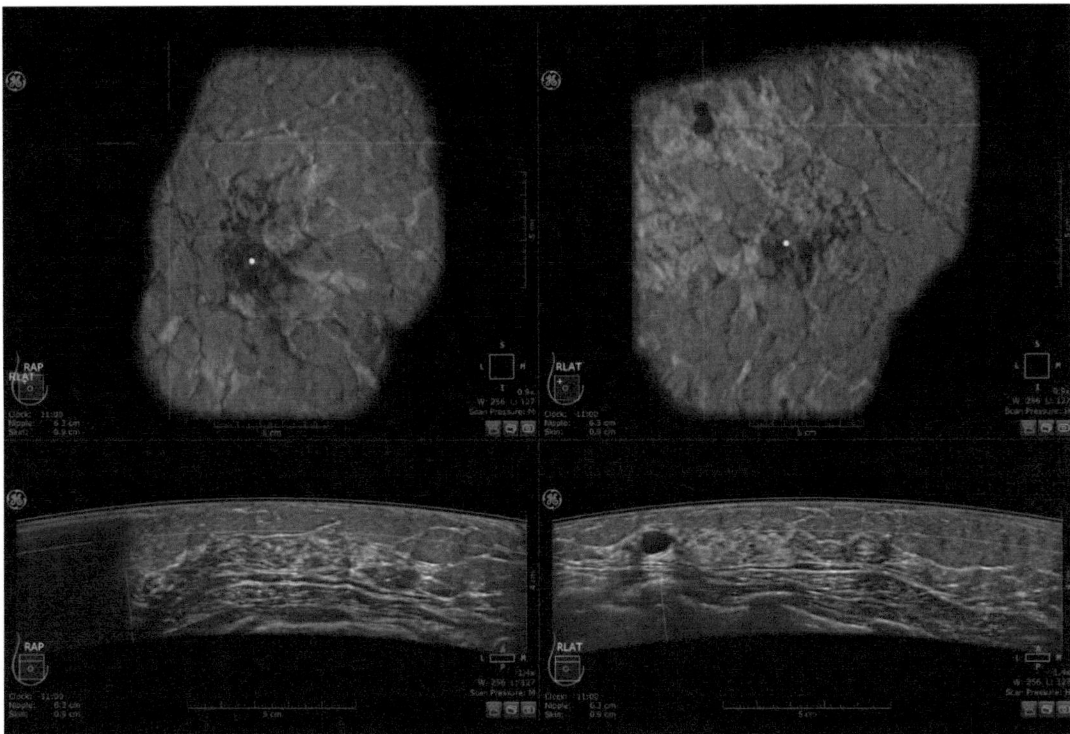

Fig. 35.6 ABUS allows for multiplanar visualization of an anechoic breast cyst in a dense breast, allowing for better characterization and diagnostic accuracy

with dense breasts. Also, there are no contrast or radiation risks involved with this technique.

Limitations: The major disadvantages of ABUS are related to increased false-positive recall rate especially due to the technique-related artifacts. Small invasive cancers may be easily overlooked when interpreting large breast imaging volume on ABUS.ABUS requires training in image acquisition and interpretation of multiplanar US images. Pitfalls in acquisition technique and lesion interpretation also can lead to increased false-positive recalls. In situ breast cancers are rarely detected with supplemental ABUS. There is also additional equipment cost and cost of training staff in ABUS image acquisition.

35.6 Elastography

Elastography has been developed as a complementary technique to standard B mode ultrasound [12, 13]. It utilizes the principle of estimating velocity of acoustic impulse inside a lesion to assess its stiffness and is mainly used as a supplemental tool to characterize a lesion that has already been detected in B mode. Its main use is in determining the true nature of an indeterminate or cystic breast lesion prior to biopsy. Shear waves are not induced when the ultrasound beam encounters a pure cyst, which helps in differentiation of solid and cystic lesions.

Technique: Elastography mode is activated on the keyboard while the B mode image is centrally located on the screen. In shear wave elastography, acoustic radiation force impulse (ARFI) mode is used to generate the impulse. The image generated is an elastogram, which can be displayed differently based on the manufacturer, either as a color or a black and white on the image and with differences in elasticity measurement depicted as speed level (ARFI, Siemens®) or as kPa (Aixplorer, SuperSonic Imagine®).A value of over 80 kPa (SWE) or velocity results of over 2 m/s are considered as suspicious. Color ARFI mode indicates stiffness of a lesion.

Limitations of elastography include false negatives in soft breast cancers such as mucinous carcinoma, carcinoma with an inflammatory stroma etc. Equally false positives can be seen in poorly deformable benign lesions such as old fibroadenomas. Despite the ability to enhance characterization, elastography is not yet sufficient to preclude the necessity of fine needle aspiration or core biopsy if cases where standard ultrasound features remain suspicious.

35.7 Contrast-Enhanced Ultrasound in Breast Using Microbubble

In patients with invasive breast cancer, the axillary lymph node (ALN) status plays a vital role in staging the breast cancer, assessing prognosis and influences on the treatment decisions. Earlier ALN dissection used to be the gold standard technique to clear nodal metastasis; however, this technique had significant morbidity due to lymphedema. With the advent of the national level screening programs and high-quality advanced imaging techniques, patients are now being diagnosed with smaller/early tumors even before nodal metastasis. Almost two-third of the breast cancers now are diagnosed without axillary metastasis [14].

Sentinel lymph node (SLN) being the first node that drains the breast cancer, its histological status from the SNL biopsy gives a reliable indicator of the lymph node status. Blue dye with gamma camera has been very widely used in the past for intraoperative identification of the SLN and were surgically excised. About 50% of the SLN-positive patients required a second surgery for complete axillary lymph nodes clearance. This was an important drawback of intraoperative SLN biopsy. Clinical examination and gray scale ultrasound imaging of the axillary lymph nodes were also not very sensitive in diagnosing nodal metastasis, especially in case of micrometastasis.

Contrast-enhanced ultrasound (CEUS) has been in clinical practice for a long time now. Ultrasound contrast agents are composed of microbubbles which are smaller the size of the RBC and disperse in the blood reflecting the ultrasound beam. After successful injection of microbubble in swan model, percutaneous injection of the microbubble was found to enter the lymphatic system and can be used in breast cancer patients to identify the SLN preoperative.

Technique: After administrating local anesthesia, about 0.2–0.5 mL of microbubble reconstituted in 5 mL of saline is injected just underneath the skin of the areolar in the upper outer quadrant. After injection of the microbubbles, lymphatic channels were visualized immediately on contrast pulse sequencing and were tracked into the axilla. Areas of contrast agent accumulation were then imaged with grayscale or were simultaneously viewed on live dual images to confirm the presence of an architecturally defined lymph node. 14/16 G core biopsy is performed on these nodes.

Advantage of CESU with microbubble in assessing the SLN status is that in case of macrometastasis after the microbubble SLN biopsy, gives the surgeon to plan for axillary nodal clearance (ANC) in the same setting as the breast surgery. Also, early recognition of SLN metastasis helps in starting the patient on neoadjuvant chemotherapy rather than surgery.

Limitations: It is a newer technique and requires further multicentric meta-analysis to implement into a standard clinical practice. In a study by Cox et al. [15], about 8% of patients who has benign SLN where found to have macro metastasis on subsequent axillary node dissection.

35.8 Advances in Breast Intervention

35.8.1 Vacuum-Assisted Biopsy (VAB)

VAB has been used as a first-line or second-line diagnostic procedure in breast lesions for over a decade. More recently, this interventional technique has been increasingly used to excise benign breast lesions (therapeutic) under image guidance thereby reducing the need for open surgical excision (Fig. 35.7). Current evidence appears to support its use provided that consent, audit, and clinical governance are in place. The diagnostic procedure utilizing this technique is often referred

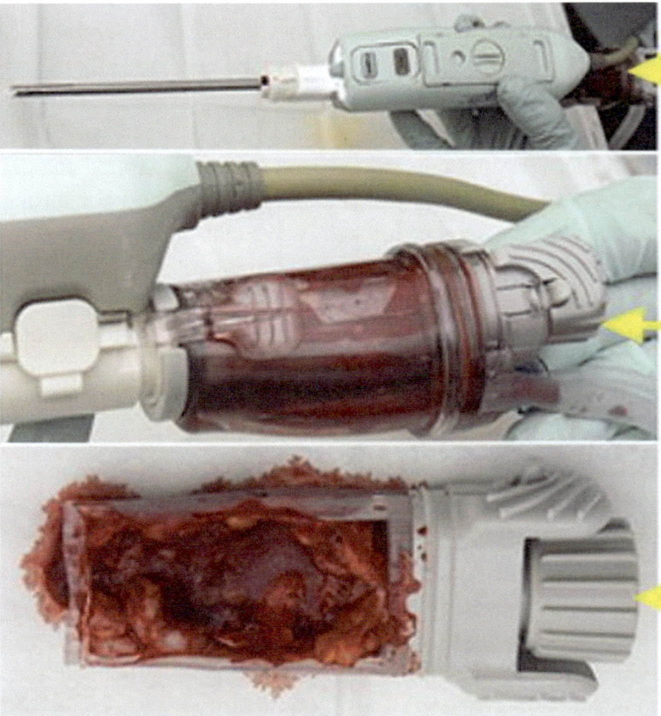

Fig. 35.7 Demonstrates the VAB needle in its holder and maneuvering of collection chamber to retrieve the samples from a vacuum biopsy needle. Image courtesy Dr. Caroline Parkin, Manchester, UK

to as vacuum assisted biopsy (VAB) while the excision of lesion with this is referred to as vacuum-assisted excision (VAE). While the aim of VAB is to obtain adequate number of samples to make a diagnosis, VAE aims at sufficient sampling of the lesion to replace the surgical diagnostic biopsy (min 4 g tissue).

Common indications for VAE include benign breast masses, B3 lesions without atypia and debulking of lesions in patients not suitable for surgery.

Technique: VAB and VAE can be undertaken under any imaging guidance including mammography, US, and MRI as long as the apparatus is compatible. The procedure is usually carried out under local anesthesia. A small incision is made in the breast, and a probe between 7 and 11 gauge is inserted through the lesion. Needle probe device is then attached to vacuum/suction. As the probe is drawn into the lesion, small amounts of tissue are continuously aspirated until the lesion disappears. At the end of procedure, compression is used to contain bleeding and skin is secured using with adhesive sutures if required. The procedure takes between 15 and 60 min, depending on the size of lesion being removed.

35.8.1.1 Limitations

Procedural hematoma is a well-recognized complication and can occur in in 10–20% cases. Complete removal may sometimes not be possible due to location or size of the abnormality. Such incompletely excised lesions may still require open surgery excision or follow up. Benign lesions such as fibroadenomas can recur even after complete excision and patients should be made aware of this.

35.8.2 Non-wire Breast Localizations

Breast conservation surgery often requires the use of an imaging-guided preoperative localization, and traditionally this was undertaken in the form of wire localization. This meant that image guided wire is placed in the breast percutaneously so that distal wire segment positioned adjacent to the abnormality and the proximal wire segment remains outside the breast. This had to be typically undertaken very close to or on the day of surgery to avoid wire displacement and it was necessary for the patient to be compliant and careful. Furthermore, wire entry site was determined by the radiologist, and this did not necessarily correspond with the ideal surgical incision site. Additional risks of wire transection and migration further complicated the issue. Non-wire localizations were developed to address these issues.

Types of non-wire localization devices that are currently available include:

- Radioactive seeds.
- Magnetic seeds.
- Radar reflectors.
- Radiofrequency identification tags.

Technique: Non-wire localization systems have three main components, which include a single-use 5–12 mm device with 12–18-gauge introducer, a small reusable console and an intraoperative detection probe.

Sterile localization device is introduced into the breast via the introducer following local anesthetic infiltration. Localization devices send and receive signal at a specific wavelength in the electromagnetic spectrum. A designated detection probe is used in the theater to identify the localization device. The detection console aids in identification of lesion location by emitting real-time audio and visual feedback to the surgeon as they dissect and advance closer to the target.

Advantages of non-wire localizations include improved patient experience with no wire (s) coming out of breast and less chance of migration. Non wire localizers (NWL) can be placed in advance of the surgery date giving flexibility of scheduling for radiologist and surgeon. Additional flexibility in surgical incision site for the surgeon has an advantage of improved cosmesis. There is also potential to remove less nontarget tissue because of intraoperative real time feedback for accuracy of lesion location. This technique has also shown improved access for targeted axillary node dissection which was not feasible with wire-guided localization technique.

35.8.2.1 Limitations

The disadvantages of non-wire localizations include the fact that once deployed they cannot be repositioned. If incorrectly positioned, placement of a second device is required, and this result in the removal of nontargeted tissue to retrieve the incorrectly positioned device. Minimum spacing of the devices is a necessary in bracketing (min 2 cm) to avoid signal interference. NWL devices cannot yet be placed under MRI guidance and detectability of nonradioactive devices limited by the depth from the skin.

Radioactivity from radioactive seeds caused additional limitations on people contact. Also, in these cases, once the seed is retrieved from the excised specimen, it must be placed in a lead container and sent back to the nuclear medicine service for safe disposal.

Further limitations pertaining to magnetic seeds (Magseed), which was introduced in 2016, are that it cannot be used with a pacemaker or implanted chest wall device and can cause susceptibility artifact on breast MRI. The depth detection is limited to 4 cm and therefore not suitable for deeper lesions or in big breasts. There is also a risk of ferromagnetic interference with the signal, so nonferromagnetic surgical instruments are necessary when operating on these patients.

35.9 Advances in Breast Imaging Interpretation

With the growth of machine learning applications, the radiology practice is evolving. Computer-aided detection (CAD) is a software technology that has been developed particularly to aid in breast cancer screening to improving earlier mammographic detection. Many studies have assessed the diagnostic accuracy of CAD, but its adaptation in clinical setting is yet to be widely implemented [16].

References

1. World Health Organization (WHO). Global health estimates 2020: deaths by cause, age, sex, by country and by region, 2000–2019. 2020. Accessed 11 Dec 2020.
2. Nyström L, Andersson I, Bjurstam N, Frisell J, Nordenskjöld B, Rutqvist LE. Long-term effects of mammography screening: updated overview of the Swedish randomised trials. Lancet. 2002;359(9310):909–19.
3. Kolb TM, Lichy J, Newhouse JH. Comparison of the performance of screening mammography, Physical examination, and breast US and evaluation of factors that influence them: an analysis of 27,825 patient evaluations. Radiology. 2002;225(1):165–75.
4. Vedantham S, Karellas A, Vijayaraghavan GR, Kopans DB. Digital breast tomosynthesis: state of the art. Radiology. 2015;277:663–84.
5. Sechopoulos I, Suryanarayanan S, Vedantham S, D'Orsi C, Karellas A. Computation of the glandular radiation dose in digital tomosynthesis of the breast. Med Phys. 2007;34(1):221–32.
6. Roth RG, et al. Digital breast tomosynthesis: lessons learned from early clinical implementation. Radiographics. 2014;34(4):18.
7. Zuley ML, Bandos AI, Abrams GS, et al. Time to diagnosis and performance levels during repeat interpretations of digital breast tomosynthesis: preliminary observations. Acad Radiol. 2010;17(4):450–5.
8. Kuhl CK, Schrading S, Strobel K, Schild HH, Hilgers RD, Bieling HB. Abbreviated breast magnetic resonance imaging (MRI): first postcontrast subtracted images and maximum-intensity projection-a novel approach to breast cancer screening with MRI. J Clin Oncol. 2014;32(22):2304–10.
9. Ghaderi KF, et al. Contrast-enhanced mammography: current applications and future directions. Radiographics. 2019;39(7):1907–20.
10. Patel BK, Naylor ME, Kosiorek HE, et al. Clinical utility of contrast-enhanced spectral mammography as an adjunct for tomosynthesis-detected architectural distortion. Clin Imaging. 2017;46:44–52.
11. van Zelst JCM, Man RM. Automated three-dimensional breast US for screening: technique, artifacts, and lesion characterization. Radiographics. 2018;38(3):663–83.
12. Balleyguier C, Canale S, Ben Hassen W, Vielh P, Bayou EH, Mathieu MC, et al. Breast elasticity: principles, technique, results: an update and overview of commercially available software. Eur J Radiol. 2013;82(3):427–34.
13. Balleyguier L, Ciolovan S, Ammari S, Canale S, Sethom S, RAI R, Vielh P, Dromain C. Breast elastography: the technical process and its applications, diagnostic and interventional. Diagn Interv Imaging. 2013;94(5):503–13. ISSN 2211–5684.
14. Silverstein MJ, Skinner KA, Lomis TJ. Predicting axillary nodal positivity in 2282 patients with breast carcinoma. World J Surg. 2001;25:767–77.
15. Cox K, et al. Validation of a technique using microbubbles and contrast enhanced ultrasound (CEUS) to biopsy sentinel lymph nodes (SLN) in pre-operative breast cancer patients with a normal grey-scale axillary ultrasound. Eur J Surg Oncol. 2013;39(7):760–5.
16. Masud R, Al-Rei M, Lokker. Computer-aided detection for breast cancer screening in clinical settings: scoping review. JMIR Med Inform. 2019;7(3):e12660.

Artificial Intelligence in Breast Imaging

36

Almir Bitencourt and Katja Pinker

Abstract

The use of artificial intelligence (AI) in breast imaging is rapidly evolving, with many possible applications, including improved image acquisition, more accurate detection and diagnosis of breast lesions, breast cancer risk assessment, and the development of new imaging biomarkers to predict treatment response and clinical outcomes. The application of AI tools in breast imaging offers an unprecedented opportunity to better derive clinical value from imaging data and reshape the way we care for our patients. This chapter discusses AI applications for mammography, breast ultrasound, and magnetic resonance imaging.

A. Bitencourt
Department of Imaging, A.C. Camargo Cancer Center, Sao Paulo, SP, Brazil

Department of Radiology, Breast Imaging Service, Memorial Sloan Kettering Cancer Center, Weill Medical College of Cornell University, New York, NY, USA

K. Pinker (✉)
Department of Radiology, Breast Imaging Service, Memorial Sloan Kettering Cancer Center, Weill Medical College of Cornell University, New York, NY, USA
e-mail: pinkerdk@mskcc.org

Keywords

Artificial Intelligence · Deep learning · Breast cancer · Mammography · Ultrasound · Magnetic resonance imaging

36.1 Introduction

One of the most promising areas of innovation in health care is the application of artificial intelligence (AI) in biomedical imaging. Of the myriad potential applications for AI in radiology, breast cancer screening is perhaps the best known and most researched case. Mammography was one of the first imaging modalities to incorporate AI techniques, beginning with traditional computer-aided detection (CAD), which have been available for over a decade. Significant advances in imaging analysis and the development of high-throughput methods have allowed the rapid and simultaneous extraction and correlation of multiple imaging parameters that are beyond what the human eye can detect [1–3]. Due to the non-invasive nature of medical imaging and its ubiquitous use in clinical practice, the field of AI is rapidly evolving in breast imaging [4–7].

Breast imaging is an ideal platform for AI since it mitigates a relevant clinical problem—big datasets—and applies algorithms to the workflow [8]. The analysis of large amounts of

B. Dev, L. D. Joseph (eds.), *Holistic Approach to Breast Disease*,
https://doi.org/10.1007/978-981-99-0035-0_36

imaging data has become a challenge, and the demand for breast radiologists has dramatically increased. A labor shortage of breast radiologists and high prevalence of burnout [9, 10] compounds this problem. AI is well suited to handle repetitive work processes and to manage large amounts of data; hence, it could be used to enhance breast imaging efficiency and overcome workload problems. With the continuous advances in radiomics analysis and machine learning (such as deep learning), we are now on the cusp of providing more effective, more efficient, and even more patient-centric breast cancer care than ever before.

AI in breast imaging offers many possible applications, including improved image acquisition, more accurate detection and diagnosis of breast lesions, and the development of new imaging biomarkers. AI can also be applied to different imaging modalities and clinical scenarios, which will be discussed in this chapter.

36.2 Basic Concepts for AI Studies

In AI studies, either traditional machine learning (ML) or more recently deep learning (DL) techniques are employed. The first AI models in breast imaging were computer-aided design (CAD) models, which have been studied since the 1960s. CAD uses hand-crafted radiomics coupled with ML to extract patterns such as shape, margin, or texture of a lesion based on a large number of examples and then defines algorithms to aid the radiologist. However, its performance in studies was limited, which in turn hampered clinical implementation. The early CAD systems for screening relied on machine learning with human-coded feature engineering, and their performance was generally limited. Recently, DL has been increasingly studied in breast imaging, owing to advances in computing power. DL is based on the structure of neural networks akin to those in the human brain, allowing computers to autonomously learn to identify patterns in a set of images, without the need for predefined characteristics. The convolutional neural network (CNN) is currently the most used DL architecture in image analysis and has been successfully applied to imaging analysis in various areas of knowledge. Recent advances in both software and hardware have enabled CNN models to surpass human performance in many situations.

DL studies must pass through rigorous validation steps including defining the imaging data sets (training, validation, and test sets), defining the "ground truth" reference standard, having a detailed description of the training approach and metrics of model performance, and having validation or testing of the algorithm with external data [11, 12]. Three independent data sets (the aforementioned training, validation, and test sets) are needed: first, AI algorithms are trained on an initial set of images according to a reference standard; second, the final algorithm is validated on a separate set of images; and third, an external set of images is used to report the final statistical results of the algorithm [11].

36.3 AI in Mammography

Mammography is the current gold standard in screening to detect early breast cancer, when treatment can achieve better outcomes. One limitation of screening mammography is the relatively high number of missed cancers; in the general screening population, mammography has a sensitivity ranging from 75% to 85%, but this sensitivity is significantly reduced among women with dense breasts [13]. Additionally, this technique has a high rate of false positives and therefore comes with a high recall rate. Thus, AI in mammography has been mainly used to increase the detection of significant cancer and reduce the recall rate [14].

The most recent AI studies in mammography have focused on using CNN to increase screening accuracy by characterizing mammographic abnormalities (Figs.36.1 and 36.2). Different frameworks have been trained, used, and com-

Fig. 36.1 The outline of the Faster R-CNN model for CAD in mammography. Reprinted under a Creative Commons Attribution 4.0 International (CC BY 4.0) license from: Ribli D, Horváth A, Unger Z, et al. (2018.) Detecting and classifying lesions in mammograms with deep learning. Sci Rep. 8: 4165. https://doi.org/10.1038/s41598-018-22437-z

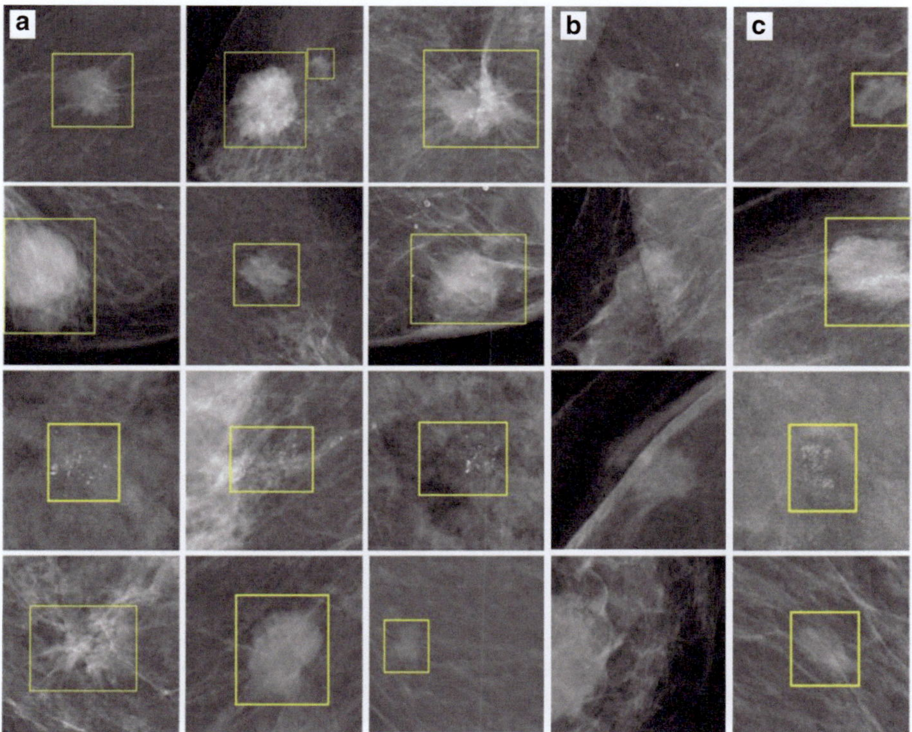

Fig. 36.2 Detection examples: The yellow boxes show the lesion proposed by the model. The threshold for these detections was selected to be at lesion detection sensitivity = 0.9. (**a**) Correctly detected malignant lesions. (**b**) Missed malignant lesions. (**c**) False-positive detections, courtesy of the Breast Research Group, INESC Porto, Portugal. Reprinted under a Creative Commons Attribution 4.0 International (CC BY 4.0) license from: Ribli D, Horváth A, Unger Z, et al. (2018). Detecting and classifying lesions in mammograms with deep learning. Sci Rep 8: 4165. https://doi.org/10.1038/s41598-018-22437-z

pared, and the most representative algorithms have achieved an area under the curve (AUC) of around 0.9 [15–17]. Many authors have compared AI algorithm performance in multi-reader studies and demonstrated that a hybrid model, using an AI algorithm combined with radiologist assessment, is more accurate than either one separately [18–21]. Notably, most of these studies are retrospective and cannot be directly compared with radiologist performance in a real screening scenario.

Another important goal is to increase screening efficiency. Less than 1% of screening examinations yields a cancer diagnosis; therefore, most of the workload is related to reading normal exams. In addition, double reading is standardized in several countries, lengthening reporting times. Using an ML classifier to correctly identify normal mammograms would reduce radiologist workload and improve screening mammography workflow without impacting diagnostic accuracy. AI can correctly identify a proportion of screening mammograms as normal [22–25] and can safely reduce the screening workload by up to 70% for digital mammography and digital breast tomosynthesis-based programs without reducing the sensitivity by 5% or more (Figs. 36.3 and 36.4) [26].

AI has also been used as a tool for breast cancer risk prediction based on mammography image analysis, which could be an essential foundation for the implementation of personalized screening. High mammographic breast density is known to be an independent risk factor for the development of breast cancer [27], and using AI for automated quantitative assessment of breast density has proven to be superior to human evaluation in several studies [28, 29]. DL density-

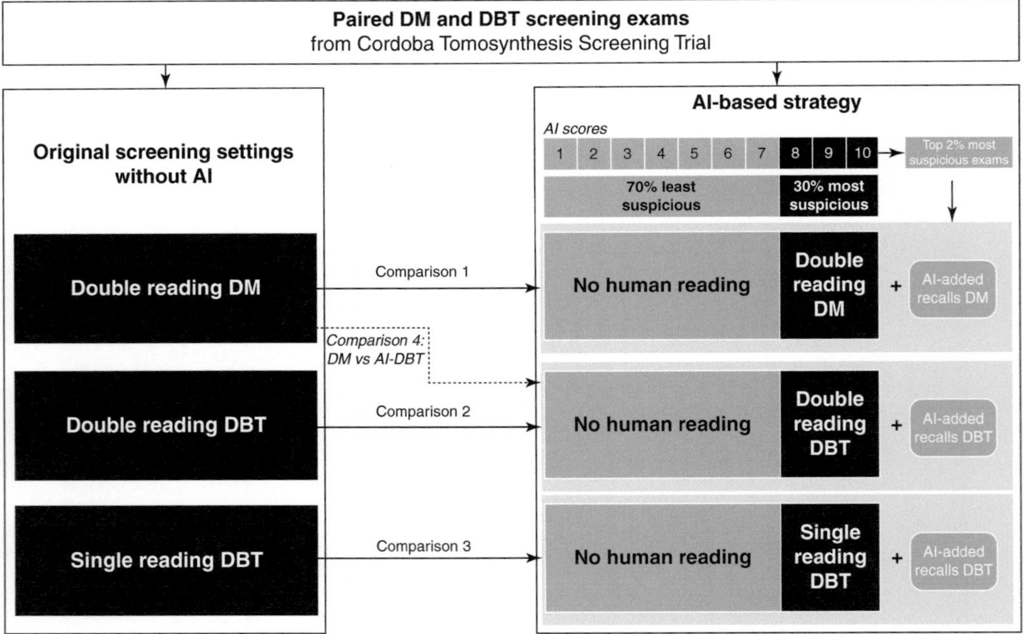

Fig. 36.3 Flowchart of the original screening strategies and how they were compared with the artificial intelligence (AI)-based screening strategy. If the original setting used digital mammography (DM), AI scores computed on DM images were used. Similarly, if the original setting used digital breast tomosynthesis (DBT), the AI scores computed on only DBT images were used. Cases were considered very likely normal if the AI score was 7 or lower (approximately 70% of screening volume). Additionally, the examinations not recalled by radiologists but with an AI score among the 2% most suspicious examinations in the cohort were considered automatically recalled. Reprinted under a Creative Commons Attribution 4.0 International (CC BY 4.0) license from: Raya-Povedano JL, Romero-Martín S, Elías-Cabot E, et al. (2021). AI-based strategies to reduce workload in breast cancer screening with mammography and tomosynthesis: A retrospective evaluation. Radiology 300(1): 57–65. https://doi.org/10.1148/radiol.2021203555

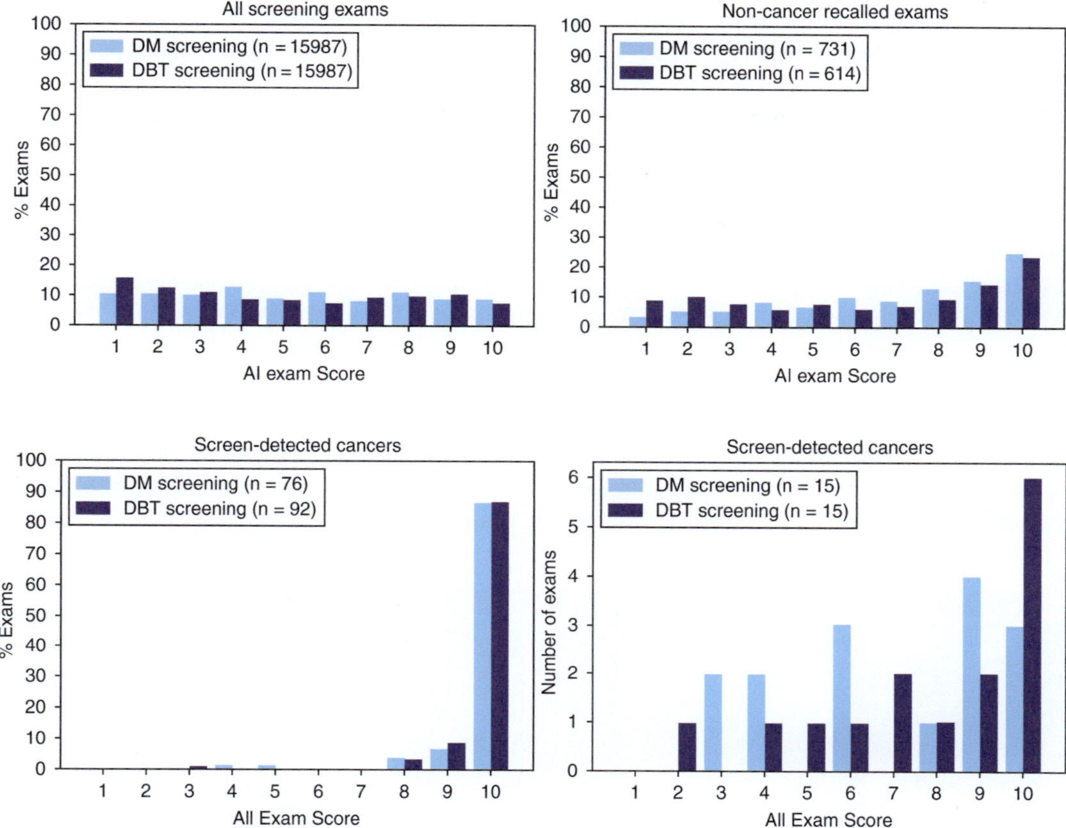

Fig. 36.4 Bar graphs show distribution of artificial intelligence (AI) examination scores across different groups of examinations in the paired digital mammography (DM)-digital breast tomosynthesis (DBT) cohort (all examinations, non-cancer recalled examinations, screening-detected cancers, and interval cancers). AI scores were computed for DM and DBT examinations independently. The ground truth was computed for DM-based screening outcomes and for DBT-based screening outcomes (which includes DBT plus DM and DBT plus synthetic mammography workflows). For interval cancers, the only difference is whether the AI scores were computed for DM or DBT images. Reprinted under a Creative Commons Attribution 4.0 International (CC BY 4.0) license from: Raya-Povedano JL, Romero-Martín S, Elías-Cabot E, et al. (2021). AI-based strategies to reduce workload in breast cancer screening with mammography and tomosynthesis: A retrospective evaluation. Radiology 300(1): 57–65. https://doi.org/10.1148/radiol.2021203555

based models combining traditional risk factors could be more accurate than density-based models and the established risk models currently used in clinical practice alone for breast cancer risk prediction. Dembrower et al. [30] developed a DL risk score that predicts women's risk for future breast cancer more accurately than density-based models, with a lower false-negative rate for aggressive cancers. Yala et al. [31] developed three full-field mammography-based DL breast cancer risk models to determine breast cancer risk within 5 years by using traditional risk factors, mammographic density alone, and a hybrid DL model that used both traditional risk factors and mammograms. The latter yielded the best AUC (0.70) compared to the other two models as well as the clinically established Tyrer–Cuzick (version 8) model.

36.4 AI in Breast Ultrasound

Ultrasound (US) has shown more sensitivity than mammography for breast cancer detection regardless of age group. However, its specificity remains lower than that of mammography, especially for women aged 50 years or older [32]. Thus, the main interest of AI in breast US has been the differentiation of benign and malignant breast masses based on B-mode features [33–35]. Several groups have investigated these AI models in multi-reader studies [36–39], showing that AI accuracy for breast cancer diagnosis is comparable to that of radiologists and allows for a better and faster learning curve than a human reader without prior experience (Fig. 36.5). DL algorithms have been recently incorporated in US devices to assist radiologists in decision-making based on static B-mode images for the assessment of focal breast lesions [40–42]. Although some of these AI-based decision support systems are approved by regulators in different countries, there are still no guidelines to recommend the application of AI with US in clinical practice.

36.5 AI in Breast Magnetic Resonance Imaging (MRI)

Breast MRI has a high sensitivity for breast cancer diagnosis and can provide quantitative biomarkers for breast cancer assessment. Therefore, breast MRI is probably the imaging modality with the most data available from AI studies on different applications, mainly for lesion detection and classification [43]. Fully automated detection of breast cancer on screening MRI using CNN has been shown to be possible, not only for sys-

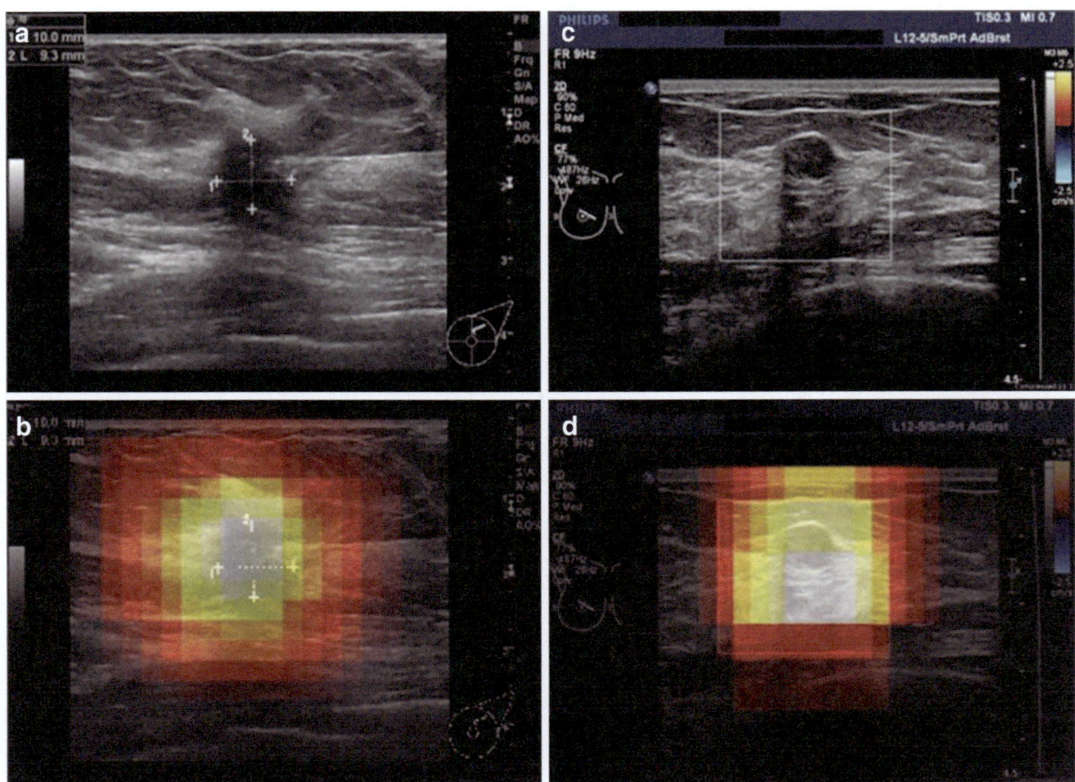

Fig. 36.5 (**a**, **b**) Ultrasound (US) image of a lesion in a female patient from the internal test dataset (age 58). The lesion was histologically proven as invasive-ductal breast cancer and classified as BI-RADS 5 in the radiological report and by both readers. The lesion was correctly identified by the deep convolutional neural network (dCNN) via the sliding window approach and was analyzed. (**c**, **d**) US image of a fibroadenoma confirmed via stable follow-up examinations from the external test dataset. Despite the different vendors and institutions, the dCNN was able to correctly identify and classify the lesion. Reprinted with permission from: Ciritsis A, Rossi C, Eberhard M, et al. (2019) Automatic classification of ultrasound breast lesions using a deep convolutional neural network mimicking human decision-making. Eur Radiol 29: 5458–5468. https://doi.org/10.1007/s00330-019-06118-7

tematic diagnostic interpretation [44] but also for identifying tumor-containing slices stored on picture archiving and communication systems [45]. This can be particularly useful for non-systematic image review, such as for research purposes or interdisciplinary tumor board meetings.

The more extensive use of breast MRI for both screening and conventional imaging problem-solving purposes has posed significant challenges in clinical practice due to the high number of detected lesions. Hence, different approaches have been tested to help classify breast lesions identified on MRI as benign or malignant, which could reduce the number of unnecessary breast biopsies. Models using both dynamic contrast enhancement (DCE) and diffusion-weighted imaging (DWI) have achieved AUCs of up to 0.88 [46–52]. This is particularly important in the setting of challenging lesions such as sub-centimeter lesions, non-mass-like lesions, or those pertaining to high-risk patient groups [53–55].

Another reported application beyond lesion classification and detection is the prediction of breast cancer molecular subtype. It has been shown that specific molecular subtypes seem to carry radiomics signatures on DCE-MR images that can be used to accurately classify lesions with respect to receptor status and molecular subtypes (Fig. 36.6) [56–68]. Although radiomics and AI are unlikely to replace invasive tissue sampling, these signatures may have the potential to provide prognostic indicators derived from the whole tumor, while biopsy sampling, currently used for molecular subtyping, only provides a snapshot of the bigger picture. This could be especially useful for monitoring changes in biology during treatment.

AI-enhanced MRI has also been used to predict response to neoadjuvant chemotherapy

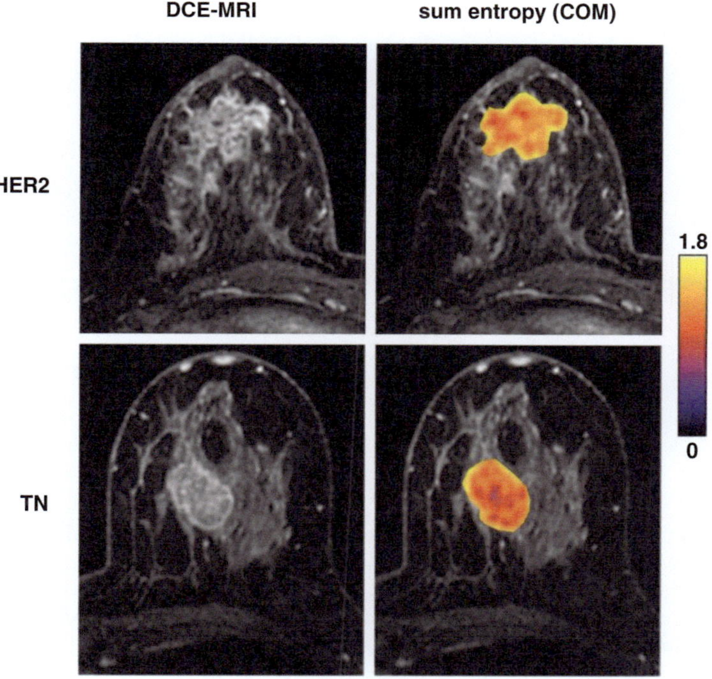

Fig. 36.6 Original CE-MRI images and corresponding color-coded sum entropy feature map as overlay of the tumor area of triple-negative (TN) and HER2-enriched (HER2) breast cancer. TN shows a clearly lower sum entropy than HER2. Reprinted under a Creative Commons Attribution 4.0 International (CC BY 4.0) license from: Leithner D, Horvat J V., Marino MA, et al. (2019). Radiomic signatures with contrast-enhanced magnetic resonance imaging for the assessment of breast cancer receptor status and molecular subtypes: initial results. Breast Cancer Res 21: 106. https://doi.org/10.1186/s13058-019-1187-z

(NAC) at an early stage or even prior to commencing NAC (Fig. 36.7) [69, 70]. This application of AI would help avoid administering ineffective and potentially toxic therapies and help expedite surgery in patients who would not benefit from NAC. Furthermore, surgery can be potentially avoided in patients with pathologic complete response (pCR) after NAC. ML with multiparametric MRI allowed early prediction of pCR after only two cycles of NAC (AUC of 0.86) and of survival outcomes with high accuracy [71–76].

The prediction of cancer recurrence is another relevant clinical query. Currently, this is assessed through recurrence score genetic testing, which is relatively costly and not always available. AI-enhanced MRI has shown to be potentially useful for recurrence prediction [77–83]. Lastly, breast MRI has also been proposed as a tool for breast cancer risk prediction, which might have relevant implications for personalized breast câncer screening. Portnoi et al. [84] developed an image-based DL model to predict the 5-year breast cancer risk on the basis of a single breast MRI from a screening examination and showed that this model improved individual risk discrimination when compared with a state-of-the-art risk assessment model.

36.6 Conclusions

The field of AI-enhanced breast imaging is rapidly evolving, with many potential applications, such as breast cancer risk prediction, lesion detection and classification, radiogenomics, and prediction of treatment response and clinical outcomes. The application of AI tools in breast imaging offers an unprecedented opportunity to better derive clinical value from imaging data and reshape the way we care for our patients. Currently, the main challenges for implementing AI techniques in the clinical setting are the lack of standardization and small sample sizes. Collaboration among different institutions and independent testing to validate results will be key for achieving the necessary milestones for meaningful clinical implementation.

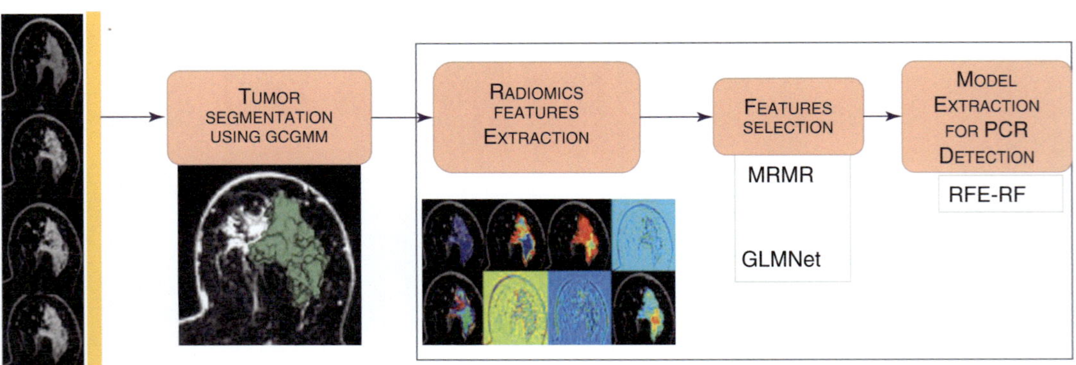

Fig. 36.7 Framework for radiomics analysis. The Grow Cut Gaussian Mixture Model was used to generate volumetric tumor segmentation from the T1w DCE-MRI. Next, radiomics analysis was performed to extract the texture measures from the segmented volumes followed by machine learning analysis consisting of feature pre-filtering using Maximum Relevance Minimum Redundancy (MRMR) and generalized linear regression with elastic net constraints feature selection (GLMNet), followed by a recursive feature elimination random forest (RFE-RF) classifier for extracting a model for detecting a pCR. Reprinted under a Creative Commons Attribution 4.0 International (CC BY 4.0) license from: Sutton EJ, Onishi N, Fehr DA, et al. (2020). A machine learning model that classifies breast cancer pathologic complete response on MRI post-neoadjuvant chemotherapy. Breast Cancer Res 22: 57. https://doi.org/10.1186/s13058-020-01291-w

References

1. Gillies RJ, Kinahan PE, Hricak H. Radiomics: images are more than pictures, they are data. Radiology. 2016;278:563–77. https://doi.org/10.1148/radiol.2015151169.
2. Lambin P, Leijenaar RTH, Deist TM, et al. Radiomics: the bridge between medical imaging and personalized medicine. Nat Rev Clin Oncol. 2017;14:749–62. https://doi.org/10.1038/nrclinonc.2017.141.
3. Pinker K, Chin J, Melsaether AN, et al. Precision medicine and Radiogenomics in breast cancer: new approaches toward diagnosis and treatment. Radiology. 2018;287:732–47. https://doi.org/10.1148/radiol.2018172171.
4. Chartrand G, Cheng PM, Vorontsov E, et al. Deep learning: a primer for radiologists. RadioGraphics. 2017;37:2113–31. https://doi.org/10.1148/rg.2017170077.
5. Giger ML. Machine learning in medical imaging. J Am Coll Radiol. 2018;15:512–20. https://doi.org/10.1016/j.jacr.2017.12.028.
6. Hosny A, Parmar C, Quackenbush J, et al. Artificial intelligence in radiology. Nat Rev Cancer. 2018;18:500–10. https://doi.org/10.1038/s41568-018-0016-5.
7. Yamashita R, Nishio M, Do RKG, Togashi K. Convolutional neural networks: an overview and application in radiology. Insights Imaging. 2018;9:611–29. https://doi.org/10.1007/s13244-018-0639-9.
8. Morgan MB, Mates JL. Applications of artificial intelligence in breast imaging. Radiol Clin N Am. 2021;59:139–48. https://doi.org/10.1016/j.rcl.2020.08.007.
9. Parikh JR, Sun J, Mainiero MB. Prevalence of burnout in breast imaging radiologists. J Breast Imaging. 2020;2:112–8. https://doi.org/10.1093/jbi/wbz091.
10. Wing P, Langelier MH. Workforce shortages in breast imaging: impact on mammography utilization. Am J Roentgenol. 2009;192:370–8. https://doi.org/10.2214/AJR.08.1665.
11. Bluemke DA, Moy L, Bredella MA, et al. Assessing radiology research on artificial intelligence: a brief guide for authors, reviewers, and readers—from the radiology editorial board. Radiology. 2020;294:487–9. https://doi.org/10.1148/radiol.2019192515.
12. Mongan J, Moy L, Kahn CE. Checklist for artificial intelligence in medical imaging (CLAIM): a guide for authors and reviewers. Radiol Artif Intell. 2020;2:e200029. https://doi.org/10.1148/ryai.2020200029.
13. Domingo L, Hofvind S, Hubbard RA, et al. Cross-national comparison of screening mammography accuracy measures in U.S., Norway, and Spain. Eur Radiol. 2016;26:2520–8. https://doi.org/10.1007/s00330-015-4074-8.
14. Geras KJ, Mann RM, Moy L. Artificial intelligence for mammography and digital breast tomosynthesis: current concepts and future perspectives. Radiology. 2019;293:246–59. https://doi.org/10.1148/radiol.2019182627.
15. Chougrad H, Zouaki H, Alheyane O. Deep convolutional neural networks for breast cancer screening. Comput Methods Prog Biomed. 2018;157:19–30. https://doi.org/10.1016/j.cmpb.2018.01.011.
16. Lee RS, Gimenez F, Hoogi A, et al. A curated mammography data set for use in computer-aided detection and diagnosis research. Sci Data. 2017;4:170177. https://doi.org/10.1038/sdata.2017.177.
17. Ribli D, Horváth A, Unger Z, et al. Detecting and classifying lesions in mammograms with deep learning. Sci Rep. 2018;8:4165. https://doi.org/10.1038/s41598-018-22437-z.
18. Kim HE, Kim HH, Han BK, et al. Changes in cancer detection and false-positive recall in mammography using artificial intelligence: a retrospective, multi-reader study. Lancet Digit Health. 2020;2:e138–48. https://doi.org/10.1016/S2589-7500(20)30003-0.
19. Rodríguez-Ruiz A, Krupinski E, Mordang J-J, et al. Detection of breast cancer with mammography: effect of an artificial intelligence support system. Radiology. 2019;290:305–14. https://doi.org/10.1148/radiol.2018181371.
20. Schaffter T, Buist DSM, Lee CI, et al. Evaluation of combined artificial intelligence and radiologist assessment to interpret screening mammograms. JAMA Netw Open. 2020;3:e200265. https://doi.org/10.1001/jamanetworkopen.2020.0265.
21. Wu N, Phang J, Park J, et al. Deep neural networks improve radiologists' performance in breast cancer screening. IEEE Trans Med Imaging. 2020;39:1184–94. https://doi.org/10.1109/TMI.2019.2945514.
22. Kyono T, Gilbert FJ, van der Schaar M. Improving workflow efficiency for mammography using machine learning. J Am Coll Radiol. 2020;17:56–63. https://doi.org/10.1016/j.jacr.2019.05.012.
23. Lång K, Dustler M, Dahlblom V, et al. Identifying normal mammograms in a large screening population using artificial intelligence. Eur Radiol. 2021;31:1687–92. https://doi.org/10.1007/s00330-020-07165-1.
24. McKinney SM, Sieniek M, Godbole V, et al. International evaluation of an AI system for breast cancer screening. Nature. 2020;577:89–94. https://doi.org/10.1038/s41586-019-1799-6.
25. Yala A, Schuster T, Miles R, et al. A deep learning model to triage screening mammograms: a simulation study. Radiology. 2019b;293:38–46. https://doi.org/10.1148/radiol.2019182908.
26. Raya-Povedano JL, Romero-Martín S, Elías-Cabot E, et al. AI-based strategies to reduce workload in breast cancer screening with mammography and tomosynthesis: a retrospective evaluation. Radiology. 2021;300(1):57–65. https://doi.org/10.1148/radiol.2021203555.

27. Vourtsis A, Berg WA. Breast density implications and supplemental screening. Eur Radiol. 2019;29:1762–77. https://doi.org/10.1007/s00330-018-5668-8.
28. Sartor H, Lång K, Rosso A, et al. Measuring mammographic density: comparing a fully automated volumetric assessment versus European radiologists' qualitative classification. Eur Radiol. 2016;26:4354–60. https://doi.org/10.1007/s00330-016-4309-3.
29. Sprague BL, Conant EF, Onega T, et al. Variation in mammographic breast density assessments among radiologists in clinical practice. Ann Intern Med. 2016;165:457. https://doi.org/10.7326/M15-2934.
30. Dembrower K, Liu Y, Azizpour H, et al. Comparison of a deep learning risk score and standard mammographic density score for breast cancer risk prediction. Radiology. 2020;294:265–72. https://doi.org/10.1148/radiol.2019190872.
31. Yala A, Lehman C, Schuster T, et al. A deep learning mammography-based model for improved breast cancer risk prediction. Radiology. 2019a;292:60–6. https://doi.org/10.1148/radiol.2019182716.
32. Tan KP, Mohamad Azlan Z, Rumaisa MP, et al. The comparative accuracy of ultrasound and mammography in the detection of breast cancer. Med J Malaysia. 2014;69:79–85.
33. Han S, Kang HK, Jeong JY, et al. A deep learning framework for supporting the classification of breast lesions in ultrasound images. Phys Med Biol. 2017;62:7714–28. https://doi.org/10.1088/1361-6560/aa82ec.
34. Niu S, Huang J, Li J, et al. Application of ultrasound artificial intelligence in the differential diagnosis between benign and malignant breast lesions of BI-RADS 4A. BMC Cancer. 2020;20:959. https://doi.org/10.1186/s12885-020-07413-z.
35. Shen W-C, Chang R-F, Moon WK, et al. Breast ultrasound computer-aided diagnosis using BI-RADS features. Acad Radiol. 2007;14:928–39. https://doi.org/10.1016/j.acra.2007.04.016.
36. Becker AS, Mueller M, Stoffel E, et al. Classification of breast cancer in ultrasound imaging using a generic deep learning analysis software: a pilot study. Br J Radiol. 2017;91(1083):20170576. https://doi.org/10.1259/bjr.20170576.
37. Ciritsis A, Rossi C, Eberhard M, et al. Automatic classification of ultrasound breast lesions using a deep convolutional neural network mimicking human decision-making. Eur Radiol. 2019;29:5458–68. https://doi.org/10.1007/s00330-019-06118-7.
38. Li J, Bu Y, Lu S, et al. Development of a deep learning–based model for diagnosing breast nodules with ultrasound. J Ultrasound Med. 2021;40:513–20. https://doi.org/10.1002/jum.15427.
39. O'Connell AM, Bartolotta TV, Orlando A, et al. Diagnostic performance of an artificial intelligence system in breast ultrasound. J Ultrasound Med. 2021;41(1):97–105. https://doi.org/10.1002/jum.15684.
40. Di Segni M, de Soccio V, Cantisani V, et al. Automated classification of focal breast lesions according to S-detect: validation and role as a clinical and teaching tool. J Ultrasound. 2018;21:105–18. https://doi.org/10.1007/s40477-018-0297-2.
41. Kim K, Song MK, Kim E-K, Yoon JH. Clinical application of S-detect to breast masses on ultrasonography: a study evaluating the diagnostic performance and agreement with a dedicated breast radiologist. Ultrasonography. 2017;36:3–9. https://doi.org/10.14366/usg.16012.
42. Mango VL, Sun M, Wynn RT, Ha R. Should we ignore, follow, or biopsy? Impact of artificial intelligence decision support on breast ultrasound lesion assessment. Am J Roentgenol. 2020;214:1445–52. https://doi.org/10.2214/AJR.19.21872.
43. Meyer-Bäse A, Morra L, Meyer-Bäse U, Pinker K. Current status and future perspectives of artificial intelligence in magnetic resonance breast imaging. Contrast Media Mol Imaging. 2020;2020:1–18. https://doi.org/10.1155/2020/6805710.
44. Dalmış MU, Vreemann S, Kooi T, et al. Fully automated detection of breast cancer in screening MRI using convolutional neural networks. J Med Imaging. 2018;5:1. https://doi.org/10.1117/1.JMI.5.1.014502.
45. Eskreis-Winkler S, Onishi N, Pinker K, et al. Using deep learning to improve nonsystematic viewing of breast cancer on MRI. J Breast Imaging. 2021;3:201–7. https://doi.org/10.1093/jbi/wbaa102.
46. Bickelhaupt S, Paech D, Kickingereder P, et al. Prediction of malignancy by a radiomic signature from contrast agent-free diffusion MRI in suspicious breast lesions found on screening mammography. J Magn Reson Imaging. 2017;46:604–16. https://doi.org/10.1002/jmri.25606.
47. Dalmiş MU, Gubern-Mérida A, Vreemann S, et al. Artificial intelligence–based classification of breast lesions imaged with a multiparametric breast MRI protocol with ultrafast DCE-MRI, T2, and DWI. Investig Radiol. 2019;54:325–32. https://doi.org/10.1097/RLI.0000000000000544.
48. Dietzel M, Baltzer PAT, Dietzel A, et al. Artificial neural networks for differential diagnosis of breast lesions in MR-mammography: a systematic approach addressing the influence of network architecture on diagnostic performance using a large clinical database. Eur J Radiol. 2012;81:1508–13. https://doi.org/10.1016/j.ejrad.2011.03.024.
49. Herent P, Schmauch B, Jehanno P, et al. Detection and characterization of MRI breast lesions using deep learning. Diagn Interv Imaging. 2019;100:219–25. https://doi.org/10.1016/j.diii.2019.02.008.
50. Ji Y, Li H, Edwards AV, et al. Independent validation of machine learning in diagnosing breast cancer on magnetic resonance imaging within a single institution. Cancer Imaging. 2019;19:64. https://doi.org/10.1186/s40644-019-0252-2.
51. Pötsch N, Dietzel M, Kapetas P, et al. An A.I. classifier derived from 4D radiomics of dynamic contrast-enhanced breast MRI data: potential to avoid unnecessary breast biopsies. Eur Radiol. 2021;31:5866. https://doi.org/10.1007/s00330-021-07787-z.

52. Truhn D, Schrading S, Haarburger C, et al. Radiomic versus convolutional neural networks analysis for classification of contrast-enhancing lesions at multiparametric breast MRI. Radiology. 2019;290:290–7. https://doi.org/10.1148/radiol.2018181352.
53. Lo Gullo R, Daimiel I, Rossi Saccarelli C, et al. Improved characterization of sub-centimeter enhancing breast masses on MRI with radiomics and machine learning in BRCA mutation carriers. Eur Radiol. 2020a;30:6721–31. https://doi.org/10.1007/s00330-020-06991-7.
54. Lo Gullo R, Vincenti K, Rossi Saccarelli C, et al. Diagnostic value of radiomics and machine learning with dynamic contrast-enhanced magnetic resonance imaging for patients with atypical ductal hyperplasia in predicting malignant upgrade. Breast Cancer Res Treat. 2021;187:535. https://doi.org/10.1007/s10549-020-06074-7.
55. Meyer-Base A, Morra L, Tahmassebi A, et al. AI-enhanced diagnosis of challenging lesions in breast MRI: a methodology and application primer. J Magn Reson Imaging. 2020;54(3):686–702. https://doi.org/10.1002/jmri.27332.
56. Fan M, Li H, Wang S, et al. Radiomic analysis reveals DCE-MRI features for prediction of molecular subtypes of breast cancer. PLoS One. 2017;12:e0171683. https://doi.org/10.1371/journal.pone.0171683.
57. Grimm LJ, Zhang J, Mazurowski MA. Computational approach to radiogenomics of breast cancer: luminal a and luminal B molecular subtypes are associated with imaging features on routine breast MRI extracted using computer vision algorithms. J Magn Reson Imaging. 2015;42:902–7. https://doi.org/10.1002/jmri.24879.
58. Holli-Helenius K, Salminen A, Rinta-Kiikka I, et al. MRI texture analysis in differentiating luminal a and luminal B breast cancer molecular subtypes - a feasibility study. BMC Med Imaging. 2017;17:69. https://doi.org/10.1186/s12880-017-0239-z.
59. Leithner D, Bernard-Davila B, Martinez DF, et al. Radiomic signatures derived from diffusion-weighted imaging for the assessment of breast cancer receptor status and molecular subtypes. Mol Imaging Biol. 2020a;22:453–61. https://doi.org/10.1007/s11307-019-01383-w.
60. Leithner D, Horvat JV, Marino MA, et al. Radiomic signatures with contrast-enhanced magnetic resonance imaging for the assessment of breast cancer receptor status and molecular subtypes: initial results. Breast Cancer Res. 2019;21:106. https://doi.org/10.1186/s13058-019-1187-z.
61. Leithner D, Mayerhoefer ME, Martinez DF, et al. Non-invasive assessment of breast cancer molecular subtypes with multiparametric magnetic resonance imaging Radiomics. J Clin Med. 2020b;9:1853. https://doi.org/10.3390/jcm9061853.
62. Mazurowski MA, Zhang J, Grimm LJ, et al. Radiogenomic analysis of breast cancer: luminal B molecular subtype is associated with enhancement dynamics at MR imaging. Radiology. 2014;273:365–72. https://doi.org/10.1148/radiol.14132641.
63. Sun X, He B, Luo X, et al. Preliminary study on molecular subtypes of breast cancer based on magnetic resonance imaging texture analysis. J Comput Assist Tomogr. 2018;42:531–5. https://doi.org/10.1097/RCT.0000000000000738.
64. Sutton EJ, Dashevsky BZ, Oh JH, et al. Breast cancer molecular subtype classifier that incorporates MRI features. J Magn Reson Imaging. 2016;44:122–9. https://doi.org/10.1002/jmri.25119.
65. Wang Q, Mao N, Liu M, et al. Radiomic analysis on magnetic resonance diffusion weighted image in distinguishing triple-negative breast cancer from other subtypes: a feasibility study. Clin Imaging. 2021;72:136–41. https://doi.org/10.1016/j.clinimag.2020.11.024.
66. Wu J, Sun X, Wang J, et al. Identifying relations between imaging phenotypes and molecular subtypes of breast cancer: model discovery and external validation. J Magn Reson Imaging. 2017;46:1017–27. https://doi.org/10.1002/jmri.25661.
67. Xie T, Zhao Q, Fu C, et al. Differentiation of triple-negative breast cancer from other subtypes through whole-tumor histogram analysis on multiparametric MR imaging. Eur Radiol. 2019;29:2535–44. https://doi.org/10.1007/s00330-018-5804-5.
68. Zhang Y, Zhu Y, Zhang K, et al. Invasive ductal breast cancer: preoperative predict Ki-67 index based on radiomics of ADC maps. Radiol Med. 2020;125:109–16. https://doi.org/10.1007/s11547-019-01100-1.
69. Ha R, Chin C, Karcich J, et al. Prior to initiation of chemotherapy, can we predict breast tumor response? Deep learning convolutional neural networks approach using a breast MRI tumor dataset. J Digit Imaging. 2019b;32:693–701. https://doi.org/10.1007/s10278-018-0144-1.
70. Lo Gullo R, Eskreis-Winkler S, Morris EA, Pinker K. Machine learning with multiparametric magnetic resonance imaging of the breast for early prediction of response to neoadjuvant chemotherapy. Breast. 2020b;49:115–22. https://doi.org/10.1016/j.breast.2019.11.009.
71. Bitencourt AGV, Gibbs P, Rossi Saccarelli C, et al. MRI-based machine learning radiomics can predict HER2 expression level and pathologic response after neoadjuvant therapy in HER2 overexpressing breast cancer. EBioMedicine. 2020;61:103042. https://doi.org/10.1016/j.ebiom.2020.103042.
72. Braman N, Prasanna P, Whitney J, et al. Association of peritumoral radiomics with tumor biology and pathologic response to preoperative targeted therapy for HER2 (ERBB2)–positive breast cancer. JAMA Netw Open. 2019;2:e192561. https://doi.org/10.1001/jamanetworkopen.2019.2561.
73. Ha R, Chang P, Karcich J, et al. Predicting post neoadjuvant axillary response using a novel convolutional neural network algorithm. Ann Surg Oncol. 2018;25:3037–43. https://doi.org/10.1245/s10434-018-6613-4.

74. Liu Z, Li Z, Qu J, et al. Radiomics of multiparametric MRI for pretreatment prediction of pathologic complete response to neoadjuvant chemotherapy in breast cancer: a multicenter study. Clin Cancer Res. 2019;25:3538–47. https://doi.org/10.1158/1078-0432.CCR-18-3190.
75. Sutton EJ, Onishi N, Fehr DA, et al. A machine learning model that classifies breast cancer pathologic complete response on MRI post-neoadjuvant chemotherapy. Breast Cancer Res. 2020;22:57. https://doi.org/10.1186/s13058-020-01291-w.
76. Tahmassebi A, Wengert GJ, Helbich TH, et al. Impact of machine learning with multiparametric magnetic resonance imaging of the breast for early prediction of response to neoadjuvant chemotherapy and survival outcomes in breast cancer patients. Investig Radiol. 2019;54:110–7. https://doi.org/10.1097/RLI.0000000000000518.
77. Ashraf AB, Daye D, Gavenonis S, et al. Identification of intrinsic imaging phenotypes for breast cancer tumors: preliminary associations with gene expression profiles. Radiology. 2014;272:374–84. https://doi.org/10.1148/radiol.14131375.
78. Dialani V, Gaur S, Mehta TS, et al. Prediction of low versus high recurrence scores in estrogen receptor–positive, lymph node–negative invasive breast cancer on the basis of radiologic-pathologic features: comparison with oncotype dx test recurrence scores. Radiology. 2016;280:370–8. https://doi.org/10.1148/radiol.2016151149.
79. Ha R, Chang P, Mutasa S, et al. Convolutional neural network using a breast MRI tumor dataset can predict Oncotype dx recurrence score. J Magn Reson Imaging. 2019a;49:518–24. https://doi.org/10.1002/jmri.26244.
80. Li H, Zhu Y, Burnside ES, et al. MR imaging Radiomics signatures for predicting the risk of breast cancer recurrence as given by research versions of mamma print, oncotype DX, and PAM50 gene assays. Radiology. 2016;281:382–91. https://doi.org/10.1148/radiol.2016152110.
81. Sutton EJ, Oh JH, Dashevsky BZ, et al. Breast cancer subtype intertumor heterogeneity: MRI-based features predict results of a genomic assay. J Magn Reson Imaging. 2015;42:1398–406. https://doi.org/10.1002/jmri.24890.
82. Tokuda Y, Yanagawa M, Minamitani K, et al. Radiogenomics of magnetic resonance imaging and a new multi-gene classifier for predicting recurrence prognosis in estrogen receptor-positive breast cancer. Medicine (Baltimore). 2020;99:e19664. https://doi.org/10.1097/MD.0000000000019664.
83. Wan T, Bloch BN, Plecha D, et al. A radio-genomics approach for identifying high risk estrogen receptor-positive breast cancers on DCE-MRI: preliminary results in predicting oncotype DX risk scores. Sci Rep. 2016;6:21394. https://doi.org/10.1038/srep21394.
84. Portnoi T, Yala A, Schuster T, et al. Deep learning model to assess cancer risk on the basis of a breast MR image alone. Am J Roentgenol. 2019;213:227–33. https://doi.org/10.2214/AJR.18.20813.

Artificial Intelligence in Breast Pathology

37

Nermeen Chaudhry, Zaibo Li, and Anil Parwani

Abstract

As the most common cancer and second leading cause of cancer-related death worldwide, efficient and accurate diagnosis of breast cancer are foundational in improving outcomes. Breast cancer diagnosis, and subsequent therapy and prognosis, is based on manual histopathological examination. Traditional methods of pathology slide-interpretation are both time-consuming and subjective, with inevitable interobserver variability. Advancements at the intersection of technology and research have provided an opportunity to make the diagnostic process more streamlined and precise. From digitized whole-slide imaging, to artificial intelligence that can detect, stage, and predict therapeutic response, there are opportunities to improve clinical workflow efficiency, diagnostic quality, and ultimately optimize patient care and accessibility globally.

Keywords

Breast cancer · Digital pathology · Whole slide imaging · Artificial intelligence

N. Chaudhry · Z. Li · A. Parwani (✉)
Department of Pathology, The Ohio State University, Columbus, OH, USA
e-mail: Anil.Parwani@osumc.edu

37.1 Digital Pathology as a Foundation to Artificial Intelligence

In order to understand artificial intelligence (AI) and how algorithms work, it is firstly important to understand what they are analyzing: digitized pathology slides. Digital pathology includes the process of using whole-slide scanners to digitize histopathology, immunohistochemistry and cytology slides, and the subsequent analysis and management of the images using computational approaches. The digital data can be stored in a cloud-based system, allowing for remote review by a pathologist. A 2018 study by Mukhopadhyay et al. showed diagnostic performance with whole-slide imaging (WSI) techniques was almost equal to traditional microscopy across a wide variety of organ systems and specimen types [1]. The study was pivotal in the FDA approval of the Philips IntelliSite Pathology Solution for primary diagnosis, the first digital pathology system on the market. Since then, the FDA has approved another system, Leica Biosystems' scanner Aperio AT2 DX, and developed a digital pathology program dedicated to regulatory research of digital pathology devices. Further studies have validated the use of WSI for primary diagnosis in surgical pathology, in addition to providing economic and turnaround time

B. Dev, L. D. Joseph (eds.), *Holistic Approach to Breast Disease*,
https://doi.org/10.1007/978-981-99-0035-0_37

advantages [2]. Benefits of WSI integration include risk reduction of patient and slide misidentification and tissue damage, easier retrieval of archives, and increased workflow efficiency via direct effects on time-per-slide. Additionally, widespread implementation of WSIs provide materials and data for AI training and validation. However, successful implementation is dependent upon proper training and integration into existing workflows [3].

37.2 Methods of AI and Machine Learning in Pathology

Digital image analysis and WSI make it possible for AI to be applied in pathology. AI is a computational science that generates algorithms to analyze data either through manual annotation of predefined parameters or by machine learning (ML). Examples of predefined inputs include 3D shape of a tumor, intratumoral texture, or distribution of pixel intensities. Inspired by neural networks in the human brain, deep learning is a subset of ML, which can approximate complex nonlinear relationships, self-ascertain patterns, and predict outcomes independent of explicit feature definition. This means the trained algorithm can learn new representations of data without being reprogrammed. The neural networks are composed of three functional layers of artificial neurons called "nodes," which include an input layer, multiple hidden layers, and an output layer. For recognizing distinct visual patterns, convolutional neural networks (CNNs) augment data to extract features of interest and create pooling layers in order to reduce dimensions and noise, which allow for improved analysis and accuracy. In pathology, manually annotated WSIs are used to train CNNs to process, quantitatively assess, and classify data into known categories, that is, cancerous versus noncancerous (Fig. 37.1). Then large amounts of raw data can be input and subsequently annotated and categorized by the trained CNN, which can go on to be reviewed by pathologists to aid in diagnosis, or for further analysis using computer software (Fig. 37.2).

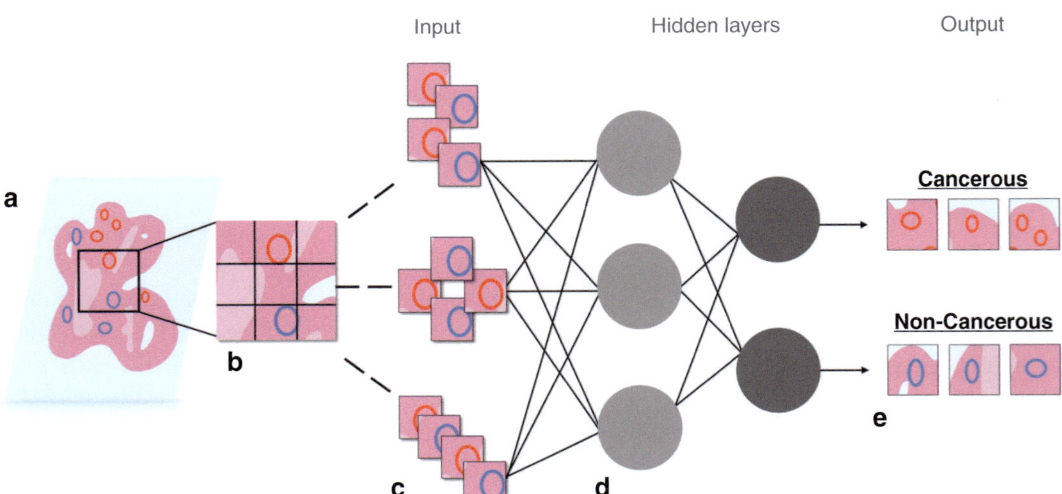

Fig. 37.1 Overview of algorithm training. (**a**) Manually annotated WSI, (**b**) image tiling, (**c**) data augmentation through rotation, mirroring, cropping, (**d**) hidden layers in CNN, (**e**) output distinguishing feature-classified areas

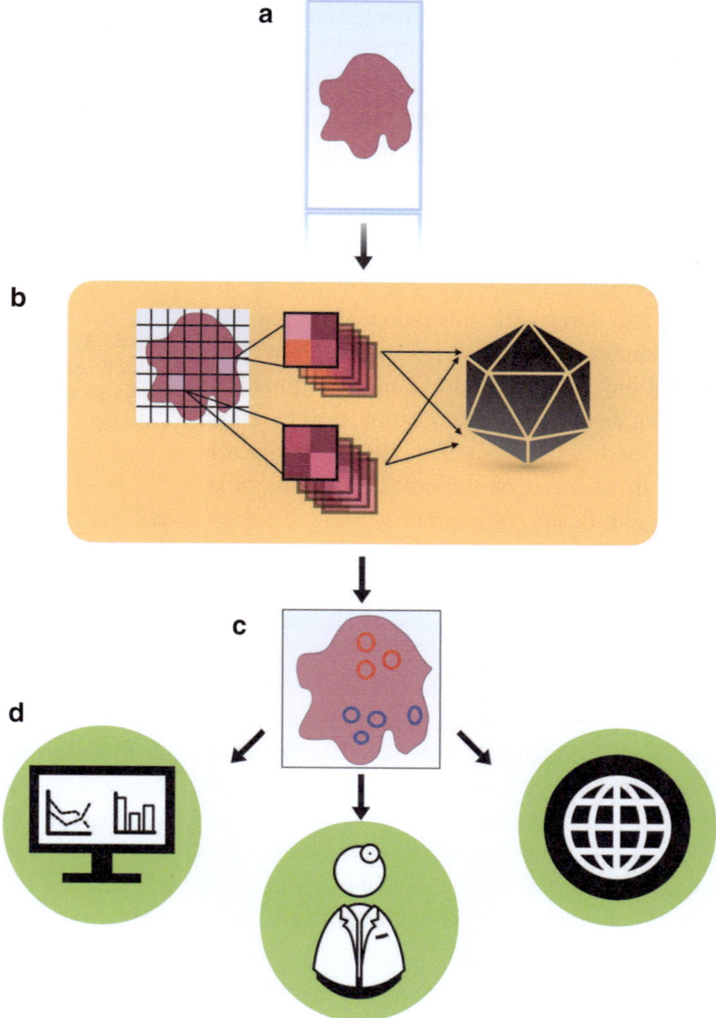

Fig. 37.2 Algorithm usage in pathology workflow. (**a**) Unmarked WSI, (**b**) patch feature extraction and pooling by trained CNN, (**c**) colorized output based on known categories, (**d**) diagnosis via data analysis, pathologist review, and consultation

37.3 Diagnostic Applications

37.3.1 Tumor Detection and Grading

During initial breast cancer diagnosis the detection of invasive tumor cells, characterization of tumor type, and quantification of tumor extent are paramount. CNN-based approaches have shown 93.2% accuracy in distinguishing between eight classes of benign and malignant breast cancer tumors [4]. Another important application of AI is determining lymph node metastasis, a critical step in breast cancer evaluation. The primary advantage of computational pathology is not just accurate diagnosis to reduce errors in diagnosis and classification found in traditional methods but also make pathologists more efficient by reducing their workload, such as help identifying metastases in lymph nodes, which is a tedious, time-consuming process. The 'CAncer MEtastases in LYmph nOdes challeNge' (CAMELYON16) was a worldwide machine learning-based competition aimed at evaluating new algorithms for the detection of lymph node metastases in hematoxylin and eosin (H&E)-stained WSI [5]. The algorithms were found to outperform a panel of pathologists in a simulated time-constrained diagnostic setting, with a 92.4% sensitivity in tumor detection rate compared to 73.2% sensitivity achieved by pathologists [6]. Furthermore, studies found significantly shorter average review time of digitized slides with AI assistance than without [7]. The Galen™ Breast system by Ibex became one of the first commercially available algorithms for screening breast biopsy specimens, aimed at providing accurate diagnosis, enhanced lab efficiency and quality control. After becoming CE marked in 2021, the solution has been implemented in diagnostic workflow across Europe and was recently granted the Breakthrough Device Designation by the Food and Drug Administration (FDA) to fast track clinical review and regulatory approval.

Not only have AI and ML methods proven to be accurate in tumor identification, they have also been used to characterize and histologically grade invasive breast tumors. Despite the prognostic significance of accurate grading, the methods used to segment and analyze slides are liable to inter- and intra-observer variability and low concordance rates due to the subjective visual examination of various cell and tissue-level features. The three components of the Nottingham grading system are nuclear pleomorphism, tubule formation, and mitotic count [8]. Most advances thus far have been in mitosis detection due to the laborious nature and high prognostic value. Preliminary studies have shown promising results using CNN-based ML to annotate PHH3 stains, which can detect mitosis with high sensitivity, suggesting AI assistance to improve concordance rates [9]. Newer strategies aim to increase the accuracy and reliability via deep-learning that removes clearly non-mitotic objects in a WSI and a preprocessing technique to increase the intensity difference between mitosis cell pixels and background [10]. Ongoing research is also being conducted for automated detection of tubular formation and nuclear grade, as well as detection and segmentation of tubule nuclei [11, 12]. QuPath is an open-source digital image analysis (DIA) software made specifically to analyze WSIs (Fig. 37.3). By defining regions of interest as "objects" and using built-in segmentation commands to identify features such as individual nuclei or cells, pathologists can rapidly view a quantitative cell map that can be selected and filtered to produce additional image data (Fig. 37.4).

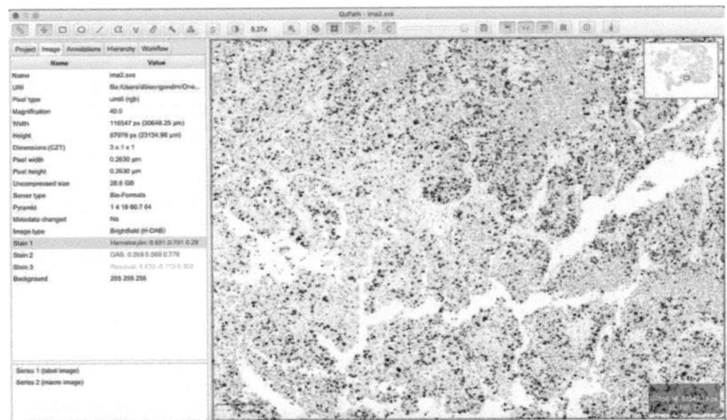

Fig. 37.3 Layout of WSI in QuPath. Image can then go on to be annotated either manually or automatically, and subsequently analyzed. (Image courtesy of Dr. Dibson Dibe Gondim, MD)

37.3.2 Quantification of Breast Cancer Biomarkers

Breast cancer biomarker status is an essential part of breast cancer diagnosis as they are predictive of therapeutic response. Specific antibodies and enzymes stain and visualize specific antigen sites and tissues, with varying intensities that can be compared against a set of biomarker-specific scoring systems. Though manual comparison and scoring of immunohistochemistry (IHC) staining is well-validated, ML-based systems offer an opportunity to decrease inter-observer variability for quantifying biomarker expression.

Overexpression of HER2 is associated with aggressive biological behavior and poor clinical outcome. Treatment with antibody-based therapy with trastuzumab can be effective when taken alone or in combination with chemotherapeutic agents. Studies using algorithms have demonstrated accurate assessment of HER2 IHC in breast carcinoma, and accurate discrimination between HER2 fluorescence in situ hybridization (FISH) positive and negative breast carcinoma cases [13, 14]. One study has shown excellent concordance between HER2 FISH manual scoring and automated analysis with an overall concordance of 98.4% [15]. Of note, a recent study used computational approaches to quantify HER2 IHC results to predict response to anti-HER2 neoadjuvant chemotherapy in HER2-

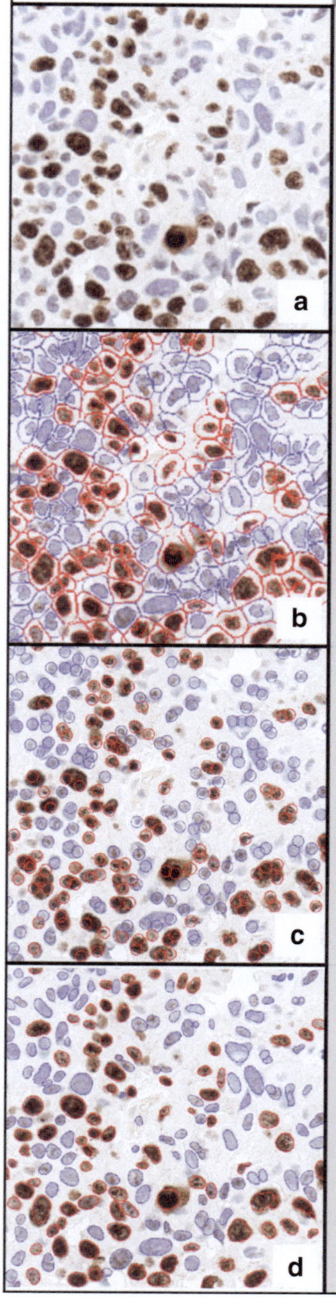

	Method	Positive%	Number Positive	Total Cells
a	Manual Counting	39%	78	200
b	Positive Cell Detection DOB Mean	44%	92	207
c	Fast cell detection DOB Mean	47%	126	267
d	StartDist DOB Mean	41%	78	213

Fig. 37.4 Different methods of QuPath cell detection using H&E and DAB staining. (**a**) Manual counting of region of interest (ROI), (**b**) positive cell detection, (**c**) fast cell detection, (**d**) StarDist based on deep-learning. (Image courtesy of Dr. Dibson Dibe Gondim, MD)

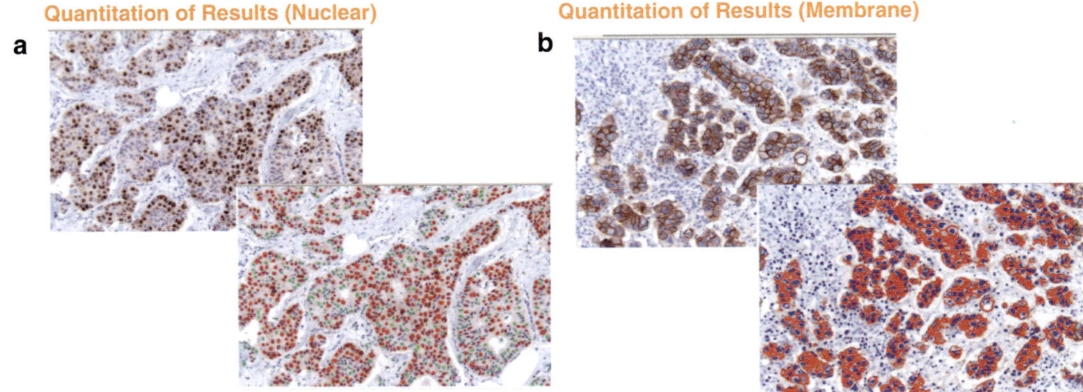

Fig. 37.5 Quantification of IHC by Digital Image Analysis (DIA). (**a**) Quantification of the intensity and amount of staining in cell nuclei, (**b**) identification of staining specific to the cell membrane. (Image courtesy of Dr. Dibson Dibe Gondim, MD)

positive breast cancer patients, which is becoming increasingly more important as research shows that stratifying patients based on HER2 expression level may identify patients who will benefit from targeted therapy [16].

Additional biomarkers predictive of therapeutic response include estrogen receptor (ER) and progesterone receptor (PR) expression. Breast cancers with "hormone-positive" expression are likely to respond to endocrine therapies that can be taken orally and reduce the chance of recurrence by nearly half. A recent study compared two different computational pathology platforms' performance in measuring ER and PR expression: one using user-supervised workflow and the other using an automated workflow [17]. They found that ER and PR measurements from these two platforms agreed well with one another, although the user-supervised platform yielded better classification accuracy than the automated platform. ImmunoRatio, a free web application, has been used to quantify ER and PR, and the results have exhibited excellent correlation with pathologists' manual scoring [18].

Ki-67 is a protein involved in ribosomal RNA transcription and is predictive of tumor aggressiveness. Ki-67 algorithms usually identify tumor nuclei based on both the size and morphology of the nuclei, detect the number of positively stained nuclei based on their color, and then calculate the percentage of positively stained nuclei. Multiple studies have demonstrated that ML algorithms are able to provide a more accurate and reproducible assessment of Ki-67 IHC than human reads [19–24]. In addition, algorithms like QuPath are capable of analyzing greater spatial coverage, which may contribute to their high accuracy as suggested in one study comparing single-field hot-spot analysis with whole section analysis [25] (Fig. 37.5).

37.4 Prognostic Applications

Early stage ER+ breast cancers with a high risk of recurrence are typically treated with both adjuvant chemotherapy and hormonal therapy; these patients are subject to significant side effects. Therefore, being able to quantitatively determine recurrence risk level can help plan treatment effectively and avoid toxic side effects in low-risk patients. American Society of Clinical Oncology Clinical Practice Guideline recommends the clinician may use Oncotype DX (Genomic Health, Redwood City, CA) recurrent score (RS) to guide decisions on adjuvant systemic chemotherapy if a patient has ER-positive, HER2-negative breast cancer. The Oncotype DX assay assesses the expression of 21 genes involved in proliferation, invasion, estrogen, and HER2 pathways to generate an RS to predict possibility of recurrence and chemotherapy benefit [26, 27]. However, multiple studies have suggested that standard histopathologic variables (including tumor grade, tubule formation, nuclear pleomorphism, and mitotic activity) together with breast cancer biomarkers (ER, PR, HER2) can provide information similar to that provided by the Oncotype DX RS [28–31]. The abovementioned histopathologic variables (tumor grade, tubule formation, nuclear pleomorphism, and mitotic activity) are routinely assessed by pathologists in a subjective manner, and interobserver variability does occur, whereas convolutional neural network model (CNN) can automatically and accurately assess these histopathologic variables [32]. A 2018 study by Whitney et al. used ML techniques to extract nuclear morphology features from H&E stained WSI in ER+ patients to predict risk categories from Oncotype DX [33].

Recurrence risk was also predicted in a retrospective cohort of patients with ductal carcinoma in situ using an ML pipeline that first annotated areas of stroma, normal ducts, cancer ducts, dense lymphocyte regions, and blood vessels. Next, a recurrence risk classifier was trained on eight various architectural and spatial organization features from the annotated areas and accurately (85%) predicted 10-year recurrence risk, in addition to identifying patients that may benefit from additional therapy. Importantly, the recurrence-risk classifier showed significantly higher accuracy, specificity, positive predictive value, concordance, and hazard ratios compared to tested clinicopathological variables in predicting recurrences [34].

Additionally, structure and organization of tumor-infiltrating lymphocytes (TILs) are prognostic of clinical outcome in response to neoadjuvant chemotherapy. For triple negative breast cancer, an active immune response has been associated with favorable prognosis. Studies identified three different categories of lymphocytes according to their proximity to cancer cells, and subsequent statistical analysis found the ratio of intratumoral lymphocytes to cancer cells was independently prognostic of survival, along with a correlation to CTLA-4 expression [35]. Further investigative studies found spatial distribution of immune cells was also associated with late recurrence in ER+ breast cancer [36]. A classical ML-based approach was used to count features on breast cancer biopsies and predict neoadjuvant response, specifically finding lymphocyte density in surrounding tissue to be the biggest predictor [37].

37.5 Limitations to AI Application

There are several key factors that impede the adoption of AI in breast pathology currently. First, an AI-based approach is dependent on the quantity and quality of data available for the initial annotation of the training set. Due to the various file formats for digitized slides, scanner quality and multiple information systems used across institutions, additional time is required when inputting initial parameters. Manual selection of artifact-free, clean, and proper quality images must be used in training of an algorithm in order to develop a comprehensive model. Furthermore, steps during slide preparation such as folded tissue section during cutting, staining variation, and air bubbles can cause unreliable data and skew results. Therefore, successful adaptation of AI in digital pathology relies on standardization and normalization methods at each step of raw data preparation.

Importantly, trust is another key limitation in employing AI in real-world applications. Many of the uses of ML in pathology workflow are as tools to be used in tandem with human evaluation. As such, the interpretability of the model becomes paramount. If the pathologist working with a model does not understand why an algorithm makes its decisions, they may be less inclined to accept the results and either spend more time double checking the slides or ignoring the model altogether. This remains a challenge for the medical community and AI community, as it becomes difficult to explain clearly what features trigger ML and how the neural networks piece together specific information. Proper interpretability relies on the communication between statisticians, bioinformaticians, and clinicians. Lastly, trust in the security of data is critical in applying AI. As cybersecurity becomes an increasing threat, sensitive health information from computational pathology will require more regulation and protection of privacy. This becomes challenging given how AI data sets are incredibly large and how they work better when they have more data available from more sources to learn from. The creation of regulatory policies and pathology-related security are important to mitigate ethical concerns but must be carefully navigated to not limit innovation in the process.

37.6 Future of AI in Breast Pathology and beyond

As more data sets become available to train algorithms, more studies are showing reliable and consistent results. Furthermore, as CNN-based approaches learn from exposure to new images over time, "pre-screening" accuracy will increase, and the number of flags for manual review will decrease. With the adaptation of ML in the workflow, the potential for collaboration between pathologists across different institutions will allow for better care of patients globally, at lower costs and quicker turnaround time. Additionally, as it becomes easier for multiple clinicians to evaluate the same data, AI results help produce reproducible assessments and be robust against inter-reader variability. Lastly, computational pathology has implications for changing the current medical system into a pathologist-centered system. As pathology assessment is critical in accurate diagnosis and subsequent prognosis of breast cancer, and as ML becomes better able to predict therapeutic response, the care plan will be driven by the AI and pathology analysis. And as health apps become more popular in tracking real-time data, there are future applications of AI extending into primary care, which can then be incorporated into an algorithm predicting treatment, and create a revolutionary way of practicing personalized medicine.

References

1. Mukhopadhyay S, Feldman MD, Abels E, Ashfaq R, Beltaifa S, Cacciabeve NG, et al. Whole slide imaging versus microscopy for primary diagnosis in surgical pathology: a multicenter blinded randomized noninferiority study of 1992 cases (pivotal study). Am J Surg Pathol. 2018;42(1):39–52. https://doi.org/10.1097/PAS.0000000000000948.
2. Retamero JA, Aneiros-Fernandez J, Del Moral RG. Complete digital pathology for routine histopathology diagnosis in a multicenter hospital network. Arch Pathol Lab Med. 2020;144(2):221–8. https://doi.org/10.5858/arpa.2018-0541-OA.
3. Mills AM, Gradecki SE, Horton BJ, Blackwell R, Moskaluk CA, Mandell JW, Mills SE, Cathro HP. Diagnostic efficiency in digital pathology: a comparison of optical versus digital assessment in 510 surgical pathology cases. Am J Surg Pathol. 2018;42(1):53–9. https://doi.org/10.1097/PAS.0000000000000930.
4. Han Z, Wei B, Zheng Y, Yin Y, Li K, Li S. Breast cancer multi-classification from histopathological images with structured deep learning model. Sci Rep. 2017;7(1):4172. https://doi.org/10.1038/s41598-017-04075-z.
5. Ehteshami Bejnordi B, Veta M, Johannes van Diest P, van Ginneken B, Karssemeijer N, Litjens G, et al. Diagnostic assessment of deep learning algorithms for detection of lymph node metastases in women with breast cancer. JAMA. 2017;318(22):2199–210. https://doi.org/10.1001/jama.2017.14585.
6. Liu Y, Gadepalli K, Norouzi M, Dahl GE, Kohlberger T, Boyko A, et al. Detecting cancer metastases on gigapixel pathology images. Arxiv 2017. https://arxiv.org/abs/1703.02442.
7. Steiner DF, Mac Donald R, Liu Y, Truszkowski P, Hipp JD, Gammage C, et al. Impact of deep learning assistance on the histopathologic review of lymph nodes for metastatic breast cancer. Am J Surg Pathol. 2018;42(12):1636–46. https://doi.org/10.1097/PAS.0000000000001151.
8. Rakha EA, Reis-Filho JS, Baehner F, Dabbs DJ, Decker T, Eusebi V, Fox SB, Ichihara S, Jacquemier J, Lakhani SR, Palacios J, Richardson AL, Schnitt SJ, Schmitt FC, Tan PH, Tse GM, Badve S, Ellis IO. Breast cancer prognostic classification in the molecular era: the role of histological grade. Breast Cancer Res. 2010;12(4):207. https://doi.org/10.1186/bcr2607.
9. Tellez D, Balkenhol M, Otte-Holler I, van de Loo R, Vogels R, Bult P, et al. Whole-slide mitosis detection in H&E breast histology using PHH3 as a reference to train distilled stain-invariant convolutional networks. IEEE Trans Med Imaging. 2018;37:2126. https://doi.org/10.1109/TMI.2018.2820199.
10. Nateghi R, Danyali H, Helfroush MS. A deep learning approach for mitosis detection: application in tumor proliferation prediction from whole slide images. Artif Intell Med. 2021;114:102048. https://doi.org/10.1016/j.artmed.2021.102048.
11. Romo-Bucheli D, Janowczyk A, Gilmore H, Romero E, Madabhushi A. Automated tubule nuclei quantification and correlation with oncotype DX risk categories in ER+ breast cancer whole slide images. Sci Rep. 2016;6:32706. https://doi.org/10.1038/srep32706.

12. Veta M, Kornegoor R, Huisman A, Verschuur-Maes AHJ, Viergever MA, Pluim JPW, et al. Prognostic value of automatically extracted nuclear morphometric features in whole slide images of male breast cancer. Mod Pathol. 2012;25(12):1559–65. https://doi.org/10.1038/modpathol.2012.126.
13. Skaland I, Øvestad I, Janssen EA, Klos J, Kjellevold KH, Helliesen T, Baak JP. Comparing subjective and digital image analysis HER2/neu expression scores with conventional and modified FISH scores in breast cancer. J Clin Pathol. 2008;61(1):68–71. https://doi.org/10.1136/jcp.2007.046763.
14. Hartage R, Li AC, Hammond S, Parwani AV. A validation study of human epidermal growth factor receptor 2 immunohistochemistry digital imaging analysis and its correlation with human epidermal growth factor receptor 2 fluorescence *in situ* hybridization results in breast carcinoma. J Pathol Inform. 2020;11:2. https://doi.org/10.4103/jpi.jpi_52_19.
15. Furrer D, Jacob S, Caron C, Sanschagrin F, Provencher L, Diorio C. Validation of a new classifier for the automated analysis of the human epidermal growth factor receptor 2 (HER2) gene amplification in breast cancer specimens. Diagn Pathol. 2013;8:17. https://doi.org/10.1186/1746-1596-8-17.
16. Li AC, Zhao J, Zhao C, Ma Z, Hartage R, Zhang Y, et al. Quantitative digital imaging analysis of HER2 immunohistochemistry predicts the response to anti-HER2 neoadjuvant chemotherapy in HER2-positive breast carcinoma. Breast Cancer Res Treat. 2020;180(2):321–9. https://doi.org/10.1007/s10549-020-05546-0.
17. Ahern TP, Beck AH, Rosner BA, Glass B, Frieling G, Collins LC, et al. Continuous measurement of breast tumour hormone receptor expression: a comparison of two computational pathology platforms. J Clin Pathol. 2017;70(5):428–34. https://doi.org/10.1136/jclinpath-2016-204107.
18. Tuominen VJ, Ruotoistenmäki S, Viitanen A, Jumppanen M, Isola J. Immuno ratio: a publicly available web application for quantitative image analysis of estrogen receptor (ER), progesterone receptor (PR), and Ki-67. Breast Cancer Res. 2010;12(4):R56. https://doi.org/10.1186/bcr2615.
19. Stålhammar G, Fuentes Martinez N, Lippert M, Tobin NP, Mølholm I, Kis L, et al. Digital image analysis outperforms manual biomarker assessment in breast cancer. Mod Pathol. 2016;29(4):318–29. https://doi.org/10.1038/modpathol.2016.34.
20. Ács B, Madaras L, Kovács KA, Micsik T, Tőkés AM, Győrffy B, et al. Reproducibility and prognostic potential of Ki-67 proliferation index when comparing digital-image analysis with standard semi-quantitative evaluation in breast cancer. Pathol Oncol Res. 2018;24(1):115–27. https://doi.org/10.1007/s12253-017-0220-8.
21. Stålhammar G, Robertson S, Wedlund L, Lippert M, Rantalainen M, Bergh J, et al. Digital image analysis of Ki67 in hot spots is superior to both manual Ki67 and mitotic counts in breast cancer. Histopathology. 2018;72(6):974–89. https://doi.org/10.1111/his.13452.
22. Klauschen F, Wienert S, Schmitt WD, Loibl S, Gerber B, Blohmer JU, et al. Standardized Ki67 diagnostics using automated scoring–clinical validation in the Gepar trio breast cancer study. Clin Cancer Res. 2015;21(16):3651–7. https://doi.org/10.1158/1078-0432.CCR-14-1283.
23. Koopman T, Buikema HJ, Hollema H, de Bock GH, van der Vegt B. Digital image analysis of Ki67 proliferation index in breast cancer using virtual dual staining on whole tissue sections: clinical validation and inter-platform agreement. Breast Cancer Res Treat. 2018;169(1):33–42. https://doi.org/10.1007/s10549-018-4669-2.
24. Røge R, Riber-Hansen R, Nielsen S, Vyberg M. Proliferation assessment in breast carcinomas using digital image analysis based on virtual Ki67/cytokeratin double staining. Breast Cancer Res Treat. 2016;158(1):11–9. https://doi.org/10.1007/s10549-016-3852-6.
25. Goodell PP, Krasinskas AM, Davison JM, Hartman DJ. Comparison of methods for proliferative index analysis for grading pancreatic well-differentiated neuroendocrine tumors. Am J Clin Pathol. 2012;137(4):576–82. https://doi.org/10.1309/AJCP92UCXPJMMSDU.
26. Paik S, Shak S, Tang G, Kim C, Baker J, Cronin M, et al. A multigene assay to predict recurrence of tamoxifen-treated, node-negative breast cancer. N Engl J Med. 2004;351(27):2817–26. https://doi.org/10.1056/NEJMoa041588.
27. Sparano JA, Gray RJ, Makower DF, Pritchard KI, Albain KS, Hayes DF, et al. Prospective validation of a 21-gene expression assay in breast cancer. N Engl J Med. 2015;373(21):2005–14. https://doi.org/10.1056/NEJMoa1510764.
28. Paik S, Tang G, Shak S, Kim C, Baker J, Kim W, et al. Gene expression and benefit of chemotherapy in women with node-negative, estrogen receptor-positive breast cancer. J Clin Oncol. 2006;24(23):3726–34. https://doi.org/10.1200/JCO.2005.04.7985.
29. Albain KS, Barlow WE, Shak S, Hortobagyi GN, Livingston RB, Yeh IT, et al. Prognostic and predictive value of the 21-gene recurrence score assay in postmenopausal women with node-positive, oestrogen-receptor-positive breast cancer on chemotherapy: a retrospective analysis of a randomised trial. Lancet Oncol. 2010;11(1):55–65. https://doi.org/10.1016/S1470-2045(09)70314-6.
30. Sparano JA, Paik S. Development of the 21-gene assay and its application in clinical practice and clinical trials. J Clin Oncol. 2008;26(5):721–8. https://doi.org/10.1200/JCO.2007.15.1068.
31. Sparano JA, Gray RJ, Makower DF, Pritchard KI, Albain KS, Hayes DF, et al. Adjuvant chemotherapy guided by a 21-gene expression assay in breast cancer. N Engl J Med. 2018;379(2):111–21. https://doi.org/10.1056/NEJMoa1804710.

32. Robertson S, Azizpour H, Smith K, Hartman J. Digital image analysis in breast pathology-from image processing techniques to artificial intelligence. Transl Res. 2018;194:19–35. https://doi.org/10.1016/j.trsl.2017.10.010.
33. Whitney J, Corredor G, Janowczyk A, Ganesan S, Doyle S, Tomaszewski J, Feldman M, Gilmore H, Madabhushi A. Quantitative nuclear histomorphometry predicts oncotype DX risk categories for early stage ER+ breast cancer. BMC Cancer. 2018;18(1):610. https://doi.org/10.1186/s12885-018-4448-9.
34. Klimov S, Miligy IM, Gertych A. A whole slide image-based machine learning approach to predict ductal carcinoma in situ (DCIS) recurrence risk. Breast Cancer Res. 2019;21(1):83. https://doi.org/10.1186/s13058-019-1165-5.
35. Saltz J, Gupta R, Hou L, Kurc T, Singh P, Nguyen V, et al. Spatial organization and molecular correlation of tumor-infiltrating lymphocytes using deep learning on pathology images. Cell Rep. 2018;23(1):181–193.e7. https://doi.org/10.1016/j.celrep.2018.03.086.
36. Heindl A, Sestak I, Naidoo K, Cuzick J, Dowsett M, Yuan Y. Relevance of spatial heterogeneity of immune infiltration for predicting risk of recurrence after endocrine therapy of ER+ breast cancer. J Natl Cancer Inst. 2018;110(2). https://doi.org/10.1093/jnci/djx137.
37. Ali HR, Dariush A, Provenzano E, Bardwell H, Abraham JE, Iddawela M, et al. Computational pathology of pre-treatment biopsies identifies lymphocyte density as a predictor of response to neoadjuvant chemotherapy in breast cancer. Breast Cancer Res. 2016;18(1):21. https://doi.org/10.1186/s13058-016-0682-8.

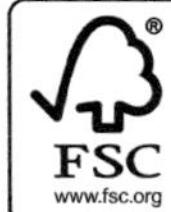

MIX
Papier aus verantwortungsvollen Quellen
Paper from responsible sources
FSC® C105338

If you have any concerns about our products,
you can contact us on
ProductSafety@springernature.com

In case Publisher is established outside the EU,
the EU authorized representative is:
Springer Nature Customer Service Center GmbH
Europaplatz 3, 69115 Heidelberg, Germany

Printed by Libri Plureos GmbH
in Hamburg, Germany